Atlas of Anatomic Hepatic Resection for Hepatocellular Carcinoma

Jiangsheng Huang · Xianling Liu · Jixiong Hu
Editors

Atlas of Anatomic Hepatic Resection for Hepatocellular Carcinoma

Glissonean Pedicle Approach

Springer

Editors
Jiangsheng Huang
Department of Minimally Invasive Surgery
The Second Xiangya Hospital
Central South University
Changsha, Hunan, PR China

Xianling Liu
Department of Oncology
The Second Xiangya Hospital
Central South University
Changsha, Hunan, PR China

Jixiong Hu
Department of Hepatobiliary Surgery and
Hunan Provincial Key Laboratory of
Hepatobiliary Disease Research
The Second Xiangya Hospital
Central South University
Changsha, Hunan, PR China

ISBN 978-981-13-0667-9 ISBN 978-981-13-0668-6 (eBook)
https://doi.org/10.1007/978-981-13-0668-6

Library of Congress Control Number: 2018952502

This Springer imprint is published by the registered company Springer Nature Singapore Pte Ltd.
The registered company address is: 152 Beach Road, #21-01/04 Gateway East, Singapore 189721, Singapore

Preface

Hepatocellular carcinoma (HCC) is the most common primary tumor of the liver. It currently is the fifth most common cancer worldwide and is the third most frequent cause of cancer death, with an annual incidence of over 0.5 million worldwide. Unfortunately, half of these cases and deaths happen in China. Currently, curative-intent treatment options for HCC include liver resection, liver transplantation, and regional ablative therapies. In strictly selected patients, reasonable and comprehensive use of these treatment options can reach 5-year overall survival of 50–75%. Unluckily, only a small number of patients with HCC are fit to be chosen for all of these treatment modalities. Hepatic resection, however, is a well-applied treatment modality for the bulk of patients with various stages of HCC, in case the patient has enough compensated liver function. Besides, hepatic resection has been reported to be a cost-effective surgical option for HCC that can reach satisfactory oncological outcomes.

The extent of hepatic resection for HCC has been a topic of lasting interest. In recent years, it is suggested by some authors that segment-based anatomical resection, which is defined as the removal of a hepatic segment including tumor-bearing portal tributaries as well as major branch of the portal vein and hepatic artery, is preferable to nonanatomic resection for HCC. Many techniques of segment-based systematic liver resection have been developed. In this book, we just in detail discuss the most valuable one of these techniques: segment-based liver resections by the Glissonean pedicle approach. This concept was introduced by Couinaud and Takasaki in the early 1980s and then developed by Sugioka A and Machado MA. The pedicles can be isolated, looped, divided, and suture-ligated as one of the bundles. Consequently, any anatomical hepatectomy may be carried out using this technique.

To our knowledge, up to now, no clinical book focusing on Glissonean pedicle transection method for hepatic resection for HCC has been published. The only book focusing on Glissonean pedicle transection method for hepatic resection for HCC was written by Takasaki and published in 2011 in English, but this book is just comprised of hand-drawn schematic diagrams describing the surgical proceedings using Glissonean pedicle approach, without describing clinical and actual surgical proceedings.

This book aims to provide a fully updated knowledge in concisely describing the application of liver resections by the Glissonean pedicle approach, as well as our modifications of this technique and the application of methylene blue staining technique. Our modifications include the following maneuvers: (1) No need of isolating and dividing the right-sided retrohepatic short veins draining into the infrahepatic inferior vena cava and mobilizing the process of the caudate lobe from the infrahepatic inferior vena cava; (2) No need of making a vertical incision perpendicular to the hepatic hilum between segment 7 and the process of the caudate lobe; (3) After lowering the hilar plate, the surgeon puts his index finger beneath the hilar plate, then a large curved clamp was inserted into the incision in front of the hilum and the clamp was vertically inserted further, until the clamp reached down to the tip of the surgeon's index finger; using the finger as a guide, the clamp was pushed out of the inferior edge of the right or the left hepatic pedicle. Thus, the right or the left hepatic pedicle was easily and rapidly isolated and then looped with a vascular tape. According to our own clinical practice, this maneuver is safe, simple, and time-saving. It is very important that the maneuver must not be forceful.

The photographs in this book are taken during our operation procedures in the past years. We wish to give our readers a precise, intuitive, and standardized description of the Glissonean pedicle transection method for hepatic resection. Most of the contributors of this book are experts of the 2nd Xiangya Hospital, Central South University, who contribute their own knowledge, experiences, research as well as cases to this book.

This book systematically presents complete technical details for anatomical segmentectomy (Couinaud's classification), sectionectomy, and hemi-hepatectomy for hepatocellular carcinoma by the modified suprahilar Glissonean approach, using the simplest, essential, and easily available surgical instruments. Meanwhile, to precisely transect the deepest hepatic parenchyma, this book also describes the methylene blue staining technique. By clearly describing our surgical proceedings, this anatomical hepatic resection technique can be easily learned and applied by unexperienced surgeon in the non-tertiary or low-volume HCC patients centers or hospitals.

The potential readers of this book include hepato-pancreato-biliary surgeons, gastrointestinal surgeons, liver disease clinicians, radiologists, and hepatobiliary surgery researchers.

Changsha, China Jixiong Hu

Acknowledgments

Our deepest gratitude goes first and foremost to all of the contributors to this book. We would like to extend our sincere gratitude to our advisors Professor Shouzhi Xiong, Professor Dewu Zhong, and Professor Xundi Xu, chairman of Hunan Provincial Key Laboratory of Hepatobiliary Disease Research, for their help in performing some surgical operations included in this book.

High tribute shall be paid to Professor Enhua Xiao and Dr. Manjun Xiao for their help in the writing of preoperative imaging chapter.

We would like to express our appreciation of our secretaries, Dr. Zhongkun Zuo and Tenglong Tang, for their help in typing the manuscript and production of the operative photographs.

We are deeply indebted to our families and coworkers for their help and great confidence in us all through these years.

Last but not least, we pay our innermost thanks to our hospital for providing all necessary conveniences to accomplish this book.

Contents

List of Contributors

Advisors

Dewu Zhong, MD Department of Hepatobiliary Surgery, The Second Xiangya Hospital, Central South University, Changsha, Hunan, PR China

Shouzhi Xiong, MD Department of Hepatobiliary Surgery, The Second Xiangya Hospital, Central South University, Changsha, Hunan, PR China

Editors

Jiangsheng Huang, MD Department of Minimally Invasive Surgery, The Second Xiangya Hospital, Central South University, Changsha, Hunan, PR China

Xianling Liu, MD Department of Oncology, The Second Xiangya Hospital, Central South University, Changsha, Hunan, PR China

Jixiong Hu, MD Department of Hepatobiliary Surgery and Hunan Provincial Key Laboratory of Hepatobiliary Disease Research, The Second Xiangya Hospital, Central South University, Changsha, Hunan, PR China

Contributors

Weidong Dai, MD Department of Hepatobiliary Surgery and Hunan Provincial Key Laboratory of Hepatobiliary Disease Research, The Second Xiangya Hospital, Central South University, Changsha, Hunan, PR China

Jiangbei Deng, MD Department of Interventional Medicine, Changsha Central Hospital, Changsha, Hunan, PR China

Wentao Fan, MD Department of Hepatobiliary Surgery and Hunan Provincial Key Laboratory of Hepatobiliary Disease Research, The Second Xiangya Hospital, Central South University, Changsha, Hunan, PR China

Guohuang Hu, MD Department of General Surgery, Affiliated Changsha Hospital, Hunan Normal University, Changsha, Hunan, PR China

Shengfu Huang, MD Department of Hepatobiliary Surgery, The Second Xiangya Hospital, Central South University, Changsha, Hunan, PR China

Chun Liu, MD Department of Hepatobiliary Surgery and Hunan Provincial Key Laboratory of Hepatobiliary Disease Research, The Second Xiangya Hospital, Central South University, Changsha, Hunan, PR China

Wei Liu, MD Department of Minimally Invasive Surgery, The Second Xiangya Hospital, Central South University, Changsha, Hunan, PR China

Tenglong Tang, MD Department of Minimally Invasive Surgery, The Second Xiangya Hospital, Central South University, Changsha, Hunan, PR China

Jilong Wang, MD Department of Hepatobiliary Surgery, Xiangya Hospital, Central South University, Changsha, Hunan, PR China

Xianming Wang, MD Department of General Surgery, Shenzhen Second People's Hospital, Shenzhen University, Shenzhen, Guangdong, PR China

Yinhuai Wang, MD Department of Urology Surgery, The Second Xiangya Hospital, Central South University, Changsha, Hunan, PR China

Yu Wen, MD Department of Hepatobiliary Surgery and The Second Xiangya Hospital Central South University, Changsha, Hunan, PR China

Enhua Xiao, MD Department of Radiology, The Second Xiangya Hospital, Central South University, Changsha, Hunan, PR China

Hongbo Xiao, MD Department of General Surgery, Guangzhou First People's Hospital, Guangzhou Medical University, Guangzhou, Guangdong, PR China

Manjun Xiao, MD Department of Radiology, The Second Xiangya Hospital, Central South University, Changsha, Hunan, PR China

Xundi Xu, MD, PhD Department of Hepatobiliary Surgery and Hunan Provincial Key Laboratory of Hepatobiliary Disease Research, The Second Xiangya Hospital, Central South University, Changsha, Hunan, PR China

Hongliang Yao, MD Department of General Surgery, The Second Xiangya Hospital, Central South University, Changsha, Hunan, PR China

Enxiang Zhou, MD Department of General Surgery, The Second Xiangya Hospital, Central South University, Changsha, Hunan, PR China

Ning Zhou, MD Department of Hepatobiliary Surgery, Hunan Provincial Hospital, Hunan Normal University, Changsha, Hunan, PR China

Zhongkun Zuo, MD Department of Minimally Invasive Surgery, The Second Xiangya Hospital, Central South University, Changsha, Hunan, PR China

Clinical Anatomy of the Liver

Jixiong Hu, Jiangsheng Huang, Xianling Liu, and Zhongkun Zuo

General Anatomy

The liver is the largest organ, amounting to about 2–3% of average body weight. The liver has three surfaces: diaphragmatic, visceral and posterior surfaces. The liver has two hemilivers, the large right hemiliver and the smaller left hemiliver, which is generally described in two ways, by morphologic anatomy and by functional anatomy. The two hemilivers are divided on the anterior surface of the liver by the falciform ligament and on the inferior surface by the round ligament as it runs into the umbilical fissure. At the upper margin, the two layers of the falciform ligament divide from each other. On the right side, the falciform ligament attaches the right diaphragmatic peritoneum and constitutes the upper layer of the right coronary ligament, which runs inferiorly to form the right triangular ligament, and then turns backwards to constitute the lower layer of the right coronary ligament. The area between these ligaments, which is completely devoid of peritoneum, is named as the bare area. The retrohepatic inferior vena cava (IVC) locates within this bare area on the undersurface of the liver. At its left extremity, the lower layer of the right coronary ligament passes through the posterior surface of the retrohepatic inferior vena cava and connects with the peritoneal reflexion from the right boundary of the Spigelian lobe of the caudate lobe. This right-sided part of this ligament posteriorly surrounding the retrohepatic IVC was referred to as the hepatocaval ligament (Makuuchi ligament). On the left side, the other layer of the falciform ligament constitutes the anterior layer of the left triangle ligament, which reflexes backwards to form the posterior layer. At the top of the fissure for the ligamentum venosum, it constitutes the anterior layer of the gastrohepatic ligament. The posterior layer of the gastrohepatic ligament is the reflexed peritoneum from the right boundary of the top portion of the Spigelian lobe of the caudate lobe. This layer then goes around the Spigelian lobe to join the lower layer of the coronary ligament. The gastrohepatic ligament ties to the ligamentum venosum, which divides the historically defined right and left hemilivers on its posterior surface. This common early description of liver anatomy was only based on external landmarks of the liver and has no strict relationship to functional anatomy. It is well accepted that the liver does not have reliable external landmarks as guides for anatomical hepatic resection.

J. X. Hu
Department of Hepatobiliary Surgery and Hunan Provincial Key Laboratory of Hepatobiliary Disease Research, The Second Xiangya Hospital, Central South University, Changsha, Hunan, PR China
e-mail: 13908459086@163.com

J. S. Huang (✉)
Department of Minimally Invasive Surgery, The Second Xiangya Hospital, Central South University, Changsha, Hunan, PR China
e-mail: HJS13907313501@yahoo.com

X. L. Liu
Department of Oncology, The Second Xiangya Hospital, Central South University, Changsha, Hunan, PR China
e-mail: liuxianling3180@163.com

Z. K. Zuo
Department of Minimally Invasive Surgery, The Second Xiangya Hospital, Central South University, Changsha, Hunan, PR China
e-mail: arthasreal@csu.edu.cn

Functional Surgical Anatomy

Concept of Liver Sections, Sectors and Segments

Understanding the intrahepatic anatomy is crucial to perform liver resections and, in particular, parenchymal-sparing resections. The Couinaud's liver segmentation system is based on the identification of the three hepatic veins and the plane passing by the portal vein bifurcation. Nowadays, Couinaud's classification is widely used clinically, because it is best adapted for surgery and has become essential in localizing and monitoring various intrahepatic lesions.

J. S. Huang et al. (eds.), *Atlas of Anatomic Hepatic Resection for Hepatocellular Carcinoma*,
https://doi.org/10.1007/978-981-13-0668-6_1

As above-mentioned, Couinaud's portal segmentation is entirely different from the historically defined two hemilivers based on external landmarks [1, 2] and is also partially different from Healey's arteriobiliary segmentation [3]. According to Couinaud's descriptions, the right, middle and left hepatic veins divide the liver into four sectors (called suprahepatic segmentation by Couinaud), each of which is supplied by a portal pedicle that consists of a branch of the hepatic artery, portal vein and bile duct. The middle hepatic vein runs in the main portal scissura (midplane of the liver) which separates the liver into the right and the left hemiliver. The main portal scissura moves forward from the gallbladder fossa anteriorly to the left of the suprahepatic IVC posteriorly, and in clinical practice, these external landmarks may be used as external demarcation line between the functional right and left hemiliver. Both the right and left hemilivers are further separated into sectors by the right and left portal scissura holding the right and left hepatic veins separately.

In the right hemiliver, the right portal scissura divides the right hemiliver into the right anterior sector (right paramedian sector) and the right posterior sector (right lateral sector). It is noteworthy that in the right hemiliver, Healey's liver sections which he defined as segments are accurately the same as Couinaud's sectors. In the left hemiliver, the left portal scissura divides the left liver into the anterior sector (left medial sector or left paramedian sector) and the posterior sector (left posterior sector or left lateral sector). The anterior sector consists of segments 4 and 3, and the posterior sector only includes segment 2. However, in the left hemiliver, Healey's liver sections which he defined as segments are not the same as Couinaud's sectors.

In the right hemiliver, as Healey's sections are precisely the same as Couinaud's sectors, the right anterior sector (section) can be further subdivided into segment 8 superiorly and segment 5 inferiorly. The right posterior sector (Healey's section) is also further subdivided into segment 7 superiorly and segment 6 inferiorly. In the left hemiliver, Healey's sections are not the same as Couinaud's sectors. The Healey's left medial section locates between the main portal scissura and the falciform ligament, and it is comprised only of segment 4, which can further be subdivided into segment 4A superiorly and segment 4B inferiorly, while the Healey's left lateral section is comprised of segments 2 and 3, being divided by the left hepatic vein which runs in the left portal scissura.

For the Couinaud's left medial sector, it is comprised of segments 3 and 4, locating between the middle hepatic vein running in the main portal scissura and the left hepatic vein running in the left portal scissura. The falciform ligament and the umbilical fissure separate segment 4 from segment 3. The Couinaud's left lateral sector, which is located within the left territory of the left hepatic vein, is comprised only of segment 2. The caudate lobe is defined as segment 1 in both the Couinaud's portal and the Healey's arteriobiliary segmentation systems. This segment is surrounded by the major vascular structures, with the retrohepatic posteriorly, the main portal pedicle inferiorly and the hepatocaval confluence superiorly. Its inflow vasculature originates from both the right and the left portal pedicles, and its biliary drainage exists as a similar pattern. Its venous drainage directly enters into the retrohepatic IVC.

Brisbane Terminology of Liver Anatomy and Hepatic Resections

The American surgeons prefer to use the terminology proposed by Healey; however, most of the European surgeons incline to use terminology proposed by Couinaud. The term *Segment* used in Healey's segmentation system is not the same as the Couinaud's segment, and the term *Section* used in Healey's segmentation system may be the same, or different, from the term *Sector* used in Couinaud's segmentation system. There are other more confusion surrounding the terminology of liver anatomy and resections. To clarify the confusion in terminology of liver anatomy and hepatic resection, the Scientific Committee of the International Hepato-Pancreato-Biliary Association (IHPBA), at a meeting held in 1998, decided to form a Terminology Committee of international experts. Then, an alternative nomenclature was worked out by this Committee in Brisbane, Australia, in 2000 [4, 5]. To state briefly this terminology, the liver is separated into two parts: the main liver and the caudate lobe (defined as dorsal sector by Couinaud). The main liver is separated by three orders of division into the hemilivers (or livers), sections and segments, respectively. Each segment is an independent functional unit, with a separate vascular inflow supply and a separate biliary and venous drainage. Therefore, each segment can be resected individually or in combination with other segment(s). The main difference between Couinaud's portal segmentation and the Brisbane 2000 Terminology is the renaming of Couinaud's sectors as sections. In addition, the left hemiliver is not separated into two sectors based on the left hepatic vein. The left hemiliver is defined as having a left lateral section (including segments 2 and 3) and a left medial section (segment 4). This new segmentation of the left hemiliver is based on the separation of the left hemiliver by the line between the falciform ligament and the umbilical fissure. The anatomical terms, Couinaud segments and all anatomical hepatic resection terms are described in Table 1.

Table 1 Couinaud's segments, anatomical hepatic resection terms and their corresponding anatomic terms

	Anatomical term	Couinaud segments	Terms for surgical resection
First-order division	Right liver or right hemiliver	Sg5–8	Right hepatectomy or right hemihepatectomy
	Left liver or left hemiliver	Sg2–4 (±Sg1)	Left hepatectomy or left hemihepatectomy
Second-order division	Right anterior section	Sg5, 8	Right anterior sectionectomy
	Right posterior section	Sg6, 7	Right posterior sectionectomy
	Left medial section	Sg4	Left medial sectionectomy or segmentectomy 4
	Left lateral section	Sg2, 3	Left lateral sectionectomy or bisegmentectomy 2,3
	Right hemiliver plus left medial section	Sg4–8 (±Sg1)	Right trisectionectomy or extended right hepatectomy or extended right hemihepatectomy
	Left hemiliver plus right anterior section	Sg2–5, 8 (±Sg1)	Left trisectionectomy or extended left hepatectomy or extended left hemihepatectomy
Third-order division	Segments1–9	Any one of Sg1–9	Segmentectomy
	Two contiguous segments	Any two of Sg1–9 in continuity	Bisegmentectomy

Anatomy of Glissonean Sheath (Glisson's Sheath)

Couinaud described the Walaeus sheath as the most important element of the liver in his book entitled *Surgical Anatomy of the Liver Revisited* [6]. This sheath was discovered by Johannis Walaeus in 1640 [7]. Subsequently, in 1645, Glisson also described the connective tissue capsule wrapping the liver tissue—which bears his name. Glisson's capsule contracts around the hilar triad as they enter into the liver parenchyma; and each bile duct, hepatic artery and portal vein unit is wrapped by a fibrous sheath named the Glissonean or Walaeus sheath. Generally, this term 'Glissonean sheath' is referred to the portion of the intrahepatic Glissonean pedicle.

In the portion of the 'Glissonean pedicle' outside the liver, the hepatic pedicle is also wrapped by connective tissues and peritoneum up to the hepatic hilum. The intrahepatic and extrahepatic of the hepatic pedicle have the same anatomical structures. That is to say, the intrahepatic and extrahepatic hepatic pedicle can be seen as parts of the same Glissonean pedicle tree.

The main pattern of the intrahepatic Glissonean pedicle tree has been used by the Brisbane 2000 Terminology to separate the liver into hemilivers, sections (sectors) and segments (see section "Functional Surgical Anatomy"). The anatomic variations inherent to the intrahepatic vasculature and biliary tract entail dissection of the intrahepatic individual structures technically demanding and even dangerous. However, any portal pedicle entering the hepatic parenchyma takes a sheath, which goes with the pedicle up to the sinusoids. All anatomical variations in the branching of the sectional and segmental pedicles are within the Glissonean sheath, which includes the exact components supplying the hepatic parenchyma entered by this sheath; at this level, dissection of any individual sheath is technically simple and safe [8].

The union of Glisson's capsule with connective tissue sheaths wrapping the biliary tract and vasculature at the inferior surface of the liver makes up the hilar plate system. This plate system also includes a large member of lymphatics and nerves and a small vascular network. The hepatic hilar plate system is comprised of the hilar plate above the biliary confluence, the cystic plate related to the gallbladder bed, the umbilical plate located above the umbilical portion of the left portal vein and the Arantian plate wrapping the ligamentum venosum [9].

Hepatic Vascular Anatomy

Hepatic Artery

The hepatic artery originates from the celiac trunk in more than 80% of cases and becomes the proper hepatic artery after sending out the gastroduodenal and right gastric arteries. The proper hepatic artery accompanies the portal vein and the common bile duct to form the portal triad. It then branches off the right hepatic artery after the left hepatic artery. The left hepatic artery stretches out towards the base of the umbilical fissure and emits branches to the Spigelian lobe of the caudate lobe and segments 2–4. Usually the left hepatic artery breaks into medial and lateral branches extrahepatically that supply segment 4 and segments 2 and 3, respectively. The segment 4 branch can also originate from the right hepatic artery and was historically defined as the middle hepatic artery. The right hepatic artery arises from the proper hepatic artery in more than 80% of cases. It crosses posterior to the common bile duct in 65% of cases, anteriorly in about 10–20% of cases. The right hepatic artery classically breaks into an anterior and posterior branch, which often occurs extrahepatically.

The most common variations in hepatic arterial anatomy are replaced or accessory right or left hepatic arteries, which originate from the superior mesenteric or left gastric arteries, respectively. An aberrant hepatic artery is referred to a branch that does not originate from its usual origin. An accessory vessel is defined as an aberrant origin of a branch that is in addition to the normal branching pattern. A replaced vessel is defined as an aberrant origin of a branch that substitutes for the lack of the normal branch. Aberrant arterial anatomy is present in about 40% of cases, and almost any combination of aberrant arterial branches can be encountered. The left hepatic artery originates from the proper hepatic artery in more than 80% of individuals. In approximately 10–20% of individuals, there is a replaced left hepatic artery that usually originates from the left gastric artery. The replaced left hepatic artery passes in the gastrohepatic ligament and can be injured when incising the gastrohepatic ligament without noticing its existence. An accessory left hepatic artery may be encountered in up to 35% of cases. Replaced and accessory left hepatic arteries can usually be found out by carefully palpating the gastrohepatic ligament. A replaced right hepatic artery passes laterally to the common bile duct and can be easily injured when dissecting the hepatoduodenal ligament without noticing its existence. In slightly more than 5% of cases, there is an accessory right hepatic artery that may originate from the superior mesenteric artery. Replaced and accessory right hepatic artery can be discovered by carefully palpating the hepatoduodenal ligament. The common hepatic artery can also arise from the superior mesenteric artery and pass in the same plane as a replaced right hepatic artery.

Portal Vein

The portal vein has a segmental intrahepatic distribution, and it closely runs alongside the hepatic artery. The portal vein is made by the confluence of the splenic and superior mesenteric veins behind the neck of the pancreas. It goes up posterior to the common bile duct and the hepatic artery into the hepatic hilum. After its entry through hilum, the main portal vein (MPV) bifurcates into a larger right portal vein (RPV) and a small left portal vein (LPV). The RPV then bifurcates into right anterior portal sectoral vein (RAPV), supplying segments 5 and 8 and right posterior portal vein (RPPV) supplying segments 6 and 7. The LPV passes horizontally to left and then turns medially, supplying segments 2, 3 and 4 and a branch to the Spigelian lobe of the caudate lobe. This prevailing branching pattern was present in about 65–80% of individuals.

Variations of the main portal vein at the hepatic hilum were seen in 20–35% of the individuals [10], less frequently compared with those of the hepatic arteries and hepatic veins. The most common variant is the portal trifurcation in which the MPV is separated into the RAPV, RAPP and LPV, all originating from a common place, and was observed in 10.9–15% of the cases. The second commonest variant is that the RPPA originates early directly from the MPA, which then bifurcates into the RAPP and LPV. This pattern was observed in 0.3–7.0% of the population. The third pattern of variation is the origin of the RAPP from the LPV. This pattern was seen in 2.9–4.3% of the persons. In these persons, the MPV separates into the RPPV and the LPV. The RAPV arises directly from the LPV.

Hepatic Vein

Most often, there are three hepatic veins (right, middle and left) that drain into the suprahepatic inferior vena cava (IVC). The left hepatic vein is formed by the union of drainage veins of segments 2 and 3 [11], giving rise to a short and posterior venous trunk. The left hepatic vein also receives two main branches within the hepatic parenchyma; one is the umbilical vein which runs in the umbilical fissure draining parts of segments 4 and 3. This vein is not always present, occurring in less than 60% of the population. Another is the accessory segment 4 vein which drains into the left hepatic vein in 57.5% of individuals. Attention should be paid not to confuse the umbilical portion of the left portal vein with the umbilical vein. The left hepatic vein runs in the left portal scissura, firstly in the intersegmental plane between segments 3 and 2, and then in the posterior part of the fissure for the ligamentum venosum which constitutes a portion of the intersectional plane between the left medial and lateral section. The left hepatic is located in the cranial 2 cm of this fissure which separates segment 4 from segment 2, and it constitutes a portion of the posterior margin of the left liver. At this point, this vein is wrapped only by the lower layer of the left triangular ligament. The vein subsequently goes transversely and posteriorly towards the left-side wall of the suprahepatic IVC, crossing over the top margin of the Spigelian lobe of the caudate lobe. The vein forms a common trunk with the middle hepatic vein in 60–95% of the population before draining in the suprahepatic IVC [12, 13].

The ligamentum venosum often adheres to the left and posterior aspects of the common trunk. Dissection and division of this ligament at this site facilitate to extrahepatically isolate and loop the common trunk [14].

The middle hepatic vein runs in the middle or main portal scissura, dividing the left hemiliver from the right hemiliver. It drains segment IV and sometimes receives branches from segment 5 or 8 [11]. A considerable amount of venous drainage from segment 6 drains into the middle hepatic vein in 25% of the population [14]. In 9% of the persons, a venous branch from segment 8 drains in the middle hepatic vein and may lead to venous congestion, necrosis and atrophy of this segment if injured during hepatic resection [15, 16].

The middle hepatic vein enters as a single entity in the suprahepatic inferior vena cava in only approximately 3–15% of the population [14]. In most cases, it makes up a common trunk with the left hepatic vein, and the common trunk drains in the suprahepatic inferior vena cava. This trunk is often 5 mm or less in length. It is not rare that no common trunk exists but there is a common wall between the roots of the middle and the left hepatic veins. Consequently, it must be kept in mind as a strict surgical rule that there are only two major hepatic veins draining in the suprahepatic inferior vena cava—the right hepatic vein and the common trunk of the middle and left hepatic veins. Any attempt to extrahepatically separate the middle hepatic vein from the left hepatic vein is rude, unwise and even lethal as any injury to the common trunk or the common wall can cause massive bleeding [14].

In addition, the main pattern of the common trunk of the middle and left hepatic veins is that the trunk is headed to the right. In rare cases, the common trunk is headed to the left, or the trunk can be completely devoid. In the latter situation, the middle and the left hepatic veins arise from the suprahepatic inferior vena cava in a Y pattern.

The vein(s) draining the cranial (or posterior) portion of segment 4 (defined as segment 4A) is(are) a short hepatic vein(veins) that insert(s) into the middle and/or the left hepatic vein. Segment 4A is small and its volume is only about 20% of the segment 4 [6]. The traditional quadrate lobe is defined as segment 4B by some surgeons, and its draining vein is long, tenuous and sagittal and inserts into the middle hepatic vein in the main pattern. This vein is named segment 4 vein or accessory segment 4 vein by some surgeons. This vein can also enter into the common trunk of the middle/left hepatic veins, into the left hepatic vein, or even directly into the retrohepatic inferior vena cava.

The right hepatic vein is the largest. It runs in the right portal scissura or the right intersectional plane and drains all of the veins of segments 6 and 7 and some of the veins of segments 5 and 8 [11]. It attaches to the right border of the suprahepatic inferior vena cava, laterally and below the middle hepatic vein. The variations of the hepatic vein include the following: (1) the right hepatic vein has only a short main trunk, and early separates into a posterior branch which drains all of segments 6 and 7, and an anterior branch which drains some of segments 5 and 8; (2) a small right hepatic vein, associated with a large and stout middle hepatic vein; (3) a small right hepatic vein, accompanied by a large right inferior hepatic vein (RIHV); and (4) a small right hepatic vein, coexisting with an accessory right hepatic vein [14].

There are inconsistent and classical several retrohepatic short veins that drain directly from the caudate lobe into the retrohepatic inferior vena cava.

Biliary Anatomy

The individual biliary drainage pursues a considerably similar anatomical pathway as the portal venous supply [17]. The right anterior sectional branches, with a more vertical course, and the right posterior sectional branch, with an almost horizontal course, combine to make up the right hepatic duct, which has a short extrahepatic course (about 1 cm) before fusing with the left hepatic duct at the biliary confluence to form the common hepatic duct. The left hepatic duct is made up by segmental branches draining segments 2–4, and it has a much longer extrahepatic course (about 2–3 cm) than the right hepatic duct. The bile duct draining the caudate lobe usually enters into the origin sites of the right or left hepatic duct. By convention, the common hepatic duct is renamed as the common bile duct below the site of entry of the cystic duct.

Common variations in biliary anatomy include [17] (1) a triple confluence. There are two types of triple confluence. One is the confluence of the right anterior and posterior sectional ducts and the left hepatic duct, occurring in about 10–15% of the persons. Another is the confluence of a right (anterior or posterior) sectional duct directly inserting into the common bile duct in 20% of the persons; (2) ectopic drainage of either of the right sectional branches into the left hepatic duct; (3) absence of the confluence; and (4) absence of the right hepatic duct and drainage of the right posterior duct into the cystic duct.

The Hjortsjo crook exists in the majority of the individuals [18]. As the right posterior sectional bile duct traverses superiorly, dorsally and inferiorly to the right branch of the portal vein and takes hold of the original portion of the right anterior sectional portal vein, right anterior sectionectomy may cause injury to the right posterior bile duct in the case of transecting the right anterior pedicle too close to its origin. In order to avoid this mistake, transection of the right anterior pedicle should be carried out as distal as possible.

References

1. Couinaud C. Anatomic principles of left and right regulated hepatectomy: technics. J Chir. 1954;70(12):933.
2. Lau WY, et al. Chapter 2. Liver segments. In: Lau WY, editor. Applied anatomy in liver resection and liver transplantation. Beijing: People's Medical Publishing House; 2011. p. 7–21.
3. Healy JE Jr, Schroy PC. Anatomy of the biliary ducts within the human liver: analysis of the prevailing pattern of branchings and the major variations of the biliary ducts. Arch Surg. 1953;66(5):599.
4. Strasberg SM. Nomenclature of hepatic anatomy and resections: a review of the Brisbane 2000 system. J Hepatobiliary Pancreat Surg. 2005;12(5):351–5.
5. Terminology committee of the IHPBA. The Brisbane 2000 terminology of liver anatomy and resections. HPB (Oxford). 2000;2:333–9.
6. Couinaud C. Surgical anatomy of the liver revisited. Paris: Self-printed; 1989.
7. Yamamoto M, Katagiri S, Ariizumi S, Kotera Y, Takahashi Y, Egawa H. Tips for anatomical hepatectomy for hepatocellular carcinoma by the Glissonean pedicle approach (with videos). J Hepatobiliary Pancreat Sci. 2014;21(8):E53–6.
8. Launois B, Tay KH. Intrahepatic glissonian approach. In: Lau WY, editor. Hepatocellular carcinoma. Singapore: World Scientific Publishing; 2008. p. 429–46.
9. Lau WY, et al. Chapter 6. Hepatic hilar plate system. In: Lau WY, editor. Applied anatomy in liver resection and liver transplantation. Beijing: People's Medical Publishing House; 2011. p. 31–40.
10. Iqbal S, Iqbal R, Iqbal F. Surgical implications of portal vein variations and liver segmentations: a recent update. J Clin Diagn Res. 2017;11(2):AE01–5.
11. Dina C, Bordei P, Beşleagă A, Bordei L. Aspects de la vascularisation segmentaire veineuse du foie. Morphologie. 2005;89(287):176.
12. Sahani D, Mehta A, Blake M, Prasad S, Harris G, Saini S. Preoperative hepatic vascular evaluation with CT and MR angiography: implications for surgery. Radiographics. 2004;24(5):1367.
13. Soyer P, Bluemke DA, Choti MA, Fishman EK. Variations in the intrahepatic portions of the hepatic and portal veins: findings on helical CT scans during arterial portography. Am J Roentgenol. 1995;164(1):103–8.
14. Lau WY, et al. Chapter 7. Anatomy of the abdominal inferior vena cava and its suprarenal branches. In: Lau WY, editor. Applied anatomy in liver resection and liver transplantation. Beijing: People's Medical Publishing House; 2011. p. 60–7.
15. Erbay N, Raptopoulos V, Pomfret EA, Kamel IR, Kruskal JB. Living donor liver transplantation in adults: vascular variants important in surgical planning for donors and recipients. Am J Roentgenol. 2003;181(1):109.
16. Kamel IR, Lawler LP, Fishman EK. Variations in anatomy of the middle hepatic vein and their impact on formal right hepatectomy. Abdom Imaging. 2003;28(5):668.
17. Blumgart LH, Hann LE. Liver, biliary, and pancreatic anatomy and physiology. In: Jarnagin WR, editor. Blumgart's surgery of the liver, pancreas and biliary tract. 5th ed. Philadelphia: Elsevier Saunders; 2012. p. 31–57.
18. Hjortsjo CH. The topography of the intrahepatic duct systems. Acta Anat. 1952;11(4):599–615.

Preoperative Preparations for Patients with Hepatocellular Carcinoma

Jiangsheng Huang, Jixiong Hu, Xianling Liu, Zhongkun Zuo, and Tenglong Tang

Preoperative Imaging

Enhua Xiao, Manjun Xiao and Shanshan Chen

Introduction

- As the most common primary hepatic malignant tumor, hepatocellular carcinoma (HCC) is related to chronic liver disease (CLD) and cirrhosis. The main risk factors of HCC are chronic hepatitis B and hepatitis C.
- The diagnosis of HCC may be established noninvasively on imaging, and treatment may be initiated without confirmation of biopsy [1].
- At present, major clinical practice guidelines approve dynamic computed tomography (CT) and magnetic resonance (MR) imaging using the extracellular contrast agent as the preferred choice of HCC detection. Unenhanced, hepatic arterial, portal venous, and delayed phase should be included in these examinations. Both patterns show an excellent sensitivity for HCC nodules >2 cm, moderate for HCCs sized 1–2 cm, and poor for HCCs <1 cm, and which pattern is superior is not yet clear.
- Imaging staging refers to the size and number of HCC lesions, the presence of macrovascular invasion and extrahepatic metastases based on imaging examinations, it is very important in clinical decision making and treatment strategies optimizing.

CT and MR Imaging Appearances of Precursor Nodules and HCC

- Typically, HCC develops in a stepwise manner. The carcinogenesis of HCC is orderly termed regenerative nodule (RN), dysplastic nodule (DN), which includes low-grade dysplastic nodule (LGDN) and high-grade dysplastic nodule (HGDN), early HCC and progressed HCC [2, 3].

Regenerative Nodules (RNs)

- CLD leads to hepatocyte injury and the formation of RNs plays as a repair mechanism to replace the damaged hepatocytes and hepatic tissue.
- RNs are areas of the cirrhotic hepatic parenchyma surrounded by fibrosing scar. Typically, they are well-defined and rounded.
- RNs are normal in nature and are generally recognized as benign nodules.
- Compared to background hepatic parenchyma, RNs are typically iso- or hyperattenuating on pre-enhanced CT image and T1 weighted image (T1WI), and hypoattenuating on T2 weighted image (T2WI). Occasionally, they may demonstrate hyperattenuating on TIWI and hypoattenuating on T2WI (Fig. 1).

The corresponding author of the section "Preoperative Imaging" is Enhua Xiao, Email: cjr.xiaoenhua@vip.163.com
The corresponding author of the section "Management Before Hepatectomy for Hepatocellular Carcinoma with Cirrhosis" is Jiangsheng Huang, Email: HJS13907313501@yahoo.com

J. S. Huang
Department of Minimally Invasive Surgery, The Second Xiangya Hospital, Central South University, Changsha, Hunan, PR China
e-mail: HJS13907313501@yahoo.com

J. X. Hu
Department of Hepatobiliary Surgery and Hunan Provincial Key Laboratory of Hepatobiliary Disease Research, The Second Xiangya Hospital, Central South University, Changsha, Hunan, PR China
e-mail: 13908459086@163.com

X. L. Liu
Department of Oncology, The Second Xiangya Hospital, Central South University, Changsha, Hunan, PR China
e-mail: liuxianling3180@163.com

Z. K. Zuo (✉) · T. L. Tang
Department of Minimally Invasive Surgery, The Second Xiangya Hospital, Central South University, Changsha, Hunan, PR China
e-mail: arthasreal@csu.edu.cn; tangtenglong@csu.edu.cn

J. S. Huang et al. (eds.), *Atlas of Anatomic Hepatic Resection for Hepatocellular Carcinoma*,
https://doi.org/10.1007/978-981-13-0668-6_2

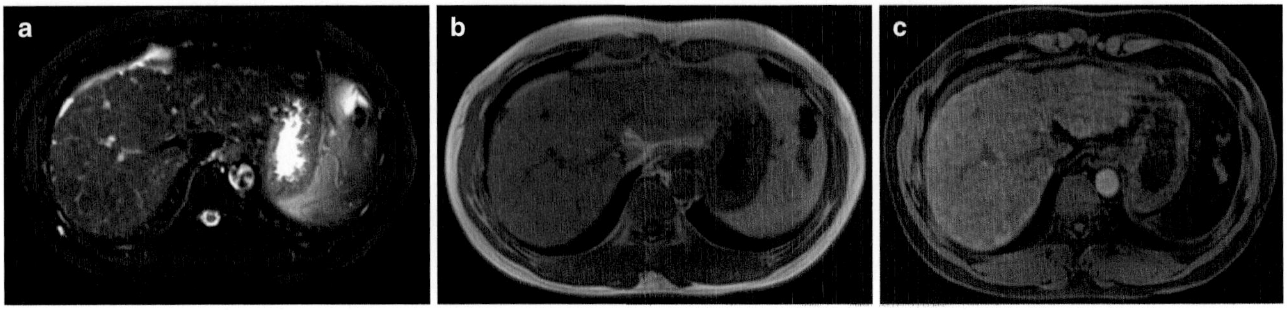

Fig. 1 MR Images of a 39-year-old man with cirrhosis show multiple RNs. (**a**) Fat-suppressed Transverse T2WI shows multiple hypointense nodules; (**b**) Transverse T1WI shows multiple nodules of iso- or hypointense; (**c**) Nodules are iso- or hyperintense on fat-suppressed T1WI

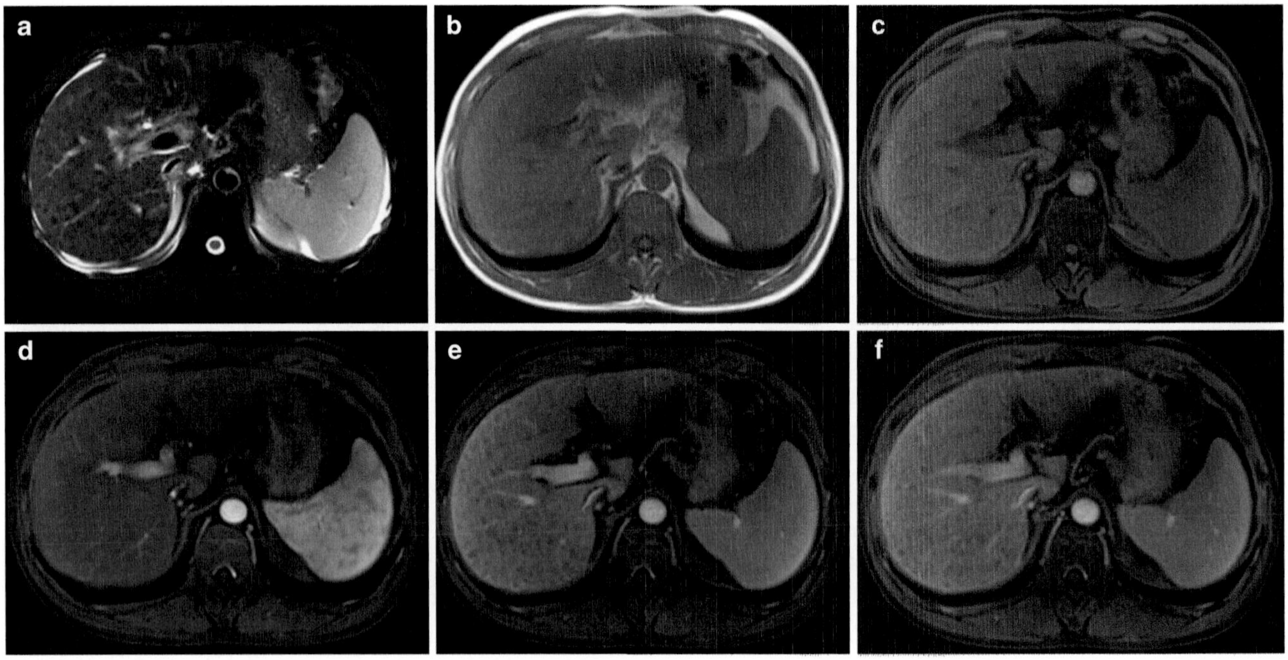

Fig. 2 MR Images of a 43-year-old man with cirrhosis show multiple RNs and DNs in the liver. (**a**) Fat-suppressed Transverse T2WI shows multiple hypointense nodules; (**b**) Transverse T1WI shows multiple iso- or hypointense nodules; (**c**) Nodules are iso- or hyperintense on fat-suppressed T1WI; (**d**) In the arterial phase, these nodules have no enhancement; (**e, f**) In the portal venous and interstitial phase, multiple RNs appear mildly hypointense relative to enhancing fibrosis, some DNs appear isointense or mildly hyperintense

- When injected with extracellular contrast, most RNs have the same enhanced degree as neighboring hepatic parenchyma or enhance slightly less, and in portal venous phase, they may appear slightly hypoattenuating relative to enhancing fibrosis (Fig. 2).

Dysplastic Nodules

- Some hepatic cells in RNs may present atypical characteristic and become dysplastic. As the number of dysplastic cells increases, RNs develop into DNs, which are precancerous lesions.
- Depending on the existence of histocytological and structural alterations, DNs are classified into low grade (LGDN) or high grade (HGDN).
- LGDNs show features similar to that of RN histologically except containing unpaired arteries and clone-like features.
- HGDNs demonstrate cellular atypia with clone-like populations, enlarged subnodules, and structural aberrations, which resemble a highly differentiated HCC. Some HGDNs may have a nodule-in-nodule architecture resulted from containing subnodules of HCC.
- In the arterial phase, portal venous phase and delayed phase of CT examination, most DNs are hypo- or isoattenuating. They are typically hyper- or isoattenuating on T1WI and iso- to hypoattenuating on T2WI (Figs. 2 and 3). Some DNs may have intracellular fat leading to intensity decrease in out-phase image relative to in-phase image. Unlike HCCs, DNs hardly show hyperintense on T2WI or restricted diffusion.

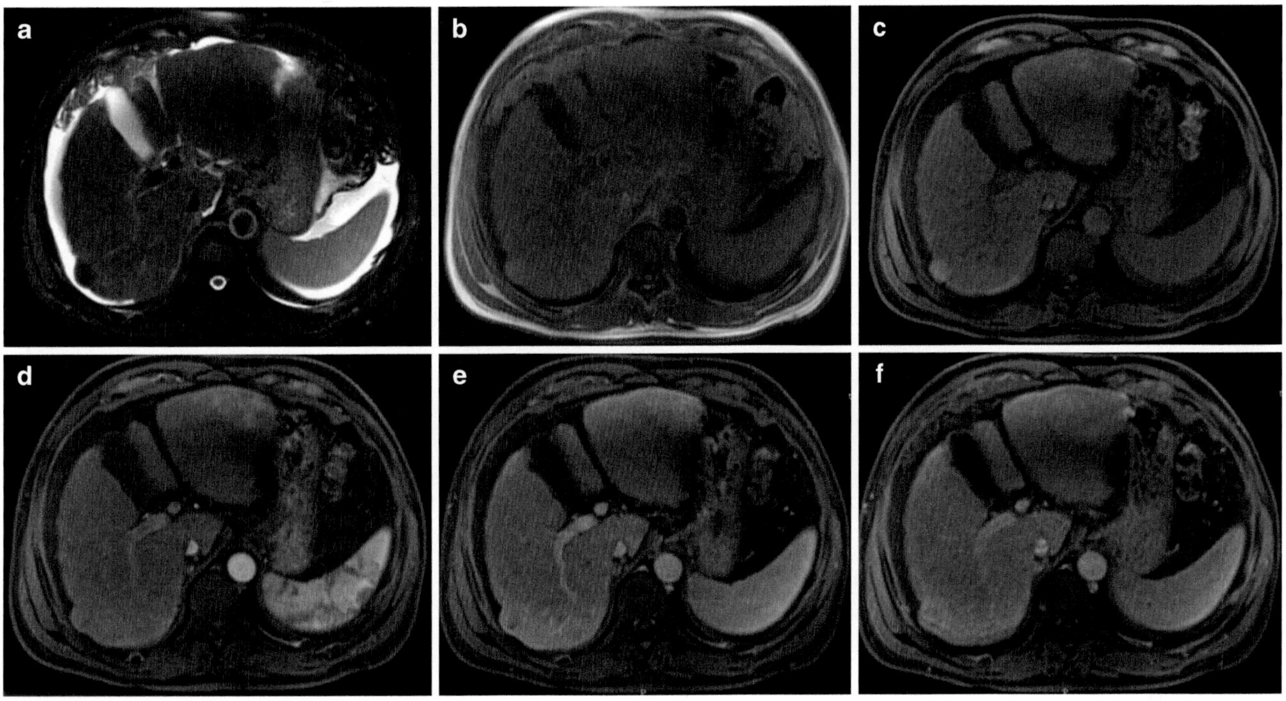

Fig. 3 MR Images of a 54-year-old man with cirrhosis show a DN in S6. (**a**) Fat-suppressed Transverse T2WI shows a hypointense nodule in S6; (**b**, **c**) The nodule is hyperintense on transverse T1WI (**b**) and on fat-suppressed T1WI (c); (**d**) In arterial phase, the nodule has no enhancement; (**e**, **f**) In the portal venous (**e**) and interstitial phase (**f**), the nodule mildly enhanced and appeared mild hyperintense. The nodule has been doubled in size since the year before, and it is an early HCC developed from DN

Early HCC

- HCC initially develops as a small focus within DNs, and then it increases in size. Neovascularity within DNs derives from branches of hepatic artery, and they immortalize the growth of these nodules and promote development into HCCs.
- Early HCC (Fig. 3) resembles carcinoma-in-situ of other organs. Early HCCs almost <2 cm and rarely displace and destroy peripheric hepatic parenchyma like progressed HCC, they gradually replace the surrounding parenchyma and grow.
- Stromal invasion of early HCC is defined as tumor cells infiltrating into fibrous tissue surrounding portal tracts, which is the main distinguishing feature of HGDNs and early HCCs.

Progressed HCC

- These lesions are significantly malignant and have a tendency to invade vessels and metastasize [4].
- Lesions <2 cm (Fig. 4) are typically well-circumscribed nodule; they expand by extending into and compressing peripheric hepatic parenchyma forming a pseudocapsule (Figs. 5, 6, 7, and 8).
- Lesions >2 cm (Figs. 5 and 9) show a more aggressive biological behavior.
- HCC may present as: Solitary (50%) (Figs. 5 and 9), Multifocal (40%) (Fig. 8), Diffuse (10%) (Figs. 10 and 11).
- Usually, HCC is a tumor of hypervascularity and blood supply of it originates from branches of hepatic artery. The most sensitive phase for small HCC detection is arterial phase because HCCs are significantly enhanced in arterial phase.
- HCCs show tendency to invade vessels, including the portal vein and hepatic veins and their branches. Compared to the hepatic veins branches, the portal vein branches are apt to be affected. Vascular invasion is infrequent in solitary and multifocal nodular HCCs, but always can be observed in diffuse HCC.

Solitary and Multifocal HCCs

- On pre-contrast CT images, HCCs are usually hypoattenuated, and sometimes may be isoattenuated.
- On dynamic enhanced CT images, enhancement features of typical HCC are as follows:
  - In arterial phase: HCCs demonstrate significant enhancement. When the lesion <3 cm, enhancement is typically homogeneous, and when the lesion >3 cm, enhancement is usually heterogeneous. Tumor capsule may present as a hypoattenuated rim (Fig. 5).

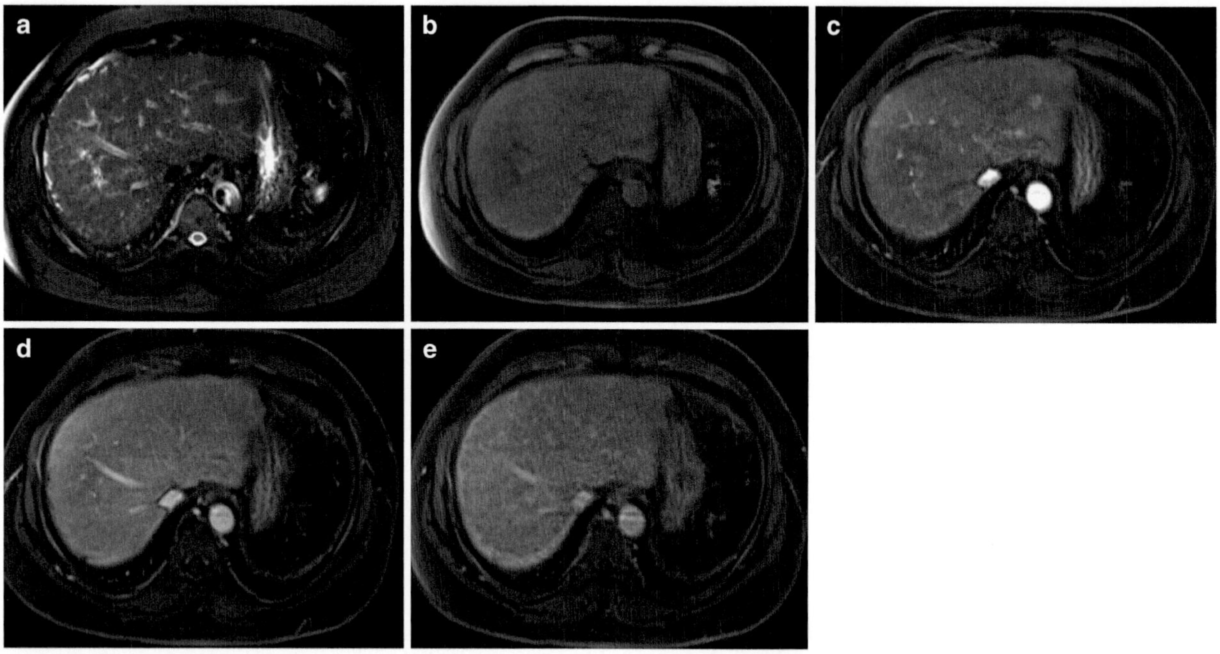

Fig. 4 MR Images of a 45-year-old man with liver cirrhosis shows a small HCC in S2. (**a**) Fat-suppressed Transverse T2WI shows a slightly hyperintense nodule in S2; (**b**) The nodule is isointense on fat-suppressed T1WI; (**c**) In arterial phase, the nodule shows significant enhancement; (**d**) In the portal venous phase, enhancement fade and subtle wash-out in the interstitial phase (**e**)

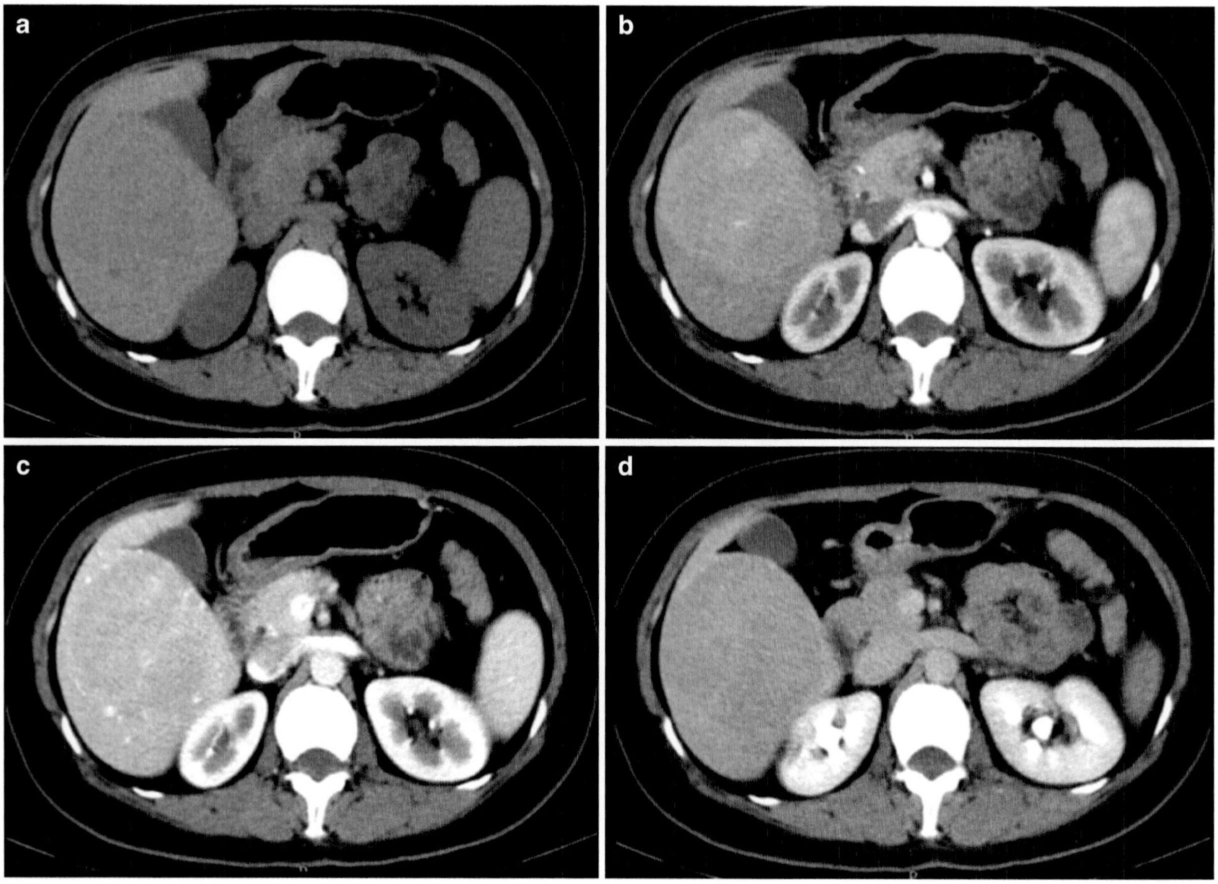

Fig. 5 CT Images of a 26-year-old woman show a large mass in right liver. The mass appears iso- or slightly hypodense relative to the peripheral liver on pre-contrast CT image (**a**), shows prominent enhancement in the hepatic arterial phase (**b**), fading in the hepatic venous phase (**c**) and subtle wash-out in the interstitial phase (**d**). Slight enhancement of capsule is noted in the interstitial phase (**d**). The mass was resected, and pathologically confirmed HCC

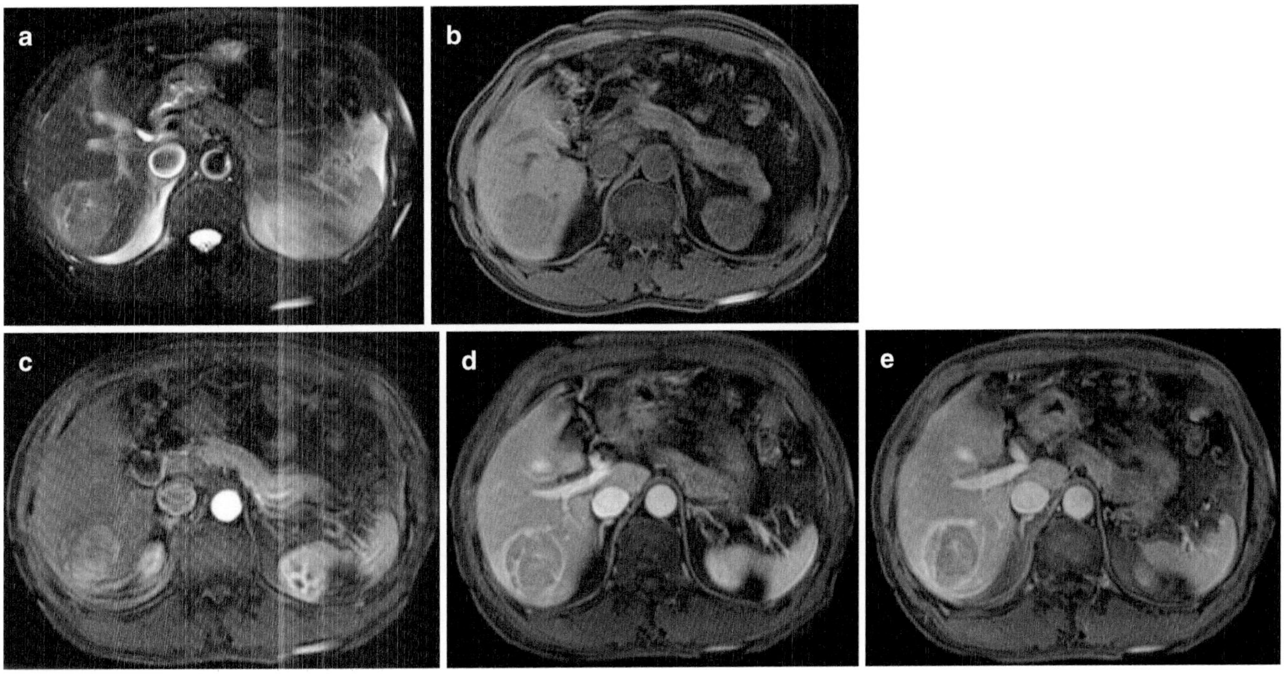

Fig. 6 MR Images of a 69-year-old man show a HCC in S6. (**a**) Fat-suppressed Transverse T2WI shows a slightly hyperintense nodule in S6; (**b**) The nodule is hypointense on fat-suppressed T1WI; (**c**) In the arterial phase, the nodule shows significant enhancement; (**d**) In the portal venous and (**e**) the interstitial phase, enhancement fade and the capsule and septa enhanced. In addition, the mass increases in size in half a year

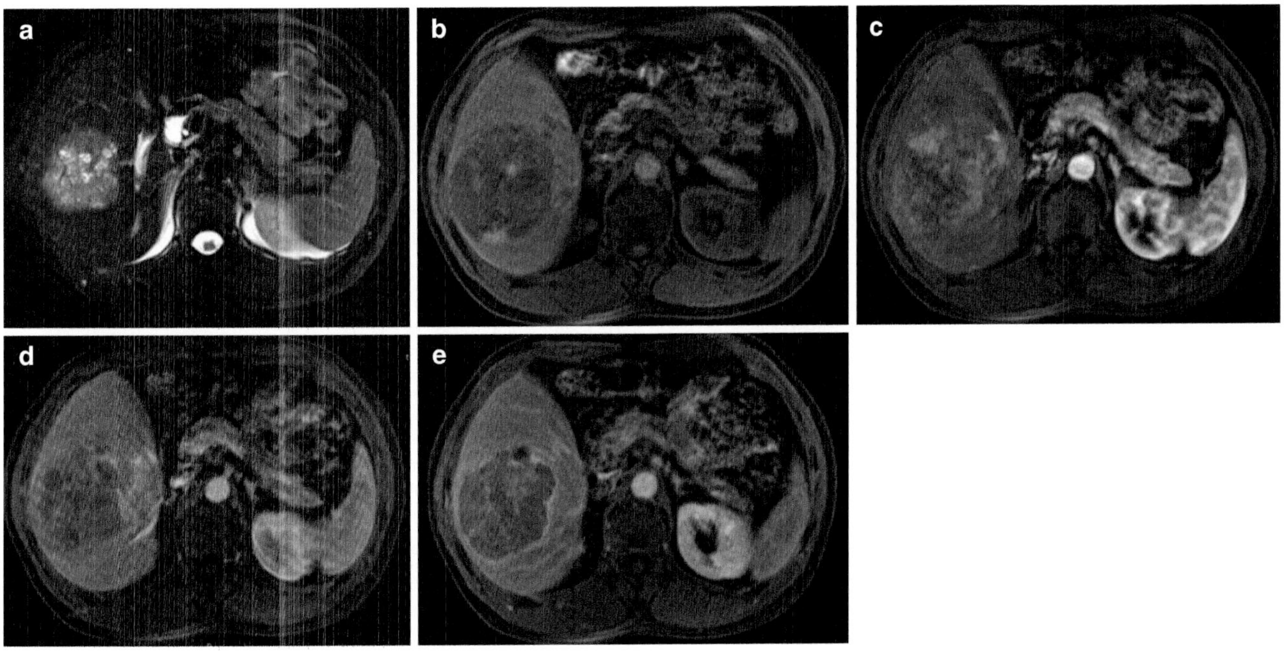

Fig. 7 MR Images of a 46-year-old man show a HCC in right liver. (**a**) Fat-suppressed Transverse T2WI shows a heterogeneous signal and major hyperintense mass in right liver lobe; (**b**) The mass is major hypointense on fat-suppressed T1WI, and there are patches of hyperintense in the lesion (hemorrhage); (**c**) In the arterial phase, the nodule appears obvious heterogeneous enhancement; (**d**) In the portal venous phase, enhancement fade and (**e**) wash-out in the interstitial phase. Capsular enhancement is noted in the interstitial phase. Mosaic appearance is noted in the portal vein phase

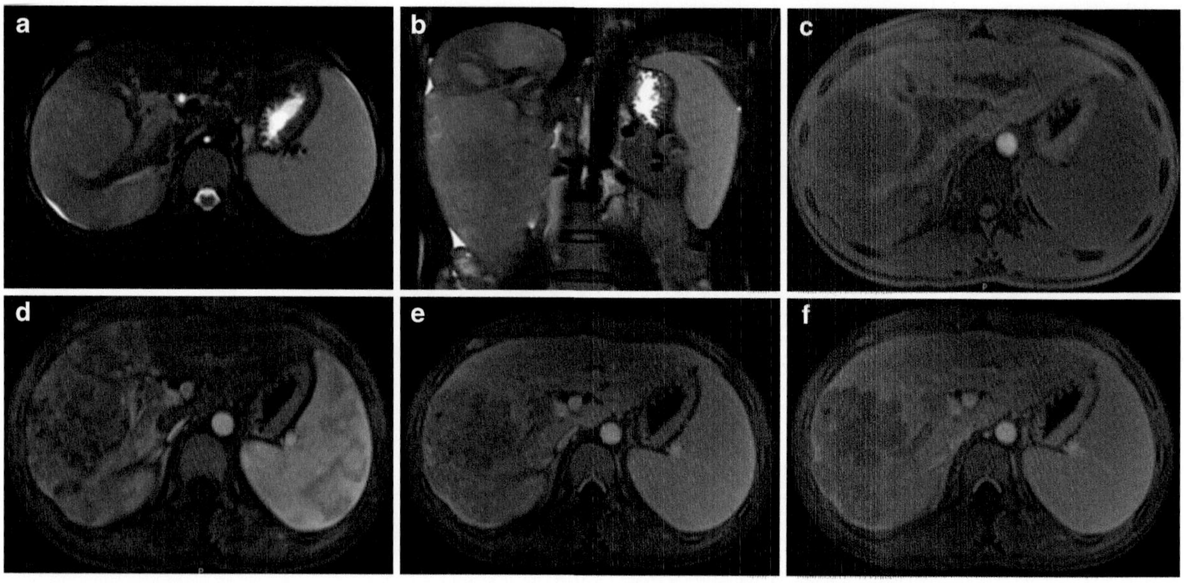

Fig. 8 MR Images of a 22-year-old man show multifocal HCCs. (**a, b**) Fat-suppressed Transverse and coronal T2WI shows multiple hyperintense mass and nodules in right liver, and hyperintense in the right portal vein; (**c**) The liver and portal vein lesions are hypointense on fat-suppressed T1WI; (**d**) In the arterial phase, the lesions (including portal vein lesion) show heterogeneous enhancement; (**e**) In the portal venous, enhancement fade, and (**f**) wash-out in the interstitial phase

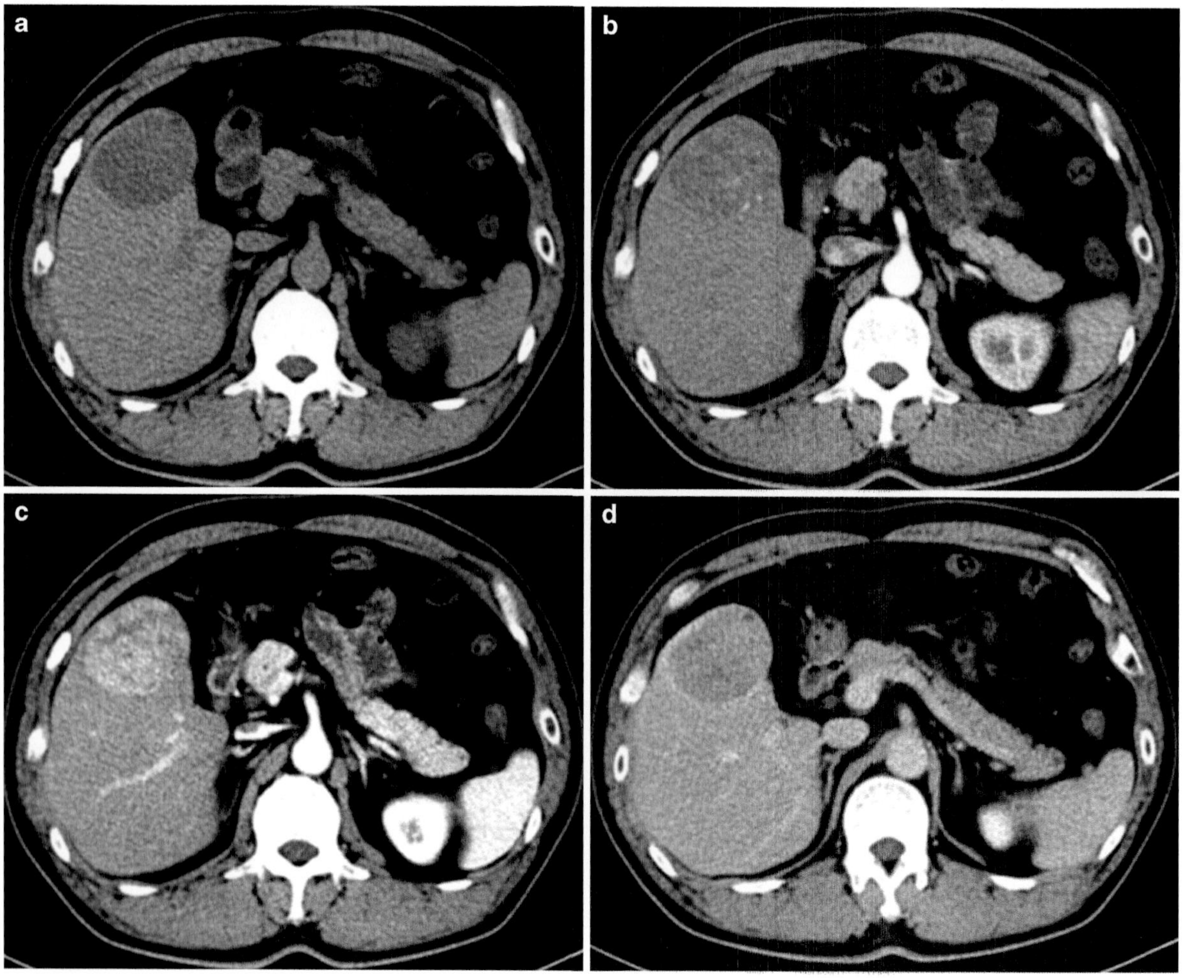

Fig. 9 CT Images of a 47-year-old man show a HCC in S4 of left liver. The lesion appears iso- or slightly hypodense relative to the surrounding parenchyma on pre-contrast CT image (**a**), shows slight enhancement in hepatic arterial phase (**b**), prominent enhancement in the hepatic venous phase (**c**) and remarkable wash-out in the interstitial phase (**d**). Slight capsular enhancement is noted in the interstitial phase (**d**). The lesion was resected, and pathologically confirmed HCC

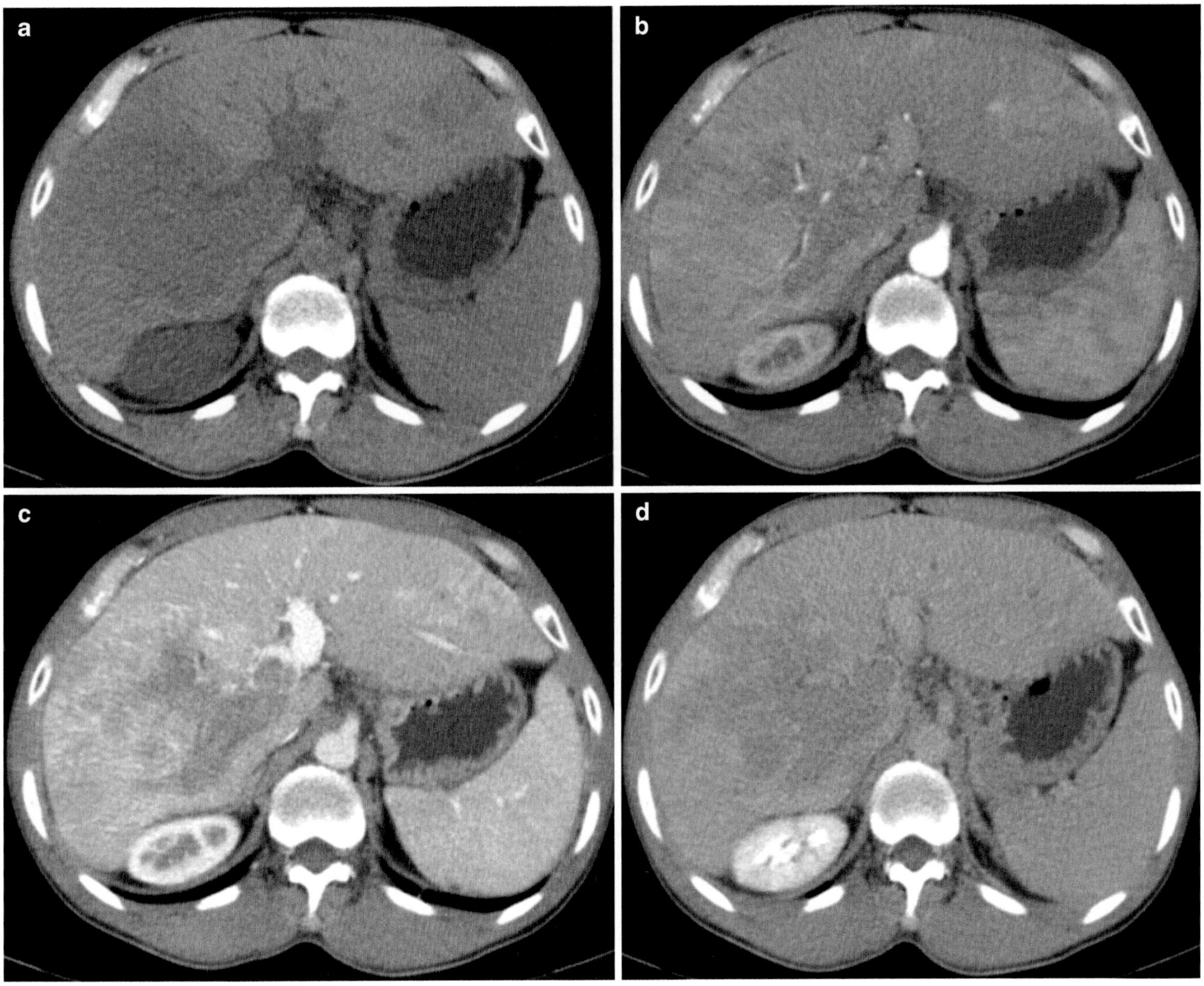

Fig. 10 CT Images of a 51-year-old man show diffuse HCC of right liver, invading the right portal vein. The lesion appears iso- or slightly hypodense compared to the liver on pre-contrast CT image (**a**), shows slight enhancement in the hepatic arterial dominant phase (**b**) and fade in the hepatic venous phase (**c**) and mild wash-out in the interstitial phase (**d**). The tumor thrombus in the right portal vein shows early enhancement (**b**) and later wash-out (**c**, **d**)

  - In venous phase: HCCs usually show wash-out and turn hypoattenuating relative to surrounding hepatic parenchyma. The capsule demonstrates enhancement. Occasionally, HCCs may also be isoattenuating in this phase (Fig. 5).
  - In delayed phase: Fibrosing areas, including tumor capsule and intratumor septa, typically show prolonged enhancement.
- On T2WI: HCCs generally show mildly high signal (Figs. 4 and 7), especially when the lesion size is >3 cm. Small HCCs (<3 cm) are commonly isoattenuating, however, they may also show mild hypo- or hyperintense.
- On T1WI: Smaller HCCs (<3 cm) are generally isoattenuating, although they may be low or high signal. Larger HCCs (>3 cm) generally show heterogeneous hypointense.
- On enhanced T1WI, typical HCCs present similar enhancement characteristics (Fig. 6).
- In solitary and multifocal HCCs, following imaging characteristics is related to poor prognosis: (1) Enlarged tumor lesion; (2) Thick ring enhancement in arterial phase; (3) Venous thrombosis; (4) Hemorrhage; (5) Large size; (6) Significantly increased size in short intervals; (6) Slight to moderate T2 hyperintensity; (7) Metastases.

Diffuse HCC (Figs. 10 and 11)

- Diffuse HCCs are usually associated with high levels of AFP, but about 1/3 patients can present normal levels of AFP.
- Characterized by an infiltrative ill-defined mass and always related to venous thrombosis.

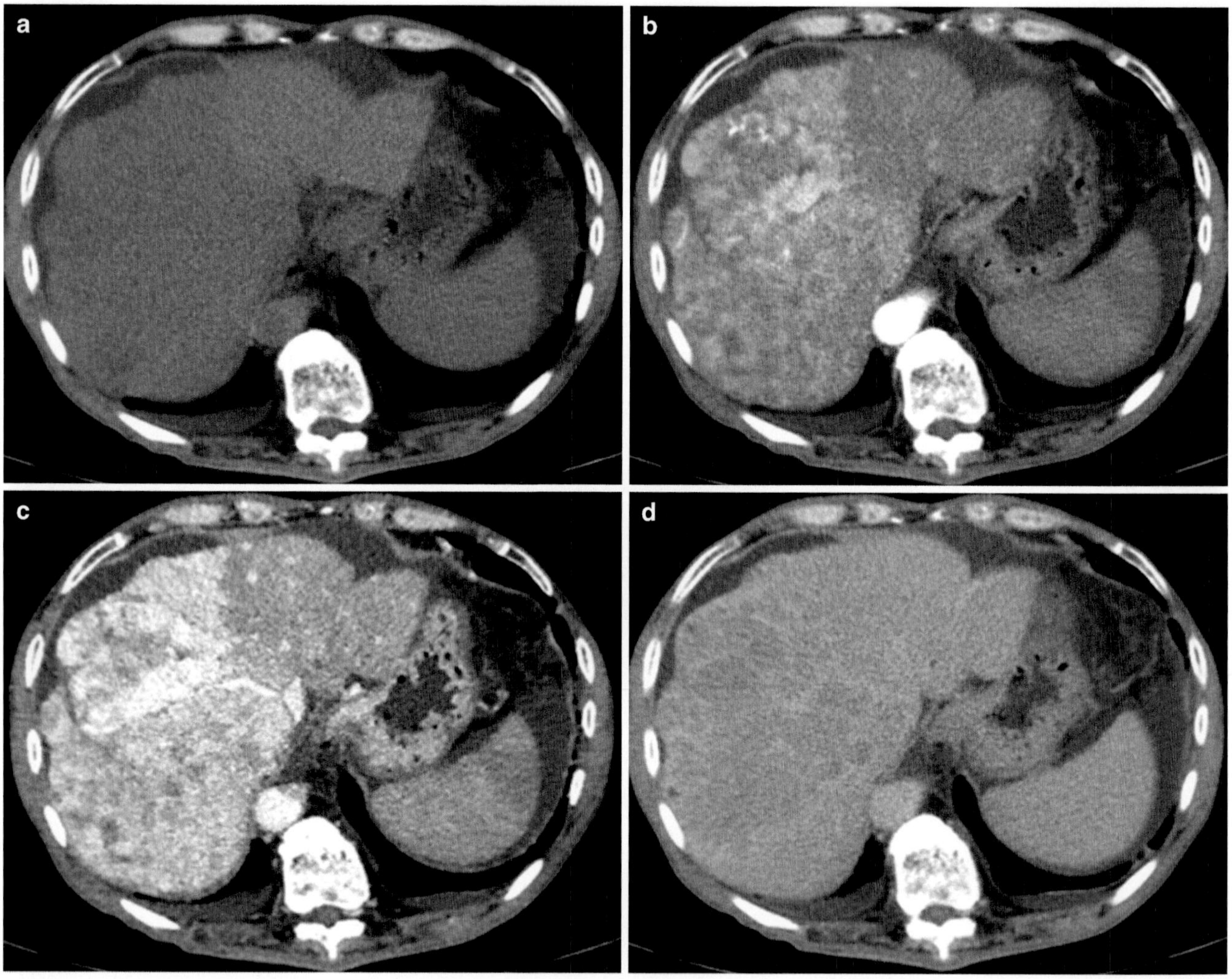

Fig. 11 CT Images of a 73-year-old man show diffuse HCC with hepatic vein invasion. The HCC involving most of the liver shows mild hypodense on pre-contrast CT image (**a**), heterogeneous prominently increased enhancement in the hepatic arterial dominant phase (**b**) and the hepatic venous phase (**c**) and wash-out in the interstitial phase (**d**). Note that the invaded right and left hepatic vein are not normally present in hepatic venous phase (**c**)

- On T2WI: amorphous, segmental or wedge-shaped, slight to moderate hyperintensity.
- On T1WI: amorphous, segmental or wedge-shaped, isointense or slight to moderate hypointense.
- On enhanced T1WI: heterogeneous wash-in in arterial phase and inhomogeneous wash-out (fading) in portal venous or delayed phases. Irregularly presented wash-out can be detected, and parts of capsules are obviously enhanced in late phase.
- Tumor thrombosis usually involves portal vein branches, while hepatic venous tumor thrombus (Fig. 11) is relatively rare, sometimes they are alone, but usually they are co-existence with thrombosis involved portal vein.
- Portal vein tumor thrombus (PVTT) (Fig. 10):
  – A well-known complication of HCC.
  – It can be more easily observed on MR than on CT.
  – Modify typical imaging features.
  – Lead to arterioportal shunting.
  – Large HCCs with PVTT less often show the typical enhancement in arterial phase and wash-out in portal venous phase.
  – PVTT expands the portal vein and itself can demonstrate arterial phase wash-in and subsequent wash-out.
  – The arterioportal shunting may also lead to lacking enhancement of peripheral hepatic tissue.
- Arterioportal shunting (Fig. 12):
  – Arterioportal shunts mostly demonstrate transient lobar, segmental or wedge-shaped enhancement near the tumor in arterial phase and fade back to isointense in portal venous or delayed phase.

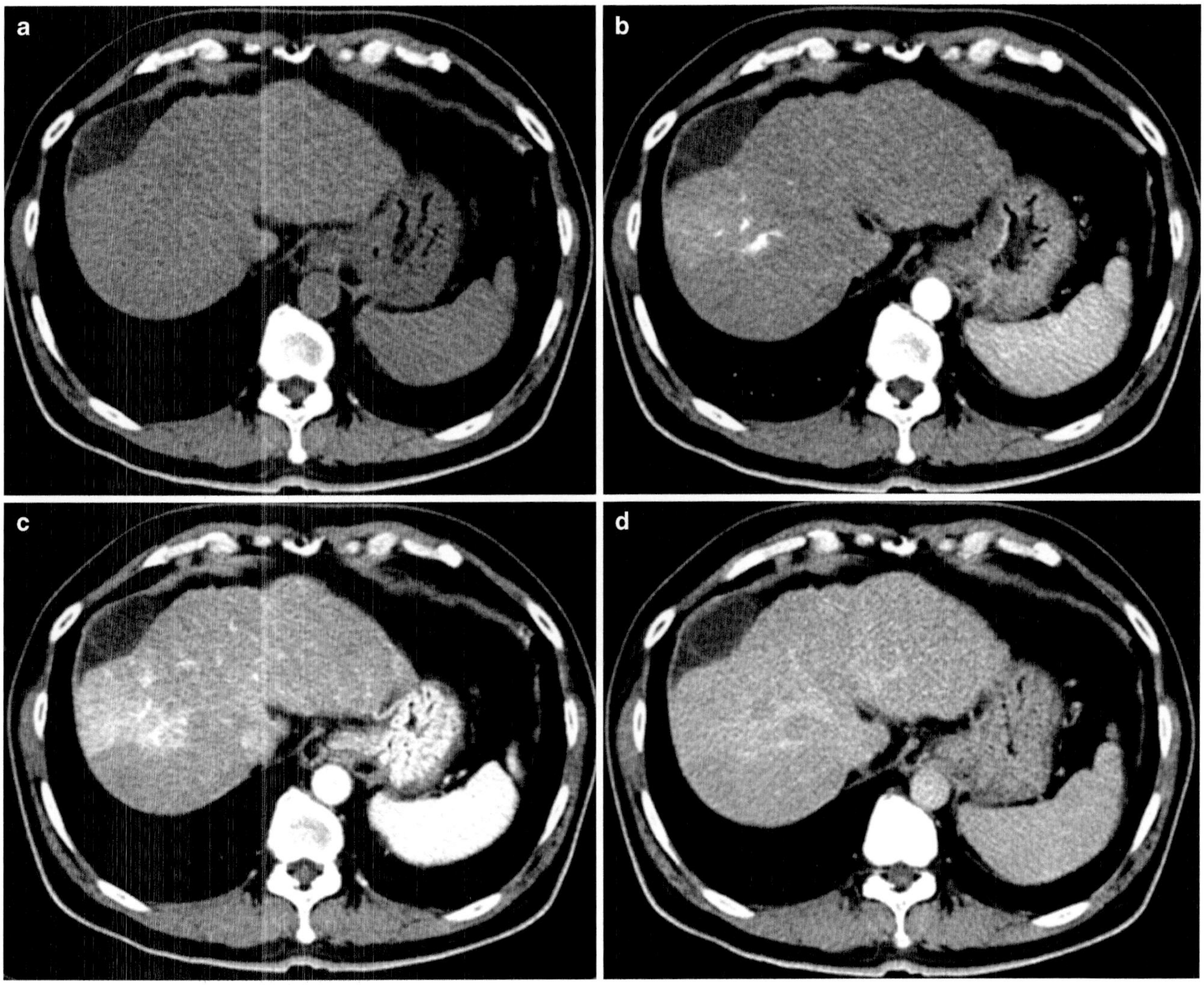

Fig. 12 CT Images of a 62-year-old man show a small HCC with arterioportal shunting, the HCC shows mild hypodense on pre-contrast CT image (**a**), heterogeneous prominently increased enhancement in the hepatic arterial dominant phase (**b**) and the hepatic venous phase (**c**) and wash-out in the interstitial phase (**d**). Transient early increased enhancement represents shunting

Diagnosis and Staging of HCC Based on CT and MR Imaging [5–9]

- Imaging may be used to confirm HCC diagnosis noninvasively, and treatment may be initiated without confirmatory biopsy:
  - In well-defined high-risk populations (e.g., patients with cirrhosis), some imaging features permit a positive predictive value approximating 100% to the diagnosis of HCC.
  - For HCC, biopsy has many limitations such as false-negative outcomes for small lesions and impracticability for evaluating multiple lesions concurrently.
  - Biopsy also has a number of attendant risks, such as bleeding and needle tract seeding complications.
  - According to the current guidelines, biopsy is reserved for suspicious nodules which don't fully satisfy HCC imaging criteria.
- Implicit in imaging-based diagnosis:
  - Differentiation of HCC from non-malignant nodules associated with cirrhosis (e.g., RN, LGDN, HGDN).
  - Benign lesions and pseudolesions encountered in cirrhotic liver (e.g., small hemangiomas, perfusion alterations, focal or confluent fibrosis).
  - Differentiation of HCC from nonhepatocellular malignant tumors that may occur in cirrhotic liver.
- Staging systems are of great importance in predicting the prognosis of HCC patients and guiding the therapeutic approach.
- To assess the prognosis of HCC patients it may be necessary to take not only the tumor stage but also liver function, physical status, and treatment efficacy into consideration.
- Conventionally HCC has been classified by the TNM (tumor-node-metastasis) or Okuda staging systems.

- The use of TNM system is limited because it is based on data from patients who underwent surgical resections and liver function is not considered.
- The Okuda grading system takes tumor size and the degree of underlying cirrhosis into account, but it has limitations in stratifying early or intermediate stage patients.

- Recently, to incorporate tumor stage, physical status, and liver function, some new systems including Barcelona Clinic Liver Cancer (BCLC) staging system have been established. The disease stage is linked to a definite treatment strategy by BCLC staging system.
  - For each stage, there is a corresponding treatment schedule ranging from curative surgery to best supportive care.
  - BCLC system does a good job in making clinical treatment strategy and especially in selecting early stage patients who could benefit from curative surgery.
  - However, a limitation of the BCLC system is lack of discrimination within the intermediate stage (BCLC-B), as this stage encompasses a broad clinical spectrum with potential for prognostic heterogeneity.
- Although there is no consensus on the best staging system, most current systems incorporate radiologic staging.
- Radiologic staging refers to the determination of the size and number of HCC nodules, macrovascular invasion and extrahepatic metastases based on imaging examinations, which plays an important part in making clinical decision, optimizing treatment strategies, and screening out patients eligible and prior for liver transplantation.
- Patients with one HCC nodule sized 2–5 cm or with 2–3 HCCs nodules measuring up to 3 cm may be prior for transplantation, while HCC patients with macrovascular involved or extrahepatic metastases are not suitable for liver transplantation
- Only nodules satisfying radiologic criteria for typical HCC or proven to be HCC by biopsy are recruited to the staging. Imaging-detected nodules indeterminate but not definite HCC are neglected for staging.
- Detection of microvascular invasion and differentiation of the two causes of multifocality (intrahepatic metastasis or multicentric carcinogenesis) are not part of routine radiologic staging, as imaging methods for these purposes have not yet been validated.
- MR imaging with hepatobiliary agents is emerging as a promising method for HCC detection, more and more evidence implies that it is the most sensitive method for small HCCs and premalignant lesions detection. Using these agents can provide hepatobiliary phase (HBP) images that offer information on hepatocellular function which cannot be provided by the vascular phases.

Diagnosis and Staging of HCC with Extracellular Agents [10]

- CT and MR imaging using extracellular agents establish assessment of HCC mainly based on tumor vascularity.
- For CT and MR imaging, the principles are essentially the same.
- Using extracellular agents, the diagnostic characteristics of HCC are arterial phase hyperenhancement followed by wash-out in portal venous or delayed phase (Figs. 13 and 14).
- Arterial phase hyperenhancement (Figs. 4, 5, 6 and 15):

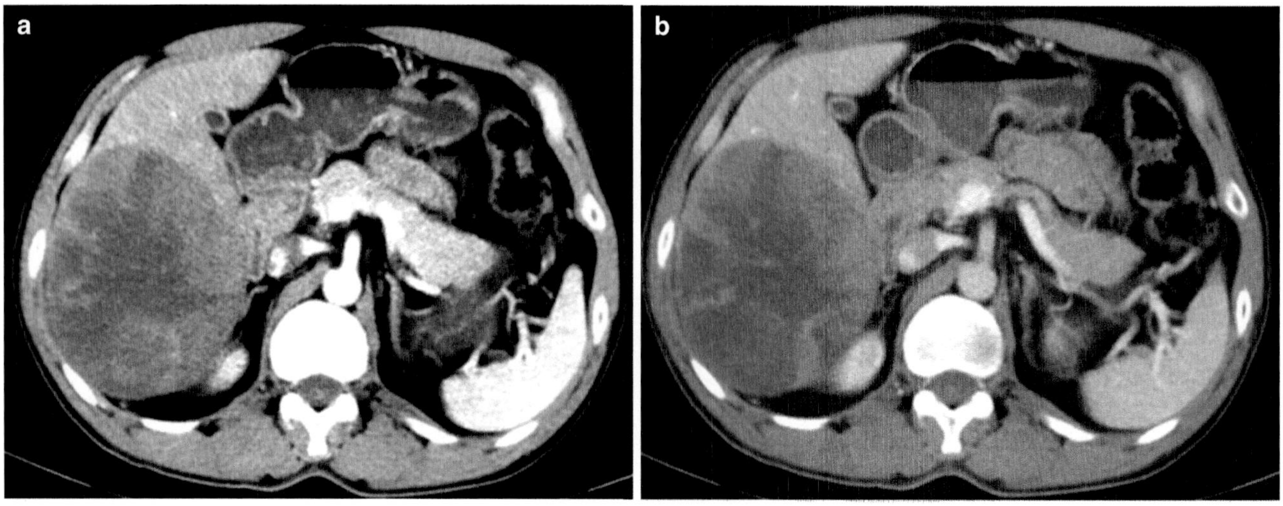

Fig. 13 CT image of a 48-year-old male with a large HCC in the right lobe of the liver shows heterogeneous enhancement in the arterial phase (**a**) and wash-out and mosaic appearance in portal venous phase (**b**)

– Defined as enhancement is greater than that of peripheral parenchyma in arterial phase, also termed arterial "wash-in" or arterial "hypervascularity."
– The pathophysiologic basis is intranodular arterial supply increases during hepatocarcinogenesis. Most RNs, DNs, and early HCCs are hypoenhancing or isoenhancing in arterial phase. Most progressed HCCs are hyperenhancing.
– It is nonspecific, it can also be observed in benign perfusion disorders, hemangiomas, focal nodular hyperplasias (FNHs), some atypical cases of focal or confluent fibrosis, some atypical RNs and DNs, and

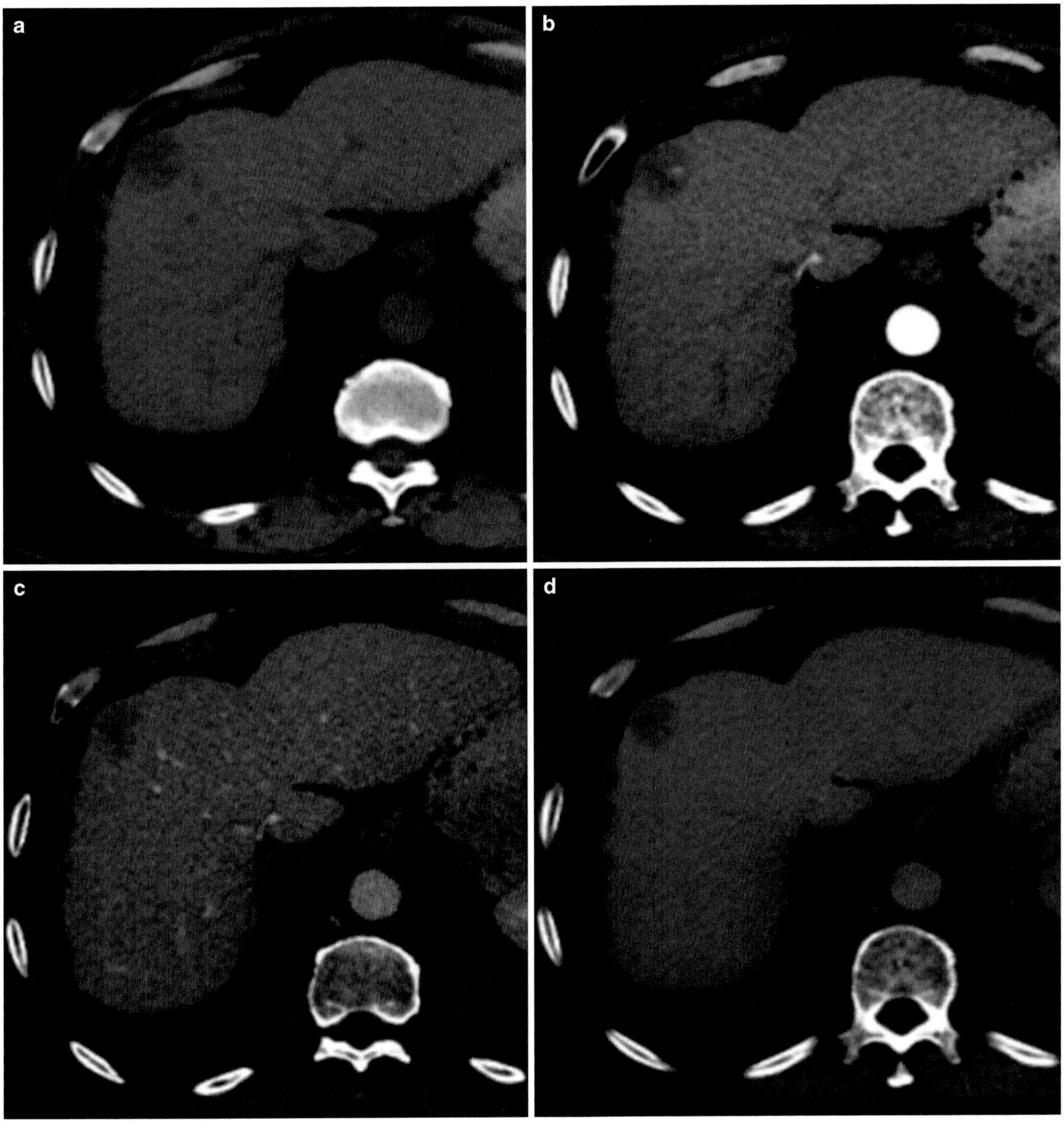

Fig. 14 Nodule-in-nodule appearance: nonenhanced CT image (**a**) showed a hypodense nodule in the right liver. A focus of arterial enhancement is within the larger hypodense nodule (**b**) which demonstrates wash-out in the portal venous (**c**) and delayed (**d**) phases suggestive of development of hepatocellular carcinoma within a pre-existing cirrhosis-related nodule

other malignant tumors such as small intrahepatic cholangiocarcinomas (ICCs) or metastases.
  - In cirrhosis or chronic hepatitis patients, small vascular pseudolesions attributable to arterioportal shunts are particularly common, and the large majority of focal enhancement seen only in arterial phase and measuring less than 2 cm are nonneoplastic, especially those that are wedge-shaped and subcapsular.
- Wash-out appearance (Figs. 4, 5, 6, and 15):
  - It is a decrease in enhancement relative to peripheral parenchyma from early to later phase, which can be visually assessed, leading to hypoenhancement in later phase.
  - The "wash-out" may be more obvious in delayed phase than in portal venous phase, and sometimes "wash-out" may be observed only in delayed phase.
  - In HCC, the mechanisms of "wash-out" are still not fully explained. The temporal decrease in enhancement relative to peripheral parenchyma may not be true wash-out, and as a result the Liver Imaging Reporting and Data System (LI-RADS) advocate the term wash-out appearance.
  - Wash-out appearance is not a specific feature for HCC, which may also be detected in RNs, DNs, and some other alterations such as architecture distortion and enhancing fibrosis.
  - Although the individual features are nonspecific, the incorporation of arterial phase hypervascularity and later phase "wash-out" show high specificity for HCC in patients at risk.
  - The high specificity of this temporal enhancement pattern results in its incorporation into all current systems developed for CT or MR imaging-based diagnosis of HCC in patients with risk factors.
  - This temporal enhancement modality is not specific for HCC diagnosis in general population, where such lesions should be differentiated from hepatocellular adenoma, metastasis, and other lesions.
- Capsule appearance (Figs. 6, 7 and 9):
  - It is another imaging feature characteristic of progressed HCC.
  - Defined as a smooth hyperenhanced peripheral rim in the portal venous or delayed phase.
  - Enhancement increases as time goes on, and the delayed phase may be better to identify this feature compared with the portal venous phase.
  - About one quarter of nodules with radiologically detected "capsules" lack a true capsule at pathologic examination but instead are surrounded by "pseudocapsules" consisting of mixed fibrous tissue and dilated sinusoids.
  - Typical capsule on MR: (1) Iso to hypointense on T2WI and unenhanced T1WI; (2) No or inappreciable arterial enhancement, and more intense later enhancement.
- Satellite nodules (Fig. 15):
  - Defined as extracapsular extension in large progressed HCC intrahepatic metastases around the main tumor within the venous drainage area.
  - Satellite nodules are progressed lesions which can invade vessels and metastasize.
  - They often present as multiple micro nodules outside the tumor outlines. They typically manifest arterial phase hyperenhancement.
  - The presence of satellite nodules has been recognized as an indication of recurrence and lower survival rate after transplantation, resection, and local ablation.
  - Satellite nodules do not help to differentiate HCC from ICC.
- For lesions that meet diagnostic criteria for HCC, careful analysis of enhancement features may provide prognostic information.
- Only HCCs satisfy the imaging criteria of arterial phase hyperenhancement as well as wash-out or capsule appearance can be definitely diagnosed. Other HCCs may be difficult to diagnose.

Diagnosis and Staging of HCC with Hepatobiliary Agents [10]

- Hepatobiliary agents permit assessment not only of tumor vascularity but also of hepatocellular function based mainly on signal intensity relative to liver parenchyma in the hepatobiliary phase (HBP).
- The signal intensity of lesions relative to the hepatic parenchyma in HBP depends on a complex interplay between numerous incompletely understood factors, the dominant determinant is OATP8 expression.
- Since OATP expression declines during hepatocarcinogenesis, the assessment of signal intensity in HPB helps to detect and characterize hepatocellular nodules in the cirrhotic liver.
- Most HCCs, including many early HCCs and some HGDNs are hypointense in HBP due to underexpression of OATP.
- Most RNs, most LGDNs, some HGDNs, and only a small number of HCCs are iso- or hyperintense due to remained expression.
- As a corollary, cirrhosis-associated nodules that are hypointense in HBP are possibly malignant or premalignant, even in the absence of arterial phase hypervascularity or later phase "wash-out" (Fig. 15).
- Perhaps the most important benefit of HBP is that it helps to identify early HCCs. These HCCs have immature neoarterialization, often are isoenhancing in vascular phases, leading to failing detection with extracellular agents.

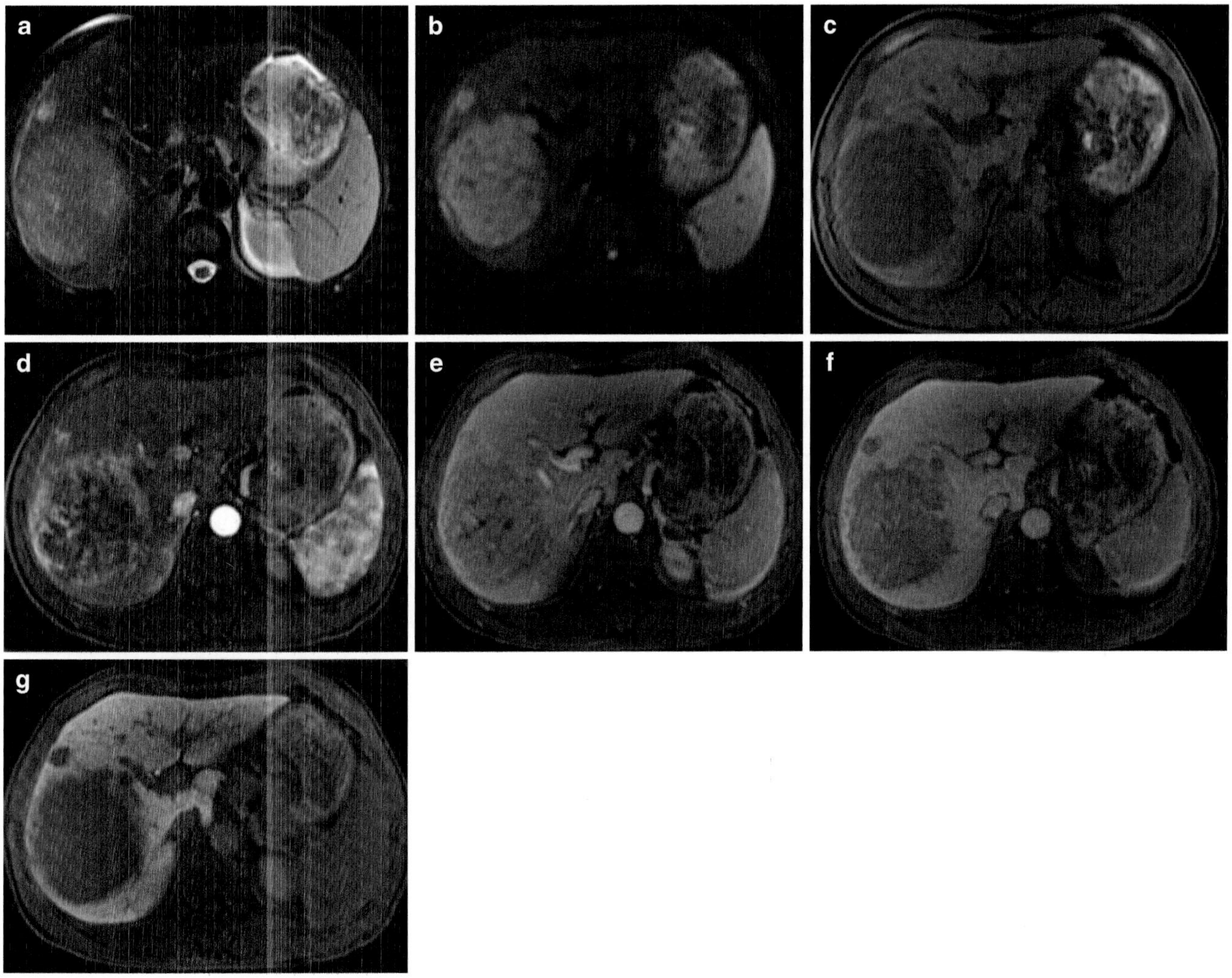

Fig. 15 MR images of a 57-year-old man with HCC show hyperintensity in the HBP. (**a**) T2WI shows a hyperintense mass in the right liver, with two hyperintense small nodules besides it. These lesions are hyperintense on DWI (**b**) and hypointense on T1WI (**c**). (**d**) Gd-EOB-DTPA–enhanced T1WI in late hepatic arterial phase shows that the mass and the two nodules are heterogeneous hyperenhanced. (**e**, **f**) Relative to liver, mass is slightly hypointense in (**e**) portal venous phase and obvious hypointense in (**f**) transitional phase. (**g**) In the hepatobiliary phase, mass is hyperintense with hypointense rim, likely representing tumor capsule. Presence of hypointense rim permits confident diagnosis of HCC despite hyperintensity of lesion. The two nodules besides the main tumor are satellite nodules

- However, since OATP8 expression decreases during hepatocarcinogenesis prior to complete neoarterialization, such HCCs may be observed in HBP as low signal nodules and some early HCCs are visible only in HBP.
- The differential diagnosis for arterial phase hypoenhancing or isoenhancing nodules with HBP hypointensity includes DNIIs, occasional DNIs, occasional large RNs, and nodular areas of fibrosis, so this appearance is not specific for HCC.
- Although most HCCs demonstrate hypointense in HBP, about 5–12% HCCs are hyperintense.
- Other HBP features that favor HCC include focal defect in contrast material uptake, presence of a hypointense rim ("capsule"), and absence of architectural features of focal nodular hyperplasia.
- The main disadvantage of HBP alone for HCC diagnosis and staging is its nonspecificity. So, HBP must be assessed in combination with other sequences and phases.
- Limitations:
  - Many conditions such as severe hepatic dysfunction or cholestasis reduce contrast between lesions and liver, thereby limiting the efficacy of HBP for lesion detection and characterization.
  - A potential pitfall unique to gadoxetate disodium is that this agent provides a transitional phase other than a conventional delayed vascular phase. Therefore, wash-out appearance probably should be estimated only in portal venous phase after injection of gadoxetate disodium.

- Another challenge associated with the transitional phase is that the "capsular" enhancement may be obscured because of relatively high enhancement of the background liver tissues.
- Other limitations unique to gadoxetate disodium-enhanced MR imaging include relatively weak arterial phase hyperenhancement and relatively high frequency of arterial phase artifacts (mainly due to transient dyspnea associated with this agent).

Ancillary Imaging Features for Diagnosis of HCC [11]

- Intralesional fat
  - Characteristic of early HCC but not specific.
  - Differential diagnosis: DNI and DNII. Some progressed HCCs also may be fatty, such as the steatohepatitic variant.
  - Limitation: value for diagnosis of HCC is limited.
- Corona enhancement
  - Characteristic of progressed, hypervascular HCC.
  - It manifests as a temporal zone or rim enhancement surrounding the HCC lesion in late arterial or early portal venous phase, and then falling to isoenhancement.
  - Helps to differentiate progressed, hypervascular HCC from vascular pseudolesions such as arterioportal shunts and thought to represent a frequent site of perilesional satellite metastases.
  - Limitations: May be difficult to recognize at CT or MR imaging; hence, incremental value of this feature for diagnosis of progressed HCC may be modest. Not characteristic of and therefore does not help in diagnosis of early HCC.
  - Pitfall: May overlap and blend with tumor enhancement.
- Nodule-in-nodule architecture (Fig. 14)
  - Nodule-in-nodule growth pattern suggests occurrence of progressed HCC within DN or early HCC.
  - Nodule-in-nodule appearance: (1) On T2WI, it manifests as a smaller focus of hyperintensity within a larger nodule of hypointensity; (2) On enhanced T1WI, it manifests as a focus in a DN, the focus shows a temporal enhancement pattern and the remaining parts enhanced like a DN.
  - Limitation: nodule-in-nodule architecture is uncommonly depicted in HCCs at CT or MR imaging; hence, its value for HCC diagnosis may be modest.
- Mosaic architecture (Fig. 13)
  - Intratumor subnodules separated by fibrous septa, hemorrhage, necrosis, and occasionally fatty degeneration make up a mosaic architecture.
  - Characteristic of and frequently observed in large HCCs.
  - Helps in the differentiation of HCC from ICC.
  - Limitation: mosaic architecture is uncommon in small HCCs; hence, incremental value of this feature for diagnosis of small HCC may be modest.

Assessment of Metastases

- Intrahepatic spread of HCC includes intrahepatic metastasis, vascular invasion, biliary invasion, tumor capsule invasion.
- Extrahepatic metastasis of HCC includes hematogenous metastasis, lymphatic metastasis, implantation metastasis, direct invasion of adjacent organs. Lymph node, adrenal gland, peritoneum, lung, pleura, and bone metastases are commonly observed.

Pre-Operative Imaging Assessment of Future Remnant Liver [12–14]

- The future remnant liver (FRL) is the main base of postoperative outcomes. Without sufficient FRL, liver resection unavoidably results in postresection liver failure.
- Although progress has been made in surgical and perioperative periods, hepatic failure remains a major problem, requiring precise methods to evaluate the function of FRL during liver resection.
- Many tests evaluating FRL has come into use over the past few years, demonstrating that the ideal approach has not yet been defined.

Volumetric Measurement Techniques

- Recently, CT volumetry is the golden standard in the preoperative evaluation of FRL volume.
- By tracing the liver margin in each image slice manually and totalizing the volume of all sections, the volume can be calculated. And then use three-dimensional reconstruction to figure up the volume of tumor, nontumorous liver, and FRL.
- In some institutes, in patients without potential parenchymal disease, an FRL volume of 25% is considered adequate. An FRL volume of at least 40% is accepted in patients with an injured liver.
- CT is noninvasive and is a commonly used method for clinical follow-up, which are the main advantages of CT volumetry.
- Important limitations of preoperative evaluation of liver function only based on CT volumetry are as follows:
  - Firstly, it is time-consuming to manually trace the liver contour.
  - Secondly, tumor characteristics, multiple lesions, and liver characteristics play an important role in CT volumetry sensitivity.
  - Thirdly, there are still no definite criteria and measuring method for minimal FRL volumes.
  - Finally, CT volumetry of FRL does not take into consideration the quality of the remaining liver parenchyma, which is the main limitation.

- Thus, a regional liver function test should be incorporated with CT volumetry to assess FRL.
- Adjustments have been made to overcome some shortcomings of conventional CT volumetric evaluation, such as standardized FRL volume.

Scintigraphic Liver Function Tests

- Scintigraphic liver function tests provide quantitative and visual information on hepatic function. Two most extensively used scintigraphy agents are 99mTc- GSA and HBS with 99mTc-IDA derivatives.
- 99mTc-GSA Scintigraphy
  - Rationale: 99mTc-GSA is an asialoglycoprotein analog labeled with 99mTc and liver is the only site to uptake it. Thus, it is considered as a perfect agent for liver function evaluation. Additionally, 99mTc-GSA scintigraphy can be used in cholestatic patients, as high serum bilirubin levels have no effect on the uptake of 99mTc-GSA.
  - Application: uptake and clearance ratios of 99mTc-GSA, the uptake index of 99mTc-GSA, combining 99mTc-GSA with SPECT-CT or PET.
- HBS with IDA Derivatives Scintigraphy
- Rationale: 99mTc-IDA agents are lidocaine analogs and bound to albumin when transported to the liver, then separate from albumin. Afterwards, hepatocytes take up the agents and then directly excreted the agents into biliary system. As a result, IDA agents are fit for hepatobiliary system imaging.
- Combining dynamic HBS with SPECT-CT can provide an accurate assess of FRL function.

Liver Function Assessment Using MRI

- Except for providing structural information, MRI can also be a probable method for preoperative evaluation of liver function. Gadolinium ethoxybenzyl diethylenetriamine pentaacetic acid (Gd-EOB-DTPA) is a liver-specific contrast agent whose pharmacokinetic properties are similar to 99mTc-HBS agents. Recently, data on liver function assessment using MRI with Gd-EOB-DTPA in humans have been published, confirming the possibility of liver function assessment using MRI.

Other Imaging Techniques for Hepatocellular Carcinoma [15]

Ultrasound (US)

US acts as a screening method for HCC detection. Patients with cirrhosis are recommended to follow up by abdominal US at 6-month intervals.

Advantages: less expensive and radiation-free.

Disadvantages: operator and body habitus dependence, low sensitivity.

Contrast-Enhanced Ultrasound (CEUS)

- Microbubbles utilized in CEUS are confined to the intravascular space and cleared in the lungs. The imaging characteristics of HCC in CEUS are hypervascularity in arterial phase and wash-out in subsequent phases.
- CEUS can be helpful in patients with renal dysfunction.
- Disadvantages: limited field of view, limited sensitivity, operator and body habitus dependence,

Ultrasound Elastography

- Ultrasound elastography allows noninvasive evaluation of tissue elasticity distribution within biological tissues.
- Malignancies are usually stiff, they are much stiffer than benign lesions and normal soft tissue. Ultrasound elastography may be a promising tool for early diagnosis of HCC noninvasively.

Acoustic Radiation Force Impulse Imaging (ARFI)

- As a new ultrasound imaging pattern, ARFI is mainly focused on the assessment of tissue stiffness.
- High ARFI values are related with malignant tumors, while low value associated with benign lesions. The study results of this method remain controversial.

Advances in CT

Conventional CT has relatively high sensitivity and specificity for HCCs detection. Nowadays, advances in CT emerge, such as perfusion CT and dual-energy CT.

Perfusion CT (PCT)

- PCT is performed by obtaining serial images after the injection of a bolus of iodinated contrast agent.
- PCT can provide quantitative information of tumor-related angiogenesis as well as arterial perfusion in early HCCs, can assess segmental hepatic function, and can evaluate tumor response to therapy. However, increased radiation and lower resolution are limitations of PCT.

Dual-Energy CT

- Dual-energy CT capacitates high resolution of tissues and materials, using two different energy spectras. This modality increases the enhancement of vascular structures while reducing radiation dose simultaneously.

MRI

Hepatocyte-Specific Contrast MR Imaging

- Hepatocyte-specific contrast of MRI has been developed to improve the sensitivity for HCC detection.
- The hepatobiliary agents have been described above.

- Superparamagnetic iron oxide (SPIO) particles are taken up by Kupffer cells resulting in significant decrease of signal intensity of the hepatic parenchyma on T2WI. As rarely Kupffer cells are present in HCCs, the tumor takes up little or no SPIO and becomes hyperattenuating relative to surrounding tissue.
- SPIO-enhanced MRI does well in noninvasive diagnosis of HCCs, especially small HCCs. However, as SPIO is not a US Food and Drug Administration-approved contrast agent, the use of it is limited.

Diffusion-Weighted MRI

- Diffusion-weighted imaging (DWI) provides information of the water composition and degree of tumor viability at the cellular level. Live tumors are rich in cells and their cell membranes are intact, which restricts the movement of water molecules, leading to DWI hyperintense and apparent diffusion coefficient (ADC) reduction.
- DWI may provide additional information to differentiate HCCs from DNs.

MR Elastography (MRE)

- MRE can measure the viscoelastic properties of tissues noninvasively, which has potential in differentiating solid malignancies from benign tumors. Hepatic malignancies present much greater mean shear stiffness compared to benign lesions, normal liver and cirrhotic liver.

MR Spectroscopy (MRS)

- Recently, MRS is mainly used in quantifying hepatic lipid contents, while the application of MRS assessment of hepatic tumors is still in the initial stage and study in this aspect is on the way.

Nuclear Imaging

- 18F-FDG and 11C-acetate PET imaging have been used for diagnosis and assessment of the HCC clinically.
- Dynamic PET has been suggested to be a promising method in the differentiation of benign tumors from liver malignancies in some recent studies.

Other Tests

- Invasive and semi-invasive examinations have gradually fallen out of favor for diagnosing purpose, such as hepatic angiography.

Surveillance of HCC

- US mainly acts as a screening method other than a diagnostic one for confirmation.
- CEUS is useful for characterization and diagnosis of hepatic nodules detected by US.
- When a screening test result of liver is abnormal, CT, MRI, or Gd-EOB-DTPA-enhanced MRI is recommended as a first-line method for HCC diagnosis.
- In dynamic CT or dynamic MRI, HCC is characterized by arterial enhancement and wash-out in the portal venous and/or delayed phases.
- The combination of dynamic and HBP of Gd-EOB-DTPA-enhanced MRI with DWI can improve the diagnostic accuracy of HCC.
- Dynamic CT or MRI, chest CT, and bone scintigraphy are recommended as a complete workup, when diagnosed HCC. PET may play a role in staging the whole body and resolving atypical and doubtful lesions.
- Diagnosis of typical HCC can be established by imaging, if demonstrating a specifically characterized imaging criteria on dynamic CT, dynamic MRI, or CEUS.
- Nodular lesions with an atypical imaging pattern should undergo further examinations.

Liver Imaging Reporting and Data System (LI-RADS) Categorization

- LI-RADS is a standardized system with terminology and criteria for CT and MRI liver examinations. Currently, LI-RADS is only suitable for patients with cirrhotic liver or other high risk of HCC. LI-RADS provides a diagnostic algorithm based on precisely defined terms and imaging features, to help radiologists improve consistency and interpretation in assigning a relative probability for HCC to untreated observations visualized in the cirrhotic liver [16, 17]

LI-RADS classification

Category	Description
LR-1	Definitely benign
LR-2	Probably benign
LR-3	Intermediate probability of HCC
LR-4	High probability of HCC, not 100%
LR-5	Definitely HCC
LR-5V	Definite venous invasion regardless of other imaging features
LR treated	LR-5 lesion status post-locoregional treatment
LR-M	Non-HCC malignancies that may occur in cirrhosis: metastases, lymphoma, cholangiocarcinoma, PTLD

Abbreviations: *LI-RADS* liver imaging reporting and data system, *HCC* hepatocellular carcinoma, *PTLD* post-transplant lymphoproliferative disorder

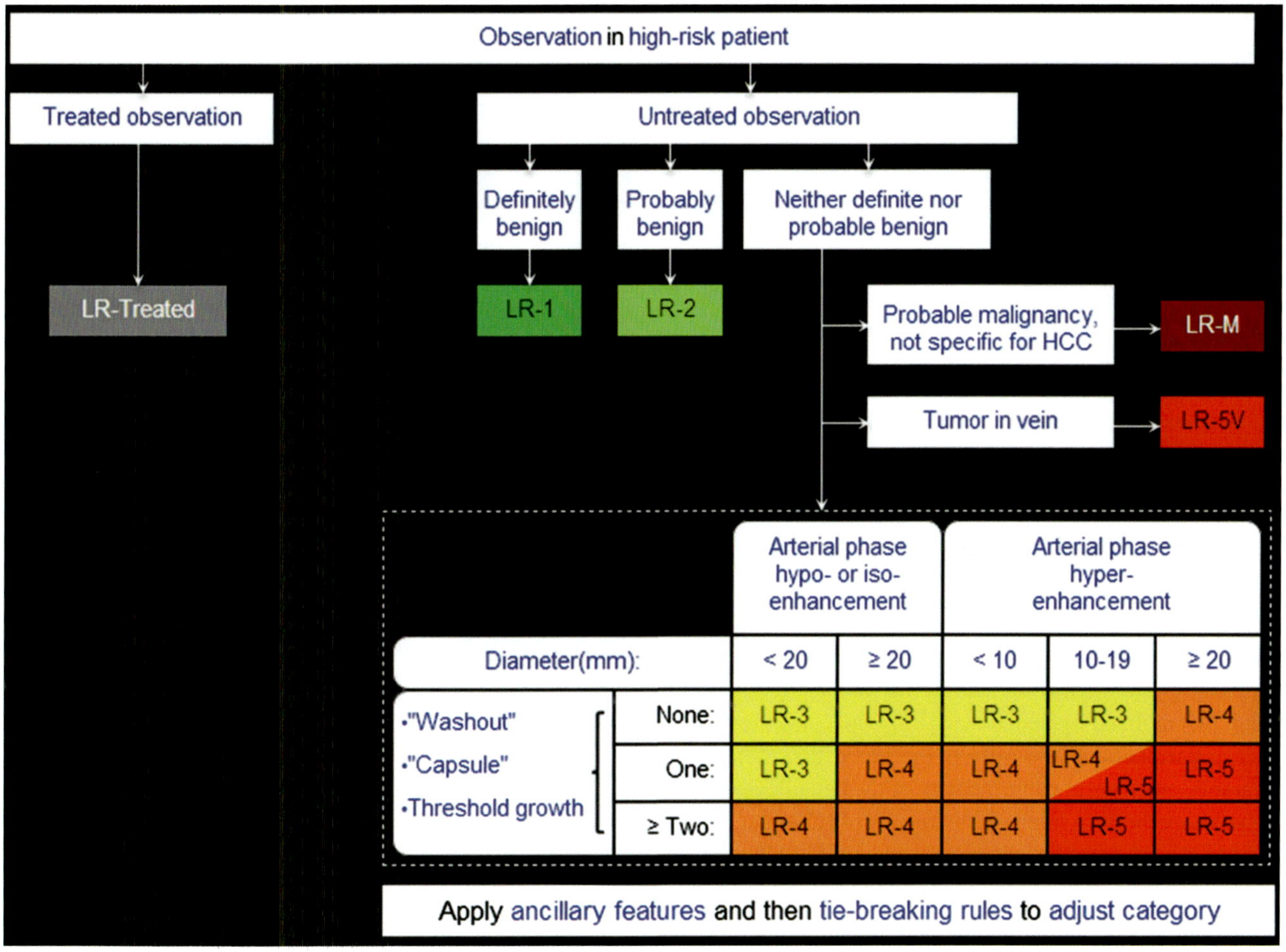

Management Before Hepatectomy for Hepatocellular Carcinoma with Cirrhosis

Jixiong Hu, Wei Liu, Xianming Wang, and Jiangsheng Huang

Liver resection is a curative procedure performed worldwide for hepatocellular carcinoma (HCC) [18]. Because most HCCs occur in patients with liver cirrhosis and poor hepatic function, there are many factors that affect survival [19]. Among them, the most important ones are the liver reserve function and the characteristics of the tumor. Inappropriate volume removal of functioning liver induces liver failure in patients with chronic liver diseases. To prevent postoperative hepatic failure, several preparations must be performed: (1) The location, number, and size of the tumor and its relationship with the intrahepatic major vascular vessels were evaluated by preoperative image. The liver reserve function was also evaluated. The combination of the tumor's characteristics and the corrected evaluation of the liver reserve function is the basis to determine the extent of hepatic resection; (2) Preoperative management of the liver, for example, in case the size of the future liver remnant is too small, it is necessary to carry out preoperative portal vein embolization supplying the tumor-bearing hemiliver; (3) If necessary, fluid infusion and drug administration was delivered to improve the liver function; (4) Evaluation of the patients general condition; (5) The evaluation of the experience of the operating team.

The Planned Hepatic Resection Was Based on the Corrected Evaluation of the Liver Reserve Function and the Tumor's Characteristics

Evaluation of the Liver Reserve Function

The preoperative evaluation of the liver reserve function was based on the following two assessment tests: a. The Child-Turcotte-Pugh (CTP) score (Table 1) was originally developed to predict the risk of mortality in patients undergoing shunting procedures for portal hypertension [20]. Later on, this score system was expanded to evaluate the liver reserve function. The parameters of this CTP score system include serum total bilirubin level, albumin level, prothrombin time, ascites, and encephalopathy. The CTP

Table 1 The Child-Turcotte-Pugh scoring system

	Child-Turcotte-Pugh scores		
Parameters	1 point	2 points	3 points
Albumin (mg/dL)	>3.5	3.5–2.8	<2.8
Bilirubin (mg/dL)	<2	2–3	>3
PT-INR	<1.7	1.7–2.3	>2.3
PT (%)	>70	40–70	<40
Ascites	None	Small or controlled	Tense
Encephalopathy	Absent	State I or II	State III or IV

Grade A: 5–6 total points, Grade B: 7–9 total points, Grade C: 10–15 total points

score is categorized into three grades: Grade A, B, and C. In the past 10 years, the CTP score system was also regarded as an indispensable evaluation tool, but two main parameters in this system were picked out as alternatives to evaluate preoperative liver reserve function. The two parameters are serum total bilirubin level and ascites. Indocyanine green (ICG) is a water-soluble tricarbocyanine dye, which distributes uniformly in blood within 3 min after intravenous injection and binds to albumin. It is exclusively taken up by hepatocytes and then excreted into the biliary tract without being metabolized by hepatocyte [21]. The concentration of ICG in peripheral blood reflects the blood flow-dependent clearance and transporting capacity of the hepatocyte. There are three methods to interpret the results of ICG tests, which include the plasma disappearance rate (ICG-PDR), retention of ICG in peripheral blood during the first 15 min (ICGR15) (expressed as percentage) and clearance of ICG at 15 min. ICGR15 is the most commonly used parameter of ICG test, and 10% of ICGR15 is used as up-limit for major hepatectomy [22, 23].

In order to prevent postoperative liver failure, although several criteria for safe liver resection have been advocated [24], Makuuchi's criteria for hepatic resection is easy to apply and well accepted [25, 26]. This criteria is comprised of two main parameters: preoperative peripheral serum total bilirubin level and ICGR15 value. No matter what the value of ICGR15 is, in patients with elevated serum total bilirubin level between 1.0 mg/dL and 2.0 mg/dL, only tumor enucleation or minor hepatic resection is recommended. In patients with serum total bilirubin level less than 1.0 mg/dL, hepatic functional parenchyma to be sacrificed is decided based on the value of ICGR15. In case of ICGR15 value less than 10%, right or left hemihepatectomy and right or left extended hemihepatectomy can be performed; in case of ICGR15 value between 10% and 19%, only left hemihepatectomy, or right anterior sectionectomy, or right posterior sectionectomy can be recommended; single segmentectomy or subsegmentectomy could be performed in case of ICGR15 value between 20% and 29%; in case of ICGR15 value between 30% and 39%, only limited (local) resection could be indicated; in case of ICGR15 value more than 40%, any resection is dangerous and intraoperative errhysis may be uncontrollable, if necessary, only just enucleation may be attempted and preoperative sufficient blood products should be prepared for probable stubborn oozing.

Evaluation of the Tumor

The intrahepatic vascular and biliary vessels are highly complex. The routine preoperative contrast ultrasound and high-resolution helical CT were employed to ascertain the location, size, number of the tumor and recognize the positional relationship between the tumor and the intrahepatic major vascular vessels. Sometimes, magnetic resonance cholangiopancreatography (MRCP) [27] is required to exclude tumor's invasion into the bile duct or to identify bile duct tumor thrombus [28, 29]. PET-CT is occasionally required to demonstrate or exclude remote metastasis. Furthermore, the liver volume to be resected and the volume of the future liver remnant must be assessed preoperatively for safe hepatic resection, especially for patients with either borderline liver function or a small-for-size future liver remnant [25, 30, 31]. For tumors located in the vicinity of or involved with the major vascular vessels, it is necessary to assess the volume of tumor-bearing area to be resected using three-dimensional (3D) image-processing software [32, 33]. Volumetric analysis facilitates selection of the optimal and precise parenchymal transection plane and estimation of the future liver remnant (FLR) volume.

Preoperative Strategy to Improve Surgical Tolerance of the Liver

Portal Vein Embolization (PVE) or Associated Liver Partition and Portal Vein Ligation for Staged Hepatectomy (ALPPS)

In case of ICGR15 less than 10% and the liver volume to be resected more than 60% of the total liver volume, or ICGR15 between 10% and 20% and planned liver volume to be sacrificed more than half of the total liver volume, portal vein embolization or ALPPS should be employed prior to liver resection. After about 14 days, 3D volumetric analysis was once more employed to assess the volume of the planned future liver remnant. In case that the volume of the planned future liver remnant is adequately increased, the proposed hepatic resection could be performed.

Hepatic Arterial Embolization

For patients with HCC with portal vein tumor thrombus, preoperative selective hepatic arterial embolization may shrink the tumor thrombus, which could decrease postoperative early recurrence.

Strategy to Reduce Jaundice

For patients with HCC associated with obstructive jaundice, percutaneous transhepatic cholangical drainage (PTCD) can drain bile to decrease jaundice. In case that patients with HCC associated with bile duct tumor thrombus (BDTT), selective hepatic arterial embolization can lead to necrosis of the tumor thrombus and enterohepatic circulation could be achieved to reduce jaundice.

Fluid Infusion and Drug Administration to Improve Liver Function

Chronic Active Hepatitis (Including Hepatitis B and C)

In China, most patients with hepatocellular carcinoma are associated with hepatitis B and/or hepatitis C. In case that patients have peripheral serum AST and ALT levels more than 150 IU/L at admission, liver protection drugs should be administered and the patients should lie silently in bed. Having lowering the levels of AST and/or ALT below 100 IU/L, the planned liver resection is indicated.

Administration of Diuretic

As above-mentioned, in China, most hepatocellular carcinomas occur in patients with cirrhosis and poor liver function. These patients are often associated with hypoalbuminemia and hyperaldosteronemia, which often lead to pleural and abdominal fluid effusion and edema. Generally, ascites and edema caused by hypoalbuminemia is temporarily contraindication for any of hepatic resection. Exogenous human albumin and diuretic should be administered to eradicate pleural and abdominal fluid effusion before liver surgery.

Evaluation of the Patient's General Condition and Co-Existing Morbidity

The evaluation of the preoperative patients' general condition and co-existing morbidity has been previously reported in our clinical studies [34–38].

References

1. Hennedige T, Venkatesh SK. Advances in computed tomography and magnetic resonance imaging of hepatocellular carcinoma. World J Gastroenterol. 2016;22(1):205–20.
2. Watanabe A, Ramalho M, AlObaidy M, Kim HJ, Velloni FG, Semelka RC, Watanabe A, Ramalho M, AlObaidy M, Kim HJ, Velloni FG, Semelka RC. Magnetic resonance imaging of the cirrhotic liver: an update. World J Hepatol. 2015;7(3):468–87.
3. Schraml C, Kaufmann S, Rempp H, Syha R, Ketelsen D, Notohamiprodjo M, Nikolaou K. Imaging of HCC-current state of the art. Diagnostics (Basel). 2015;5(4):513–45.
4. Omata M, Cheng AL, Kokudo N, Kudo M, Lee JM, Jia J, Tateishi R, Han KH, Chawla YK, Shiina S, Jafri W, Payawal DA, Ohki T, Ogasawara S, Chen PJ, Lesmana CRA, Lesmana LA, Gani RA, Obi S, Dokmeci AK, Sarin SK. Asia–Pacific clinical practice guidelines on the management of hepatocellular carcinoma: a 2017 update. Hepatol Int. 2017;11(4):317–70.
5. Kierans AS, Leonardou P, Hayashi P, Brubaker LM, Elazzazi M, Shaikh F, Semelka RC. MRI findings of rapidly progressive hepatocellular carcinoma. Magn Reson Imaging. 2010;28(8):790–6.
6. Bellissimo F, Pinzone MR, Cacopardo B, Nunnari G. Diagnostic and therapeutic management of hepatocellular carcinoma. World J Gastroenterol. 2015;21(42):12003–21.
7. Morise Z, Kawabe N, Tomishige H, Nagata H, Kawase J, Arakawa S, Yoshida R, Isetani M. Recent advances in liver resection for hepatocellular carcinoma. Front Surg. 2014;1:1–8.
8. Kanda T, Ogasawara S, Chiba T, Haga Y, Omata M, Yokosuka O. Current management of patients with hepatocellular carcinoma. World J Hepatol. 2015;7(15):1913–20.
9. Wong R, Frenette C. Updates in the management of hepatocellular carcinoma. Gastroenterol Hepatol. 2011;7(1):16–24.
10. Waghray A, Murali AR, Menon KN. Hepatocellular carcinoma: from diagnosis to treatment. World J Hepatol. 2015;7(8):1020–9.
11. Vauthey JN, Dixon E, Abdalla EK, Helton WS, Pawlik TM, Taouli B, Brouquet A, Adams RB, American Hepato-Pancreato-Biliary Association, Society of Surgical Oncology, Society for Surgery of the Alimentary Tract. Pretreatment assessment of hepatocellular carcinoma: expert consensus statement. HPB (Oxford). 2010;12(5):289–99.
12. Choi JY, Lee JM, Sirlin CB. CT and MR imaging diagnosis and staging of hepatocellular carcinoma: part I. Development, growth, and spread: key pathologic and imaging aspects. Radiology. 2014;272(3):635–54.
13. Choi JY, Lee JM, Sirlin CB. CT and MR imaging diagnosis and staging of hepatocellular carcinoma. Part II. Extracellular agents, hepatobiliary agents, and ancillary imaging features. Radiology. 2014;273(1):30–50.
14. D'Onofrio M, De Robertis R, Demozzi E, Crosara S, Canestrini S, Pozzi Mucelli R. Liver volumetry: is imaging reliable? Personal experience and review of the literature. World J Radiol. 2014;6(4):62–71.
15. Cieslak KP, Runge JH, Heger M, Stoker J, Bennink RJ, van Gulik TM. New perspectives in the assessment of future remnant liver. Dig Surg. 2014;31(4–5):255–68.
16. Mitchell DG, Bruix J, Sherman M, Sirlin CB. LI-RADS (liver imaging reporting and data system): summary, discussion, and consensus of the LI-RADS Management working group and future directions. Hepatology. 2015;61(3):1056–65.
17. Elsayes KM, Hooker JC, Agrons MM, Kielar AZ, Tang A, Fowler KJ, Chernyak V, Bashir MR, Kono Y, Do RK, Mitchell DG, Kamaya A, Hecht EM, Sirlin CB. 2017 version of LI-RADS for CT and MR imaging: an update. Radiographics. 2017;37(7):1994–2017.
18. Lai EC, Fan ST, Lo CM, Chu KM, Liu CL, Wong J. Hepatic resection for hepatocellular carcinoma. An audit of 343 patients. Ann Surg. 1995;221(3):291–8.
19. Kang KJ, Ahn KS. Anatomical resection of hepatocellular carcinoma: a critical review of the procedure and its benefits on survival. World J Gastroenterol. 2017;23(7):1139–46.
20. Pugh RN, Murray-Lyon IM, Dawson JL, Pietroni MC, Williams R. Transection of the oesophagus for bleeding oesophageal varices. Br J Surg. 1973;60(8):646–9.
21. Hoekstra LT, de Graaf W, Nibourg GA, Heger M, Bennink RJ, Stieger B, van Gulik TM. Physiological and biochemical basis of clinical liver function tests: a review. Ann Surg. 2013;257(1):27–36.
22. Sakka SG. Assessing liver function. Curr Opin Crit Care. 2007;13(2):207–14.

23. Garcea G, Ong SL, Maddern GJ. Predicting liver failure following major hepatectomy. Digestive and liver disease. Dig Liver Dis. 2009;41(11):798–806.
24. Mise Y, Sakamoto Y, Ishizawa T, Kaneko J, Aoki T, Hasegawa K, Sugawara Y, Kokudo N. A worldwide survey of the current practice of liver surgery. Liver Cancer. 2013;2(1):55–66.
25. Makuuchi M, Kosuge T, Takayama T, Yamazaki S, Kakazu T, Miyagawa S, Kawasaki S. Sugery for small liver cancers. Semin Surg Oncol. 1993;9(4):298–304.
26. Takamoto K. Chapter II.1. Preoperative management. In: Makuuchi M, editor. Makuuchi Kanzou Gekagaku(in Japanese)/(translated to Chinese by Yong Zeng). Beijing: People's Medical Publishing House; 2016. p. 45–9.
27. Wang C, Yang Y, Sun D, Jiang Y. Prognosis of hepatocellular carcinoma patients with bile duct tumor thrombus after hepatic resection or liver transplantation in Asian populations: a meta-analysis. PLoS One. 2017;12(5):e0176827.
28. Chotirosniramit A, Liwattanakun A, Lapisatepun W, Ko-Iam W, Sandhu T, Junrungsee S. A single institution report of 19 hepatocellular carcinoma patients with bile duct tumor thrombus. J Hepatocell Carcinoma. 2017;4:41–7.
29. Navadgi S, Chang CC, Bartlett A, McCall J, Pandanaboyana S. Systematic review and meta-analysis of outcomes after liver resection in patients with hepatocellular carcinoma (HCC) with and without bile duct thrombus. HPB (Oxford). 2016;18(4):312–6.
30. Abdalla EK, Denys A, Chevalier P, Nemr RA, Vauthey JN. Total and segmental liver volume variations: implications for liver surgery. Surgery. 2004;135(4):404–10.
31. Seyama Y, Kokudo N. Assessment of liver function for safe hepatic resection. Hepatol Res. 2009;39(2):107–16.
32. Mise Y, Satou S, Shindoh J, Conrad C, Aoki T, Hasegawa K, Sugawara Y, Kokudo N. Three-dimensional volumetry in 107 normal livers reveals clinically relevant inter-segment variation in size. HPB (Oxford). 2013;16(5):439.
33. Nakayama K, Oshiro Y, Miyamoto R, Kohno K, Fukunaga K, Ohkohchi N. The effect of three-dimensional preoperative simulation on liver surgery. World J Surg. 2017;41(7):1840–7.
34. Hu J, Pi Z, Yu MY, Li Y, Xiong S. Obstructive jaundice caused by tumor emboli from hepatocellular carcinoma. Am Surg. 1999;65(5):406–10.
35. Hu JX, Miao XY, Zhong DW, Dai WD, Liu W. Anterior approach for complete isolated caudate lobectomy. Hepatogastroenterology. 2005;52(66):1641–4.
36. Hu JX, Dai WD, Miao XY, Zhong DW, Huang SF, Wen Y, Xiong SZ. Anatomic resection of segment VIII of liver for hepatocellular carcinoma in cirrhotic patients based on an intrahepatic Glissonian approach. Surgery. 2009;146(5):854–60.
37. Miao XY, Hu JX, Dai WD, Zhong DW, Xiong SZ. Null-margin mesohepatectomy for centrally located hepatocellular carcinoma in cirrhotic patients. Hepatogastroenterology. 2011;58(106):575–82.
38. Dai WD, Huang JS, Hu JX. Isolated caudate lobe resection for huge hepatocellular carcinoma (10 cm or greater in diameter). Am Surg. 2014;80(2):159–65.

Basic Techniques for Hepatic Resection by the Glissonean Approach

Jixiong Hu, Jiangsheng Huang, Xianling Liu, and Zhongkun Zuo

Control of the Inflow and Outflow System During Liver Resection

Jiangsheng Huang Jixiong Hu, and Xianling Liu

Liver resection for the treatment of hepatocellular carcinoma has progressed greatly over the last 20 years. Notable advancements include increased utilization of parenchymal-preserving resections, better patient selection, use of associating liver partition and portal vein ligation for staged hepatectomy (ALPPS), use of 3D virtual resection and reconstruction technology, and improvements in perioperative management [1]. Because of these changes, the postoperative morbidity and mortality have significantly decreased [2, 3]. Even if like this, intraoperative severe hemorrhage still is a potentially lethal problem, especially in patients with HCC associated with cirrhosis [4, 5]. Moreover, perioperative blood transfusion has been found to negatively influence long-term overall and disease-free survival [6, 7]. Therefore, minimizing blood loss while performing oncologically sound hepatectomy should be the primary goals of hepatic surgeons. During liver resection, blood loss occurs due to bleeding both from the vascular inflow system and from the vascular outflow system. It is similarly crucial to occlude the inflow and outflow systems to minimize bleeding during hepatic resection.

Vascular Clamping Techniques: Inflow Occlusion

The inflow occlusion techniques can be categorized as:

1. Total inflow occlusion (Pringle maneuver)
   (a) Continuous Pringle maneuver
   (b) Intermittent Pringle maneuver
   (c) Ischemic preconditioning followed by continuous Pringle maneuver
2. Selective inflow occlusion
   (a) Hemihepatic inflow occlusion
   (b) Sectional inflow occlusion
   (c) Segmental inflow occlusion

Total Inflow Occlusion (the Vascular Clamping of the Portal Triad, Pringle Maneuver)

Pringle, in 1908, described the use of hepatoduodenal ligament clamping to control bleeding in cases of liver injury [8]. To control the vascular inflow system, the Pringle maneuver is the simplest and one of the most widely used techniques in elective liver resection (see Section "Surgical Indications for Hepatocellular Carcinoma Confined to the Caudate Lobe" in the Chapter "Other Types of Hepatic Resection for HCC").

The corresponding author of section "Control of the Inflow and Outflow System During Liver Resection" is Jiangsheng Huang, Email: HJS13907313501@yahoo.com.
The corresponding author of section "Segment-Based Hepatic Resection by the Glissonean Pedicle Approach" is Xianling Liu, Email: liuxianling3180@163.com.
The corresponding author of section "Technical Details of Suprahilar Glissonean Approach for Anatomical Hepatic Resection" is Xianling Liu, Email: liuxianling3180@163.com.

J. X. Hu
Department of Hepatobiliary Surgery and Hunan Provincial Key Laboratory of Hepatobiliary Disease Research, The Second Xiangya Hospital, Central South University, Changsha, Hunan, PR China
e-mail: 13908459086@163.com

J. S. Huang
Department of Minimally Invasive Surgery, The Second Xiangya Hospital, Central South University, Changsha, Hunan, PR China
e-mail: HJS13907313501@yahoo.com

X. L. Liu (✉)
Department of Oncology, The Second Xiangya Hospital, Central South University, Changsha, Hunan, PR China
e-mail: liuxianling3180@163.com

Z. K. Zuo
Department of Minimally Invasive Surgery, The Second Xiangya Hospital, Central South University, Changsha, Hunan, PR China
e-mail: arthasreal@csu.edu.cn

J. S. Huang et al. (eds.), *Atlas of Anatomic Hepatic Resection for Hepatocellular Carcinoma*,
https://doi.org/10.1007/978-981-13-0668-6_3

When the lesser omentum is incised, a blunt dissector or the operator's index finger may be passed through the foramen of Winslow, and thus the hepatoduodenal ligament is isolated and then encircled with a vascular tape. If necessary, the Pringle maneuver can be performed by tightening the vascular tape around the hepatoduodenal ligament en masse. It is noteworthy that active bleeding following application of the Pringle maneuver, ruling out backflow bleeding from major hepatic vein(s), often suggests an anomalous hepatic artery. The most common variations in hepatic arterial anatomy are replaced or accessory right or left hepatic artery originating from the superior mesenteric artery (SMA) or the left gastric artery, respectively [9]. When an aberrant right hepatic artery is present, it runs laterally to the common bile duct and can be occluded by the Pringle maneuver. By contrast, an aberrant left hepatic artery arising from the left gastric artery runs in the gastrohepatic ligament and requires individual clamping in order to obtain total vascular inflow occlusion.

The Pringle maneuver can cause such hemodynamic responses as a 10% increase in mean arterial pressure, a 40% increase in systemic vascular resistance, a 5% decrease in pulmonary artery pressure, and a 10% decrease in cardiac index [10]. While hepatic resection with the Pringle maneuver lasting below 30 min is generally well tolerated, prolonged period of continuous inflow occlusion may induce ischemia-reperfusion injury to the future liver remnant. Fibrotic or cirrhotic hepatic parenchyma is more vulnerable to this injury than normal liver tissue. Furthermore, prolonged hepatic parenchymal ischemia can cause pernicious effects on postoperative liver function, hepatic tissue regeneration, and short- and long-term survival [11]. Intermitted portal triad clamping (intermittent Pringle maneuver) has been used as a substitute for continuous Pringle maneuver to minimize ischemia-reperfusion injury in complex hepatic resection. This technique alternates portal triad clamping with short intervals of unclamping and portal reperfusion. It is usually performed using 15 min of occlusion/5 min of reperfusion during hepatic resection. The major shortcomings innate in this technique are the significantly higher blood loss during the period of vascular unclamping and the increased operative time when compared with the continuous Pringle maneuver.

A substitute for the intermittent Pringle maneuver is ischemic preconditioning with continuous inflow occlusion. This technique starts with a brief period of ischemia by total vascular inflow occlusion (10–15 min) followed by a short interval of reperfusion (10–15 min). Subsequently, continuous inflow occlusion is begun in the starting time of hepatic parenchymal transection and is lasting until hepatic transection has been completely performed. This technique avoids the repeated clamping-unclamping cycle, which leads to less intraoperative blood loss and a shortened hepatic parenchymal transection time. Many studies have reported that ischemic preconditioning with continuous inflow occlusion is effective for hepatic resection [12–16].

Selective Inflow Occlusion

Selective vascular inflow occlusion was defined as the clamping of pedicle which supply the hemiliver, the section, the segment, or the combination of segments that is (are) planned to be resected. The aim of this technique was as follows: (1) to limit the ischemic-reperfusion injury to the tumor-bearing liver parenchyma to be resected and (2) to accurately demarcate anatomical territory by creating ischemic demarcating boundary at the liver surface.

In 1987, Makuuchi et al. [17] first described the hemihepatic vascular inflow occlusion technique to reduce the severity of splanchnic congestion and total liver ischemia. This technique selectively occludes the vascular inflow to the right or left hemiliver. The potential advantages of this technique are preserving vascular inflow to the contralateral hemiliver and have no visceral congestion and hemodynamic disturbances. On the other hand, one of the concerns of this technique is the risk of continuous bleeding from the cut surfaces of the non-clamped remaining hemiliver. For hemihepatectomy, the surgeon can devascularize the corresponding hemiliver by dividing the unilateral portal pedicle by the Glissonean pedicle approach (see Figs. 1 and 2). Hepatic parenchymal transection can then be carried out along the ischemic demarcation line on the liver surface. Another method is composed

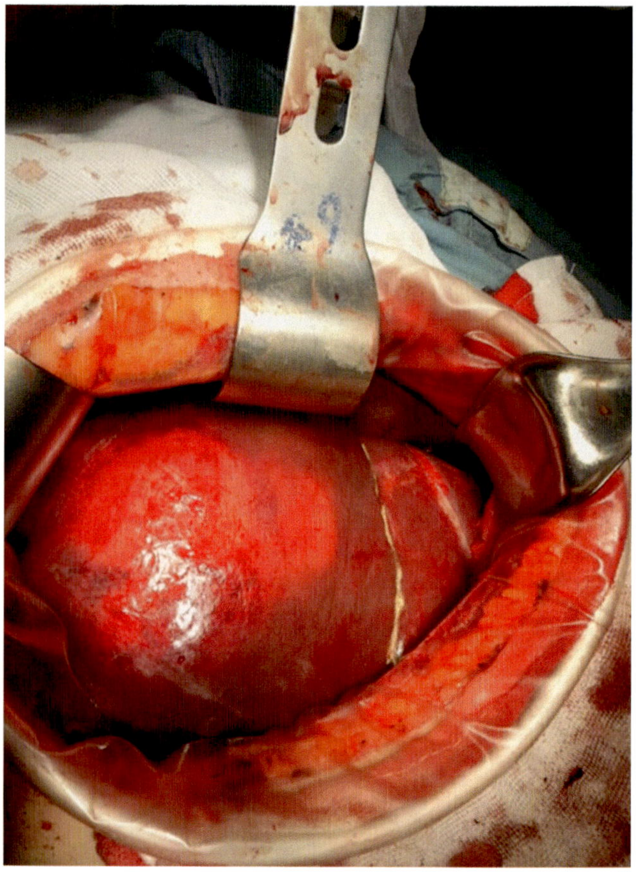

Fig. 1 Right hemiliver was occluded, and the ischemic demarcation line was marked on the liver surface with electrocautery

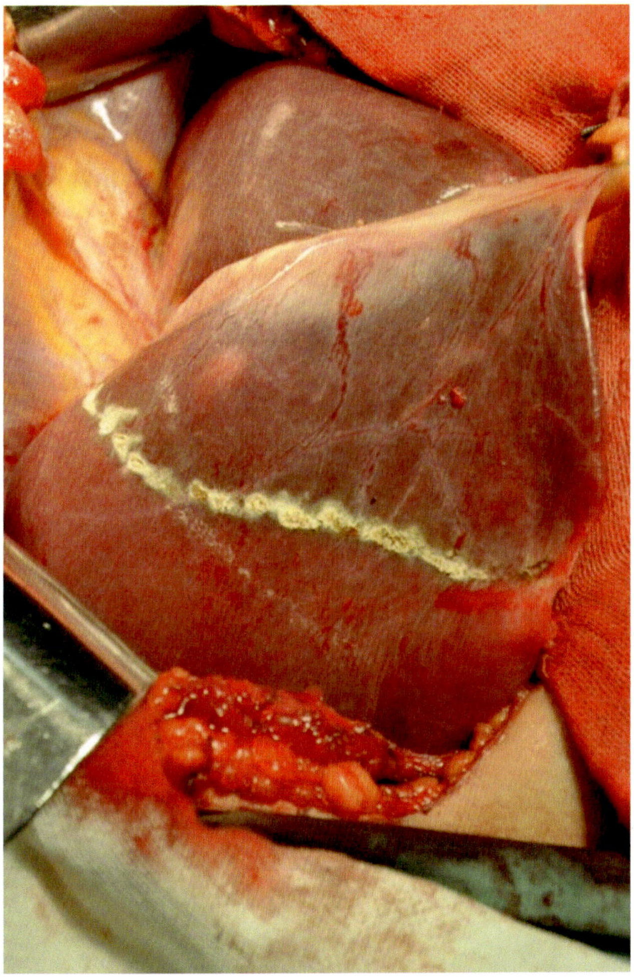

Fig. 2 Left hemiliver was occluded, and the ischemic demarcation line was marked on the liver surface with electrocautery

of initially clamping the unilateral portal pedicle and then dividing it more distally during parenchymal transection.

Selective sectoral (sectional) clamping is mainly applied in segment-oriented anatomical sectionectomies, including mesohepatectomy (see Section "Mesohepatectomy (S4+S5+S8 Resection)" in the Chapter "Types of Segment-Oriented Hepatic Resection by the Glissonean Pedicle Approach"), right anterior sectionectomy (see Section "Anatomic Right Anterior Sectionectomy Using Glissonean Pedicle Transection Method" in the Chapter "Types of Segment-Oriented Hepatic Resection by the Glissonean Pedicle Approach"), right posterior sectionectomy (see Section "Right Posterior Sectionectomy (S6+S7 Resection" in the Chapter "Types of Segment-Oriented Hepatic Resection by the Glissonean Pedicle Approach"), segmentectomy IV (see Section "Segmentectomy IV" in the Chapter "Types of Segment-Oriented Hepatic Resection by the Glissonean Pedicle Approach"), and left lateral sectionectomy (see Section "Left Lateral Sectionectomy(S2+S3 Resection)" in the Chapter "Types of Segment-Oriented Hepatic Resection by the Glissonean Pedicle Approach"). Extrahepatically, portal triad consisting of the hepatic artery, the portal vein, and the bile duct is covered by connective tissue and peritoneum (Glisson's capsule) up to the hepatic hilus; the term Glisson's sheath is retained for the Glisson's capsule which runs into the intrahepatic portion of the liver beyond the hepatic hilus. Therefore, the branches of the hepatic artery, portal vein, and bile duct are also samely enclosed by the Glissonean sheath. For the right hemiliver, further dissection distally along the right main hepatic pedicle can access the anterior sectoral (sectional) and posterior sectoral (sectional) pedicles and for the left hemiliver the medial (segment IV) and lateral sectoral (sectional) pedicles. We have previously described in detail the techniques used to obtain these sectoral (sectional) pedicles by suprahilar Glissonean approach (see Section "Technical Details of Suprahilar Glissonean Approach for Anatomical Hepatic Resection"). In addition, the right or left hepatic pedicle and the sectoral pedicle can be accessed by the intra-Glissonean dissection.

Segmental pedicle clamping was first described by Takasaki using the Glissonean pedicle approach [18]. Further dissection distally along the sectoral Glissonean pedicle was needed to access the segmental Glissonean pedicle (see Section "Technical Details of Suprahilar Glissonean Approach for Anatomical Hepatic Resection").

Vascular Clamping Techniques: Outflow Occlusion

Vascular outflow occlusion techniques can be categorized as:

1. Total vascular exclusion
2. Selective total vascular exclusion
3. Selective partial vascular exclusion

Total Vascular Exclusion (TVE)

Heaney et al. first reported hepatic resection with TVE [19]. Total vascular exclusion (TVE) combines total vascular inflow occlusion with Pringle maneuver and outflow occlusion of the liver by clamping the supra- and infrahepatic inferior vena cava (Fig. 3). It is noteworthy that outflow occlusion should always be preceded by inflow occlusion.

Variations in anatomy of the hepatic arterial branches, including an accessory or replaced artery, have been found in a large proportion of the populations (33–45%) [20]. Therefore, identification and occlusion of an accessory or replaced artery are obligatory because an incomplete inflow occlusion associated with a complete outflow occlusion causes liver congestion and hemorrhage during hepatic

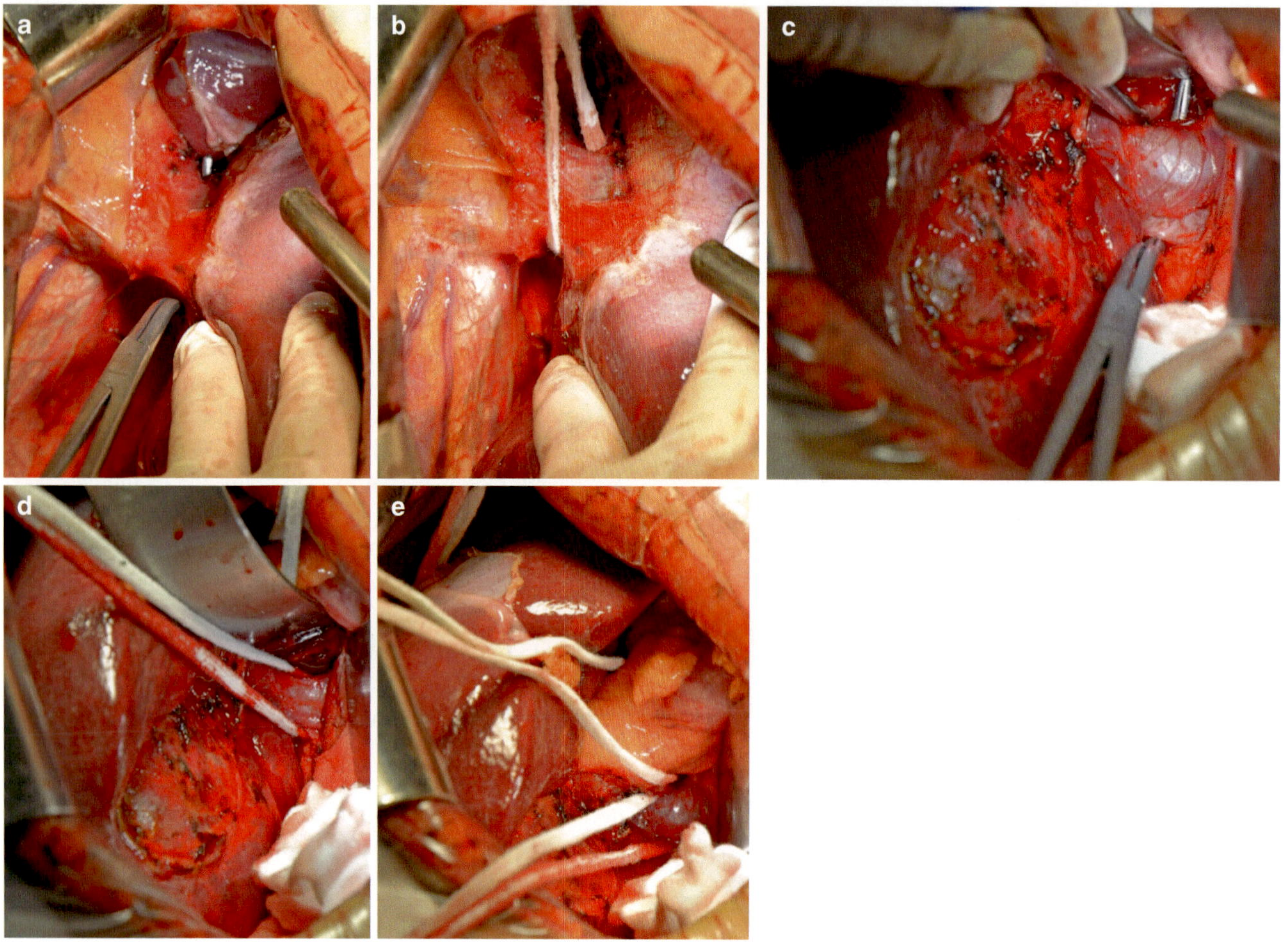

Fig. 3 Operative steps in total vascular occlusion. (**a**) The suprahepatic inferior vena cava was isolated. (**b**) The suprahepatic IVC was encircled with a vascular tape. (**c**) The infrahepatic vena cava was isolated. (**d**) The infrahepatic vena cava was looped with a vascular tape. (**e**) The hepatic pedicle and supra- and infrahepatic vena cava were pre-placed with a vascular tape, respectively; if necessary, the hepatic pedicle and then the infrahepatic vena cava can be occluded, and if tolerated by the patient, the suprahepatic vena cava was finally occluded

parenchymal transection. Supra- and infrahepatic caval clamping requires complete mobilization of the liver from its surrounding structures. The retrohepatic IVC must be freed off from the hepatic posterior plane. In addition, it is usually advisable to dissect and divide each non-hepatic venous branch, including the adrenal vein and the phrenic veins (usually 3), in order to prevent blood reflux in the excluded caval segment. Lasting bleeding during hepatic parenchymal transection suggests an incomplete TVE. Under such circumstances, hepatic transection should be stopped, and the completeness of the hepatic pedicle or caval clamping must be checked. The following order in clamping application should be followed: hepatoduodenal ligament, infrahepatic IVC, and suprahepatic IVC. If the portal triad and the infrahepatic caval occlusion can be tolerated, the suprahepatic caval occlusion is then applied. It is required that a trial of TVE for 5 min should be used before hepatic parenchymal transection is initiated.

The goals of TVE are to reduce intraoperative bleeding, avoid air embolism, and allow for a bloodless operating field during hepatic parenchymal transection. For tumors located within the paracaval portion and adjacent to or infiltrated the major hepatic veins and retrohepatic IVC, it is advisable to pre-place a vascular tape around the hepatic pedicle and the supra- and infrahepatic IVC before initiating liver resection. Severe injury to the major HV or IVC occurs during hepatic parenchymal transection; TVE can be immediately applied to prevent lethal bleeding. TVE is mainly indicated for large tumors adjacent to or infiltrating the major hepatic veins or the retrohepatic IVC. It is especially effective and even life-saving when a tumor thrombus is present in the IVC, as use of TVE prevents this thrombus migration intraoperatively. TVE also allows for safe and effective major hepatic veins or IVC repairment or reconstruction in a bloodless field. In some patients with large tumors located within the right superior portion of the right hemiliver or infiltrating the hepatocaval confluence, it is difficult to isolate and loop the suprahepatic IVC. Even under such a circumstance, a thoracoabdominal incision should not be made because thoracotomy is too much invasive and associated with much more postoperative complications and postpones the postoperative recovery. In our hospital, over the last two decades, no matter the tumors are large or located anywhere, no thoracotomy is needed to perform hepatic resection in more than 3000 patients with HCC. An alternative way to TVE is the combined use of Pringle maneuver and the infrahepatic IVC clamping to reduce bleedings during hepatic transection [21–25]. This procedure is similar to TVE with the exclusion that this method does not include cross clamping the suprahepatic inferior vena cava because of the dangers and difficulties associated with its isolation and looping. It is logically imaginable that this method has the same shortcomings of TVE.

Application of TVE may be associated with significant hemodynamic changes and requires close invasive monitoring and anesthetic expertise intraoperatively. Occlusion of IVC flow leads to significant (40–60%) reduction of venous return and cardiac output, with a compensatory 80% increase in systemic vascular resistance and 50% increase in heart rate. A fall in cardiac output exceeding 50% or a decrease in mean arterial pressure exceeding 30% (i.e., less than 80 mmHg) in a euvolemic patient is defined as hemodynamic intolerance to TVE. It has been reported that this situation occurs in 10–20% of patients and cannot be predicted preoperatively because it is a result of failure of the patient's adrenergic cardiovascular reflexes to increase cardiac output in the presence of decreased preload [26–28]. Adequate fluid expansion of the patient's blood volume before applying TVE may help the patient to well tolerate this procedure. The large volume of fluids infused before and during TVE sometimes may increase the risks of postoperative liver, renal and pulmonary dysfunction, and pulmonary fluid collection and ascites.

Having performed the hepatic parenchymal transection, the suprahepatic caval clamp is first released; any severe bleeding from the major hepatic veins or IVC is controlled by repairing the injuries occurring on these venous trunks. Then, the infrahepatic caval and hepatic pedicle clamps are released, respectively, and any further blood loss oozing from the cut surface or bleeding from the inflow system is controlled.

Our own experiences accumulated from more than 3000 patients over the past two decades showed that, if the patient cannot tolerate temporary test TVE, Pringle maneuver in combination with infrahepatic vena clamping may be a useful and effective alternative. We do not think that a venovenous bypass combined with TVE is a good choice.

Selective Total Vascular Exclusion (STVE)

STVE combines hepatic inflow vascular occlusion with extrahepatic clamping of the right and the trunk of the middle/left hepatic veins (Figs. 4, 5, and 6), respectively, which leads to total vascular isolation of the liver from the systemic circulation without interruption of the caval blood flow. Therefore, STVE is not associated with the hemodynamic and biochemical shortcomings of TVE. In addition, STVE also can overcome the shortcomings of the backflow bleeding from the major hepatic veins alone, when only the Pringle maneuver was used.

STVE requires meticulous extrahepatic dissection of the major hepatic veins, which causes the procedure to become technically difficult and potentially hazardous [29–32]. It must be kept in mind that extrahepatically dissecting and looping the major veins must not be done in a rough and forceful manner. To perform STVE, the falciform ligament is completely divided to fully expose the suprahepatic IVC and the hepatocaval confluence. After complete mobilization of the right hemiliver, the right hemiliver was lifted upward and medially; the hepatocaval ligament was isolated and divided (see Section "Right Hepatectomy (S5~S8 Resection)" in the Chapter "Types of Segment-Oriented Hepatic Resection by the Glissonean Pedicle Approach"); the right and anterior aspects of the retrohepatic IVC are dissected by division of the retrohepatic short veins separately, progressing caudal-cranially, until the right and posterior aspects of the right hepatic vein and the trunk of the middle/left hepatic vein are exposed; and then the fossa between the right hepatic vein and the trunk of the middle/left hepatic vein was dissected. At the point, the extrahepatic short root of the right hepatic vein was completely isolated and encircled with a vascular tape (Fig. 4). During the proceedings of isolating the right hepatic vein, when a right inferior hepatic vein is present, it is either preserved or isolated, divided, and suture ligated according to its size and the extent of the hepatic resection. When the planned hepatic resection includes the resection of segment I, the latter is completely dissected away from the retrohepatic IVC by division of all of its venous branches. At this point, the whole liver is connected to the IVC by the three major hepatic veins only. The isolation and looping of the trunk of the middle/left hepatic veins begin with the incision of the lesser omentum and mobilization of the left hemiliver. Then, the junction of the left hepatic vein and the suprahepatic IVC is exposed by dissecting the peritoneal reflection at the tip of the Spiegel lobe of the caudate lobe, and the ligamentum venosum is dissected near to the trunk; subsequently, the left hemiliver was rotated upward and medially, and the fossa between the right hepatic vein and the trunk was furtherly dissected. Thus, the trunk of the middle/left hepatic vein was isolated and looped with a tourniquet. In most patients, the left and middle hepatic veins form a common trunk, and the trunk is looped. Extrahepatic

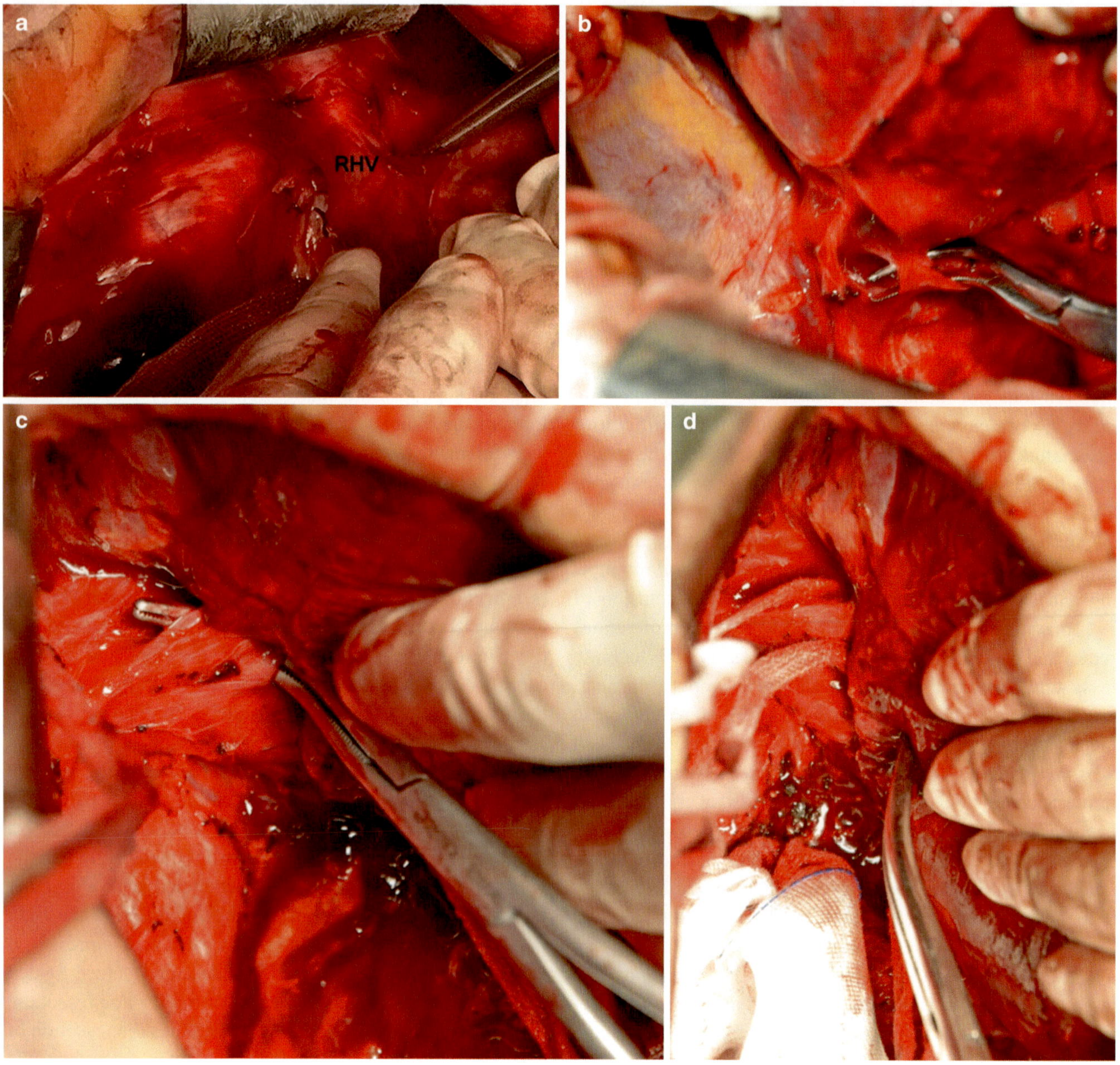

Fig. 4 Isolation of the right hepatic vein. (**a**) Dissect the fossa between the right hepatic vein and the common trunk of the middle/left vein. (**b**) Isolate and divide the hepatocaval ligament. (**c**) Isolate the right hepatic vein. (**d**) The right hepatic vein was looped with a vascular tape

isolation of the middle and the left hepatic veins is dangerous because the two veins can share a common middle wall in a significant proportion of patients. In some patients, the left and middle hepatic veins are encircled with a vascular tape, respectively (Figs. 5 and 6).

Selective Partial Vascular Exclusion

To avoid the disadvantages inherent to the selective total vascular exclusion, for hepatic resection of tumors only located within the right or left hemiliver, selective vascular exclusion could be applied on the right or left hemiliver only [11, 33]. In low-volume patients with HCC hospitals, this procedure has been uncommonly performed, probably because isolation and looping of the right hepatic vein and the trunk of the middle/left hepatic veins have been considered technically demanding and potentially dangerous. For selective vascular exclusion of the right or left hemiliver, the hilar plate is lowered (See Sections "Right Hepatectomy (S5~S8 Resection)" and "Left Hepatectomy (S2~S4 Resection)" in the Chapter "Types of Segment-Oriented Hepatic Resection by the Glissonean Pedicle Approach") to isolate and loop the right or left hepatic Glissonean pedicle. The extrahepatic isolation and looping of the right hepatic vein and the common trunk of the middle/left hepatic veins have been in detail described

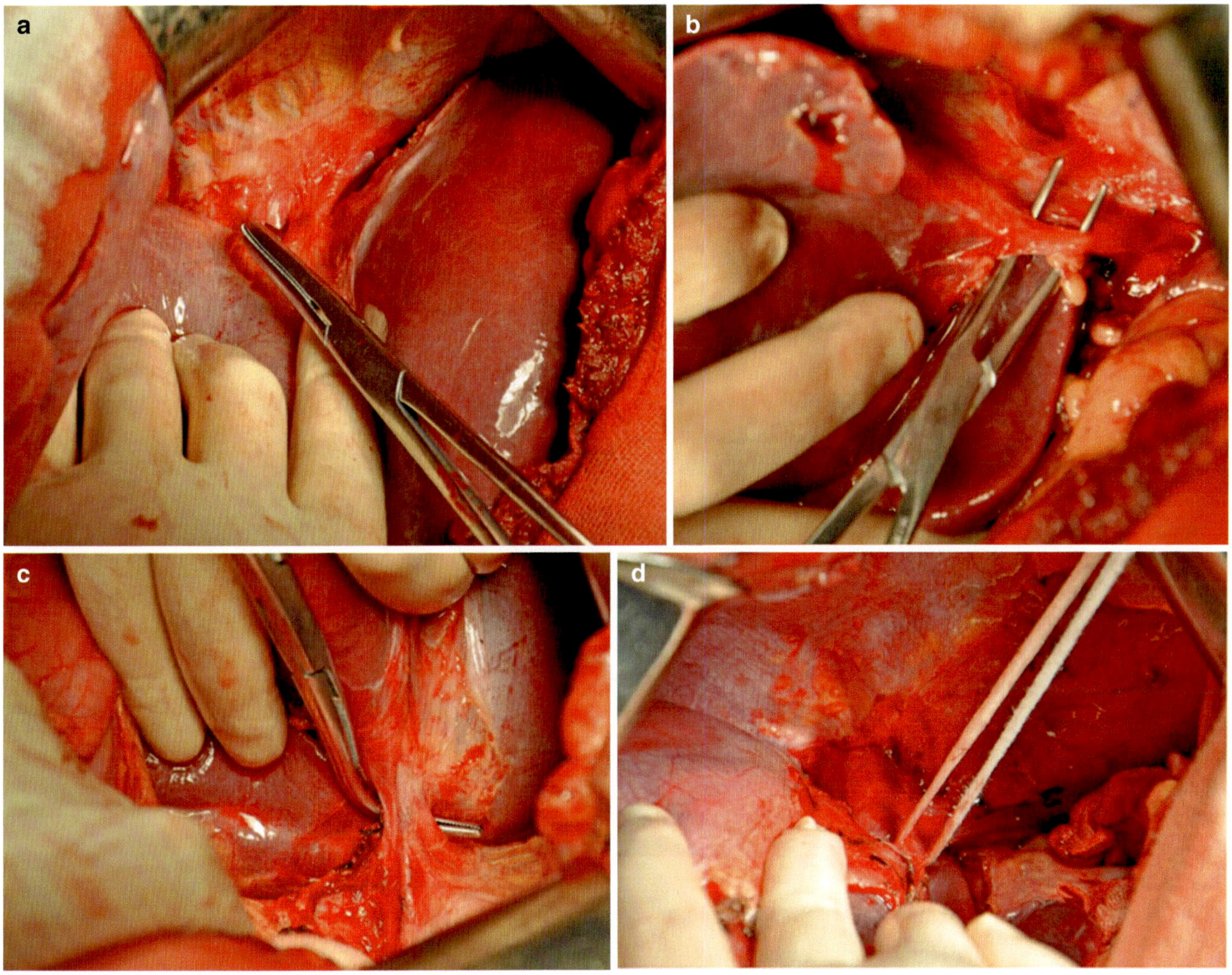

Fig. 5 Isolation of the common trunk of the middle/left hepatic vein. (**a**) Dissect the fossa between the middle hepatic vein and the left hepatic vein. (**b**) The left hemiliver is lifted upward and medially; the ligamentum venosum was isolated and divided. (**c**) The left hepatic vein is isolated. (**d**) The left hepatic vein was pre-placed with a tourniquet

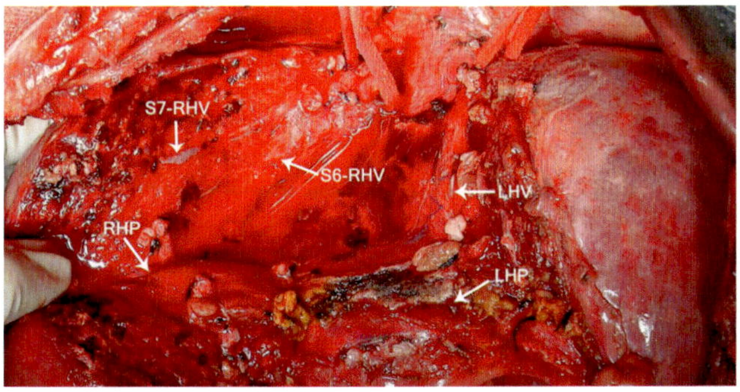

Fig. 6 Prior to mesohepatectomy, the right hepatic vein (RHV) and the left hepatic vein (LHV) were encircled with a vascular tape, respectively. Having removed the specimen, the tapes looping the RHV and LHV were unclamped. *RHP* right hepatic pedicle, *LHP* left hepatic pedicle

in the previous part of this chapter. The benefits of selective vascular on a hemiliver are the avoidance of ischemic-reperfusion injury to the remaining non-tumor-bearing hemiliver and the prevention of splanchnic congestion because of the preservation of the contralateral portal inflow. The obvious disadvantage is that bleeding can occur from the remaining hemiliver during hepatic parenchymal transection because of the persistent inflow blood supplying the remaining hemiliver.

Segment-Based Hepatic Resection by the Glissonean Pedicle Approach

Xianling Liu Jiangsheng Huang, and Jixiong Hu

Most hepatocellular carcinoma occurs in patients with liver cirrhosis and poor hepatic function representing the principal cause of death of cirrhotic patients [34, 35]. Among the local treatment modalities available for this tumor, liver surgical resection is the only potentially curative option for HCC, with a 5-year survival rate ranging from 31.8% to 59.0% [36, 37]. Theoretically, an important decision in any hepatic resection is choosing appropriate amount of hepatic parenchyma to be resected, however, which is not easy to achieve in clinical practice. Hepatic resection has its own inherent shortcomings mainly related to the unnecessary sacrifice of functioning hepatic parenchyma which is a risky point, especially in cirrhotic patients. This fact is partly explained for the still unsatisfactory postoperative morbidity and mortality reported by some authors [38]. The main problem to face when designing a hepatic resection is to find an adequately precise balance between the liver mass to be removed, which should be reduced as less as possible, and the need to perform, if possible, an anatomic resection. For the above reason, Matsue et al. [39] once reported that limited anatomic resection with no margin seems to be the best procedure for patients with tumors adjacent to the main trunk of the major hepatic vessels and with hepatic functions that do not permit wide margin resections. It is well known that intrahepatic tumor spread occurs mainly by means of portal venous invasion; thus, some authors have suggested that anatomical resection, with removal of at least the portal area including the main tumor, is preferable to non-anatomic resection for HCC, when it is being carried out with curative intent [40]. In order to uncover and identify the portal area including the main tumor to be resected, systematic segmentectomy was devised by Makuuchi et al. in the early 1980s [41]. However, this technique is technically demanding. Since then, many techniques of segment-based systematic liver resection have been developed. These techniques include (1) intraoperative ultrasound (IOUS) combined with the liver surface landmarks, (2) Glissonean pedicle approach, (3) ultrasound-guided puncture of portal vein branch and injection of dye, and (4) selective portal venous occlusion using a balloon catheter through a branch of the superior mesenteric vein. In this book, we just in detail discuss segment-based liver resections by the Glissonean pedicle approach.

Anatomical Basis for the Glissonean Pedicle Approach During Hepatectomies

Systematic segmentectomy, sectionectomy, right or left hemihepatectomy, and extended right or left hepatectomy are all called segment-based liver resections. The anatomical basis for these segment-based hepatic resections is that each Couinaud segment has its own independent inflow portal pedicle(s) and independent venous drainage and each Couinaud segment is an independent functional unit and can be resected individually or combined with adjacent segment(s). Another anatomic basis is that the Glisson's sheath originates from the vasculobiliary sheath and is not derived from the peritoneum or the capsule of the liver, which is referred to as Laennec's capsule [42]. Laennec's capsule is the proper membrane that covers not only the entire surface of the liver including the bare area but also the intrahepatic parenchyma wrapping the Glissonean pedicles. As a result, there exists a gap between the Glissonean pedicle and Laennec's capsule. Therefore, Laennec's capsule can be divided from the Glisson's sheath at the hepatic hilus, and the Glissonean pedicles condensed by the Glisson's sheath can be accessed at the hepatic hilus without parenchymal destruction. This concept was introduced by Couinaud and Takasaki in the early 1980s [43, 44] and developed by Sugioka A et al. [45]. The pedicles can be isolated, looped, divided, and suture-ligated as one of the bundles. Consequently, any anatomical hepatectomy may be carried out using this technique [46].

Our Modifications of the Methods of Applying the Glissonean Pedicle Approach and the Application of Methylene Blue Staining

Simply stated, our modifications include (1) no need of isolating and dividing the right-sided retrohepatic short veins draining into the infrahepatic inferior vena cava and mobilizing the process of the caudate lobe from the infrahepatic inferior vena cava [47]; (2) no need of making a vertical incision perpendicular to the hepatic hilum between segment 7 and the process of the caudate lobe [48, 49]; and (3) after lowering the hilar plate, the surgeon puts his index finger beneath the hilar plate, and then a large curved clamp was inserted into this incision in front of the hilum and the clamp was vertically inserted furtherly, until the clamp reached down to the tip of the surgeon's index finger; using the finger as a guide, the clamp was pushed out of the inferior edge of the right or the left hepatic pedicle. Thus, the right or the left hepatic pedicle was isolated and then looped with a vascular tape. According to our own clinical practice, this maneuver is safe, simple, and time-saving [50, 51]. It is very important that the maneuver must not be forceful.

There are currently several operative approaches for performing anatomic segment-based liver resection. In 1985, Makuuchi et al. [52] devised a method of staining the target segment by injecting methylene blue into the supplying portal vein under ultrasound guidance. Torzilli et al. [53] advocated compressing the pedicle of the target segment manually under the intraoperative US guidance, which can cause the target segment to be ischemic. Takasaki et al. [54] developed the Glissonean pedicle transection method to perform segment-based liver resection. The main goal of all these approaches to anatomic hepatic resection is to precisely identify the surgical margin of the target segment/section.

The portal venous inflow blood elute methylene blue and the latter within the target segment parenchyma are quickly washed out when applying the methods of Makuuchi et al. [52] and Torzilli et al. [53]. Consequently, the boundary of the target segment/section can only be marked on the liver surface.

It is logically similar that the ischemic boundary obtained by clamping the pedicle of the target segment is also only evident and just can be marked on the liver surface. When hepatic parenchymal transection is initiated to resect the target segment, the Pringle maneuver or occlusion of the hemiliver containing the tumor-bearing segment is usually applied, and the interface between the ischemic target segment and the uninvolved remaining segments would disappear. Simply stated, the boundary of the tumor-bearing target segment cannot be identified in the deep hepatic parenchyma by the use of either methylene blue or ischemia. It is currently known that the morphology of the individual hepatic segment is not regular and the intersegmental or intersectional plane is uneven and curved plane [55, 56]; anatomic segmentectomy or sectionectomy may not be precisely carried out just based on the boundary marking on the liver surface but without obvious boundary within the deep hepatic parenchyma.

A novel persistent methylene blue staining technique for guiding anatomical hepatic resection may solve the abovementioned problem [57]. This technique consists of immediately clamping the corresponding hepatic pedicle after directly injecting methylene blue through the portal vein branch contained within this pedicle to achieve persistent methylene blue staining in the tumor-bearing target segment/section. Not only does this method delineate the boundary of the tumor-bearing target hepatic segment on the liver surface but also facilitate to determine the intersegmental/intersectional plane within the deep hepatic parenchyma. The deep intersegmental or intersectional plane is defined as the interface between methylene blue-stained liver tissue and unstained tissue. In recent clinical practice, we modified the Glissonean pedicle approach and combined the Glissonean pedicle transection method with the methylene blue staining technology. This combined technology helps to accurately identify the intersegmental/intersectional transection plane in the deep hepatic parenchyma and facilitates to avoid injury to the major hepatic vein, which must be exposed on the cut surface in anatomic hepatic resection.

Advantage of Segment-Based Anatomical Resection

Theoretically, the advantages of segment-based hepatic resection include:

1. The hepatic parenchymal transection plane between the resected segment(s) and the remaining residual liver are not crossed by large branches of the portal pedicle; thus this transection plane is a comparative avascular plane, which facilitates parenchymal transection in a bloodless field and decreases intraoperative bleeding.
2. By preventing injury to other hepatic pedicles entering into the remaining noninvolved segments, segment-based hepatic resection prevents leaving behind devascularized hepatic parenchyma in the liver remnant, consequently reducing the risk of infection and bile leakage.
3. During division of the pedicle of the resected segment(s) prior to hepatic parenchymal transection, the cut line can be marked clearly on the liver surface, and parenchymal transection can be carried out precisely along the boundary of ischemic demarcation and/or the dye-stained liver tissue; thus an adequate surgical margin width can be obtained (unless the tumor is very close to or compresses the main trunk of the major vessel) with conserving the largest amount of non-tumorous hepatic parenchyma.
4. Just as abovementioned, segment-based hepatic resection is oncologically more radical than non-anatomic resection. Hepatocellular carcinoma usually comes into being and is limited to any single segment in its early phase. Intrahepatic dissemination occurs by portal venous invasion, firstly forming satellite metastases within the same segment and finally the involved hemiliver or the whole liver being inflicted with the tumor. It is well known that microscopic and macroscopic venous invasion and intrahepatic metastasis are the main risk factors that lead to early postoperative recurrence. In case of satellite metastasis lying in the same segment (section) as the main tumor (see Sections "Mesohepatectomy (S4+S5+S8 Resection)" and "Bisegmentectomy V–VI" in the Chapter "Types of Segment-Oriented Hepatic Resection by the Glissonean Pedicle Approach"), segment-based hepatic resection should be selected to obtain complete tumor clearance.

Technical Details of Suprahilar Glissonean Approach for Anatomical Hepatic Resection

Jiangsheng Huang Jixiong Hu, and Xianling Liu

Anatomy of Glissonean Sheath (Glisson's Sheath)

In 1640, Valoeus first described connective tissue encompassing the structures at the hilus of the liver. Soon afterward, in 1645, Glisson described the connective tissue capsule covering the liver tissue [42, 58]. Glisson's capsule contracts around the portal triads as they enter into the liver parenchyma, and each bile duct, hepatic artery, and portal vein unit is encompassed by a fibrous sheath called the Glissonean sheath. Generally, the term Glissonean sheath is used only to make reference to the intrahepatic portion of the Glissonean pedicle [59]. Meanwhile, the portal triads in the hepatoduodenal ligaments are also surrounded by connective tissues up to the hepatic hilar plate. Therefore, the intrahepatic and extrahepatic portal triads comprised of the same Glissonean pedicle system. The Brisbane 2000 Terminology used the intrahepatic Glissonean pedicle system to divide the liver into hemilivers, sections (sectors), and segments [60]. Because any portal pedicle entering a particular segment takes a sheath, if the sheath is taken, it will only contain structures entering into or passing from this segment. Therefore, isolation, division, and ligation of individual sheath are not only simpler but also safer, and any segment-based hepatic resection is feasible [43, 44, 46, 61].

A Briefing Description of Different Approaches to the Glissonean Sheaths

Traditional Hilar Dissection or Intrafascial Approach

This approach was first described by Lortat-Jocob and Robert for the first extended right hepatectomy in 1952 [62]. Vasculature and bile duct of the portal triad are extrahepatically dissected in the hilum. This dissection is technically demanding and time-consuming, and because anomalous vasculature in this region is common, there is a risk of injury of contralateral hilar structures (remnant liver). This procedure has been referred to as a controlled hepatectomy method and was recognized as the basic anatomical hepatic resection technique [63].

Extrafascial Approach

Couinaud [43] developed this extrafascial approach for left hepatectomy; thereafter, Takasaki [54] developed this surgical technique for hepatic resection in the right liver. The approaches described by Couinaud and Takasaki et al. to the Glissonean pedicles were extrahepatic approaches without liver dissection. Launois and Jamieson [64] reported the intrahepatic Glissonean pedicle approach to hepatic resection in 1992. This Glissonean pedicle approach has made various types of hepatic resection possible including hemihepatectomy [65], sectionectomy [50, 66], and Couinaud's segmentectomy [51, 67] in a cirrhotic liver. In this approach, the whole sheath of a pedicle (segment or section) is dissected directly. This isolates the portal elements of the target segment(s) exactly and so avoids any inadvertent injury. A small traverse incision was made in front of the hilum and dissection close to the hilar plate separates it from the hepatic parenchyma without bleeding. In this book, we used this approach for all hepatic resections and renamed this extrafascial approach as "suprahilar Glissonean approach" [49].

Transfissural (or Intrahepatic) Approach

This approach includes the anterior intrahepatic approach [68, 69] and the posterior intrahepatic approach [70]. The key points in the anterior intrahepatic approach that differ from the intrafascial approach are three technical aspects: first, no need of individual dissection of the extrahepatic pedicle structures (vasculature and bile duct); secondly, no "necessity" of extrahepatic isolation and division of the trunk of the hepatic veins; and, thirdly, dissection beginning with an incision along one of the scissures of the liver. The posterior intrahepatic approach may get certain advantages of the intrafascial (extrahepatic) and anterior (intrahepatic) approaches by avoiding their innate disadvantages and especially by avoiding freeing the liver from its surrounding structures.

Essential Technical Points in Suprahilar Glissonean Approach for Liver Resections

Lowering the Hilar Plate

The hilar plate was located in the hilar area of the liver. One small traverse incision (about 1.5–2.5 cm) was made in front of the hilar plate (Fig. 7a), hepatic parenchyma around this incision was pushed upward, and the hilar plate was pulled down (Fig. 7b). This maneuver was referred to as lowering of the hilar plate. It can be performed with safety because there was only exceptionally (in 1% of cases) any vasculature between the hilar plate and the inferior surface of the liver.

Isolation and Looping of the Right and Left Hepatic Pedicle

A large curved clamp was vertically inserted into this incision above the hilar plate, and the operator's left index finger was put between the undersurface of the hilar plate and the anterior wall of the retrohepatic inferior vena cava (IVC) (Fig. 8a), and then, the clamp was furtherly inserted to directly reach to the tip of the operator's left index finger,

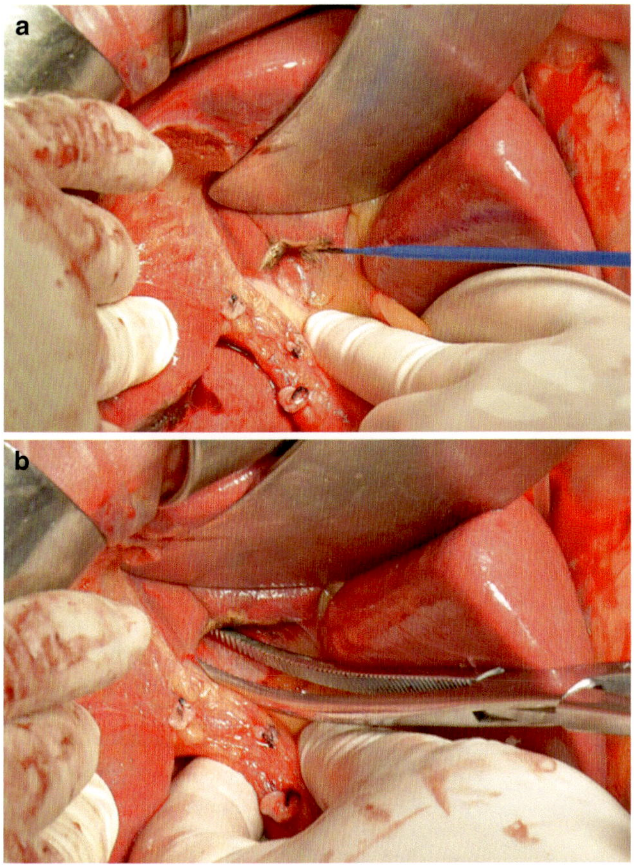

Fig. 7 Lowering the hilar plate. (**a**) One small traverse incision was made in front of the hilar plate. (**b**) The hilar plate was pulled down to exteriorize both the right and left hepatic pedicle

and using the finger as a guide, the clamp punctured through the undersurface membrane of the hilar plate and passed out of the right edge of the right hepatic pedicle (RHP) (Fig. 8b). Thus, the right hepatic pedicle was isolated and looped (Fig. 8d). If necessary, the left hepatic pedicle (LHP) was similarly isolated (Fig. 9a) and encircled (Fig. 8c). Figures 8c, e and 9b, d show schematic illustration of these procedures.

Isolation and Looping of the Right Anterior Sectional Pedicle

One small incision was made on the right edge of the gallbladder bed. Then, a large curved clamp was inserted into this incision in front of the hilus and passed out of this incision on the right edge of the gallbladder bed. Thus, the right anterior sectional Glissonean pedicle (RAP) was isolated and looped with a vascular tape (Fig. 10a, c). Figure 10b, d shows schematic illustration of this procedure.

Isolation and Looping of the Right Posterior Sectional Pedicle

A large curved clamp inserted into the incision at the right edge of the gallbladder, and meanwhile, the operator's left index finger was placed below the undersurface of the right hepatic pedicle (RHP) (Fig. 11a), and using the finger as a guide, the clamp was inserted downward and directly reached down to the fingertip and passed out of the right and inferior edge of the right hepatic pedicle (Fig. 11b). Thus, the right posterior Glissonean pedicle (RPP) was isolated and encir-

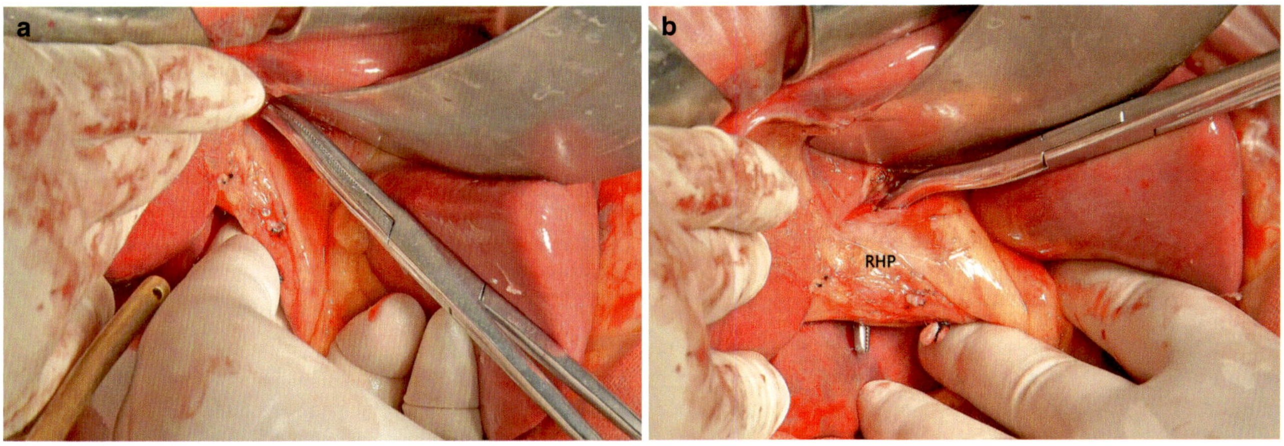

Fig. 8 Isolating the right hepatic pedicle. (**a**) A large curved clamp was inserted into this incision in front of the hilar plate. (**b**) The right hepatic pedicle was encircled by this clamp. (**c**) Schematic illustration of this procedure. (**d**) The right hepatic pedicle (RHP) was looped with a tape. (**e**) Schematic illustration of this maneuver

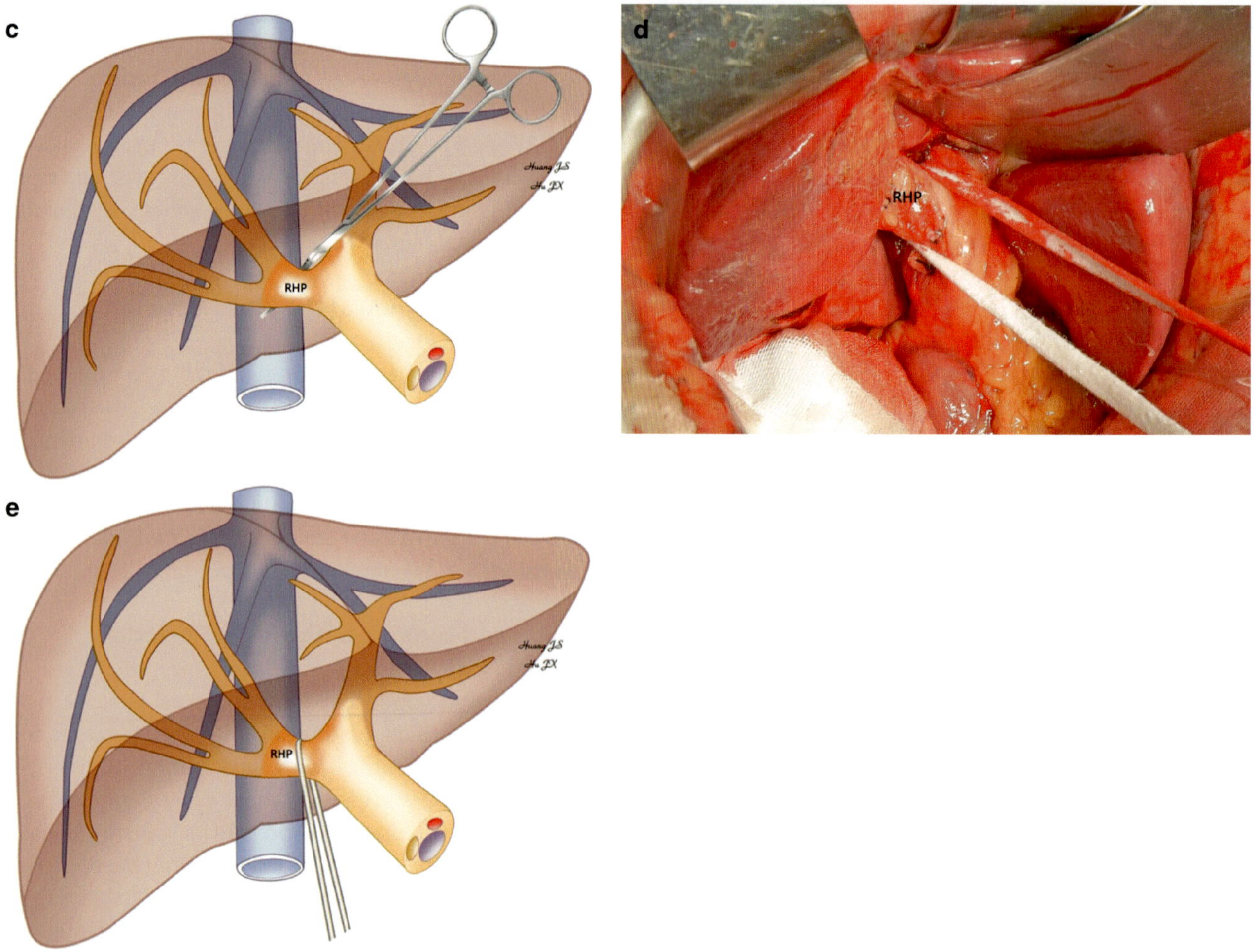

Fig. 8 (continued)

cled with a tourniquet (Fig. 11d). Figure 11c, e shows schematic illustration of this procedure.

Isolation and Looping of the Pedicle of Segment 5 and Segment 8

Further dissection is required to obtain the portal pedicle of segment 5 and segment 8. The right anterior pedicle (RAP) was dissected on its inferior, superior, and anterior surface for about 1–3 cm, where it was possible to ascertain bifurcation of segments 5 and 8. The pedicle of segment 5 and segment 8 was isolated and encircled by a vascular tape, respectively.

Isolation and Looping of the Pedicle of Segment 6 and Segment 7

The pedicle of the right posterior sector is the most deeply placed of the right pedicles. Further dissection is also required to obtain the portal pedicle of segment 6 and segment 7. The right posterior pedicle (RPP) was dissected on its anterior, superior, and inferior surface for about 1–3 cm, where it was possible to ascertain bifurcation of segments 6 and 7. The pedicle of segment 6 and segment 7 was isolated and encircled by a vascular tape, respectively. If resection of the caudate process is required, the portal pedicle entering into the process from the RPP should be ligated and divided.

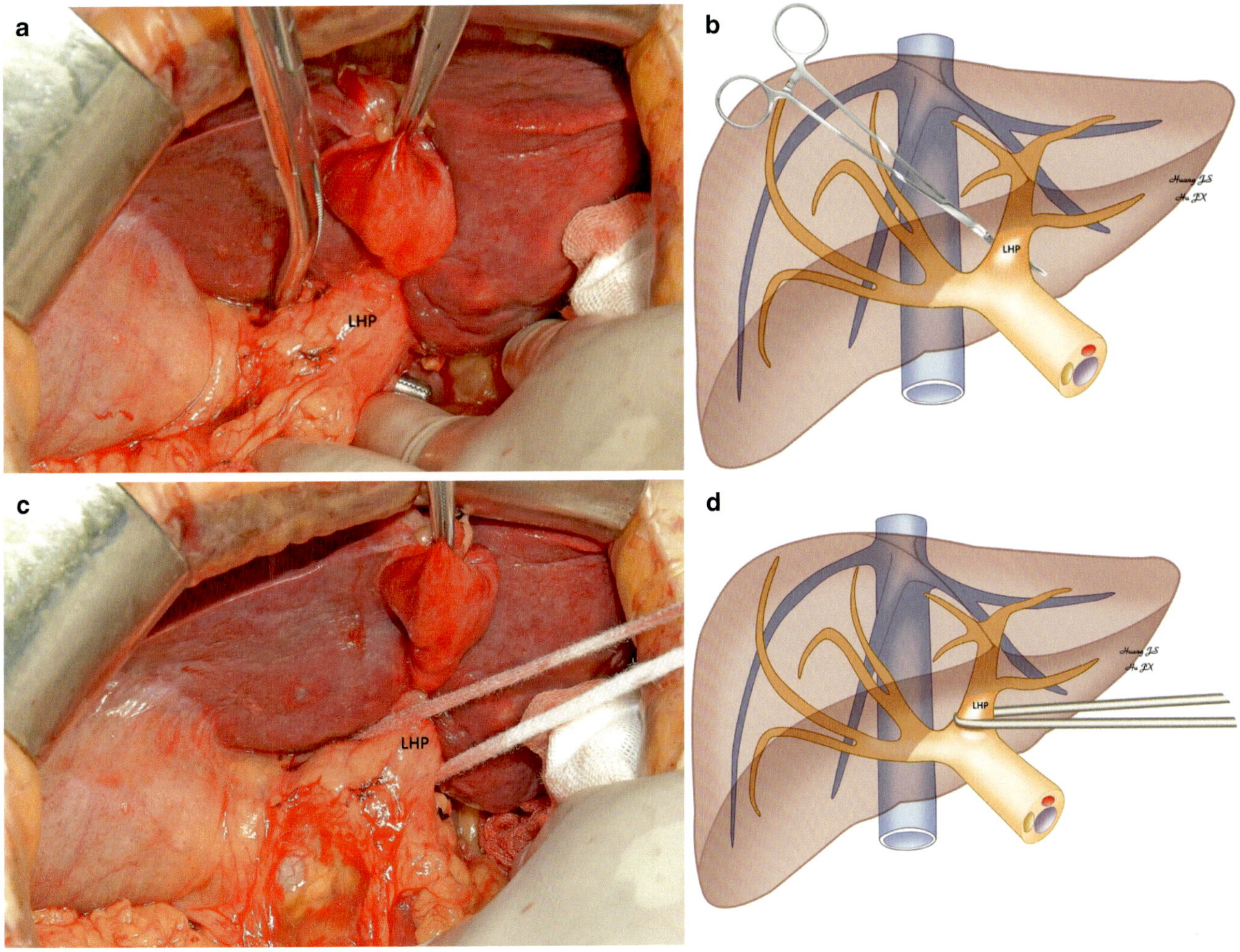

Fig. 9 Isolating the right hepatic pedicle (LHP). (**a**) The left hepatic pedicle (LHP) was encompassed by a large curved clamp. (**b**) Schematic illustration of this procedure. (**c**) The LHP was encircled with a tape. (**d**) Schematic illustration of this maneuver

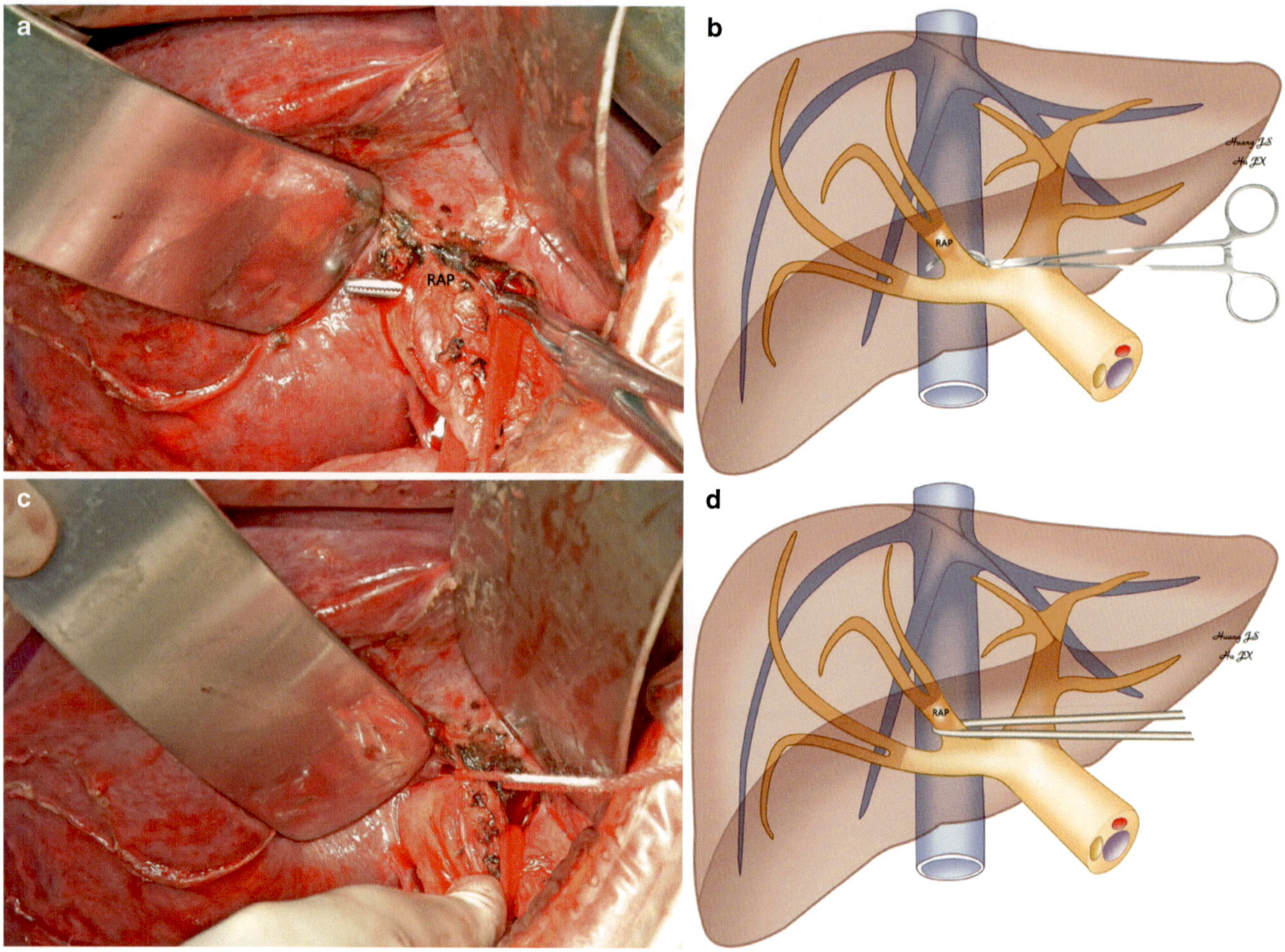

Fig. 10 Isolating the right hepatic pedicle. (**a**) The right anterior pedicle (RAP) was encircled by a large curved clamp. (**b**) Schematic illustration of this maneuver. (**c**) The RAP was encircled with a tape. (**d**) Schematic illustration

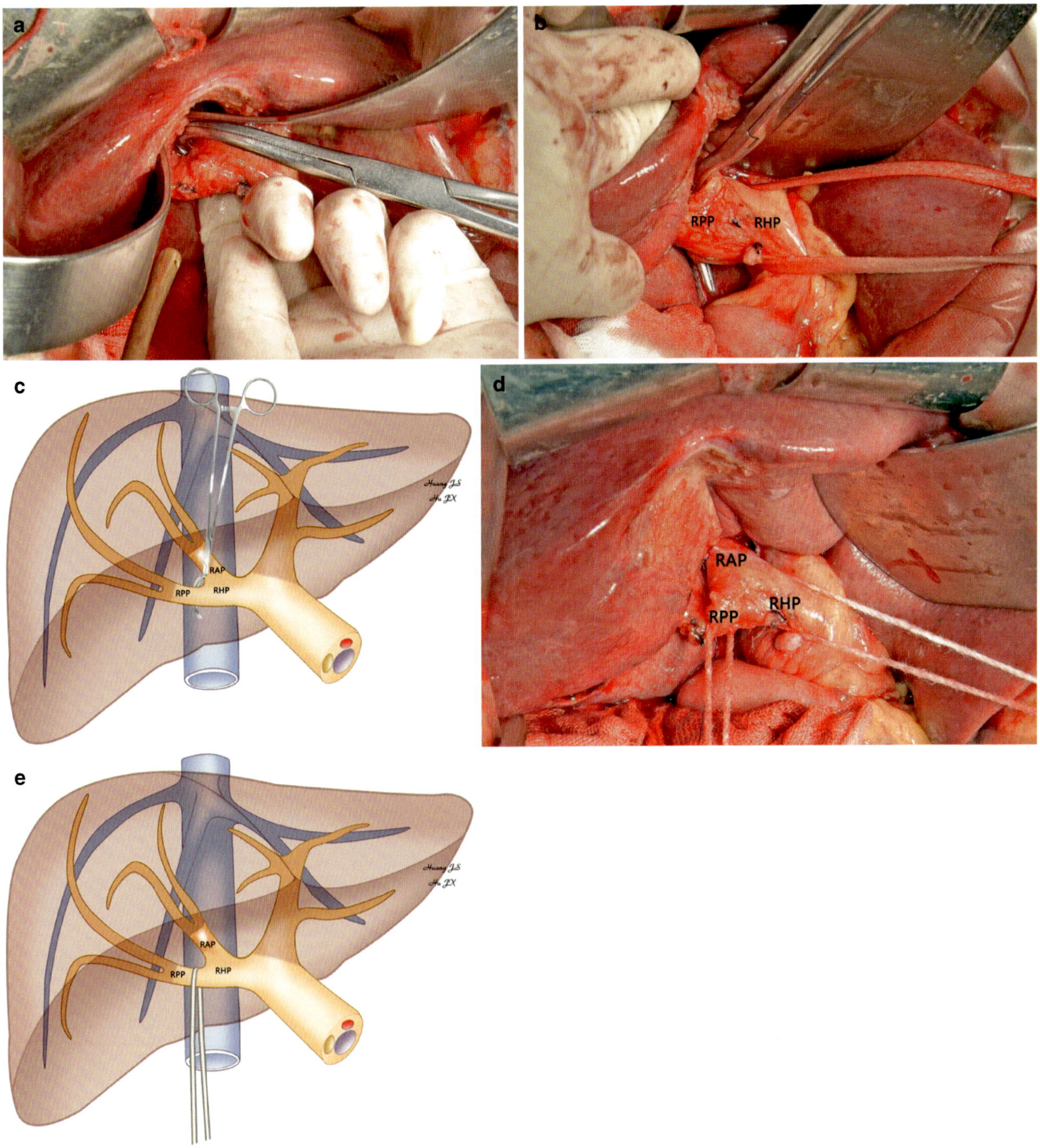

Fig. 11 Isolating the right posterior pedicle. (**a**, **b**) The right posterior pedicle (RPP) was encompassed by a large curved clamp. (**c**) Schematic illustration of these procedures. (**d**) The right posterior pedicle (RPP) was looped with a tape. (**e**) Schematic illustration of this procedure. *RAP* right anterior sectional pedicle

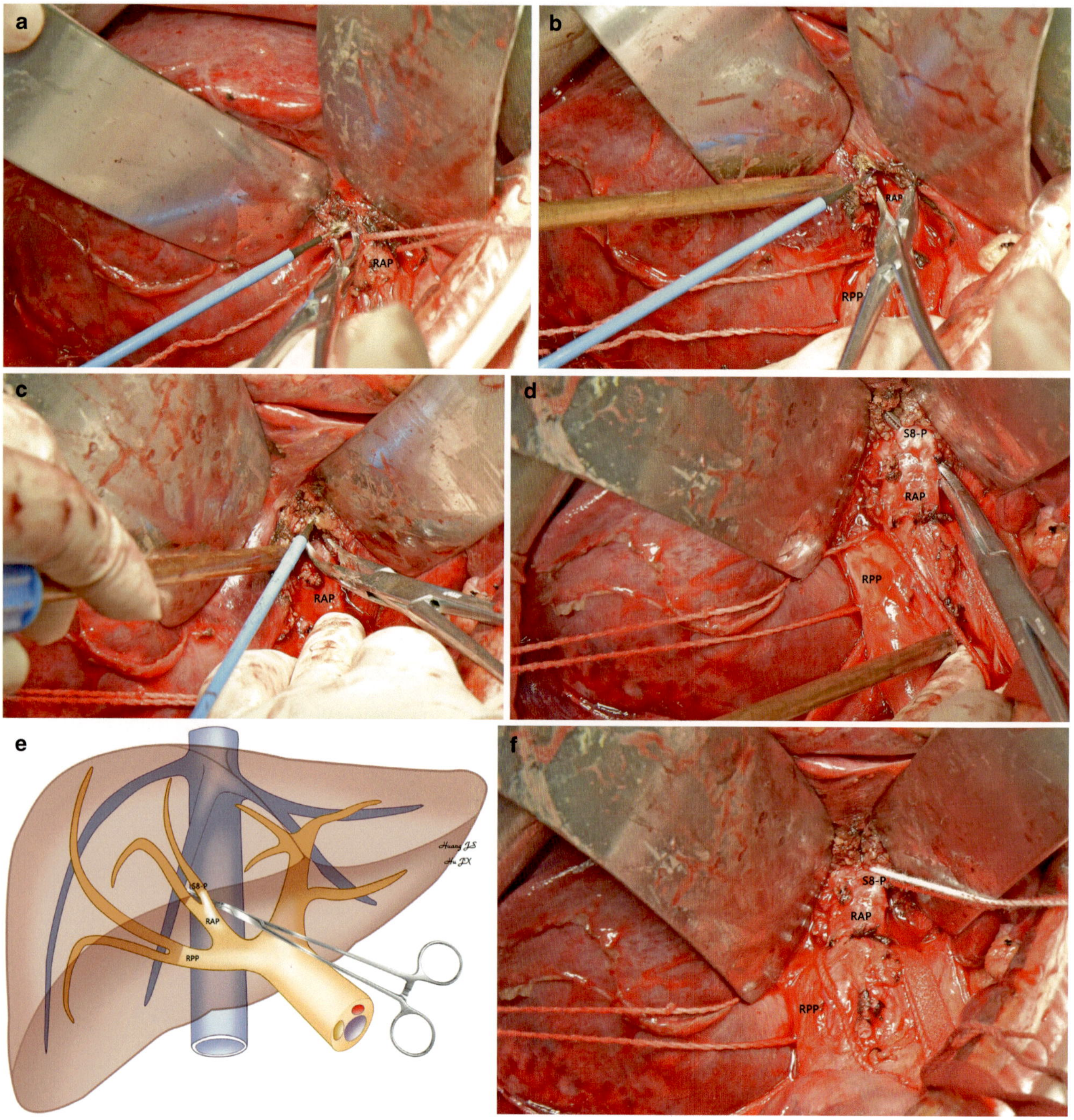

Fig. 12 (**a**) Hepatic parenchyma around the inferior surface of the right anterior pedicle (RAP) was dissected with electrocautery. (**b**) Hepatic parenchyma around the anterior surface of the right anterior pedicle (RAP) was dissected with electrocautery. (**c**) Hepatic parenchyma around the superior surface of the right anterior pedicle (RAP) was dissected with electrocautery. (**d**) The whole course of the right anterior pedicle (RAP) was exposed, and the bifurcation of segments 5 and 8 was identified. Then, the pedicle of segment 8 (S8-P) was isolated using a curved forceps; (**e**) Schematic illustration of this procedure. (**f**) The pedicle of segment 8 (S8-P) was looped with a tourniquet. (**g**) Schematic illustration of this procedure. (**h**) The pedicle of segment 5 (S5-P) was also isolated with a curved forceps. (**i**) Schematic illustration of this procedure. (**j**) The pedicle of segment 5 (S5-P) was encircled with a vascular tape. (**k**) Schematic illustration of this procedure. *RAP* right anterior pedicle, *RPP* right posterior pedicle, *S8-P* pedicle of segment 8. *RPP* right posterior pedicle, *S8-P* pedicle of segment 8, S5-P pedicle of segment 5 (Fig. 12a–k)

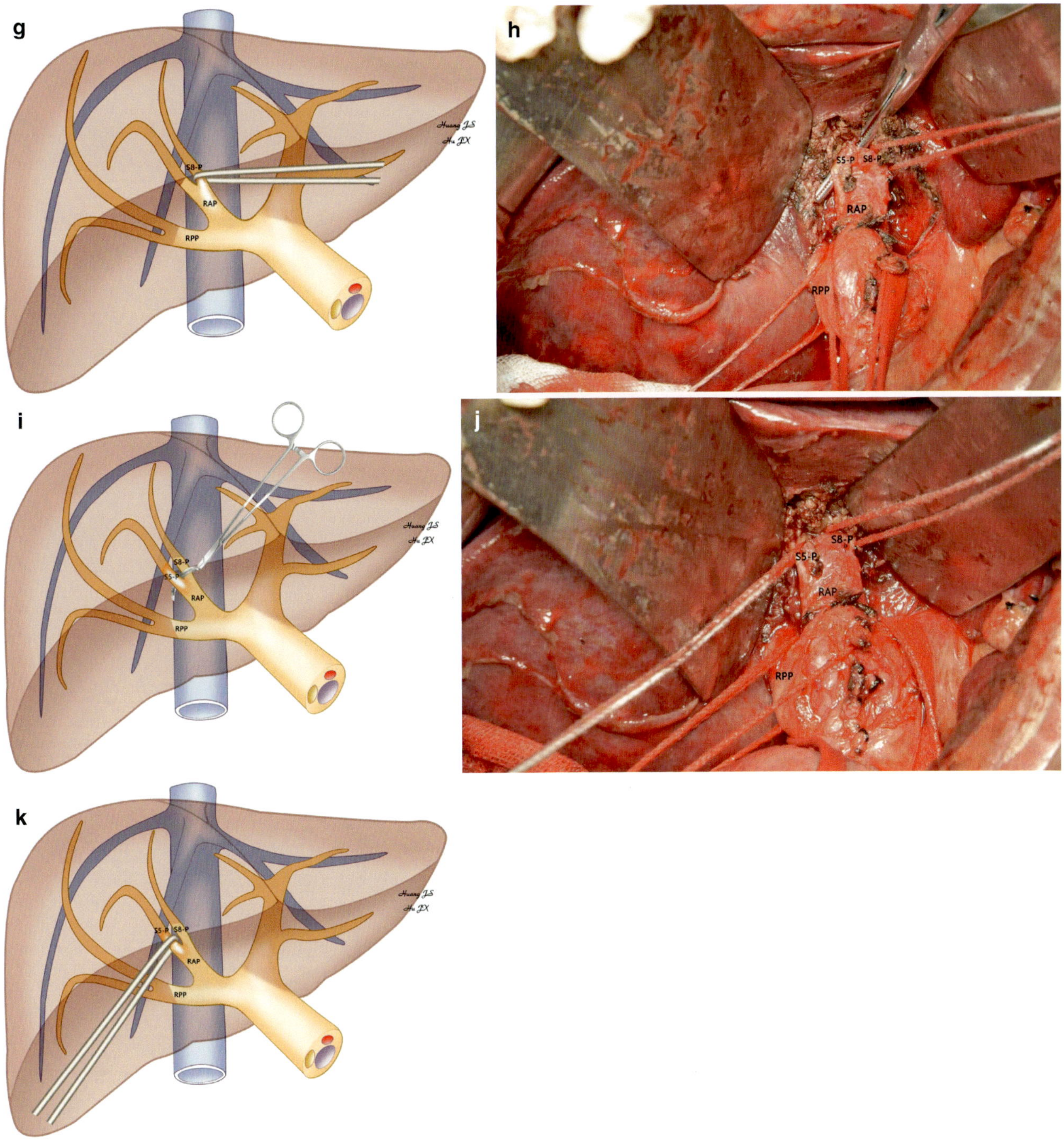

Fig. 12 (continued)

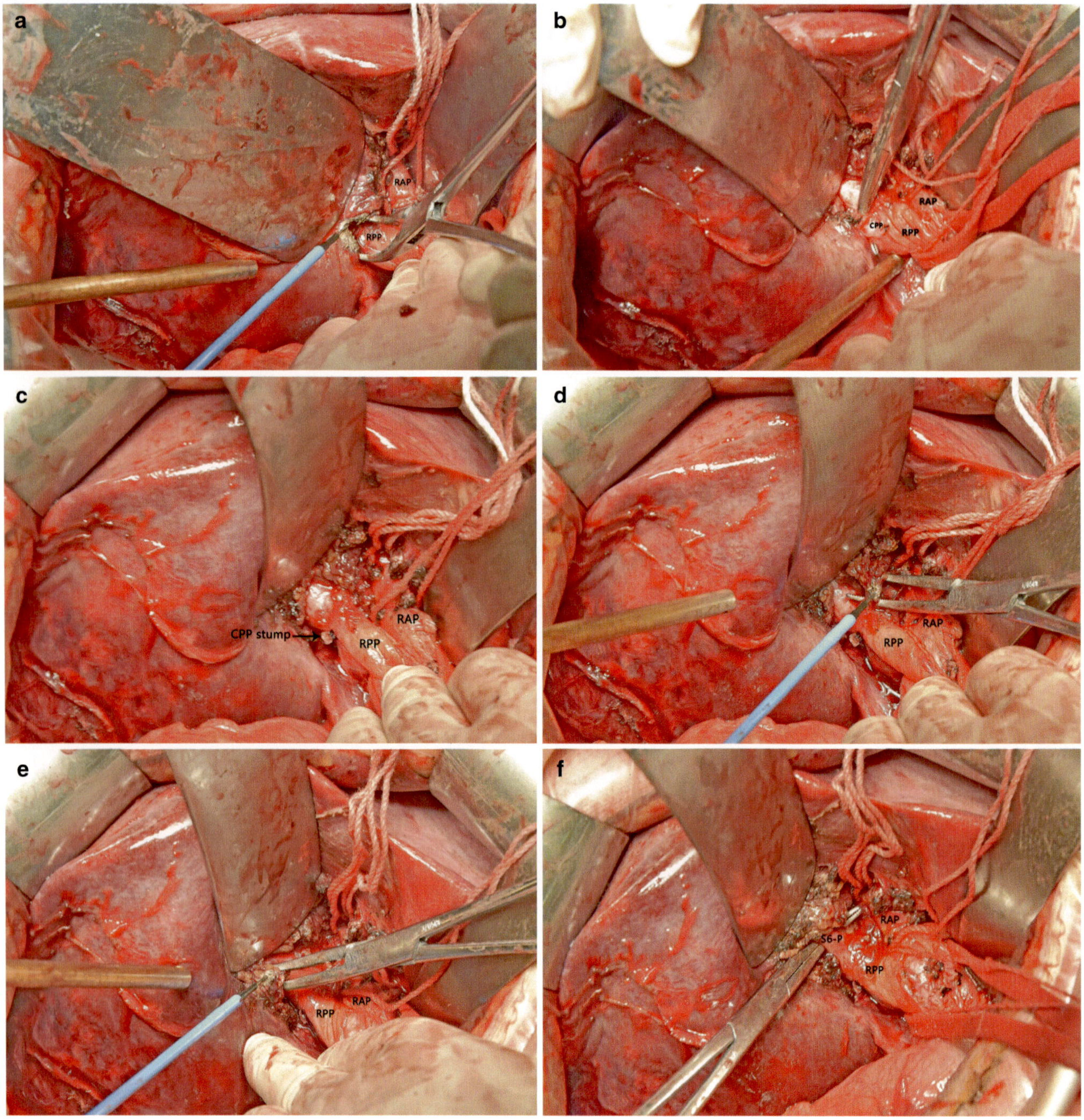

Fig. 13 (**a**) Hepatic parenchyma around the anterior surface of the right posterior pedicle (RPP) was dissected with electrocautery. (**b**, **c**) The pedicle of caudate process was isolated, clamped, divided, and suture-ligated. (**d**) Hepatic parenchyma around the superior surface of the right posterior pedicle (RPP) was dissected with electrocautery. (**e**) Hepatic parenchyma around the inferior surface of the right posterior pedicle (RPP) was dissected with electrocautery. (**f**) Up to now, the whole course of the right posterior pedicle (RPP) was exposed. The pedicle of segment 6 (S6-P) was isolated using a curved forceps. (**g**) Schematic illustration of this procedure. (**h**) The pedicle of segment 6 (S6-P) was encircled with a loop. (**i**) Schematic illustration of this procedure. (**j**) The pedicle of segment 7 (S7-P) was still deeply located within hepatic parenchyma. Hepatic parenchymal dissection around S7-P was continued. (**k**) The pedicle of segment 7 (S7-P) was fully exposed and isolated using a curved forceps. (**l**) Schematic illustration of this procedure. (**m**) The pedicle of segment 7 (S7-P) was also encircled with a tourniquet. (**n**) Schematic illustration of this procedure. *RAP* right anterior pedicle, *RPP*, right posterior pedicle, *CPP* the caudate process pedicle, *S6-P* pedicle of segment 6, *S7-P* pedicle of segment 7. *RAP*: right anterior pedicle; *CPP*: the caudate process pedicle; *S6-P* pedicle of segment 6; *S7-P* pedicle of segment 7 (Fig. 13a–n)

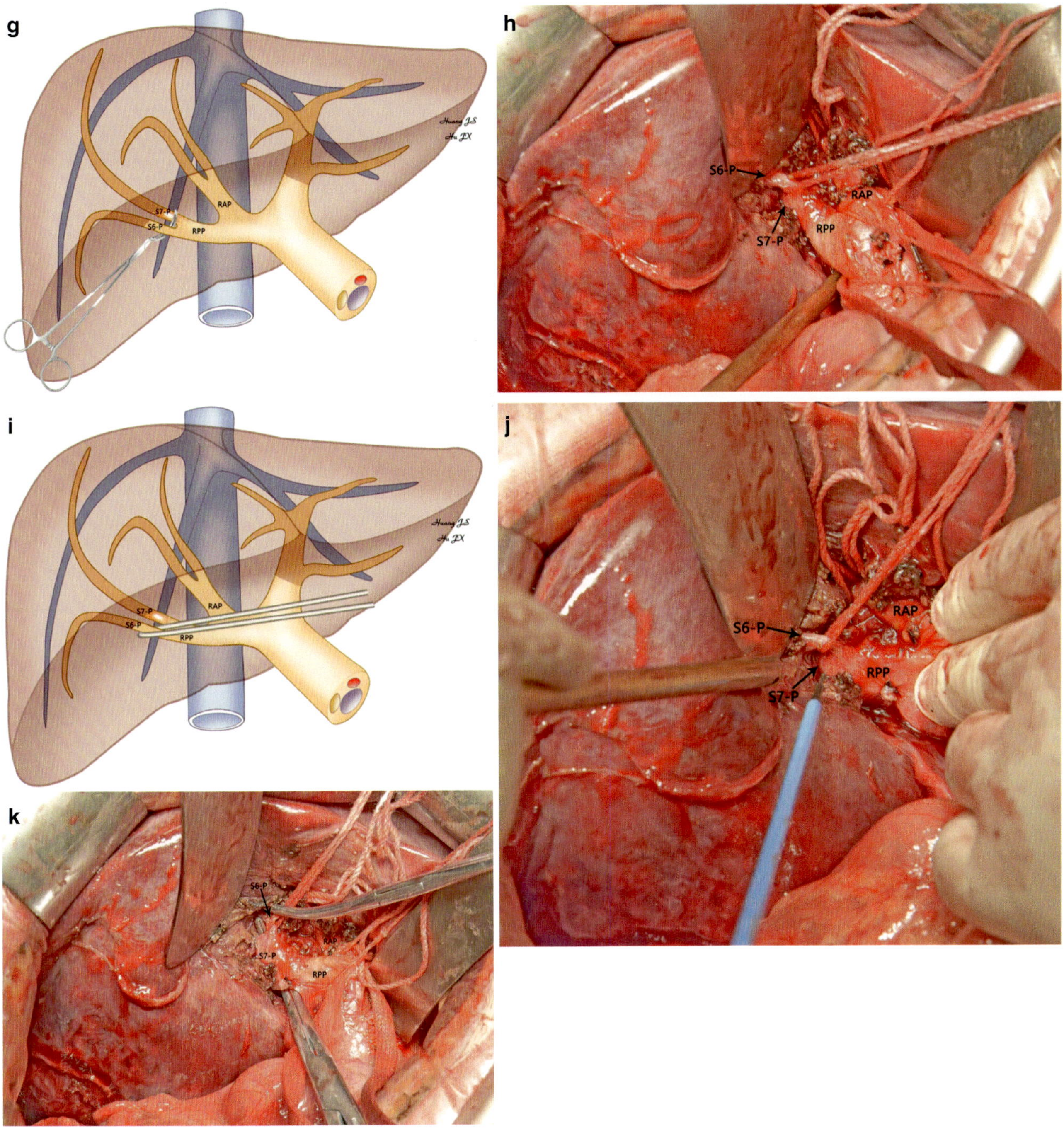

Fig. 13 (continued)

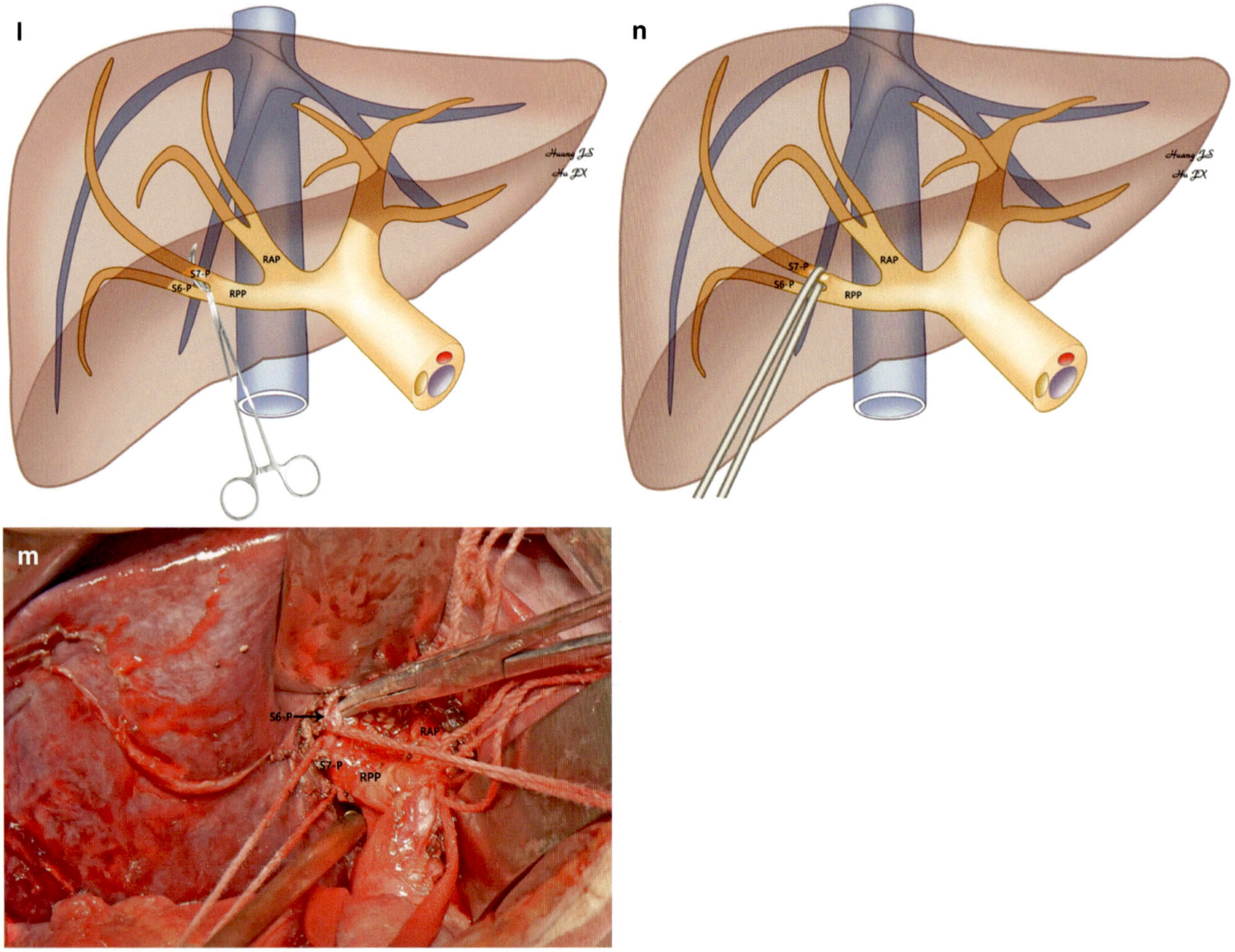

Fig. 13 (continued)

References

1. Kingham TP, Correagallego C, D'Angelica MI, Gönen M, Dematteo RP, Fong Y, Allen PJ, Blumgart LH, Jarnagin WR. Hepatic parenchymal preservation surgery: decreasing morbidity and mortality rates in 4,152 resections for malignancy. J Am Coll Surg. 2015;220(4):471–9.
2. Zimmitti G, Roses RE, Andreou A, Shindoh J, Curley SA, Aloia TA, Vauthey JN. Greater complexity of liver surgery is not associated with an increased incidence of liver-related complications except for bile leak: an experience with 2,628 consecutive resections. Gastroenterology. 2013;17(1):57–65.
3. Sadamori H, Yagi T, Shinoura S, Umeda Y, Yoshida R, Satoh D, Nobuoka D, Utsumi M, Fujiwara T. Risk factors for major morbidity after liver resection for hepatocellular carcinoma. Br J Surg. 2013;100(1):122.
4. Lau WY. A review on the operative techniques in liver resection. Chin Med J. 1997;110(7):567–70.
5. Müller MK, Petrowsky H, Clavien PA. Techniques of vascular control and protective strategies for parenchymal transection. Singapore: World Scientific Publishing; 2008.
6. Kooby DA, Stockman J, Ben-Porat L, Gonen M, Jarnagin WR, Dematteo RP, Tuorto S, Wuest D, Blumgart LH, Fong Y. Influence of transfusions on perioperative and long-term outcome in patients following hepatic resection for colorectal metastases. Ann Surg. 2003;241(2):860–9.
7. Stephenson KR, Steinberg SM, Hughes KS, Vetto JT, Sugarbaker PH, Chang AE. Perioperative blood transfusions are associated with decreased time to recurrence and decreased survival after resection of colorectal liver metastases. Ann Surg. 1988;208(6):679.
8. Pringle JH. Notes on the arrest of hepatic hemorrhage due to trauma. Ann Surg. 1908;48(4):541.
9. Lowe MC, D'Angelica MI. Anatomy of hepatic resectional surgery. Surg Clin North Am. 2016;96(2):183.
10. Belghiti J, Marty J, Farges O. Techniques, hemodynamic monitoring, and indications for vascular clamping during liver resections. J Hepatobiliary Pancreat Sci. 1998;5(1):69.
11. Lau WY, et al. Chapter 9. Hepatic vascular inflow and outflow occlusion. In: Lau WY, editor. Applied anatomy in liver resection and liver transplantation. Beijing: People's Medical Publishing House; 2011. p. 77–92.

12. Clavien PA, Yadav S, Sindram D, Bentley RC. Protective effects of ischemic preconditioning for liver resection performed under inflow occlusion in humans. Ann Surg. 2000;232(2):155.
13. Clavien PA, Selzner M, Rüdiger HA, Graf R, Kadry Z, Rousson V, Jochum W. A prospective randomized study in 100 consecutive patients undergoing major liver resection with versus without ischemic preconditioning. Ann Surg. 2003;238(6):843.
14. Chouker A, Schachtner TR, Dugas M, Lohe F, Martignoni A, Pollwein B, Niklas M, Rau HG, Jauch KW, Peter K. Effects of Pringle manoeuvre and ischaemic preconditioning on haemodynamic stability in patients undergoing elective hepatectomy: a randomized trial. Br J Anaesth. 2004;93(2):204.
15. Heizmann O, Loehe F, Volk A, Schauer RJ. Ischemic preconditioning improves postoperative outcome after liver resections: a randomized controlled study. Eur J Med Res. 2008;13(2):79–86.
16. Li SQ, Liang LJ, Huang JF, Li Z. Ischemic preconditioning protects liver from hepatectomy under hepatic inflow occlusion for hepatocellular carcinoma patients with cirrhosis. World J Gastroenterol. 2004;10(17):2580.
17. Makuuchi M, Mori T, Gunvén P, Yamazaki S, Hasegawa H. Safety of hemihepatic vascular occlusion during resection of the liver. Surg Gynecol Obstet. 1987;164(2):155.
18. Ken TMD. Glissonean pedicle transection method for hepatic resection. Tokyo: Springer; 2007.
19. Heaney JP, Stanton WK, Halbert DS, Seidel J, Vice T. An improved technic for vascular isolation of the liver: experimental study and case reports. Ann Surg. 1966;163(2):237.
20. Lau WY, et al. Chapter 6. Intrahepatic Glissonian triad: anatomy relevant to liver resection and liver transplantation. In: Lau WY, editor. Applied anatomy in liver resection and liver transplantation. Beijing: People's Medical Publishing House; 2011. p. 45–59.
21. Kato M, Kubota K, Kita J, Shimoda M, Rokkaku K, Sawada T. Effect of infra-hepatic inferior vena cava clamping on bleeding during hepatic dissection: a prospective, randomized, controlled study. World J Surg. 2008;32(6):1082–7.
22. Ueno M, Kawai M, Hayami S, Hirono S, Okada KI, Uchiyama K, Yamaue H. Partial clamping of the infrahepatic inferior vena cava for blood loss reduction during anatomic liver resection: a prospective, randomized, controlled trial. Surgery. 2017;161(6):1502–13.
23. Hamady Z, Toogood G. Infrahepatic inferior vena cava clamping for reduction of central venous pressure and blood loss during hepatic resection: a randomized controlled trial. Ann Surg. 2011;253(6):1102–10.
24. Otsubo T, Takasaki K, Yamamoto M, Katsuragawa H, Katagiri S, Yoshitoshi K, Hamano M, Ariizumi S, Kotera Y. Bleeding during hepatectomy can be reduced by clamping the inferior vena cava below the liver. Surgery. 2004;135(1):67–73.
25. Chen XP, Zhang ZW, Zhang BX, Chen YF, Huang ZY, Zhang WG, He SQ, Qiu FZ. Modified technique of hepatic vascular exclusion: effect on blood loss during complex mesohepatectomy in hepatocellular carcinoma patients with cirrhosis. Langenbecks Arch Surg. 2006;391(3):209–15.
26. Bismuth H, Castaing D, Garden OJ. Major hepatic resection under total vascular exclusion. Ann Surg. 1989;210(1):13.
27. Smyrniotis V, Farantos C, Kostopanagiotou G, Arkadopoulos N. Vascular control during hepatectomy: review of methods and results. World J Surg. 2005;29(11):1384–96.
28. Fu SY, Lau WY, Li AJ, Yang Y, Pan ZY, Sun YM, Lai ECH, Zhou WP, Wu MC. Liver resection under total vascular exclusion with or without preceding Pringle manoeuvre. Br J Surg. 2010;97(1):50.
29. Fu SY, Lai EC, Li AJ, Pan ZY, Yang Y, Sun YM, Lau WY, Wu MC, Zhou WP. Liver resection with selective hepatic vascular exclusion: a cohort study. Ann Surg. 2009;249(4):624.
30. Li AJ, Pan ZY, Zhou WP, Fu SY, Yang Y, Huang G, Yin L, Wu MC. Comparison of two methods of selective hepatic vascular exclusion for liver resection involving the roots of the hepatic veins. J Gastrointest Surg. 2008;12(8):1383–90.
31. Zhou W, Li A, Pan Z, Fu S, Yang Y, Tang L, Hou Z, Wu M. Selective hepatic vascular exclusion and Pringle maneuver: a comparative study in liver resection. Eur J Surg Oncol. 2008;34(1):49–54.
32. Miao XY, Hu JX, Dai WD, Zhong DW, Huang SF, Wen Y, Xiong SZ. Anatomic mesohepatectomy with extrahepatic control of hepatic veins. Hepatogastroenterology. 2009;56(96):1730–4.
33. Wen Y, Miao XY, Xiong L, Xiong G, Hu JX, Zhong DW, Li QL, Liu W. Application of hemihepatic vascular occlusion with hanging maneuver in hepatectomy. Hepato-gastroenterology. 2009;56(90):442–7.
34. Kang KJ, Ahn KS. Anatomical resection of hepatocellular carcinoma: a critical review of the procedure and its benefits on survival. World J Gastroenterol. 2017;23(7):1139–46.
35. Fattovich G, Giustina G, Degos F, Tremolada F, Diodati G, Almasio P, Nevens F, Solinas A, Mura D, Brouwer JT. Morbidity and mortality in compensated cirrhosis type C: a retrospective follow-up study of 384 patients. Gastroenterology. 1997;112(2):463–72.
36. Chen MF, Tsai HP, Jeng LB, Lee WC, Yeh CN, Yu MC, Hun CM. Prognostic factors after resection for hepatocellular carcinoma in noncirrhotic livers: univariate and multivariate analysis. World J Surg. 2003;27(4):443–7.
37. Hasegawa K, Makuuchi M, Takayama T, Kokudo N, Arii S, Okazaki M, Okita K, Omata M, Kudo M, Kojiro M. Surgical resection vs. percutaneous ablation for hepatocellular carcinoma: a preliminary report of the Japanese nationwide survey. J Hepatol. 2008;50(4):589–94.
38. Schroeder RA, Marroquin CE, Bute BP, Khuri S, Henderson WG, Kuo PC. Predictive indices of morbidity and mortality after liver resection. Ann Surg. 2006;243(3):373–9.
39. Matsui Y, Terakawa N, Satoi S, Kaibori M, Kitade H, Takai S, Kwon AH, Kamiyama Y. Postoperative outcomes in patients with hepatocellular carcinomas resected with exposure of the tumor surface: clinical role of the no-margin resection. Arch Surg. 2007;142(7):596.
40. Hasegawa K, Kokudo N, Imamura H, Matsuyama Y, Aoki T, Minagawa M, Sano K, Sugawara Y, Takayama T, Makuuchi M. Prognostic impact of anatomic resection for hepatocellular carcinoma. Ann Surg. 2005;242(2):252–9.
41. Makuuchi M, Hasegawa H, Yamazaki S. Intraoperative ultrasonic examination for hepatectomy. Ultrasound Med Biol. 1981;11(2):493–7.
42. Couinaud C. Surgical anatomy of the liver revisited. Paris: Self-printed; 1989.
43. Couinaud CM. A simplified method for controlled left hepatectomy. Surgery. 1985;97(3):358–61.
44. Takasaki K, Kobayashi S, Tanaka S, Saito A, Yamamoto M, Hanyu F. Highly anatomically systematized hepatic resection with Glissonean sheath code transection at the hepatic hilus. Int Surg. 1990;75(2):73–7.
45. Sugioka A, Kato Y, Tanahashi Y. Systematic extrahepatic Glissonean pedicle isolation for anatomical liver resection based on Laennec's capsule: proposal of a novel comprehensive surgical anatomy of the liver. J Hepatobiliary Pancreat Sci. 2017;24(1):17–23.
46. Yamamoto M, Katagiri S, Ariizumi S, Kotera Y, Takahashi Y. Glissonean pedicle transection method for liver surgery (with video). J Hepatobiliary Pancreat Sci. 2012;19(1):3–8.
47. Bernard L, Knoon HT. Chapter 19. Intrahepatic Glissonian approach. In: Lau WY, editor. Hepatocellular carcinoma. Singapore: World Scientific Publishing; 2008. p. 429–46.
48. Doklestić K, Djukić V, Bumbasirević V, Jovanović B, Karamarković A. Segment-oriented liver resections based on posterior intrahepatic Glissonian approach. Acta Chir Iugosl. 2012;59(3):41–8.

49. Figueroa R, Laurenzi A, Laurent A, Cherqui D. Perihilar Glissonian approach for anatomical parenchymal sparing liver resections: technical aspects: the taping game. Ann Surg. 2016;267(3):537–43.
50. Dai WD, Hu JX, Miao XY, Zhong DW, Wen Y, Xiong SZ. Intrahepatic Glissonian access for mesohepatectomy in cirrhotic patients. Hepatogastroenterology. 2008;55(85):1153–7.
51. Hu JX, Dai WD, Miao XY, Zhong DW, Huang SF, Wen Y, Xiong SZ. Anatomic resection of segment VIII of liver for hepatocellular carcinoma in cirrhotic patients based on an intrahepatic Glissonian approach. Surgery. 2009;146(5):854–60.
52. Makuuchi M, Hasegawa H, Yamazaki S. Ultrasonically guided subsegmentectomy. Surg Gynecol Obstet. 1985;161(4):346.
53. Torzilli G, Procopio F, Cimino M, Del Fabbro D, Palmisano A, Donadon M, Montorsi M. Anatomical segmental and subsegmental resection of the liver for hepatocellular carcinoma. Ann Surg. 2009;251(2):229–35.
54. Takasaki K, Kobayashi S, Tanaka S, Muto H, Watayo T, Saito A. Newly developed systematized hepatectomy by Glissonean pedicle transection method. Shujutsu. 1986;40:7–14. (in Japanese).
55. Fischer L, Cardenas C, Thorn M, Benner A, Grenacher L, Vetter M, Lehnert T, Klar E, Meinzer HP, Lamadã W. Limits of Couinaud's liver segment classification: a quantitative computer-based three-dimensional analysis. J Comput Assist Tomogr. 2002;26(6):962–7.
56. Shindoh J, Mise Y, Satou S, Sugawara Y, Kokudo N. The intersegmental plane of the liver is not always flat – tricks for anatomical liver resection. Ann Surg. 2010;251(5):917.
57. Shouwang C, Shizhong Y, Wenping L, Geng C, Wanqing G, Weidong D, Weiyi W, Zhiqiang H, Jiahong D. Sustained methylene blue staining to guide anatomic hepatectomy for hepatocellular carcinoma: initial experience and technical details. Surgery. 2015;158(1):121–7.
58. Lau WY, et al. Intrahepatic Glissonian approach. In: Lau WY, editor. Hepatocellular carcinoma. London: World Scientific Publishing; 2008. p. 429–46.
59. Lau WY, et al. Intrahepatic Glissonian triad: anatomy relevant to liver resection and liver transplantation. In: Lau WY, editor. Applied anatomy in liver resection and liver transplantation. Beijing: People's Medical Publishing House; 2010. p. 45–59.
60. Terminology Committee of the IHPBA. The Brisbane terminology of the liver anatomy and resection. HPB (Oxford). 2000;2:333–9.
61. Yamamoto M, Katagiri S, Ariizumi S, Kotera Y, Takahashi Y, Egawa H. Tips for anatomical hepatectomy for hepatocellular carcinoma by the Glissonean pedicle approach (with videos). J Hepatobiliary Pancreat Sci. 2014;21(8):E53–6.
62. Lortat-Jacob JL, Robert HG. Hepatectomie droite reglee. Presse Med. 1952;60:549–51.
63. Bismuth H. Surgical anatomy and anatomical surgery of the liver. World J Surg. 1982;6(1):3–9.
64. Launois B, Jamieson GG. The importance of Glisson's capsule and its sheath in the intrahepatic approach to resection of the liver. Surg Gynecol Obstet. 1992;174(1):7–10.
65. Katagiri S, Ariizumi SI, Kotera Y, Takahashi Y, Yamamoto M. Right hepatectomy using Glissonean pedicle transection method with anterior approach (with video). J Hepatobiliary Pancreat Sci. 2012;19(1):25–9.
66. Yamanaka J, Fujimoto J. Sectionectomy of the liver. J Hepatobiliary Pancreat Sci. 2012;19(1):54.
67. Yoshida H, Yu K, Rikiyama T, Motoi F, Onogawa T, Egawa S, Unno M. Segmentectomy of the liver. J Hepatobiliary Pancreat Sci. 2012;19(1):67–71.
68. Couinaud C. Liver anatomy: a half century investigation. In: Forni E, Mernigi F, editors. Selected topics of HPB surgery and medicine. Pavia: IRCCS; 1995. p. 33–50.
69. Belghiti J, Guevara OA, Noun R, Saldinger PF, Kianmanesh R. Liver hanging maneuver: a safe approach to right hepatectomy without liver mobilization. J Am Coll Surg. 2001;193(1):109.
70. Maddern GJ, Manganas D, Launois B. Clinical experience with the intrahepatic posterior approach to the portal triad for right hepatectomy and right segmental resection. World J Surg. 1995;19(5):764–7.

Types of Segment-Oriented Hepatic Resection by the Glissonean Pedicle Approach

Jixiong Hu, Weidong Dai, Zhongkun Zuo, and Chun Liu

Right Hepatectomy (S5–S8 Resection)

Jixiong Hu, Weidong Dai, Wengtao Fan, and Zhongkun Zuo

Surgical Indications for Right Hepatectomy

Among liver resections, right hepatectomy (RH) was defined as a major hepatectomy [1]. According to the Brisbane classification, a right hepatectomy was described as resection of the Couinaud's segments V–VIII (± segment I) [2]. Patients who required ligation of the middle hepatic vein were included only if the hepatic parenchymal transection plane containing this vein and segment IV was preserved. The volume of the right hemiliver was about 60–65% of the whole liver [3, 4]. In terms of liver function evaluation, Makuuchi criteria [5], including preoperative serum total bilirubin level, Child-Pugh classification, and the indocyanine green retention rate at 15 min (ICGR15) were used to determine the extent of safe liver resection. Right hepatectomy was indicated only for patients with Child-Pugh class A, serum total bilirubin level less than 1.0 mg/dl, and the ICGR15 less than 10%. For huge tumor confined to the right hemiliver, if the volume of the functional liver parenchymal within the right liver to be sacrificed is small, and/or the volume of the left liver is increased because of the contralateral portal vein tumor embolism, right hepatectomy can be performed even if the ICGR15 is more than 10% [3]. The patients with Child-Pugh class B and C liver function, hyperbilirubinemia, encephalopathy, hypoalbuminemia, and ascites were excluded from this procedure.

The corresponding author of "Right Hepatectomy (S5–S8 Resection)" is Jixiong Hu, Email: 13908459086@163.com.
The corresponding author of "Left Hepatectomy (S2–S4 Resection)" is Jixiong Hu, Email: 13908459086@163.com.
The corresponding author of "Anatomic Right Anterior Sectionectomy Using Glissonean Pedicle Transection Method" is Jixiong Hu, Email: 13908459086@163.com.
The corresponding author of "Right Posterior Sectionectomy (S6 + S7 Resection)" is Yinhuai Wang, Email: wangyinhuai@163.com.
The corresponding author of "Left Lateral Sectionectomy (S2 + S3 Resection)" is Zhongkun Zuo, Email: arthasreal@csu.edu.cn.
The corresponding author of "Segmentectomy IV" is Jixiong Hu, Email: 13908459086@163.com.
The corresponding author of "Mesohepatectomy (S4 + S5 + S8 Resection)" is Jixiong Hu, Email: 13908459086@163.com.
The corresponding author of "Segmentectomy VIII" is Jixiong Hu, Email: 13908459086@163.com.
The corresponding author of "Segmentectomy VII" is Tenglong Tang, Email: tangtenglong@csu.edu.cn.
The corresponding author of "Segmentectomy V" is Zhongkun Zuo, Email: arthasreal@csu.edu.cn.
The corresponding author of "Segmentectomy VI" is Jixiong Hu, Email: 13908459086@163.com.
The corresponding author of "Bisegmentectomy V–VI" is Zhongkun Zuo, Email: arthasreal@csu.edu.cn.

J. X. Hu (✉) · W. D. Dai · C. Liu
Department of Hepatobiliary Surgery and Hunan Provincial Key Laboratory of Hepatobiliary Disease Research, The Second Xiangya Hospital, Central South University, Changsha, Hunan, PR China
e-mail: 13908459086@163.com; 494489457@qq.com; liuchun504@163.com

Z. K. Zuo
Department of Minimally Invasive Surgery, The Second Xiangya Hospital, Central South University, Changsha, Hunan, China
e-mail: arthasreal@csu.edu.cn

J. S. Huang et al. (eds.), *Atlas of Anatomic Hepatic Resection for Hepatocellular Carcinoma*, https://doi.org/10.1007/978-981-13-0668-6_4

Isolated Right Hepatectomy Guided (Assisted) by Intraoperative Methylene Blue Staining (Fig. 1)

Operative Procedures	Technical Details
Laparotomy and mobilization of the liver ↓	◀The open approach was performed via a right subcostal incision. The liver was mobilized from its surrounding structures. The right adrenal gland was dissected away from the liver. The right-sided retrohepatic short veins were individually divided and ligatedcaudal-cranianally.
Hilar dissection ↓	◀After lowering the hilar plate, the right hepatic pedicle was isolated, dividedand suture-ligated using the Glissoneanpedicle transection method.
Staining the right posterior and the right anteriorsection and marking the cut line. ↓	◀Methylene blue was injecting into the right posterior and the right anterior branch of the right portal vein, respectively.
Division of the RHP and the RHV ↓	◀The right hepatic vein (RHV) andthe right hepatic pedicle(RHP) was isolated, divided and suture-ligated extrahepatically, respectively.
Parenchymal transection ↓	◀Hepatic parenchymal transection was performed from the anterior and inferior liver surface posteriorly towards the IVC and superiorly towards the hepatocaval confluence along the demarcation line by a clamp crushing method. All the small vessels were then individually ligated and divided.
Drainage and closure of the peritoneal cavity	◀A tube was placed below the right subphrenic space and secured with silk-suture.

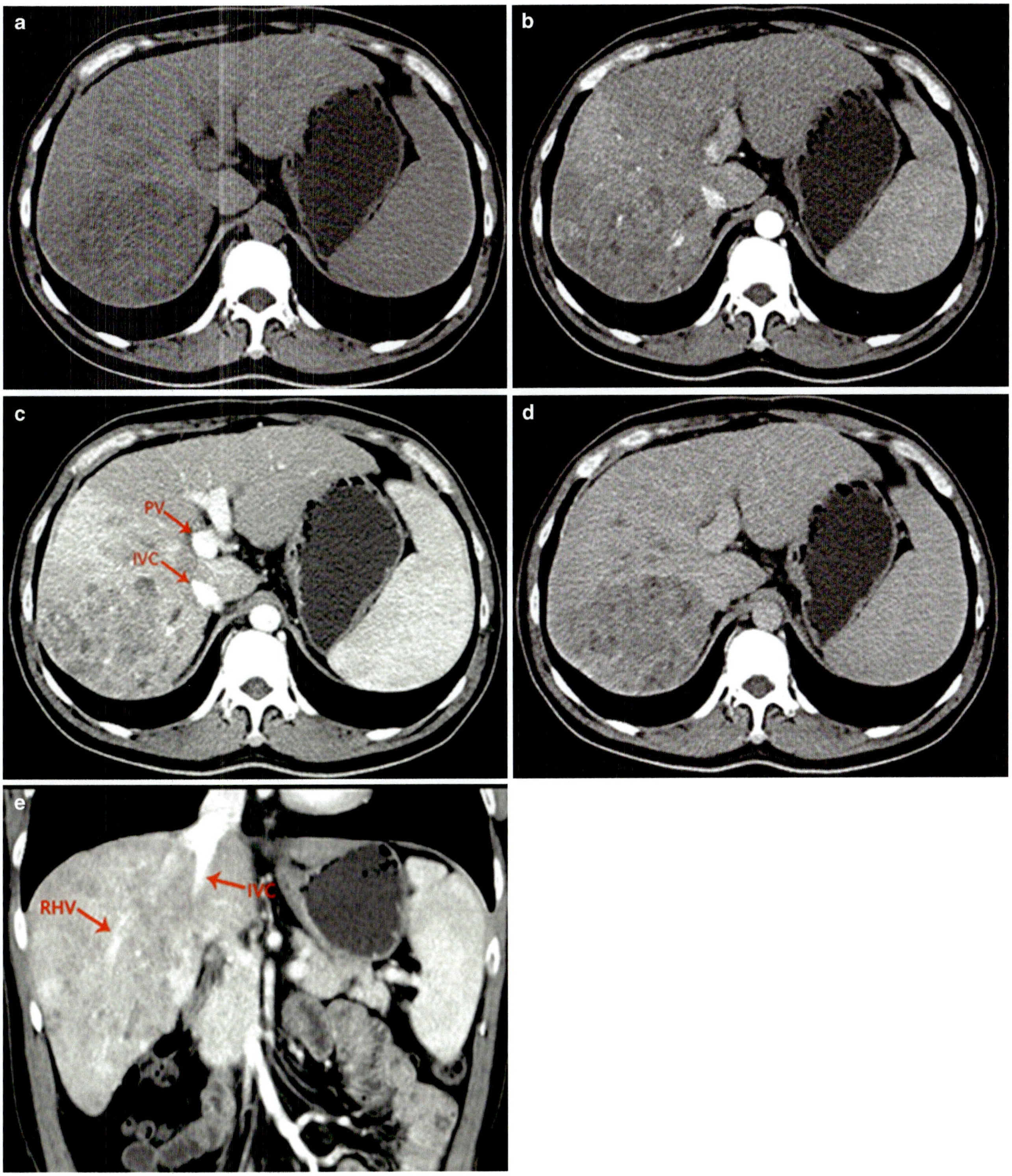

Fig. 1 (**a**) Preoperative CT (precontrast). The tumor, which appears hypodense compared to the liver, occupies the right hemiliver. (**b**) Preoperative CT (hepatic arterial phase). The tumor shows heterogeneous enhancement. (**c**) Preoperative CT (hepatic venous phase). The tumor shows enhancement fades. *PV* portal vein, *IVC* inferior vena cava. (**d**) Preoperative CT (interstitial phase). The tumor appears markedly hypodense due to washout. (**e**) The right hepatic vein (RHV), the inferior vena cava (IVC), and their relationship with the tumor

Abdominal Incision and Freeing the Right Hemiliver Away from the Surrounding Structures

(Figs. 2, 3, 4, 5, 6, 7, 8, and 9)

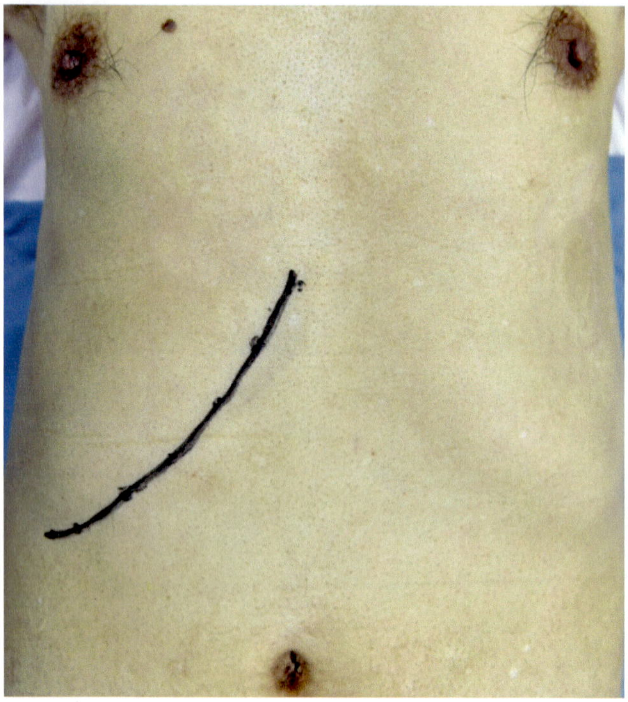

Fig. 2 The open approach was performed via a right subcostal incision

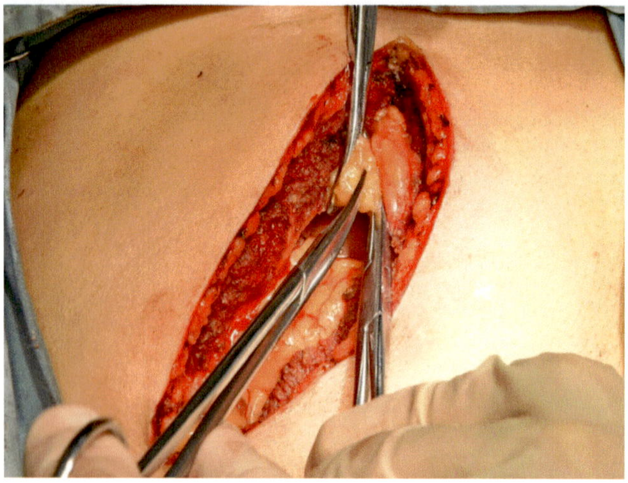

Fig. 3 The round ligament was isolated, divided, and ligated

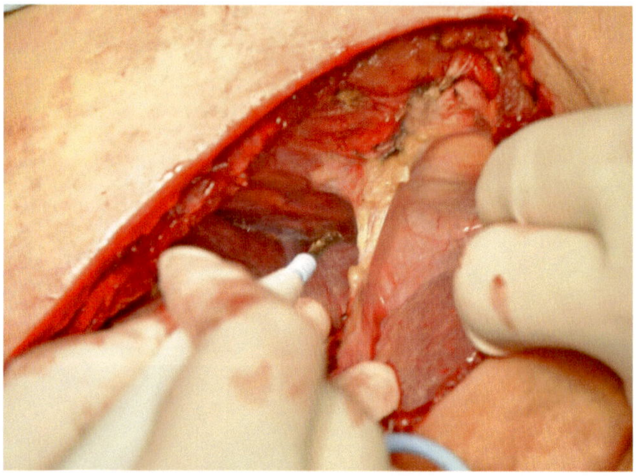

Fig. 4 The hepatocaval confluence was exposed by blunt dissection

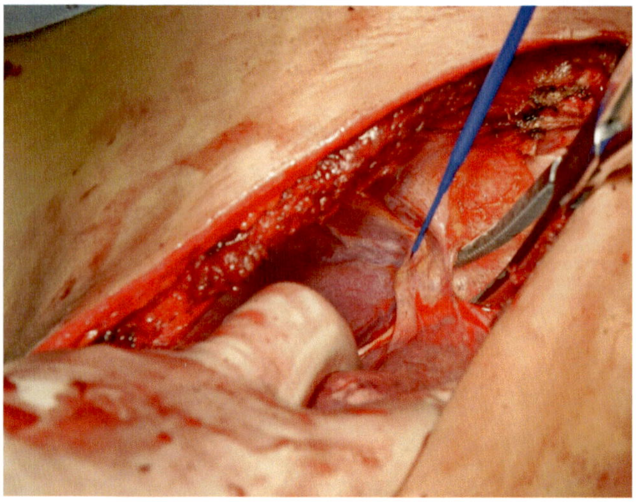

Fig. 5 The right coronary ligament was electrocauterized close to the liver surface

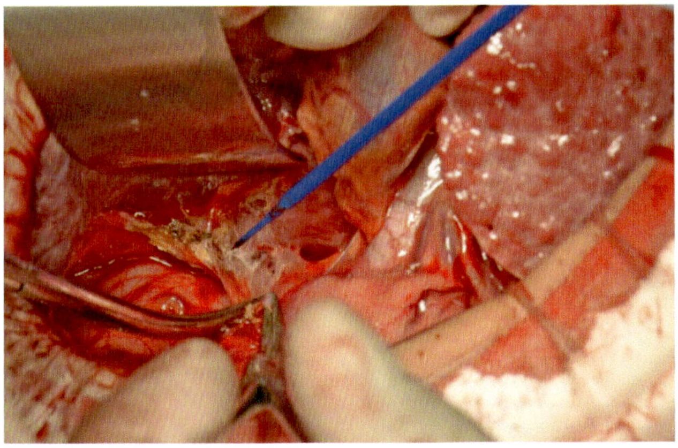

Fig. 6 The hepatocolic ligament was dissected with electrocautery

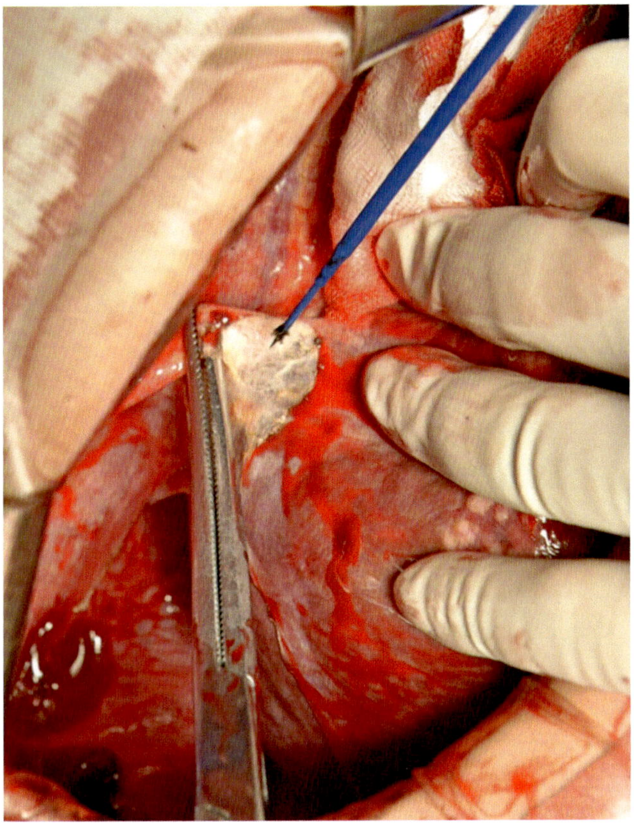

Fig. 7 The right triangular ligament was divided with electrocautery near to the hepatic parenchyma

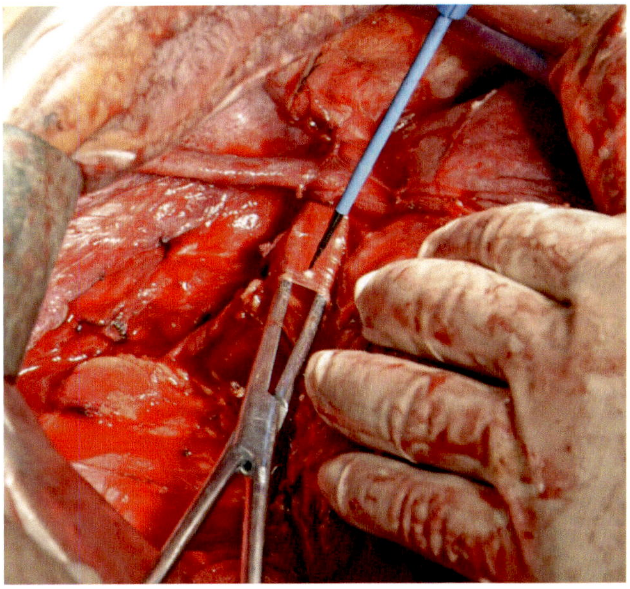

Fig. 8 The right hemiliver was rotated upwardly and medially, the right adrenal gland was dissected away from the posterior portion of the right liver, and the hepatocaval ligament was dissected to expose the retrohepatic inferior vena cava (IVC)

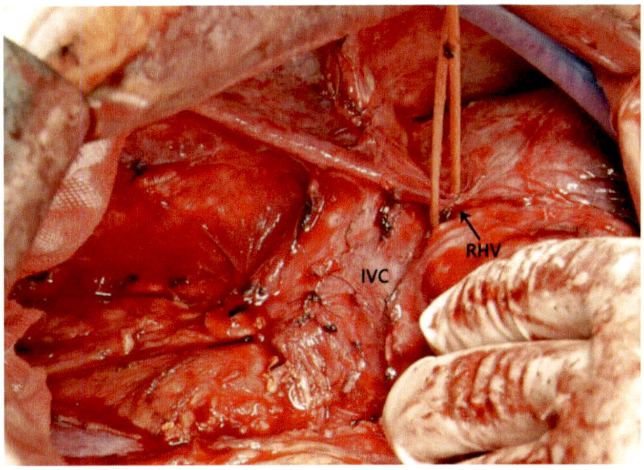

Fig. 9 Having dissected individually the right-sided retrohepatic short veins, the right hepatic vein was isolated and encircled with a vessel loop

Isolation of the Right Hepatic Pedicle (RHP) (Figs. 10, 11, and 12)

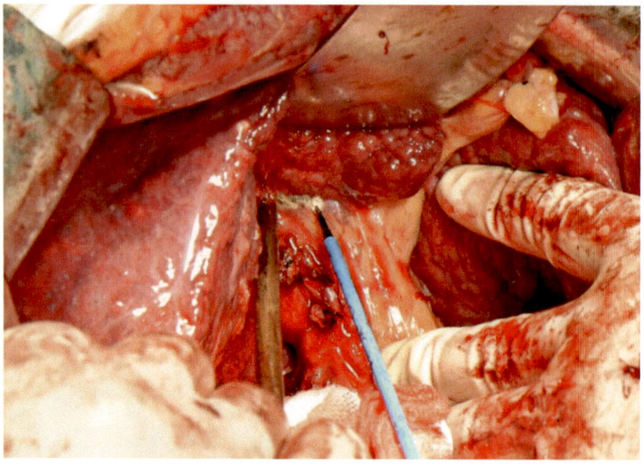

Fig. 10 One small (about 2.5 cm) traverse incision was made in front of the hilar plate, hepatic parenchyma around this incision was pushed upward, and the hilar plate was pulled down

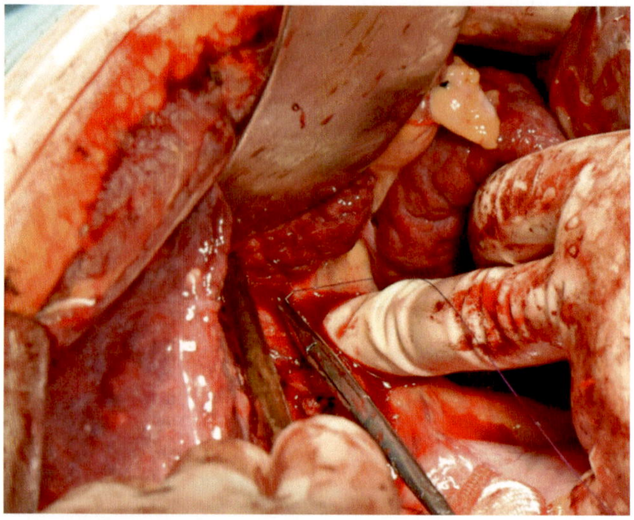

Fig. 11 During lowering the hilar plate, a dilated venous collateral caused by portal hypertension was ruptured and suture-ligated with 4-0 polypropylene

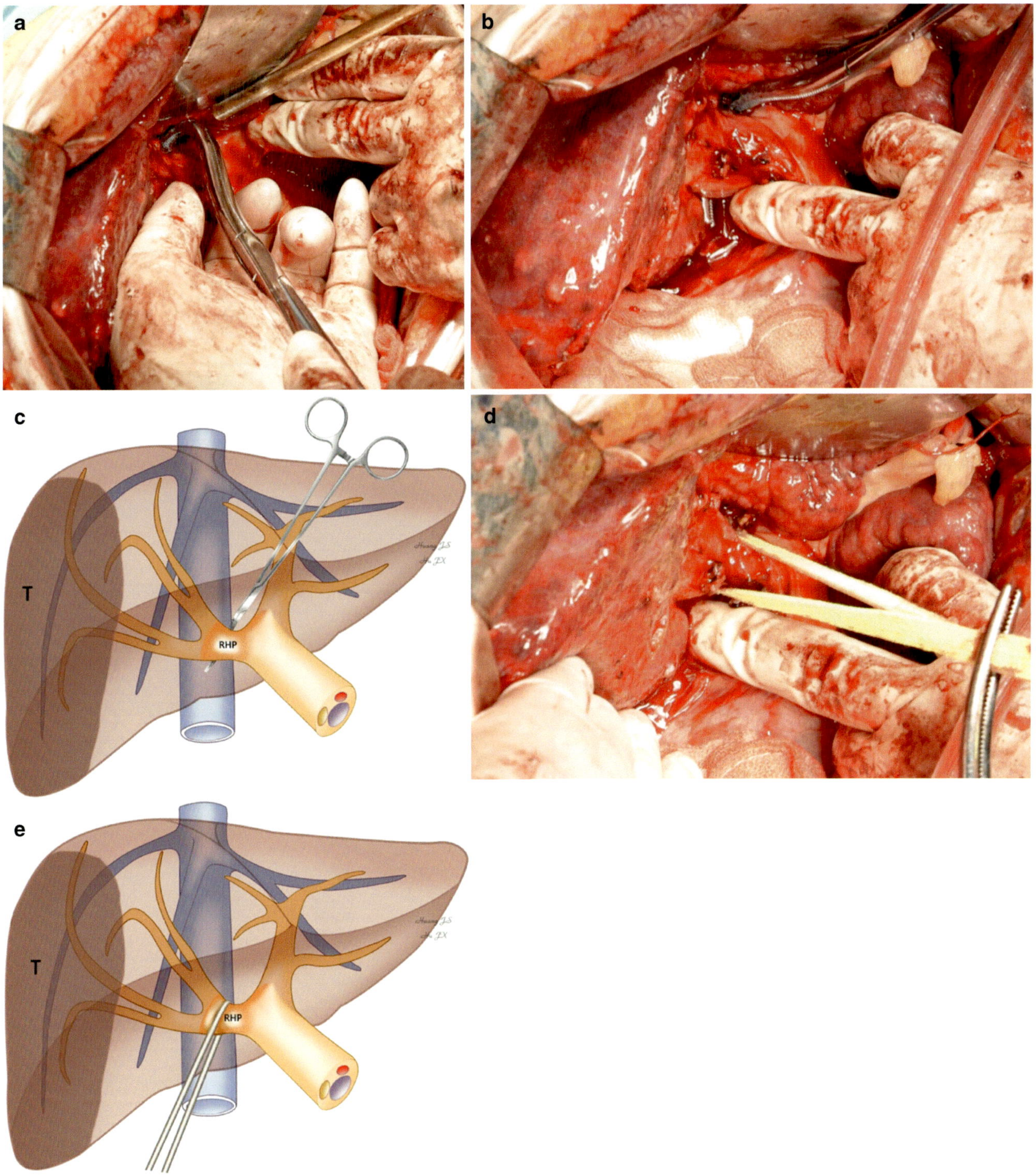

Fig. 12 (**a**, **b**) A large curved clamp was inserted vertically into this incision, and the operator's left index finger was put between the undersurface of the hilar plate and the anterior wall of the retrohepatic inferior vena cava (IVC), and then, the clamp was furtherly inserted to directly reach to the tip of the operator's left index finger, and using the finger as a guide, the clamp punctured through the undersurface membrane of the hilar plate and passed out of the posterior and inferior edge of the right hepatic pedicle. (**c**) Schematic illustration of this procedure. (**d**) Thus, the right hepatic pedicle (RHP) was isolated and looped. (**e**) Schematic illustration of this procedure

Staining the Right Hemiliver and Marking the Cut Line (Figs. 13, 14, 15, 16, and 17)

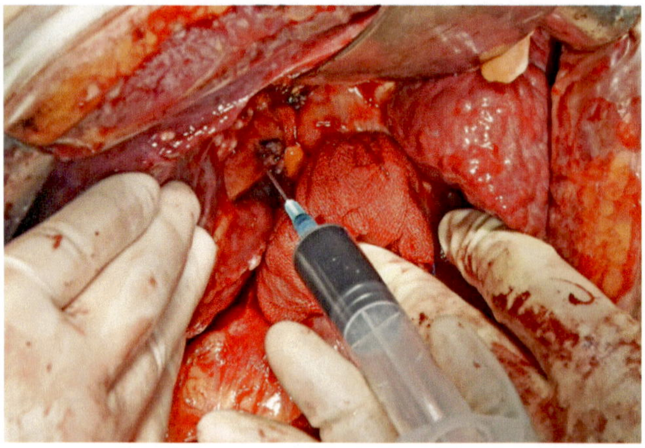

Fig. 13 Methylene blue was injected into the right posterior branch of the right portal vein

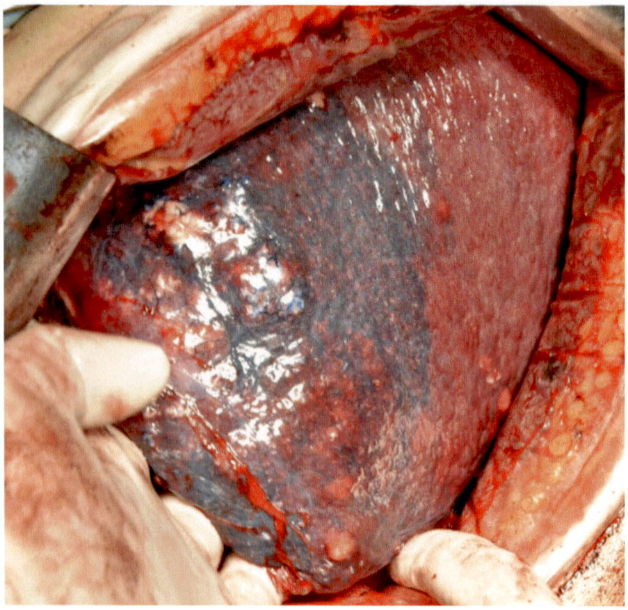

Fig. 14 The right posterior section was obviously stained

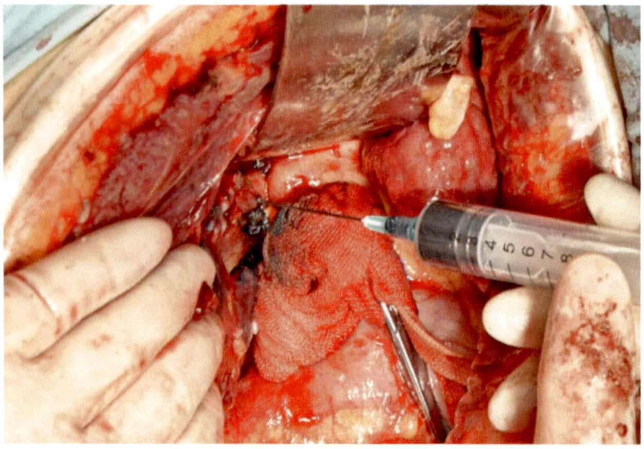

Fig. 15 Methylene blue was then injected into the right anterior branch of the right portal vein

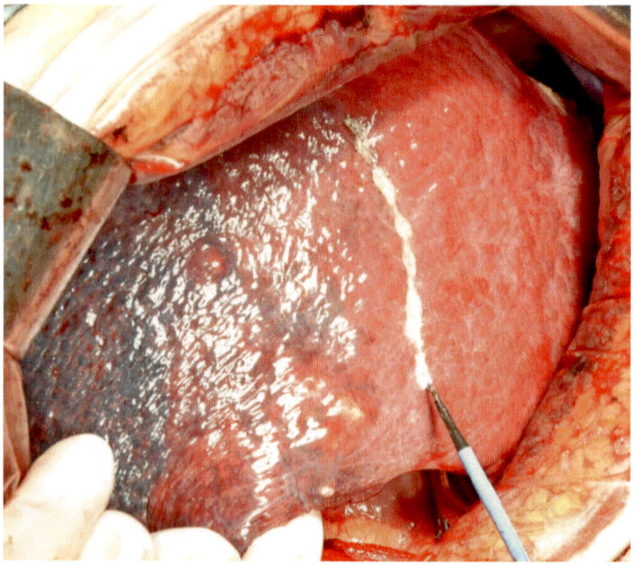

Fig. 16 The right anterior sector was also colorized. The left hemiliver was not colorized, which showed that no aberrant branch of the right portal vein supplied the left hemiliver

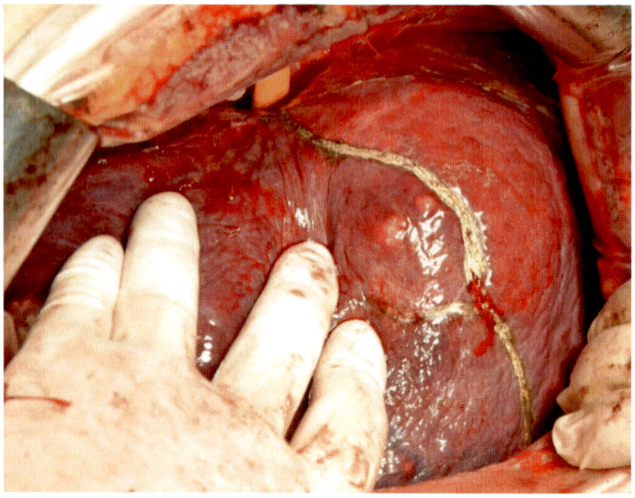

Fig. 17 The real demarcation line between the right and left hemiliver was marked on the liver surface with electrocautery

Division of the Right Hepatic Pedicle (RPP) and the Right Hepatic Vein (RHV)

(Figs. 18, 19, and 20)

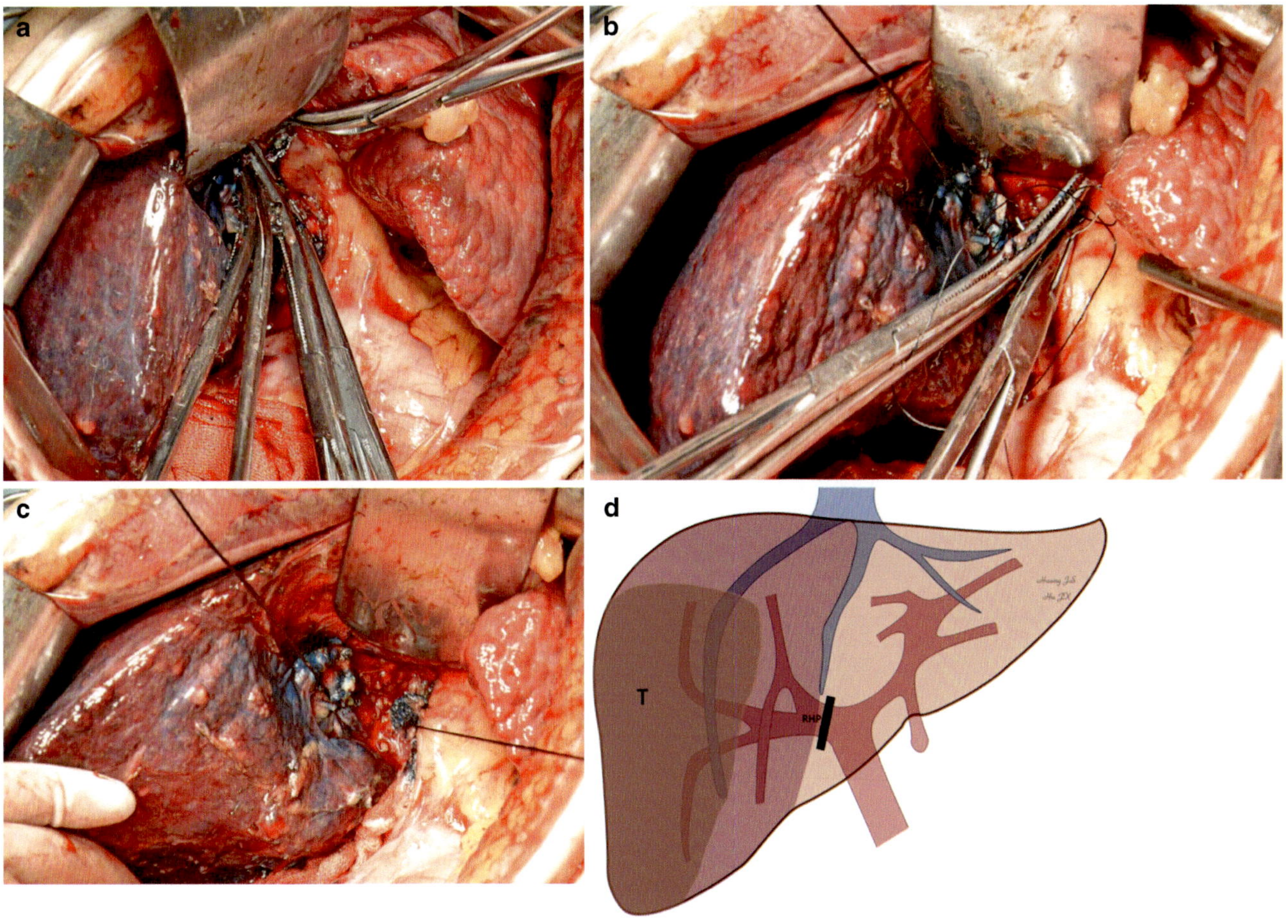

Fig. 18 The right hepatic pedicle (RHP) was clamped, divided, and suture-ligated (**a–c**). (**d**) Schematic illustration of this procedure

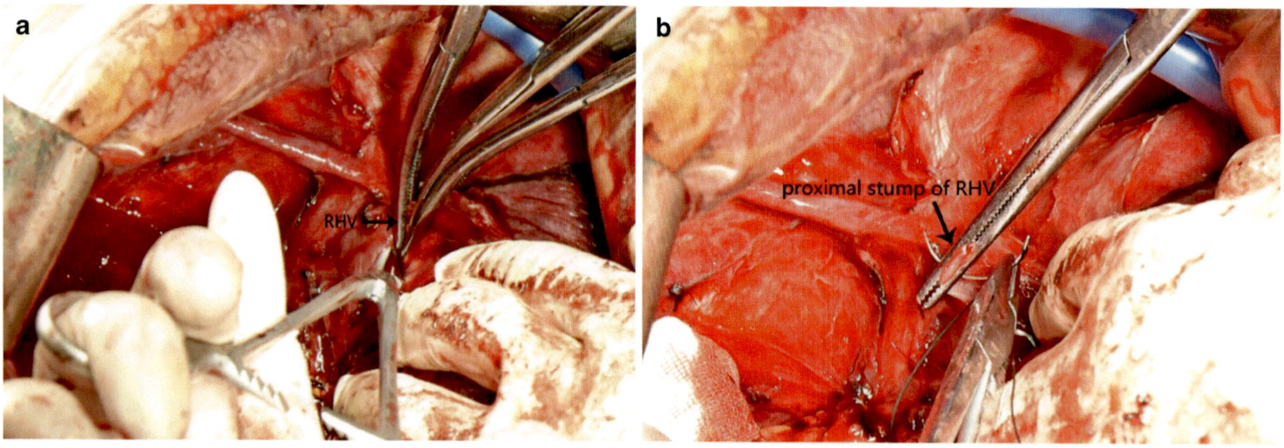

Fig. 19 (**a**, **b**) The right hepatic vein (RHV) was extrahepatically clamped, divided, and suture-ligated

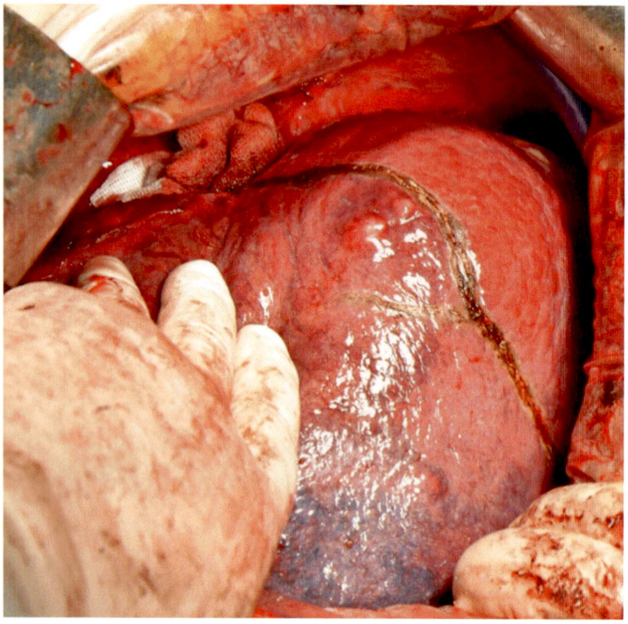

Fig. 20 Having transecting the right hepatic pedicle (RHP) and the right hepatic vein (RHV), the demarcation line between the right and left hemiliver was once more ascertained. No ischemic zone was found within the left hemiliver, which once more showed that no abnormal portal branch originated from the right portal vein

Preparation of Pringle Maneuver and Looping the Infrahepatic Inferior Vena Cava (IVC) (Fig. 21)

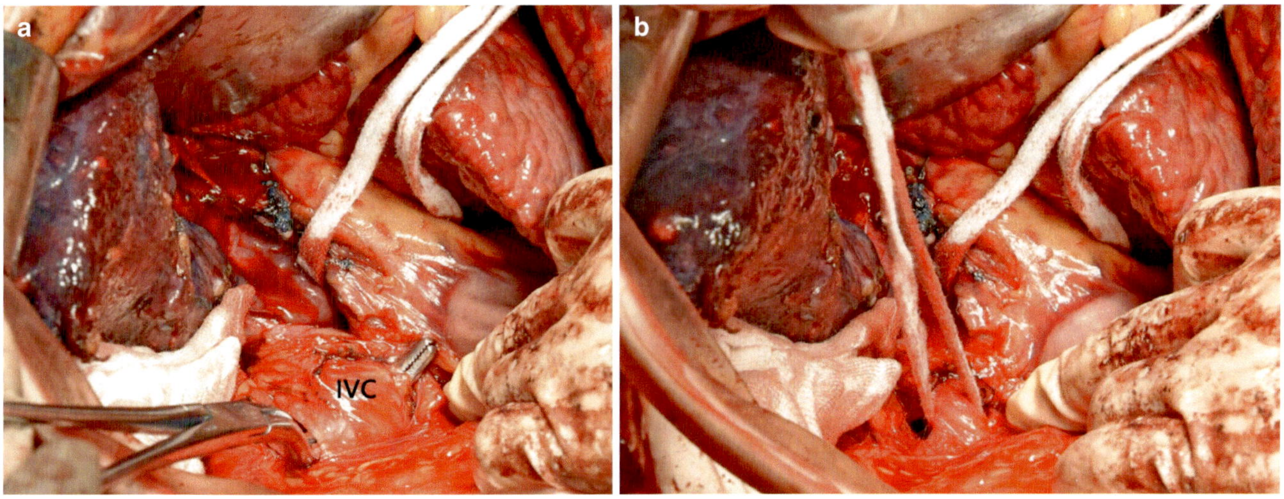

Fig. 21 (**a**) The hepatic pedicle was encircled with a loop. (**b**) The infrahepatic inferior vena cava (IVC) above the renal veins was dissected and looped with a tourniquet. If necessary, the two loops can be rapidly clamped to reduce bleeding from the remnant liver and/or the retrohepatic IVC

Hepatic Parenchymal Transection (Fig. 22)

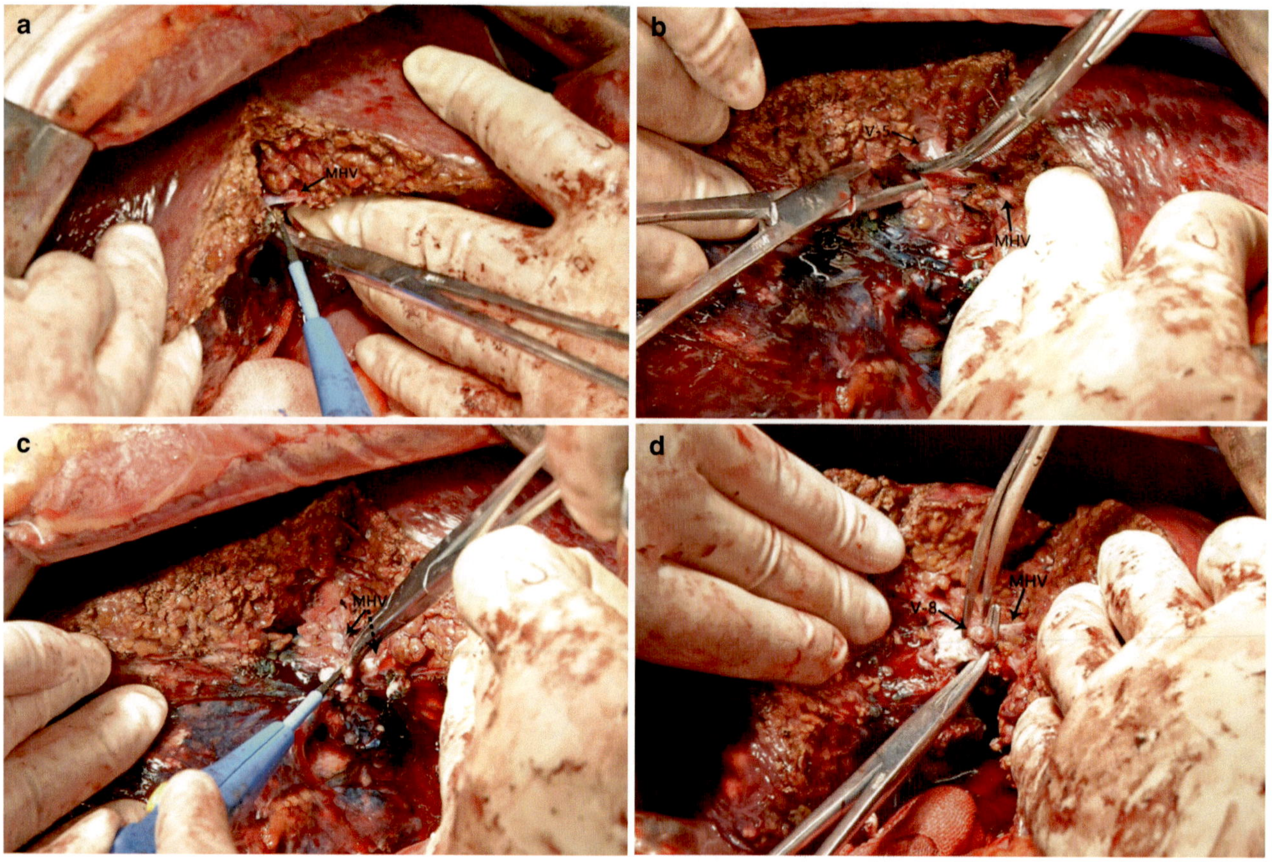

Fig. 22 (**a**) Having occluded the inflow blood system and infrahepatic IVC, hepatic parenchymal dissection was performed from the anterior and inferior liver surface posteriorly toward the retrohepatic IVC and superiorly toward the hepatocaval confluence along the demarcation line by a clamp-crushing method. (**b–d**) Large branch of the middle hepatic vein (MHV) draining segment V (V_5) and draining segment VIII (V_8) was clamped, divided, and ligated, respectively. All other relatively large vessels were also individually divided and ligated. *IVC* inferior vena cava

Management of the Cut Surface (Fig. 23)

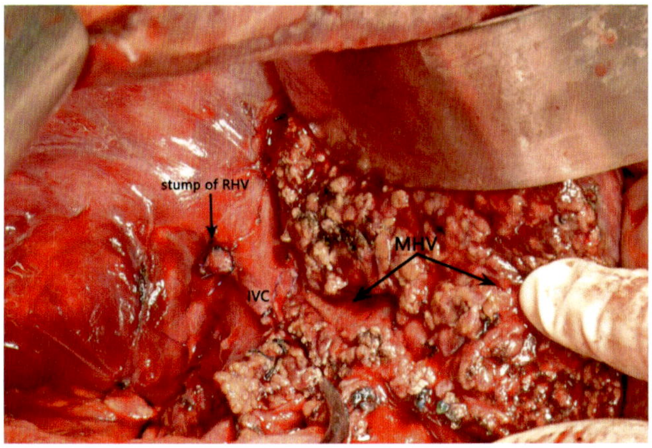

Fig. 23 The tiny holes on the middle hepatic vein (MHV) were repaired with polypropylene 5-0. Other vascular and biliary ramifications on the raw surface were sutured with silk thread and/or polypropylene 3-0. Then, the raw area of the liver remnant was covered with fibrin glue. In all cases, a drain close to the cut surface of the liver remnant was used. The MHV was completely exposed on the cut surface

The Residue Liver and the Specimen
(Figs. 24 and 25)

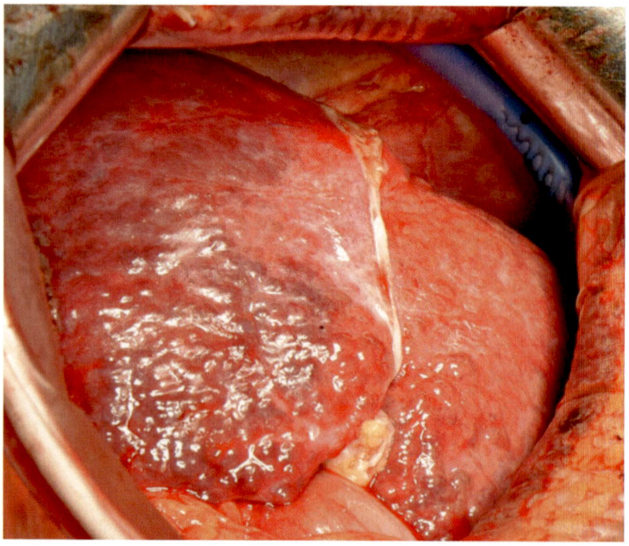

Fig. 24 The color of the liver remnant was normal, and intraoperative US verifies that inflow and outflow blood was normal. The liver remnant was secured by intermittently suturing the falciform ligament

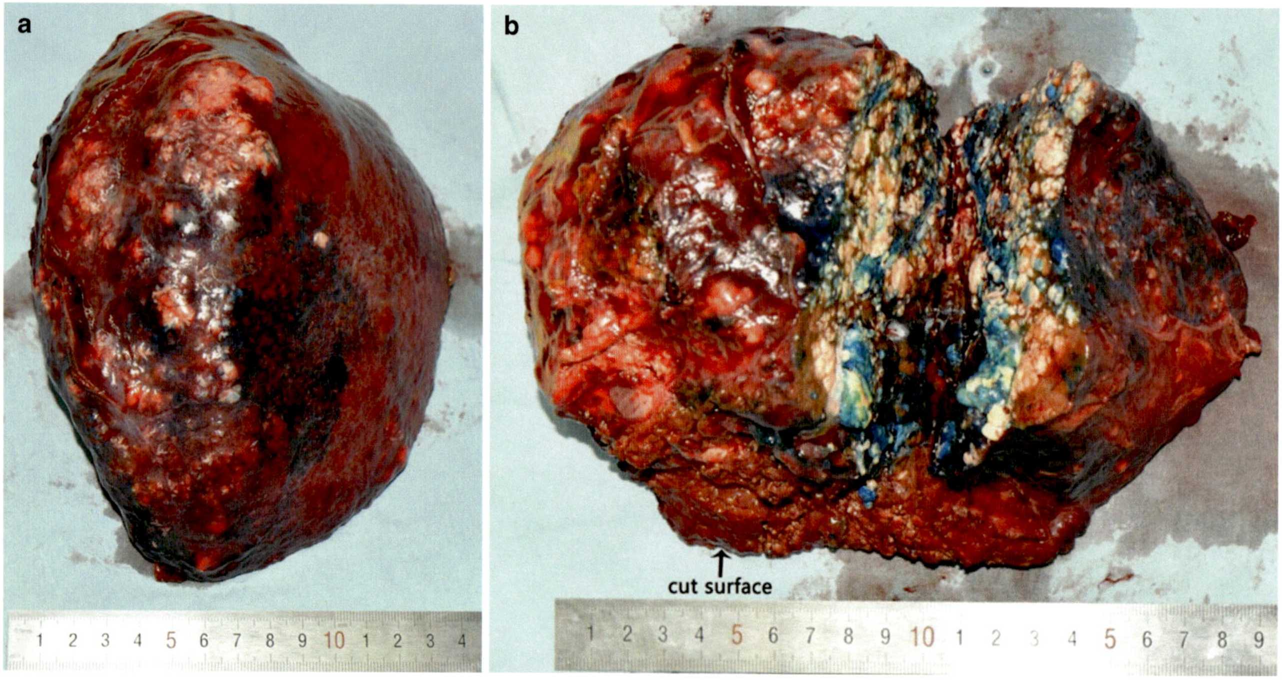

Fig. 25 (**a**, **b**) The specimen. (**a**) The anterior surface. (**b**) The surgical margin was macroscopically negative

Right Hepatectomy with Resection of the Middle Hepatic Vein (Fig. 26)

Operative Procedures	Technical Details
Laparotomy and mobilization of the liver ↓	◀ The open approach was performed via a right subcostal incision. The liver was mobilized from its surrounding structures. The right adrenal gland was dissected away from the liver. The right-sided retrohepatic short veins were individually divided and ligated.
Preparation for Total Vascular Exclusion(TVE) ↓	◀ The hepatic pedicle, the infra-and suprahepatic inferior vena cava waspre-placed witha vascular tape.
Hilar dissection ↓	◀ After lowering the hilar plate, the right hepatic pedicle was isolated, dividedand suture-ligated using the Glissonean pedicle transection method.
Division of the RHV and the RHP and marking the boundary of the right hemiliver ↓	◀ The right hepatic vein (RHV) andthe right hepatic pedicle(RHP) was isolated, divided and suture-ligated extrahepatically., respectively. The ischemic demarcation border was marked on the liver surface with electrocautery.
Parenchymal transection ↓	◀ Hepatic parenchymal transection was performed from the anterior and inferior liver surface posteriorly towards the IVC and superiorly towards the hepatocaval confluence along the demarcation line by a clamp crushing method. All the small vessels were then individually ligated and divided.The main trunk of the middle hepatic vein was transected close to its hepatocaval confluence.
Drainage and closure of the peritoneal cavity	◀ A tube was placed below the right subphrenic space and secured with silk-suture.

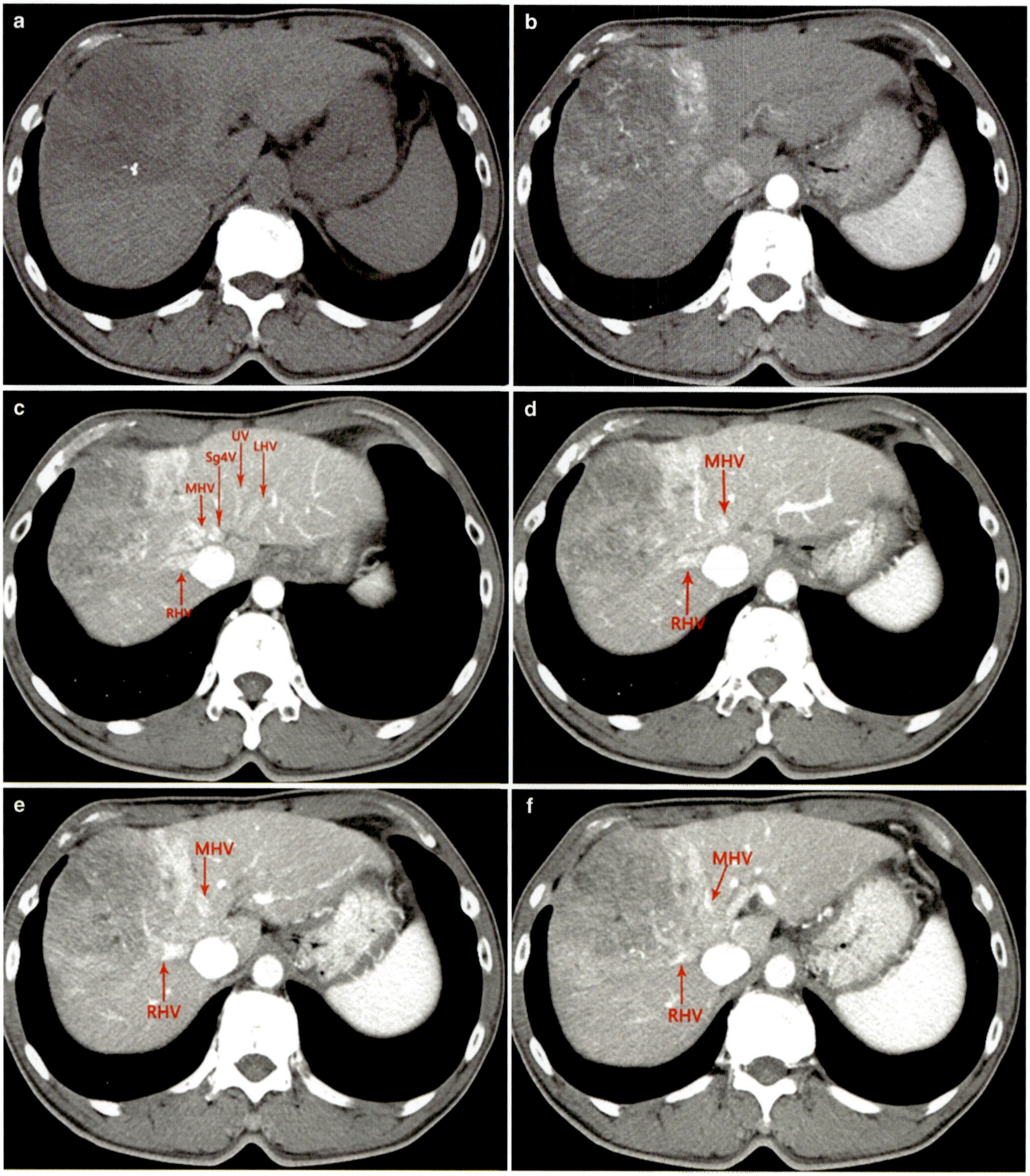

Fig. 26 (**a**) The preoperative CT (precontrast). The tumor, which appears isodense or slightly hypodense compared to the liver with dose calcification, is located in the right hemiliver. (**b**) The right hepatic vein (RHV), the inferior vena cava (IVC), and their relationship with the tumor. (**c**) The hepatic veins are shown on preoperative CT (hepatic venous phase). The tumor shows enhancement fades. (**d–f**) Preoperative CT (hepatic venous phase) shows that the main trunk of the MHV is involved with the tumor. *RHV* right hepatic vein, *MHV* middle hepatic vein, *Sg4V* segment IV vein, *UV* umbilical vein, *LHV*, left hepatic vein

Abdominal Incision and Mobilization of the Right Hemiliver (Figs. 27, 28, 29, and 30)

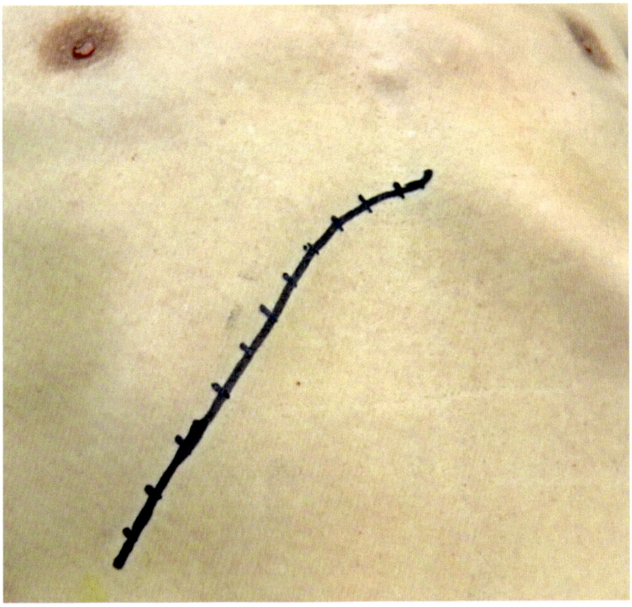

Fig. 27 The right subcostal incision was selected and made, and the right costal arch was retracted cranially with an abdominal retractor

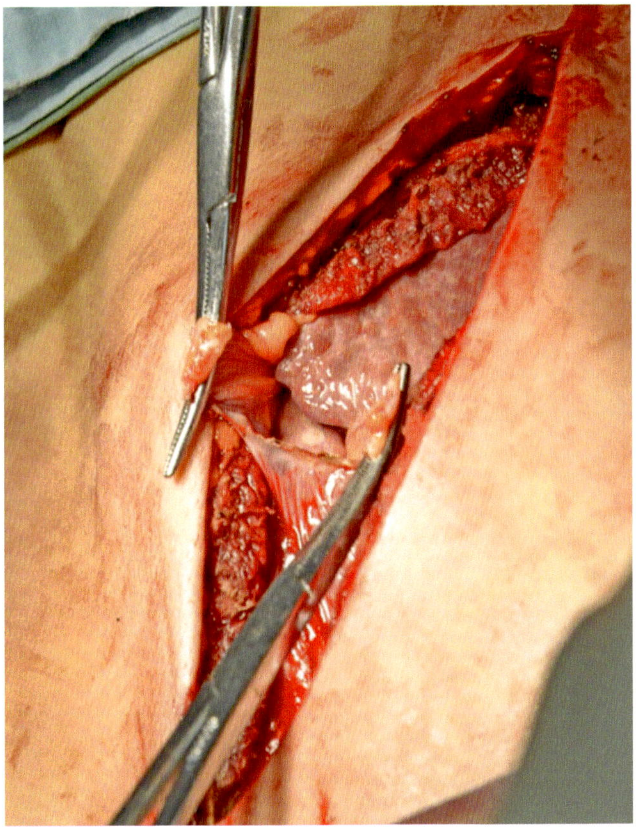

Fig. 28 The ligamentum teres was divided and ligated

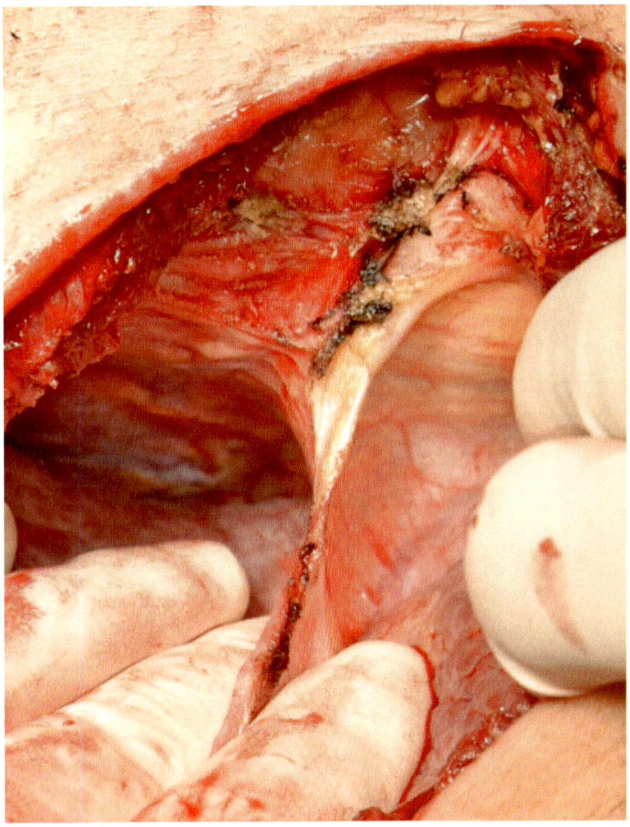

Fig. 29 Having entered into the peritoneal cavity, abdominal exploration was performed. Then, the falciform ligament was divided with electrocautery

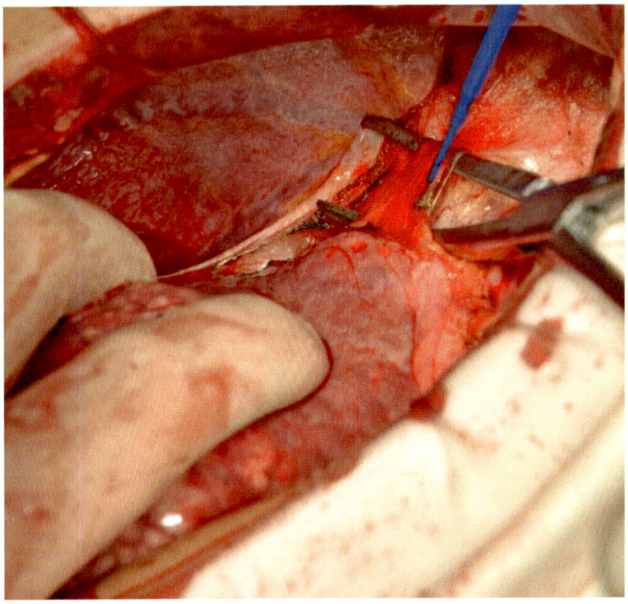

Fig. 30 The hepatocaval confluence was dissected and exposed

Preparation for Total Vascular Occlusion
(Figs. 31, 32, 33, and 34)

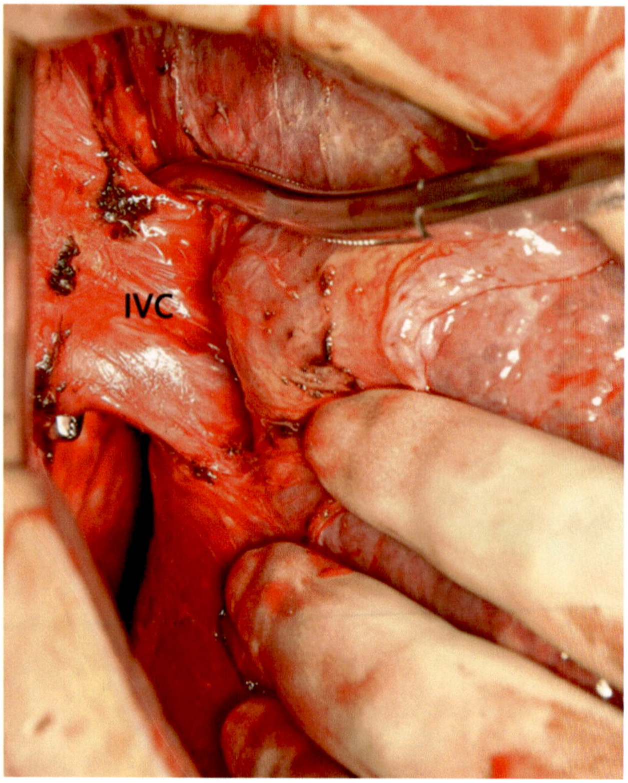

Fig. 31 A large curved clamp was inserted from the left side of the suprahepatic IVC, passed through its posterior wall and out of its right side. *IVC* inferior vena cava

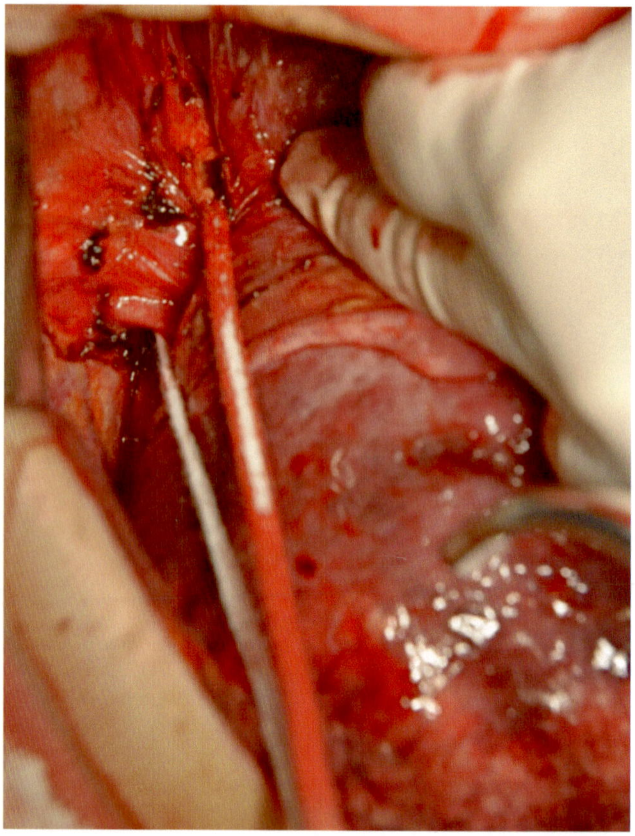

Fig. 32 A vascular tape was encircled with the suprahepatic IVC. *IVC* inferior vena cava

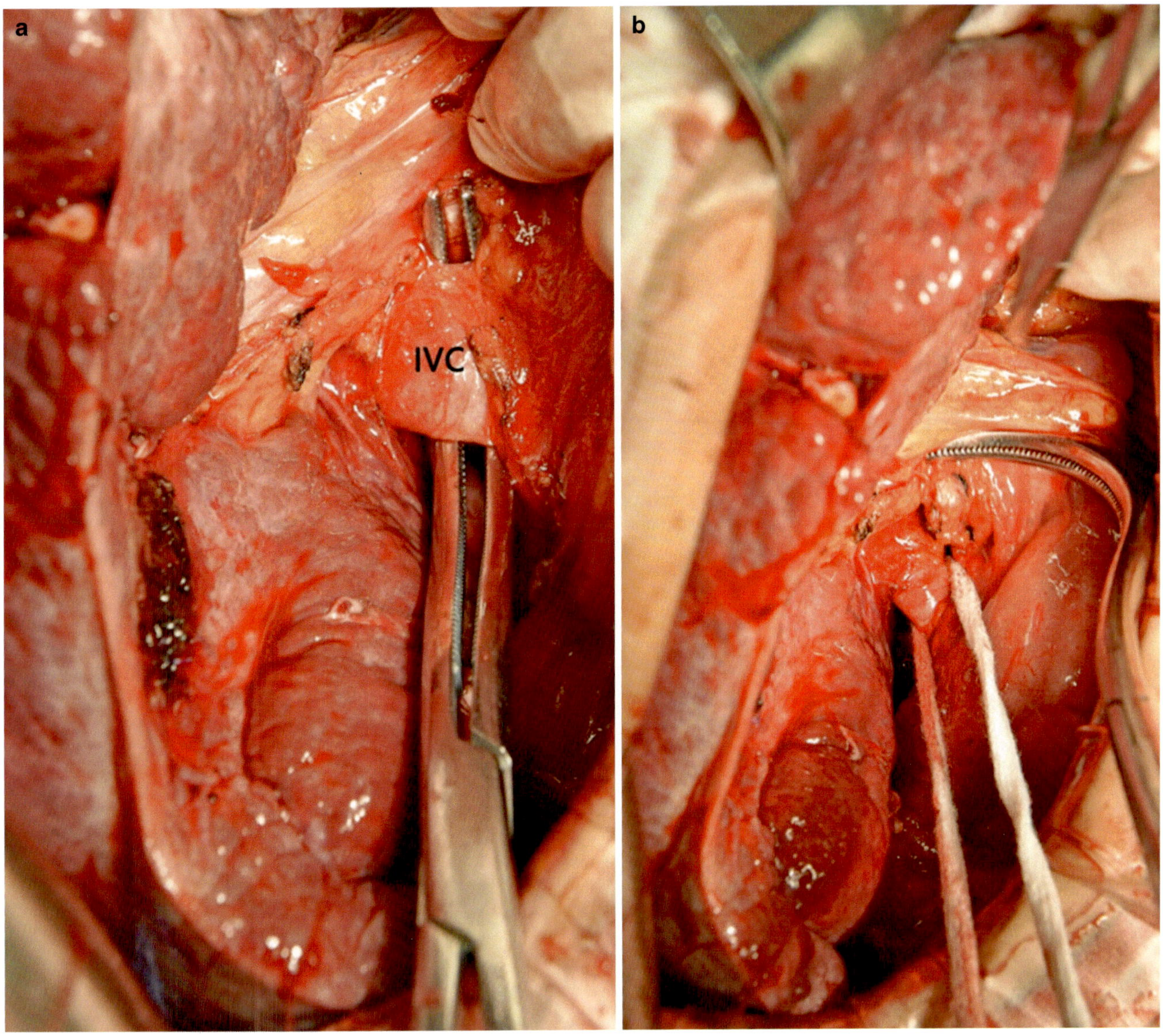

Fig. 33 (**a**, **b**) The infrahepatic IVC was isolated and encircled with a vascular tape. *IVC* inferior vena cava

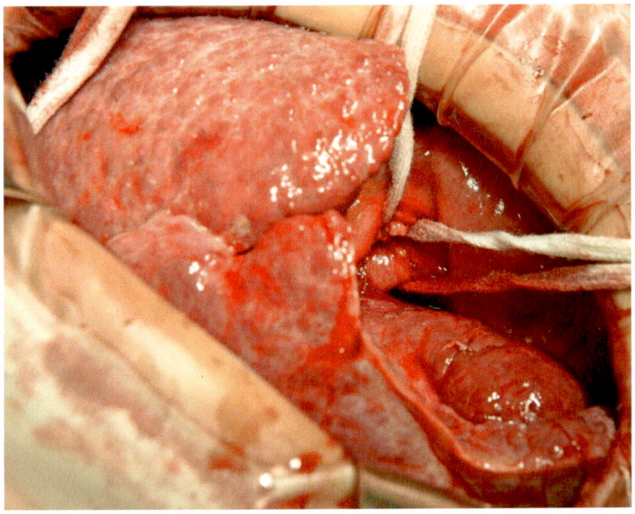

Fig. 34 The inflow and outflow blood occlusion was prepared, respectively

Extrahepatic Division of the Right Hepatic Vein (RHV) (Figs. 35, 36, 37, 38, and 39)

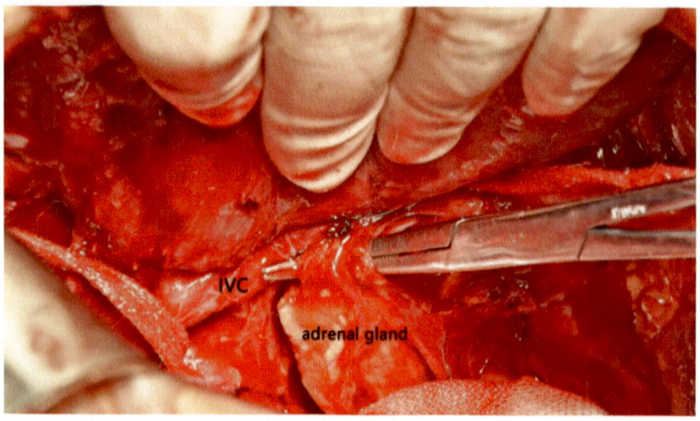

Fig. 35 The vein draining the right adrenal gland into the retrohepatic inferior vena cava (IVC) was dissected to expose the whole course of the retrohepatic IVC

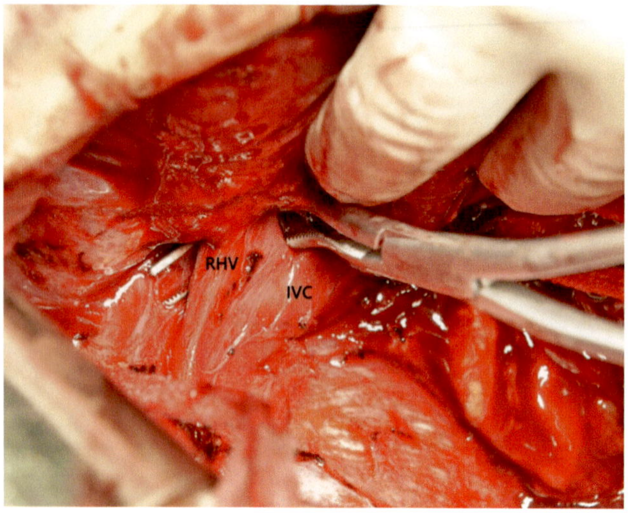

Fig. 36 The right hepatic vein (RHV) was isolated. *IVC* inferior vena cava

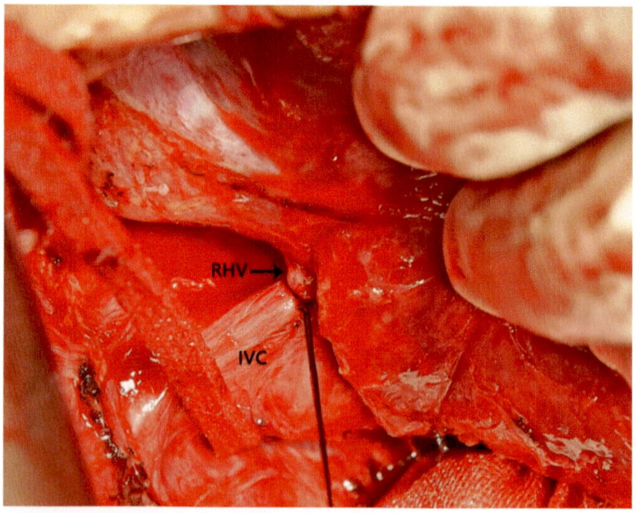

Fig. 37 The RHV was ligated at its starting point. *RHV* right hepatic vein, *IVC* inferior vena cava

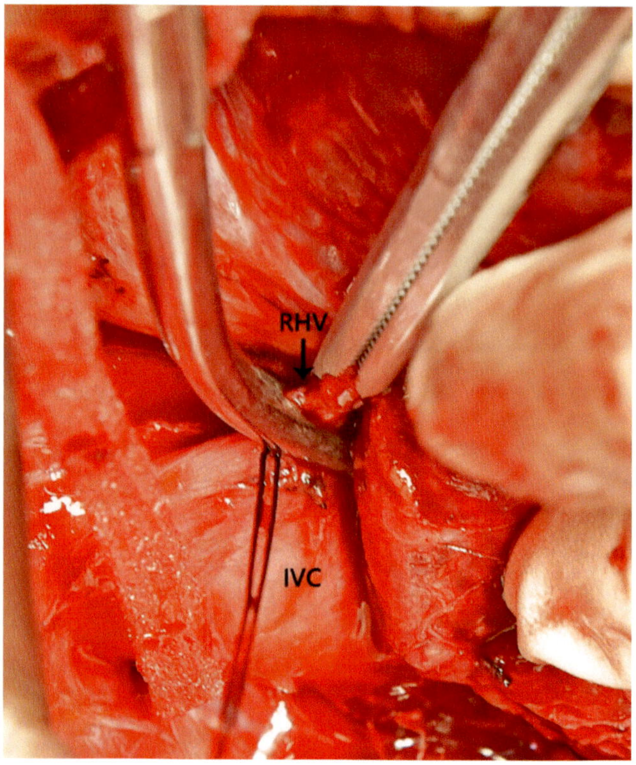

Fig. 38 The RHV was clamped and divided. *RHV* right hepatic vein, *IVC* inferior vena cava

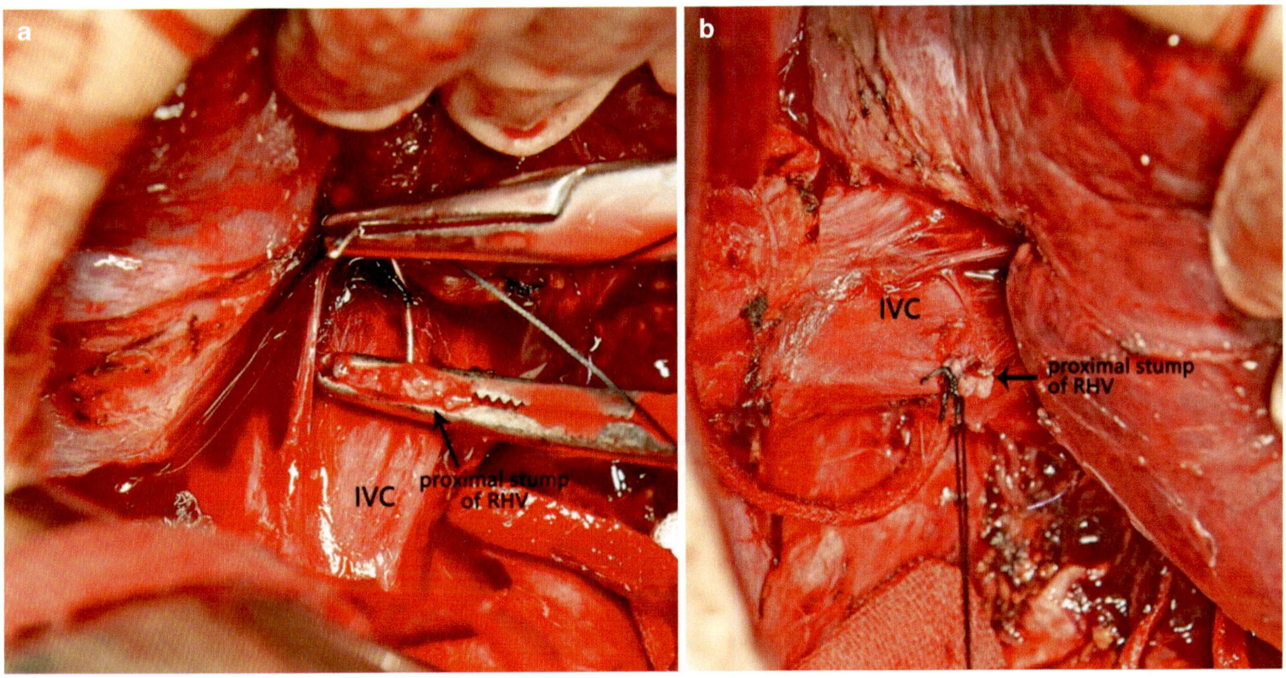

Fig. 39 (**a**, **b**) The proximal stump of the RHV was double silk-sutured. *RHV* right hepatic vein, *IVC* inferior vena cava, *IVC* inferior vena cava

Division of the Retrohepatic Short Veins (Fig. 40)

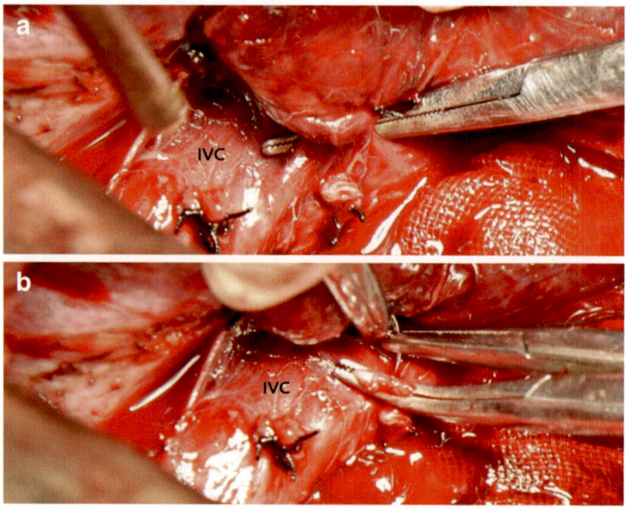

Fig. 40 (**a**, **b**) The right liver was lifted upward and medially, and the retrohepatic short veins were divided, ligated, and/or sutured one by one cranial-caudally. It should be emphasized that the proximal stumps of the retrohepatic veins must be suture-ligated to prevent the ligated-silks from sliding off. *IVC* inferior vena cava

Isolation and Division of the Right Hepatic Pedicle (RHP) and Marking the Boundary of the Right Hemiliver
(Figs. 41, 42, 43, 44, 45, 46, and 47)

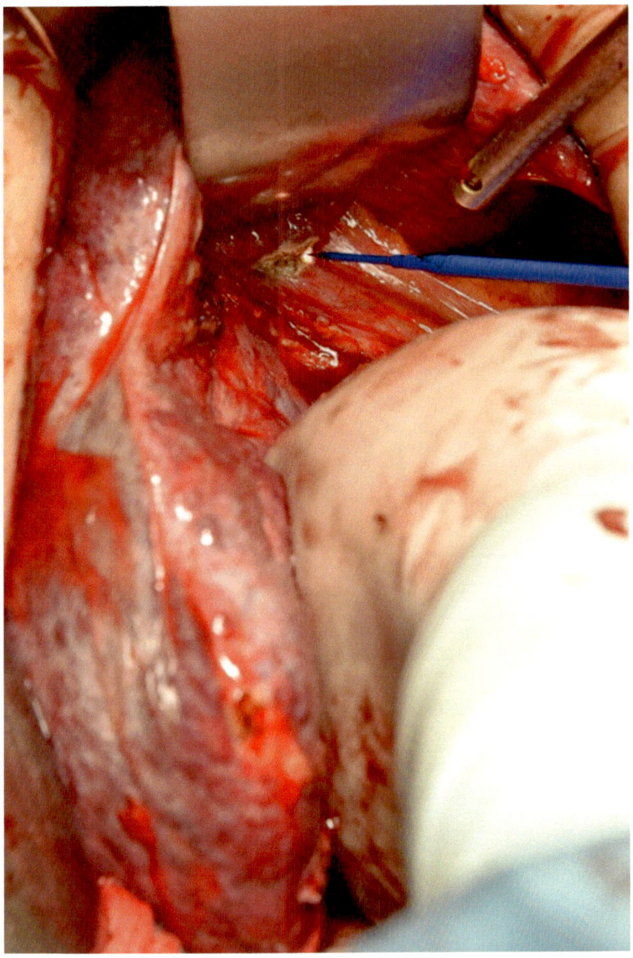

Fig. 41 One small, traverse, anterior incision was made in front of the hilus, and the hepatic parenchyma around the incision was pushed upward to expose the anterior surface of the right hepatic pedicle (RHP)

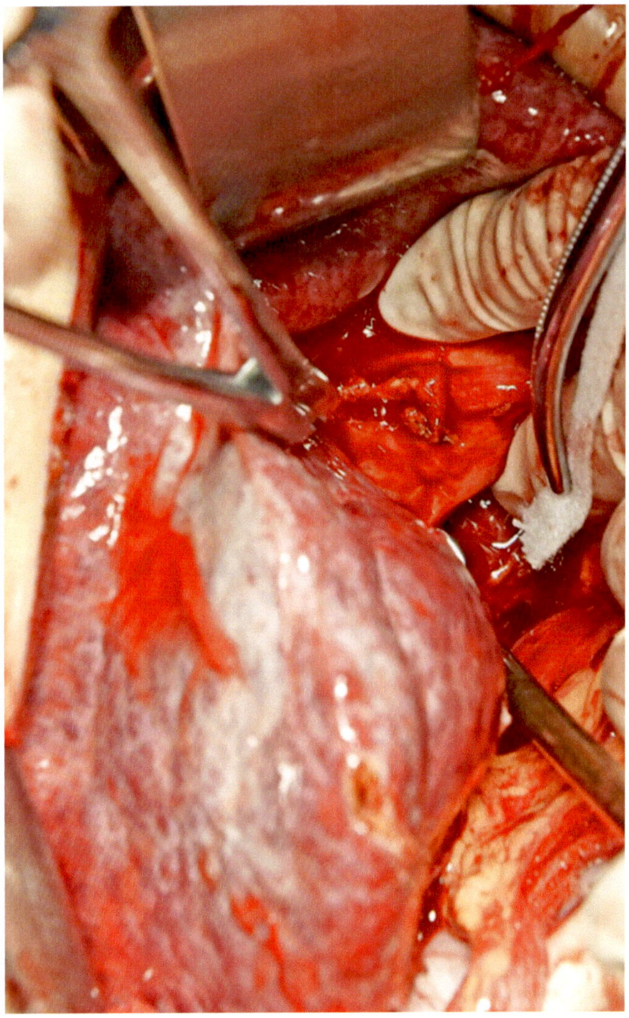

Fig. 42 The operator's index finger was put between the undersurface of the hilus and the anterior wall of the retrohepatic IVC. Then, a large curved clamp was inserting vertically into this incision and directly reached down to the tip of the index finger, using the index finger as a guide, the clamp was inserted furtherly to puncture the undersurface membrane of the hilar plate. During these surgical proceedings, attention should be paid to prevent causing injuries to the lowermost retrohepatic veins draining the caudate process and lower part of the liver into the inferior vena cava. *IVC* inferior vena cava

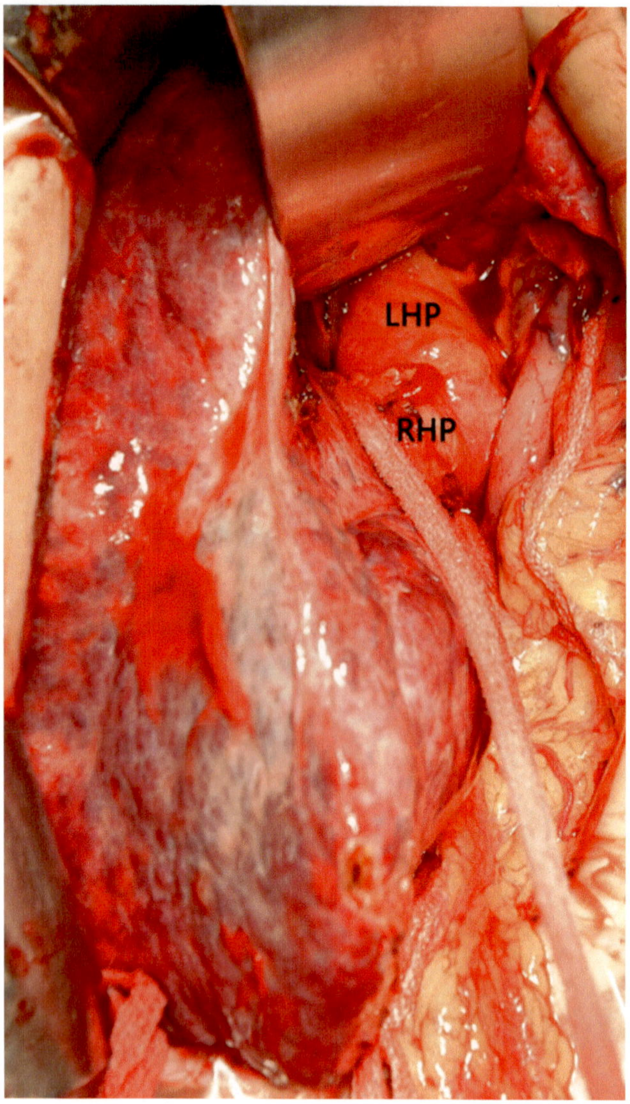

Fig. 43 A vascular tape was encircled with the right hepatic pedicle (RHP). *LHP* left hepatic pedicle

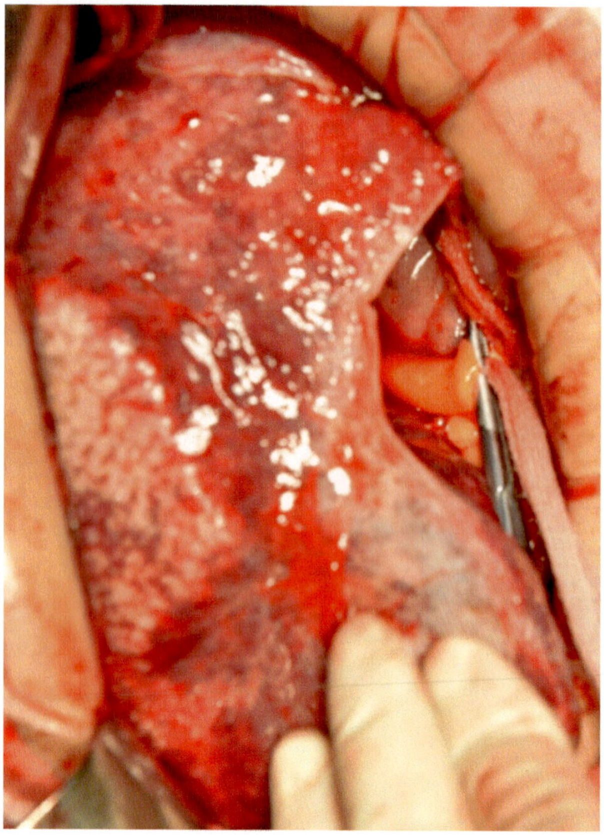

Fig. 44 The right hepatic pedicle (RHP) was clamped

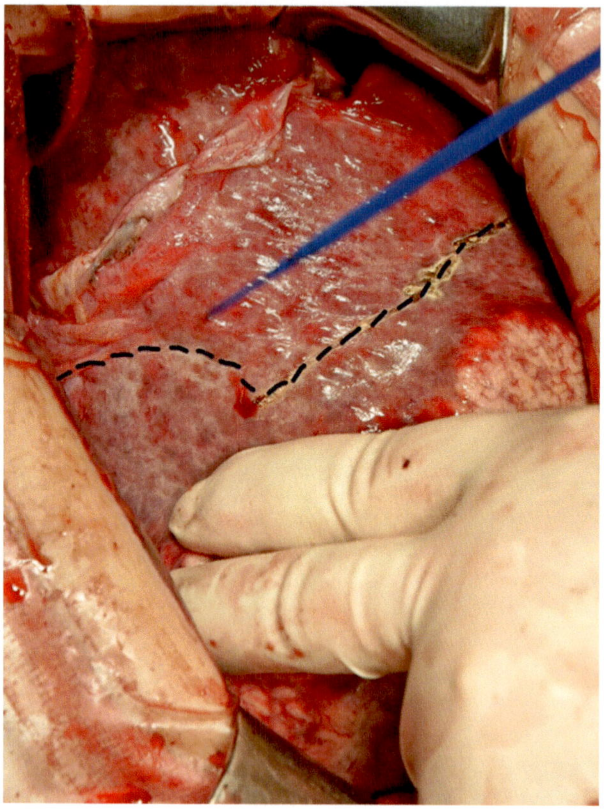

Fig. 45 The real ischemic line was marked on the liver surface with electrocautery

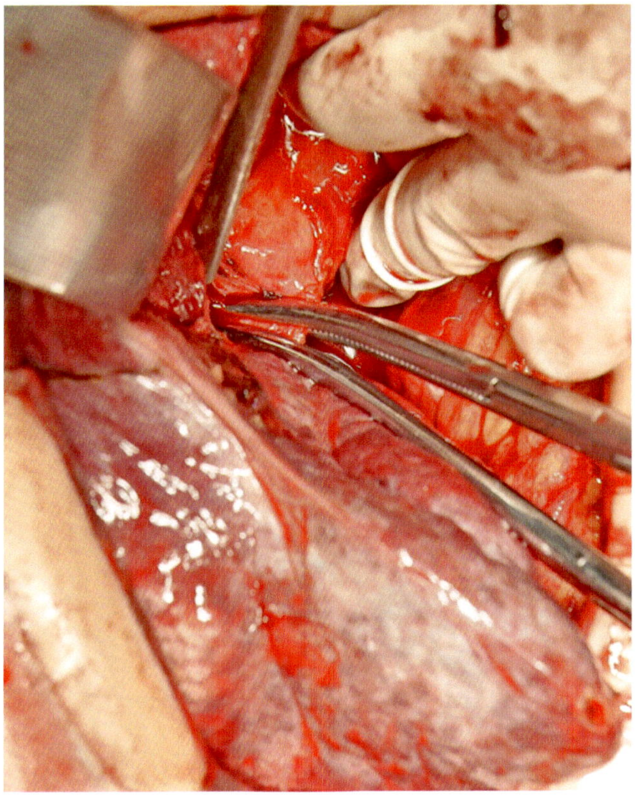

Fig. 46 To rule out anatomical variations, the right hepatic pedicle (RHP) was temporarily clamped and, if no obvious ischemic zone appeared within the left hemiliver, then, the RHP was divided

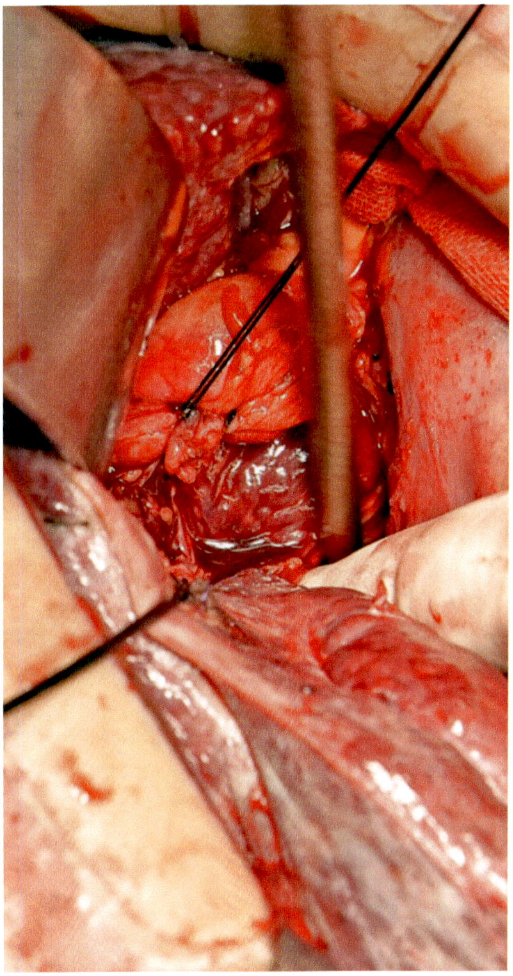

Fig. 47 The proximal and distal stump of the right hepatic pedicle has been silk-sutured

Hepatic Parenchymal Transection
(Figs. 48, 49, 50, 51, and 52)

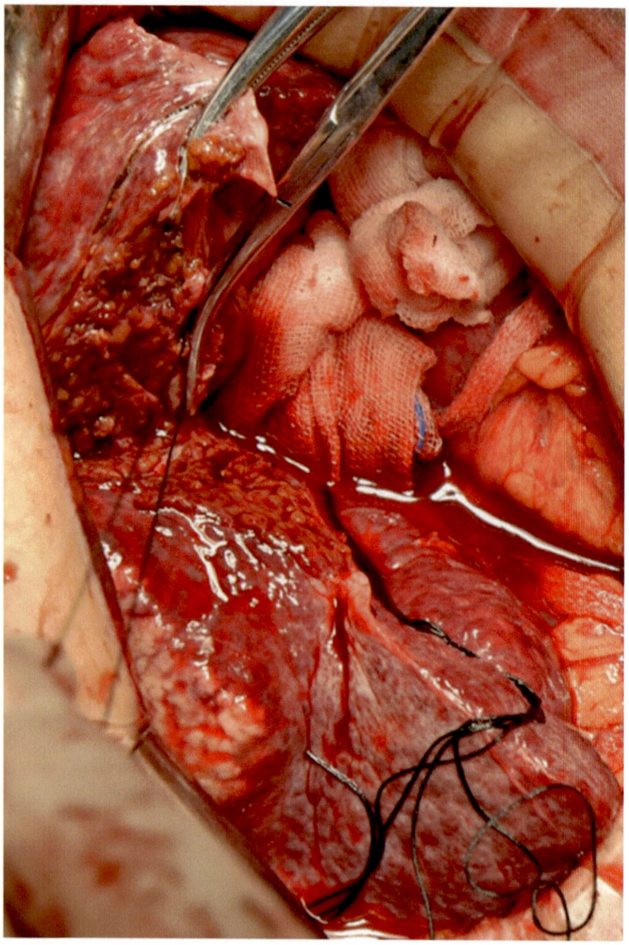

Fig. 48 The hepatic parenchymal transection was carried out caudocranially following the ischemic line using a clamp-crushing technique. Relatively large structures were ligated

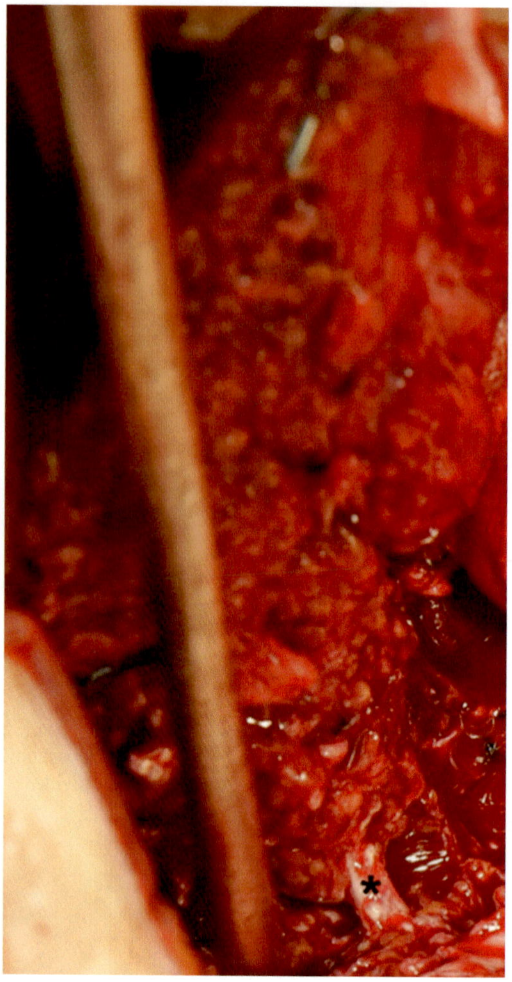

Fig. 49 Adjacent to the root of the MHV, a relatively large venous vessel (asterisk) was encountered, divided, and sutured. *MHV* middle hepatic vein

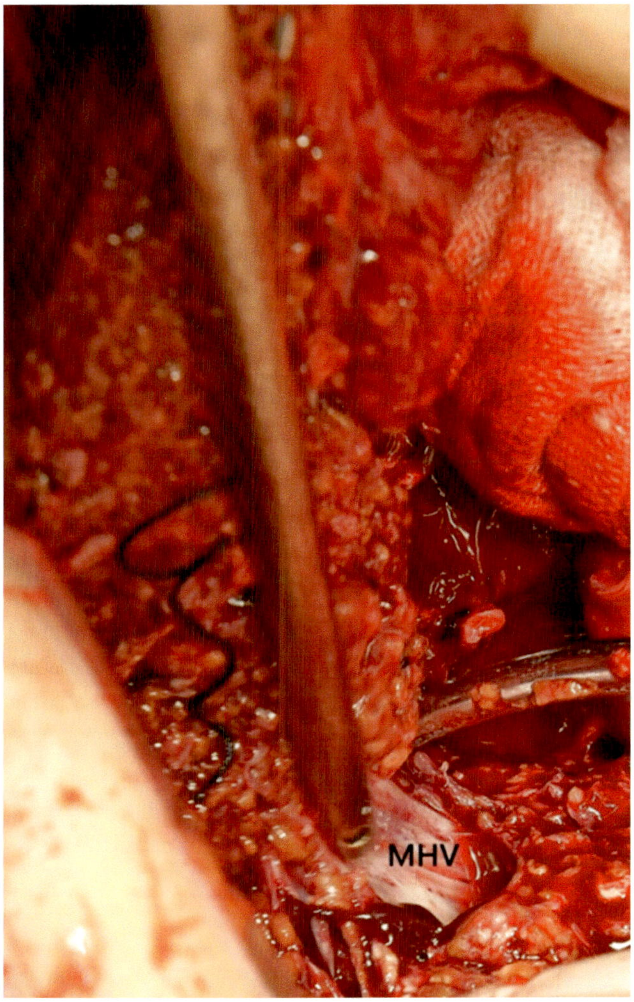

Fig. 50 Near to the hepatocaval confluence, the root of the MHV was encountered. In agreement with the preoperative CT findings (Fig. 1), the main trunk of the MHV was completely phagocytosed by the tumor. *MHV* middle hepatic vein

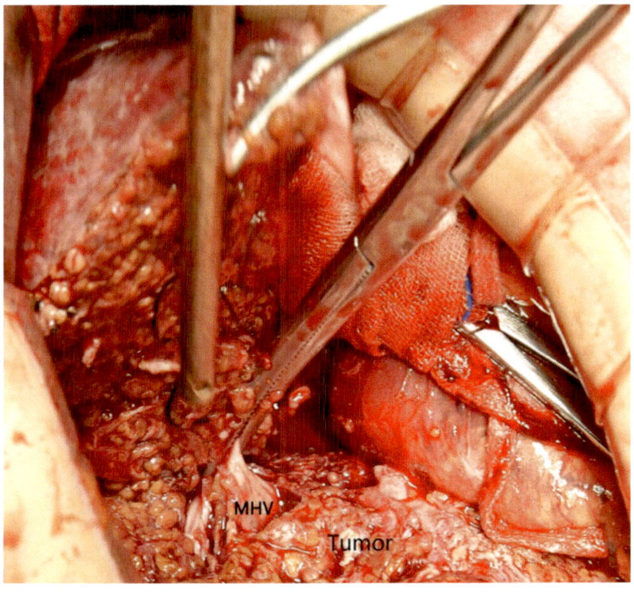

Fig. 51 The MHV was clamped proximal to its entry into the tumor. *MHV* middle hepatic vein

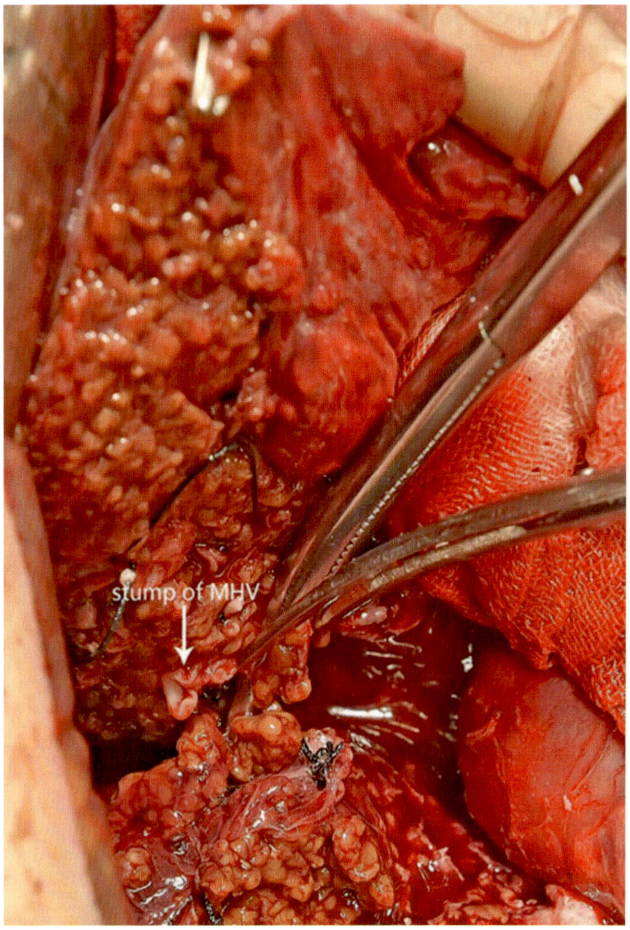

Fig. 52 The MHV was divided, and its proximal stump was double sutured. *MHV* middle hepatic vein

Raw Area of the Residue Liver and the Specimen (Figs. 53, 54, and 55)

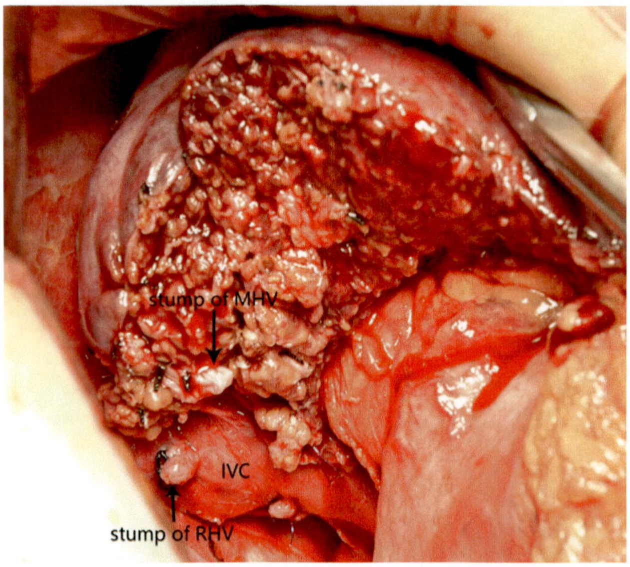

Fig. 53 Cut surface of the residual liver. *RHV* right hepatic vein, *IVC* inferior vena cava, *MHV* middle hepatic vein

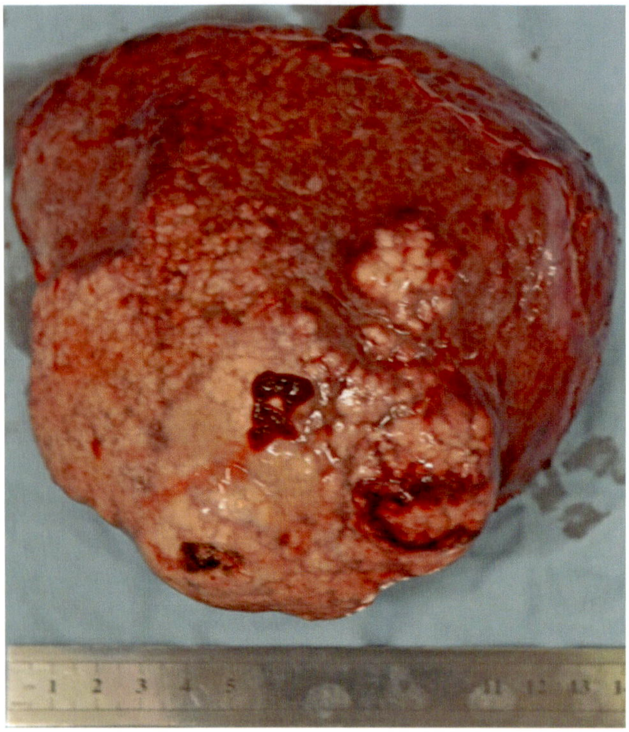

Fig. 54 Anterior view of the tumor

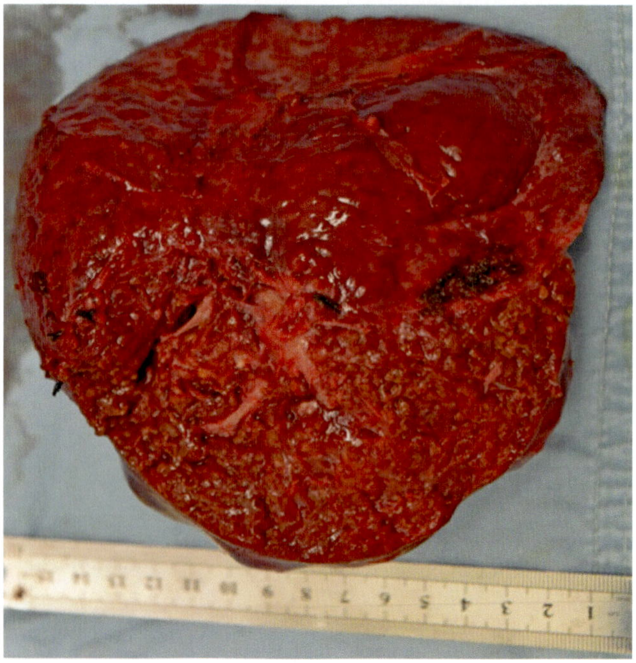

Fig. 55 Cut surface of the tumor. The surgical margin was negative

Intraoperative Key Points

1. Couinaud described that three approaches allow the control of the Glisson's pedicles [6]: (1) Intrafascial approach. The conventional dissection within the Glisson's sheath is referred to as intrafascial approach. The so-called traditional control method was first described by Honjo and Lortat-Jacob et al. in the early 1950s [7, 8]. In this traditional approach, dissection carried out under the hilar plate is sometimes time-consuming and dangerous because surgeons have to carefully identify the possible anatomic variations of the vasculatures and bile ducts, and any misidentification and injury can cause severe consequences. (2) Transfissural approach. When the main portal fissure or the left suprahepatic fissure is opened after dissecting the hepatic parenchyma, the surgeon can identify the pedicles that originate from the hilar plate or the umbilical plate. Lin et al. in the 1960s [9] and Tung et al. in the 1965s [10] described that the right main pedicle at the hepatic hilus could be approached following dissection of the parenchyma around it. (3) Extrafascial approach, which uses the Glissonean sheaths, is Takasaki's and Couinaud's procedure [6, 11, 12]. This liver resection technique using extrafascial approach (also called Glissonean pedicle transection method) was then popularized by Launois et al. [13] and Machado et al. [14] and Yamamoto et al. [15, 16]. Other authors have also reported papers focusing on the application of this technique [17–19]. Machado et al. [20] used the perihilar landmarks to make perihilar incisions in the suprahilar area, in doing so, facilitated access to the right and left main Glissonean pedicle and sectional and segmental Glissonean pedicles. The perihilar landmarks in a normal hepatic hilar anatomy are well understood by surgeons but may be misidentified by surgeons because of hepatic hilar anatomic variations. Encountering with such a circumstance, access to and division of any Glissonean pedicle may cause bleeding and biliary injury [21]. Although Katagiri S et al. [22] reported that right hepatectomy using Glissonean pedicle transection method with anterior approach is safe and effective, in clinical practice, Mouly et al. emphasized that attention should be paid to the possible hepatic hilar anatomic variations [23]. This author reported that the Glissonean approach failed in nearly 30% of patients undergoing standardized right hepatectomy, and this failure is most common associated with aberrant portal anatomy [24] (portal trifurcation, right portal trifurcation, a common trunk between the right anterior and left portal veins). The failure types of the right Glissonean pedicle clamping include extended left portal clamping (extended clamping to the left portal branch) and incomplete clamping (with the right posterior branch outside the clamping area). Figueras et al. also reported extended right Glissonean pedicle clamping to the left portal branch in 20% of patients [17]. During right hepatectomy using the Glissonean pedicle approach, extended clamping to the left portal branch is a severe technical complication. Because injury of the vascular supply to the future remaining left hemiliver is of greater consequence than incomplete right clamping, the role of careful intraoperative US of the left hemiliver after clamping the right hepatic Glissonean pedicle should be emphasized, and another technical detail should also be emphasized, which is that the right main Glissonean pedicle must be dissected furtherly to access the right anterior and right posterior Glissonean pedicles, and then, they were clamped, divided, and suture-ligated, separately. In addition, the aim of injecting the methylene blue into the right anterior and posterior portal branch is trying to find any possible portal variations and guided parenchymal transection precisely along the middle hepatic vein. Based on their experiences, Mouly et al. advocated that the Glissonean pedicle approach should be applied only in patients with normal portal vein anatomy [23].
2. Figueras et al. [18] reported a biliary fistula in 10% of patients undergoing right or left hepatectomy using the Glissonean pedicle approach. Nakai et al. [25] reported a biliary fistula rate of 14% during right hepatectomy using the Glissonean pedicle approach. It is suggested that intraoperative cholangiography should be performed to evaluate biliary anatomy before and after this resection. In addition, biliostasis should be attempted with the aid of dye injection in the biliary tree through the cystic duct catheter. When the right anterior and right posterior pedicles are divided and ligated, the transecting point should be as close to the liver parenchyma as possible. This technical detail avoids injuring the inflow vascular system that supplies another segment, section, or hemiliver [26] and prevents injuring the left hepatic duct as it originates from the common hepatic duct that can arise very close to the right inflow system [27]. If the tumor confined to the right hemiliver is huge and close to the hepatic hilum, the perihilar area is closed up, and no operative space is existing. It is difficult and dangerous to perform the extrafascial Glissonean pedicle approach. In such contexts, the transfissural approach [9, 10] can be considered as an alternative approach. Using the transfissural approach, the right anterior and posterior pedicles can be identified, isolated and looped, divided, and then suture-ligated after hepatic parenchymal dissection.
3. For cirrhotic patients undergoing right hepatectomy using Glissonean pedicle transection method, the risk of bleeding from the left liver exists during hepatic parenchymal transectional proceedings. Prior to hepatic parenchymal transection, a tourniquet was usually pre-placed to encircle the hepatic pedicle and was untightened in case of

excessive bleeding during parenchymal dissection. If preoperative imaging suggested that this tumor infiltrated or is in the vicinity of main vascular vessels, total vascular exclusion should be prepared for.

4. Once the inflow and outflow blood system of the right hemiliver was controlled, bleeding arose mainly from the middle hepatic vein (MHV) during parenchymal transection. It is well known that hepatic resection performed under low CVP (less than 5 cm H_2O) will reduce back bleeding from the hepatic venous system because the hepatic sinusoidal pressure was directly related to CVP. Traditionally, CVP was reduced by anesthesiological methods such as fluid restriction and additional administration of diuretics and nitro compounds. Nevertheless, restrictive fluid management may compromise hemodynamic stability and cause perioperative renal and heart disturbance. Infrahepatic IVC clamping is a viable option for lowering CVP without the need of systemic fluid restriction and is effective and safe in reducing bleeding from the MHV [28]. Before parenchymal dissection, the infrahepatic IVC was isolated and encircled with a vessel loop above the renal veins and was clamped in case of injuries to the MHV and severe bleeding occurring during parenchymal dissection.
5. The whole course of the main trunk of the MHV must be exposed on the cut surface of the liver remnant. The tiny holes on the wall of the MHV were individually repaired using 4-0/5-0 polypropylene. If the tumor infiltrated the middle hepatic vein close to its hepatocaval confluence, the middle hepatic vein can be taken [27].

Left Hepatectomy (S2–S4 Resection)

Jixiong Hu, Chun Liu, and Zhongkun Zuo

Left hemihepatectomy is the en bloc resection of segments II, III, and IV supplied by the left main trunk of the portal vein [27]. In cases of HCC with the left portal vein tumor thrombus or the left main trunk infiltrated by the tumor, left hemihepatectomy requires the resection of the Spiegel lobe of the caudate lobe [29]. The surgical proceedings include the following: the left perihepatic ligaments were dissected; isolation, division and suture-ligation of the left hepatic Glissonean pedicle; hepatic parenchymal transection; and isolation, division, and suture-ligation of the left hepatic vein (LHV).

Surgical Indications

Left liver includes the left lateral section (S2 + S3) and the left medial section (S4) and the Spiegel of the caudate lobe, accounting for 30–35% of the total liver volume [4]. With reference to the evaluation of the liver function, the Pugh-Child classification and the indocyanine green retention rate at 15 min (ICGR 15) were used. When the Pugh-Child classification was grade A, the serum total bilirubin level was less than 1.0 mg/dl, and ICGR 15 was less than 20%, left hemihepatectomy was considered to be a feasible procedure.

Operative Procedures	Technical Details
Laparotomy ↓	◀A right subcostal incision was made.
Mobilization of the left liver ↓	◀The left perihepatic ligaments were dissected and the hepatocaval confluence was fully exposed.
Management of the left hepatic Glissonean pedicle ↓	◀The left hepatic Glissonean pedicle was isolated, divided and suture-ligated, using the Glissonean approach.
Hepatic parenchymal transection ↓	◀The ischemic demarcation line was marked on the liver surface with electrocautery. Parenchymal transection was carried out along the cut line, using the clamp-crushing method. During the surgical proceedings, the complete course of the middle hepatic vein (MHV) was exposed on the cut surface.
Management of the left hepatic vein ↓	◀The root of the left hepatic vein (LHV) was isolated, clamped, divided and suture-ligated.
Drainage and closure of the abdominal cavity	◀A double-lumen tube was placed close to the cut surface and secured.

Operative Key Points

1. The resection of the Spiegel lobe of the caudate lobe should be decided by the tumor-related factors and the left portal vein trunk tumor thrombus [29]. If the tumor has invaded into the left portal vein trunk or the left portal vein tumor thrombus was ascertained, the resection of SL of the caudate lobe was necessary [30].
2. In case of preserving the SL, attention should be paid to keep the pedicle of the SL intact during dissecting the left hepatic pedicle. The left portal vein emits a small branch to the caudate lobe which can be recognized and conserved if possible. Just beyond the caudate branch, the ligamentum venosum infuses with the left portal vein and can be recognized with meticulous dissection. The safest place to transect the left hepatic Glissonean pedicle is between the caudate branch and the infusion site of the ligamentum venosum.
3. During hepatic parenchymal transection proceedings, care must be taken to prevent injury to the middle hepatic vein (MHV) and expose its whole course.
4. The right posterior sectoral duct puts in the left bile duct in 20% of patients, and the right anterior sectoral bile duct exists so in 6% [31]. A right sectoral bile duct putting into the left bile duct to the left side of the midplane is in the risk of injury during left hepatectomy. Figuera et al. reported a biliary fistula in 10% of patients undergoing right or left hepatectomy using the Glissonean pedicle approach [18]. Nakai et al. reported that a biliary fistula occurred more often in the Glissonean pedicle transection method group than in traditionally controlled method group and was also encountered more common in patients who underwent a left hepatectomy than in those who underwent a right hepatectomy; both left and right hepatectomies were performed by the Glissonean pedicle transection method [25, 32]. It is suggested that preoperative MRCP should be a necessary workup for patients with HCC who would undergo a major hepatectomy. Meanwhile, intraoperative cholangiography should be performed to evaluate biliary anatomy in case of doubting injury to the biliary tract. In addition, biliostasis can be attempted with the aid of dye injection in the biliary tree through the cystic duct catheter [23] (Fig. 56).

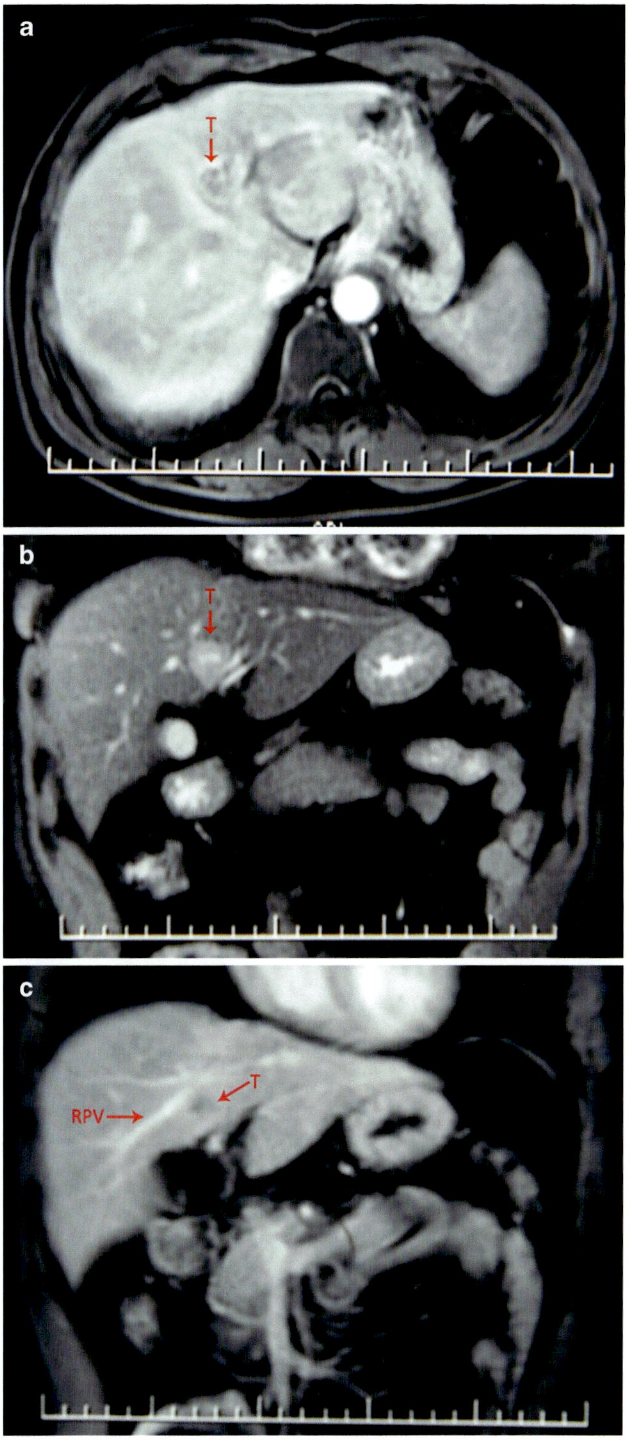

Fig. 56 (**a**) Preoperative MRI. T1 contrast hepatic venous phase. The tumor, which shows heterogeneous enhancement, is located in segment IVB. (**b**) Preoperative MRI. T2 coronal section, the tumor demonstrates high signal. (**c**) Preoperative MRI. T1 contrast venous phase. The tumor is adjacent to the right portal vein (RPV). *RPV* right portal vein, *T* tumor

Abdominal Incision and Mobilization of the Left Hemiliver (Figs. 57, 58, 59, 60, 61, 62, 63, and 64)

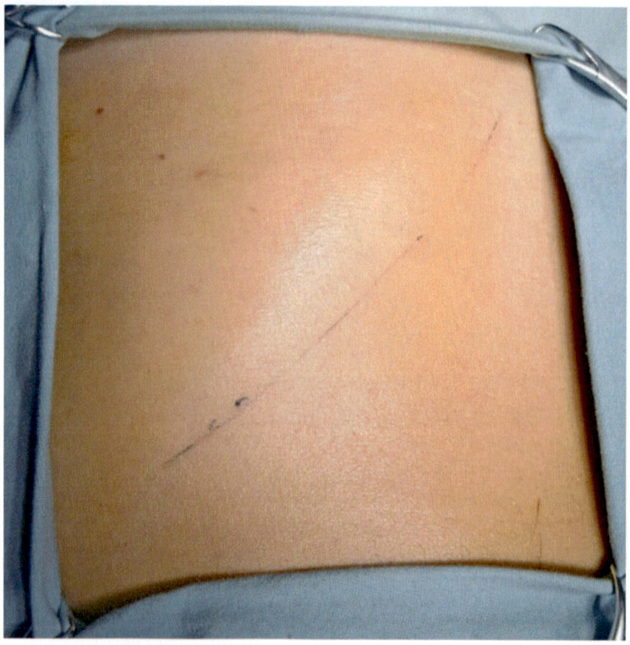

Fig. 57 A right subcoastal incision was selected

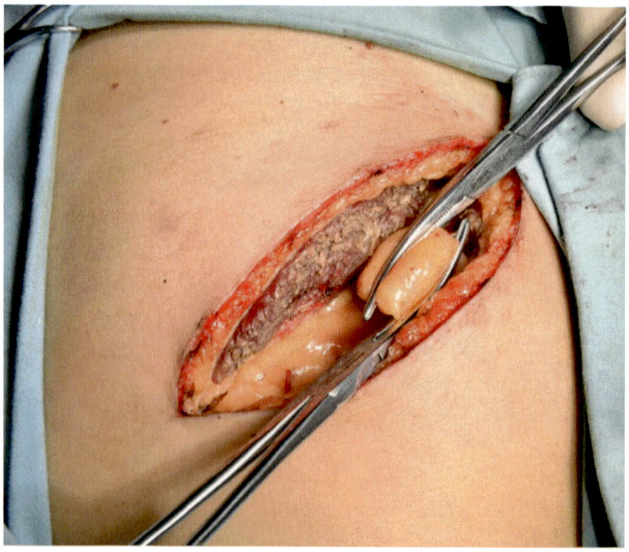

Fig. 58 The peritoneal cavity was entered into and the round ligament was divided and ligated

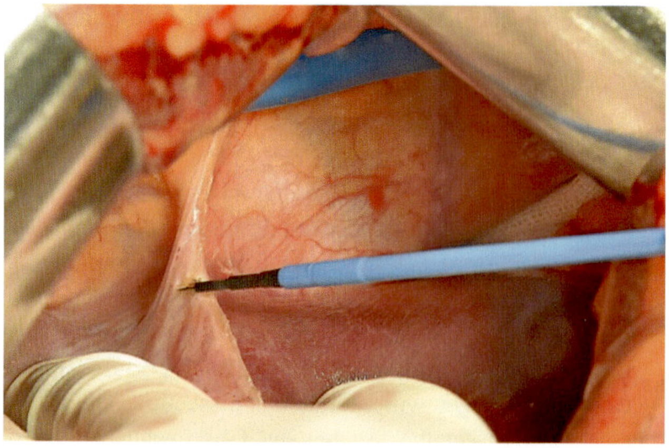

Fig. 59 The falciform ligament was divided with electrocautery

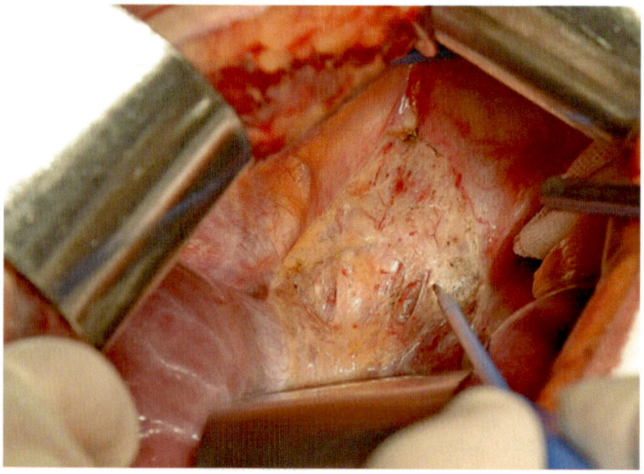

Fig. 60 Hepatocaval confluence was dissected

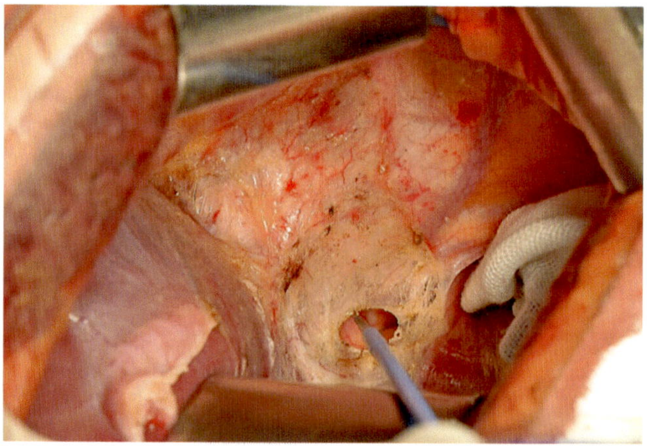

Fig. 61 The left coronary ligament was electrocauterized

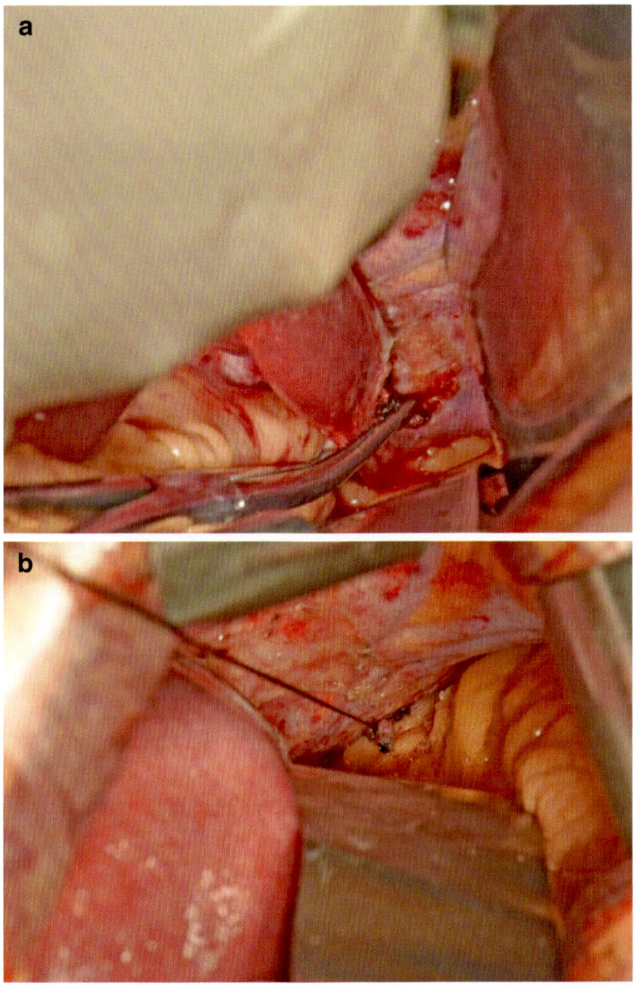

Fig. 62 (**a**, **b**) The left triangular ligament was clamped, divided, and ligated

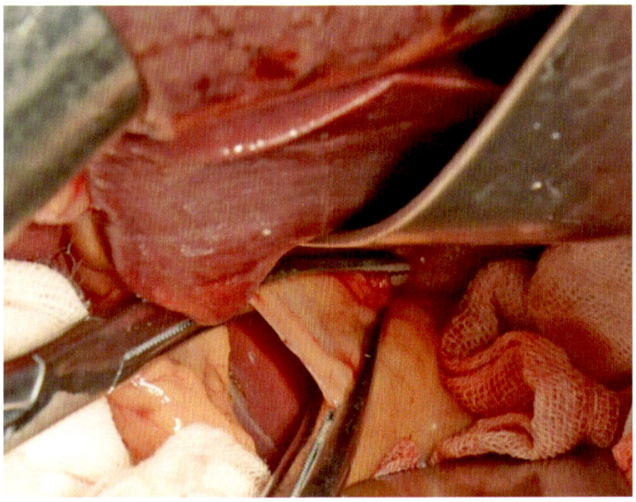

Fig. 63 The hepatogastral ligament was clamped, divided, and ligated

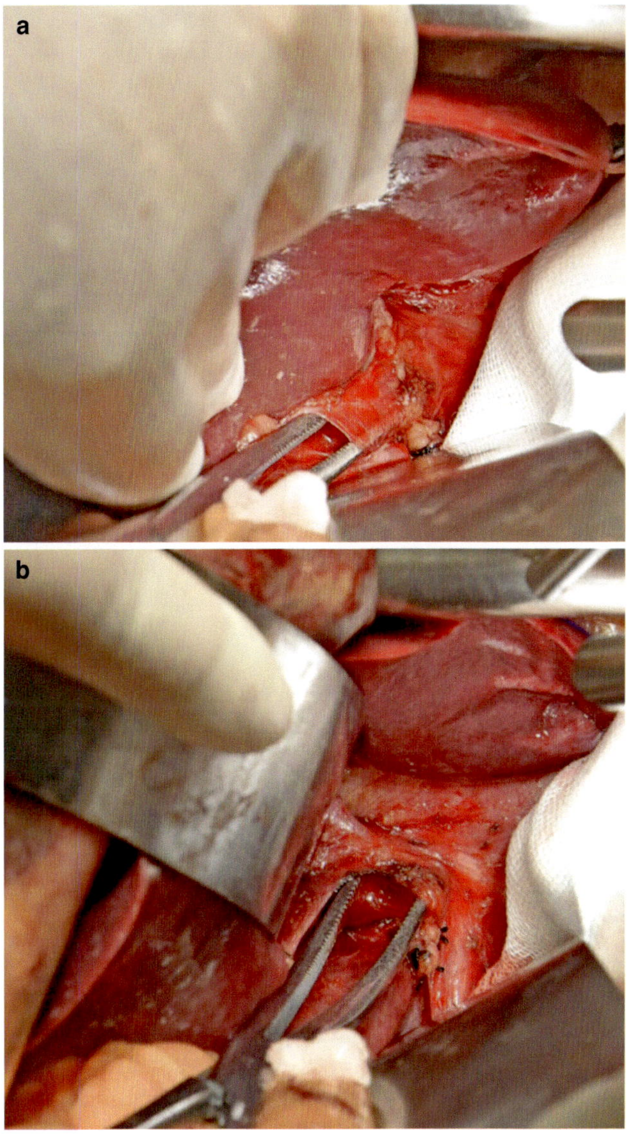

Fig. 64 (**a**, **b**) The ligamentum venosum was dissected

Isolation and Division of the Left Hepatic Pedicle (RHP) and Marking the Cut Line
(Figs. 65, 66, 67, 68, and 69)

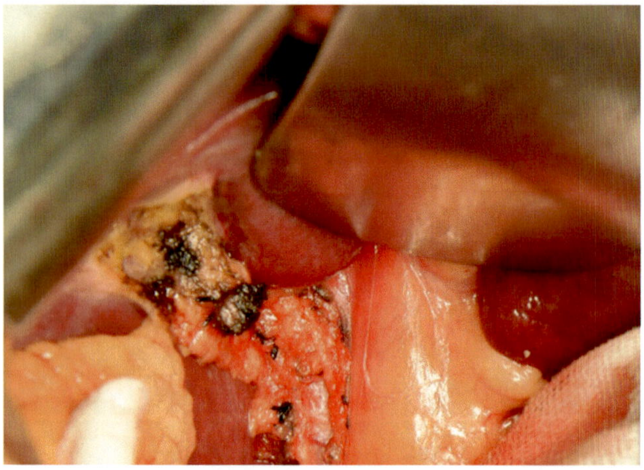

Fig. 65 Cholecystectomy was performed

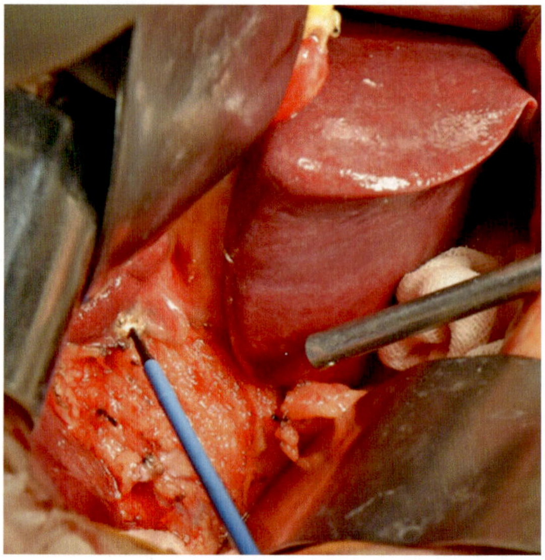

Fig. 66 A small traverse incision was made in front of the hilus

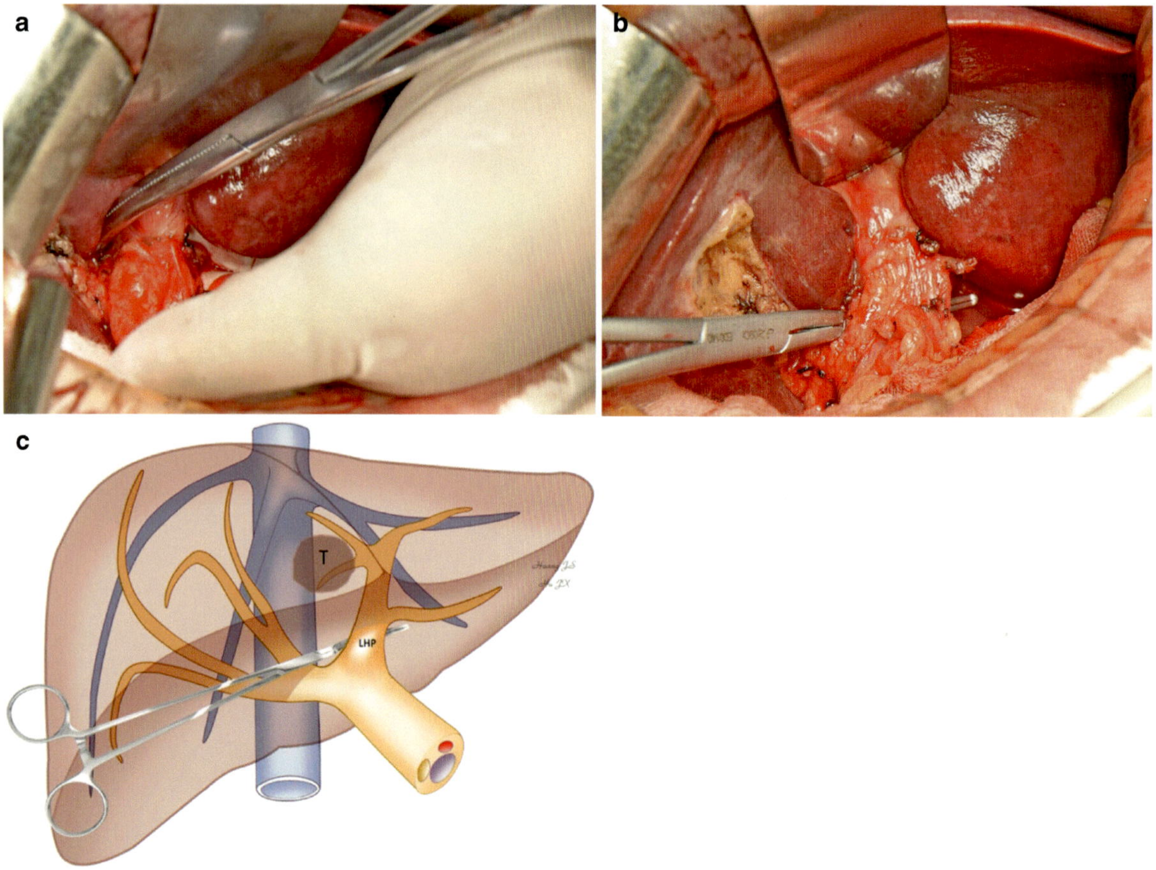

Fig. 67 (**a**) The operator's left index finger was put between the undersurface of the hilus and the anterior wall of the retrohepatic IVC. (**b**) Then, a large curved clamp was inserted vertically into this incision and directly reached down to the tip of index finger; using the index finger as a guide, the clamp was inserted furtherly to puncture through the undersurface membrane of the hilar plate. Thus, the left hepatic pedicle (LHP) was isolated. (**c**) Schematic illustration of this procedure

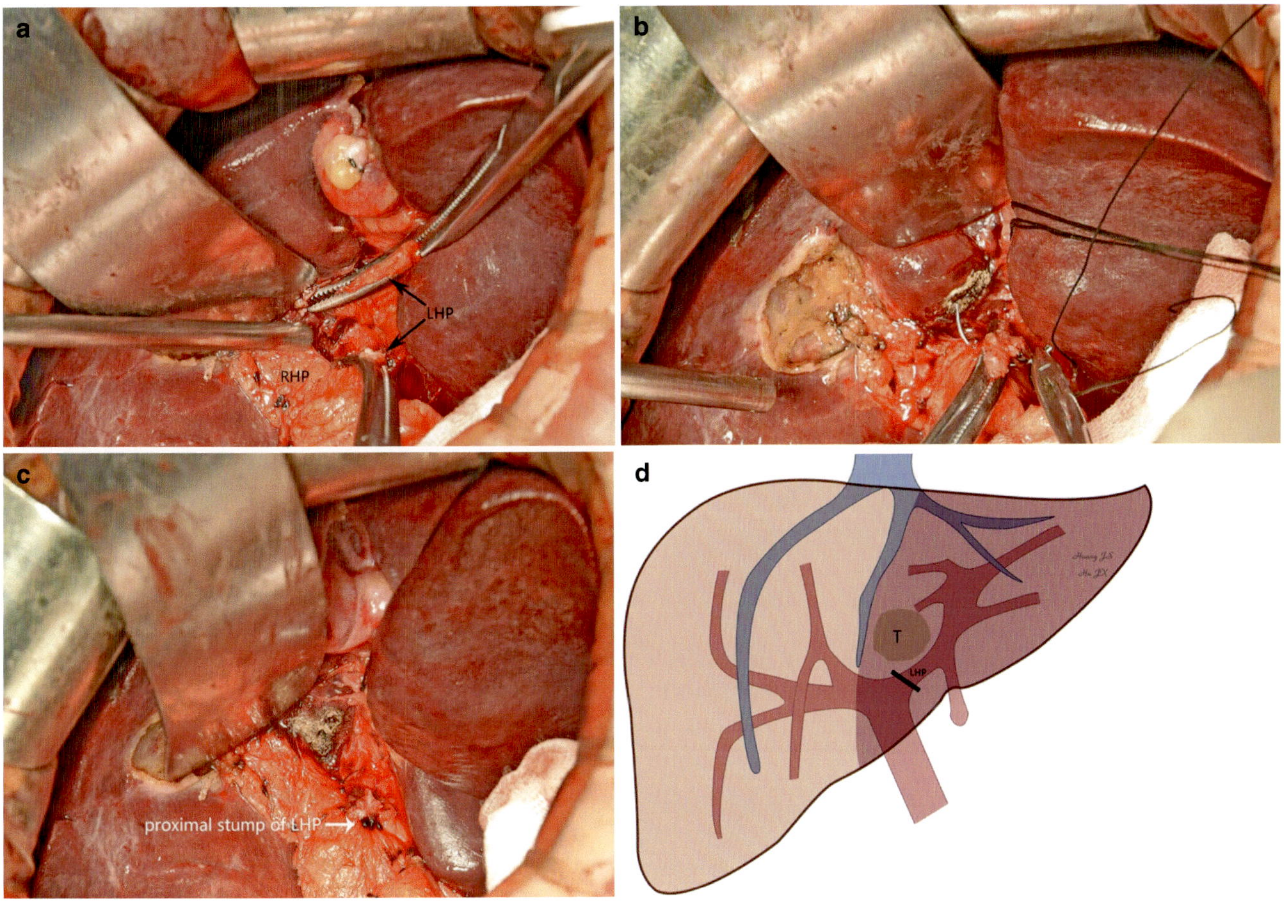

Fig. 68 (**a–c**) The left hepatic pedicle (LHP) was clamped, divided, and suture-ligated. (**d**) Schematic illustration of this procedure

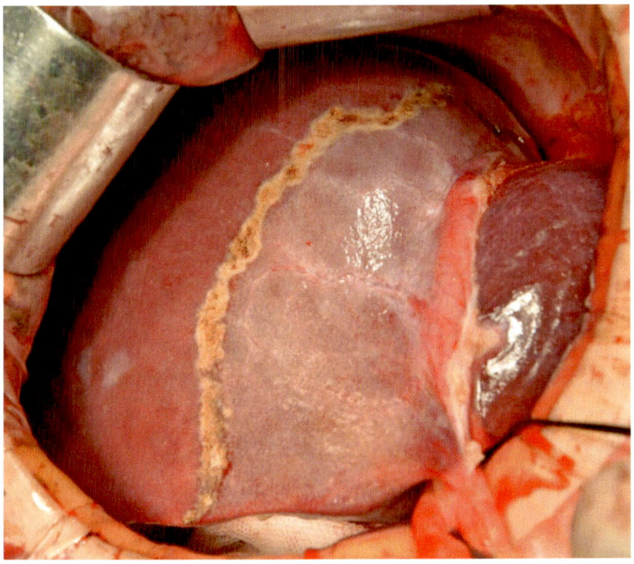

Fig. 69 The parenchymal transection line was electrocauterized on the liver surface corresponding to the ischemic line

Hepatic Parenchymal Transection
(Figs. 70, 71, 72, 73, 74, 75, and 76)

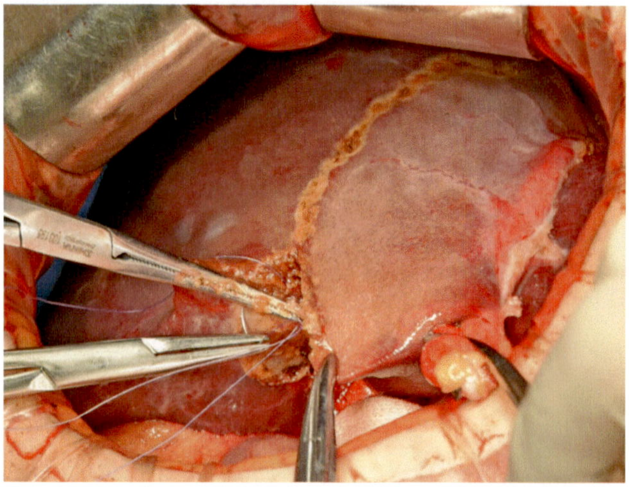

Fig. 70 Hepatic parenchymal transection was carried out caudo-cranially, using clamp-crushing method. Large vascular and biliary branches were suture-ligated

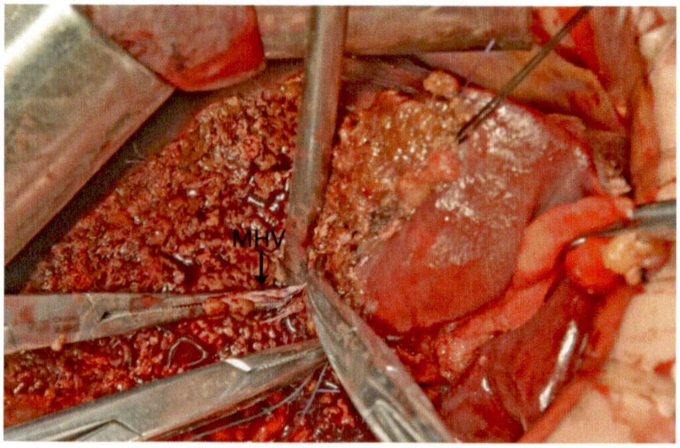

Fig. 72 The tiny holes on the wall of the middle hepatic vein (MHV) were repaired with 4-0 polypropylene

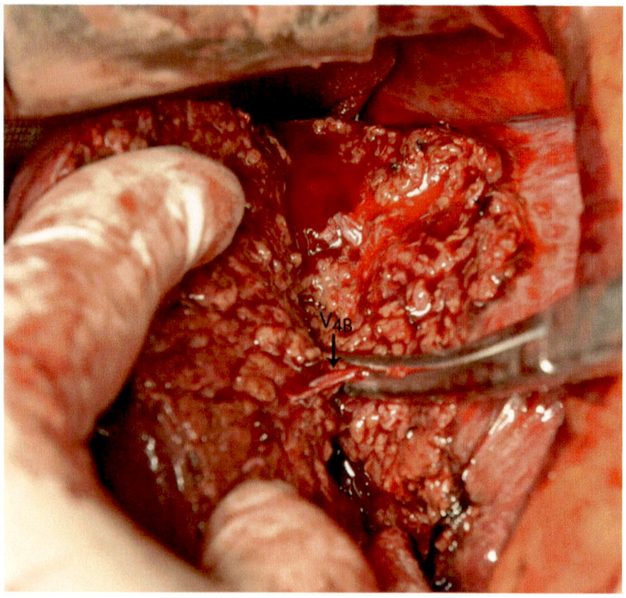

Fig. 71 V_{4B} of the middle hepatic vein (MHV) was clamped, divided, and ligated. *MHV* middle hepatic vein, V_{4B} venous branch of the MHV draining segment IVB

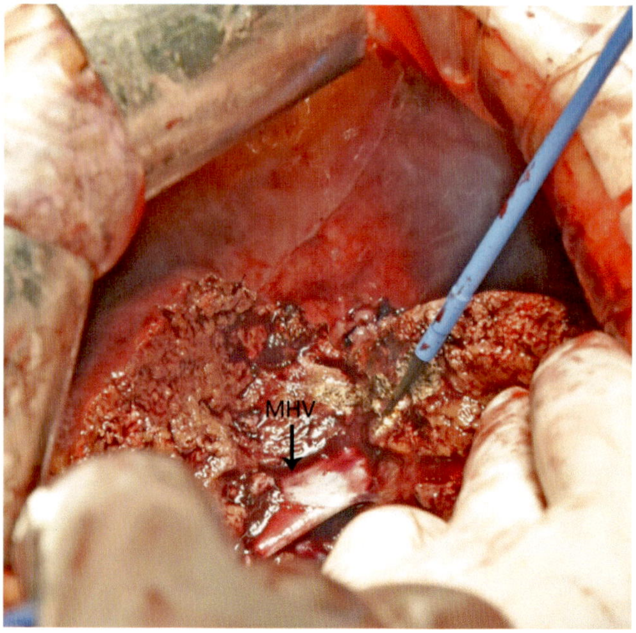

Fig. 73 The main trunk of the middle hepatic vein (MHV) was exposed

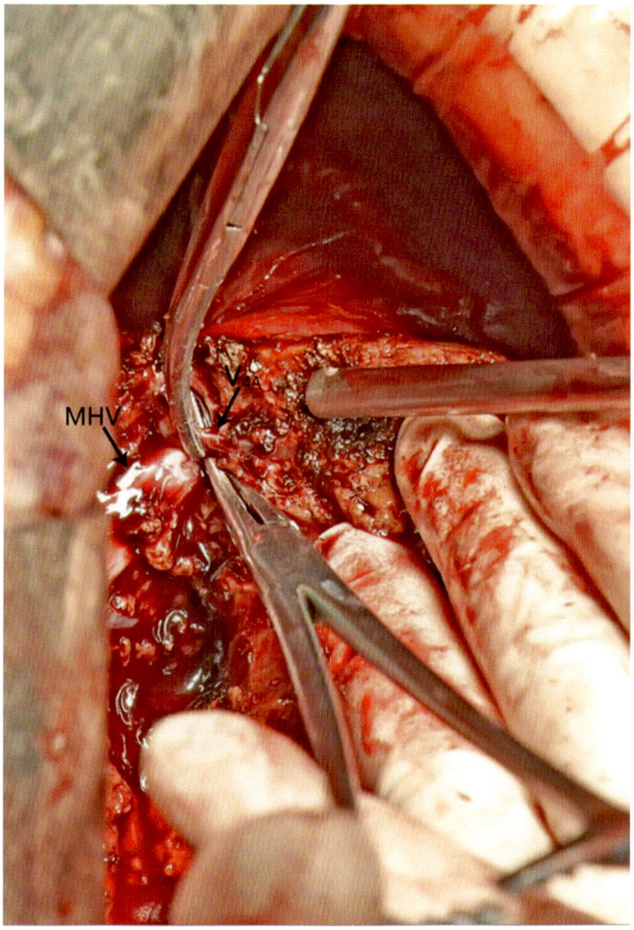

Fig. 74 V_{4A} of the middle hepatic vein (MHV) draining segment IVA was isolated, divided, and suture-ligated

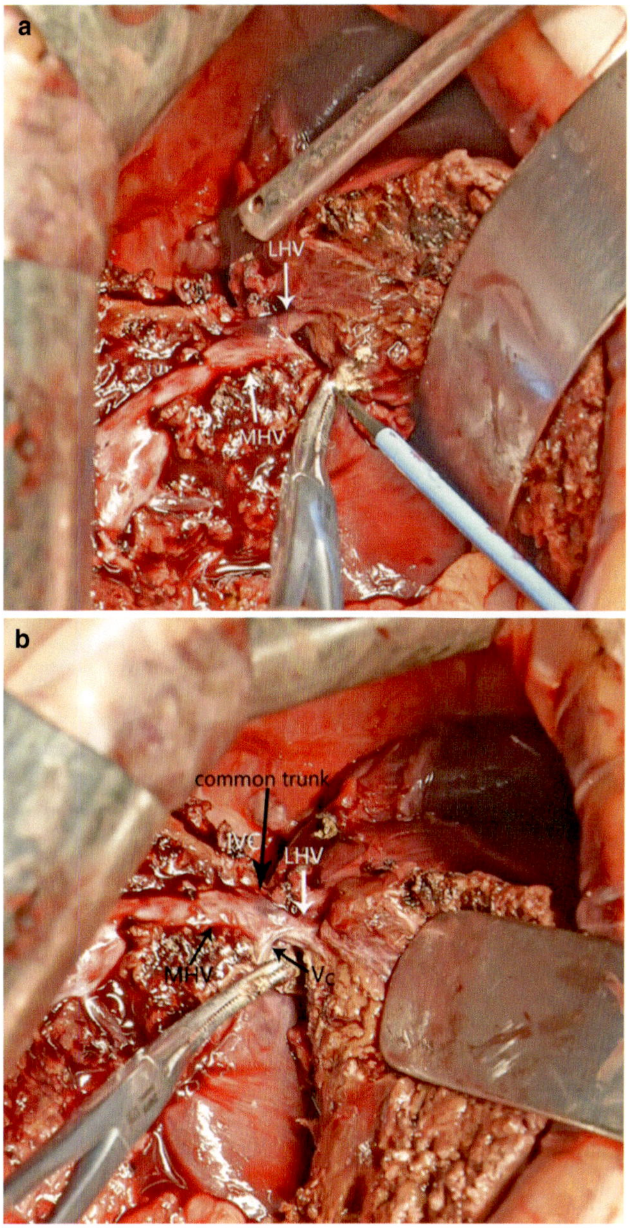

Fig. 75 (**a**, **b**) The root of the MHV and the LHV was exposed. The MHV and LHV emerged into a common trunk. *MHV* middle hepatic vein, *LHV* left hepatic vein, *IVC* inferior vena cava, V_C vein draining the proper portion of the caudate lobe

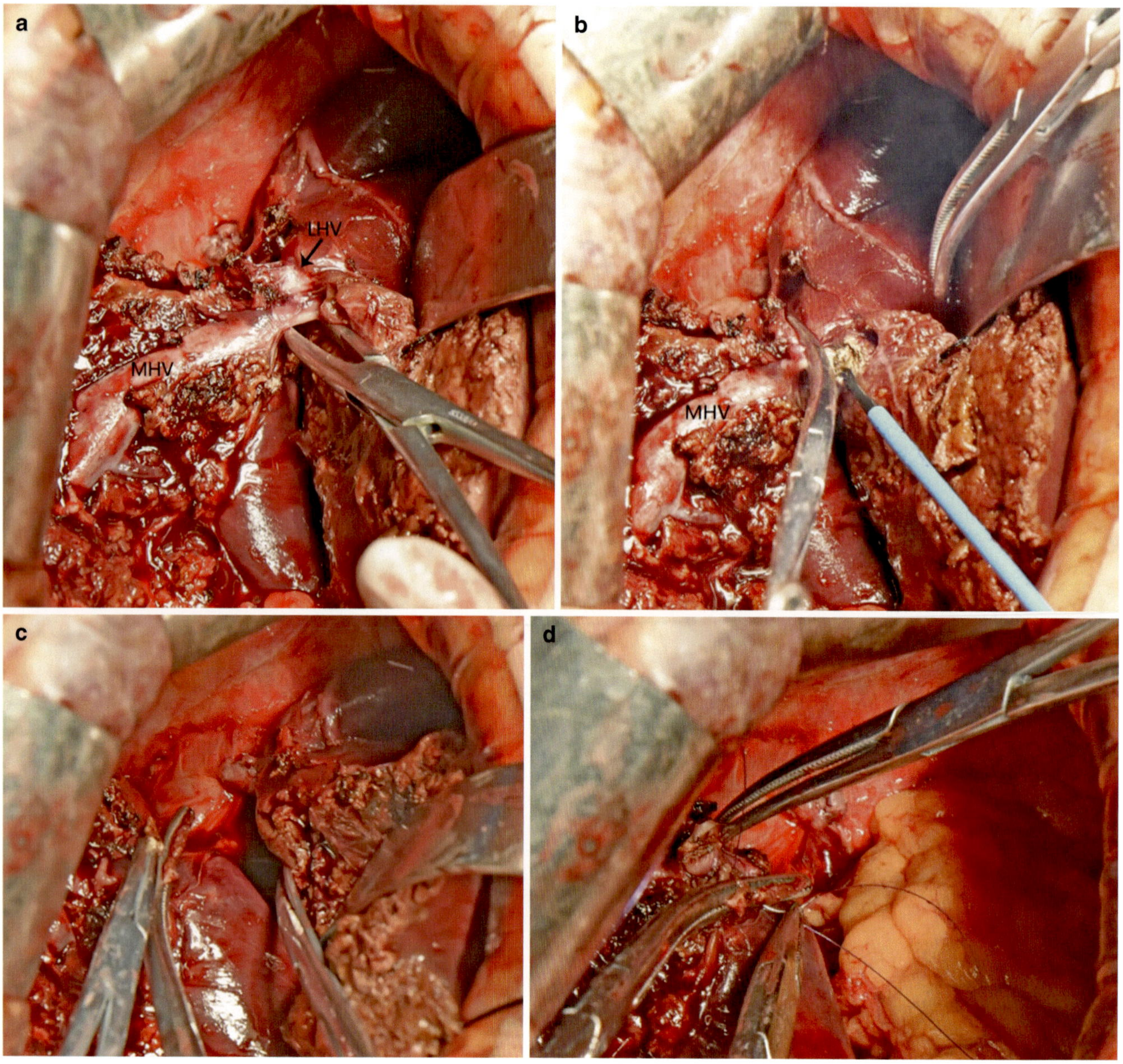

Fig. 76 (**a**–**d**) The LHV was isolated, clamped, divided, and suture-ligated at the side of its entry into the common trunk. *LHV* left hepatic vein

Cut Surface of the Remnant Liver and the Specimen (Figs. 77, 78, and 79)

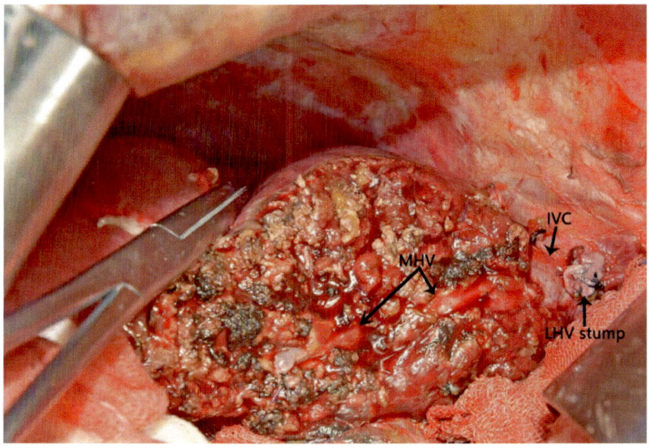

Fig. 77 The whole course of the middle hepatic vein (MHV) was clearly exposed on the cut surface. *IVC* inferior vena cava, *LHV stump* stump of left hepatic vein

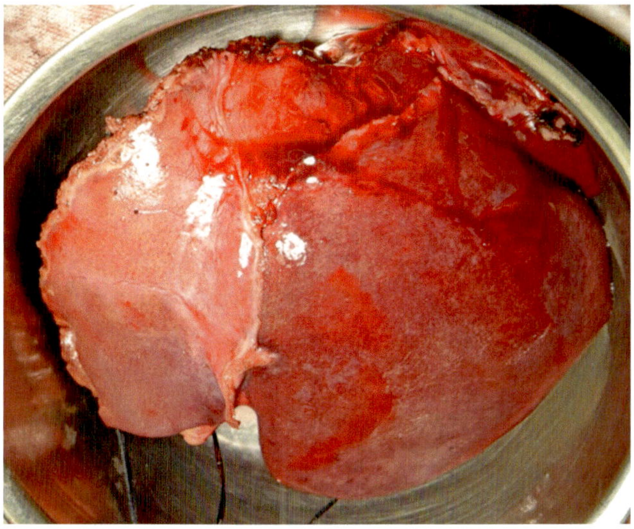

Fig. 78 Bird view of the specimen

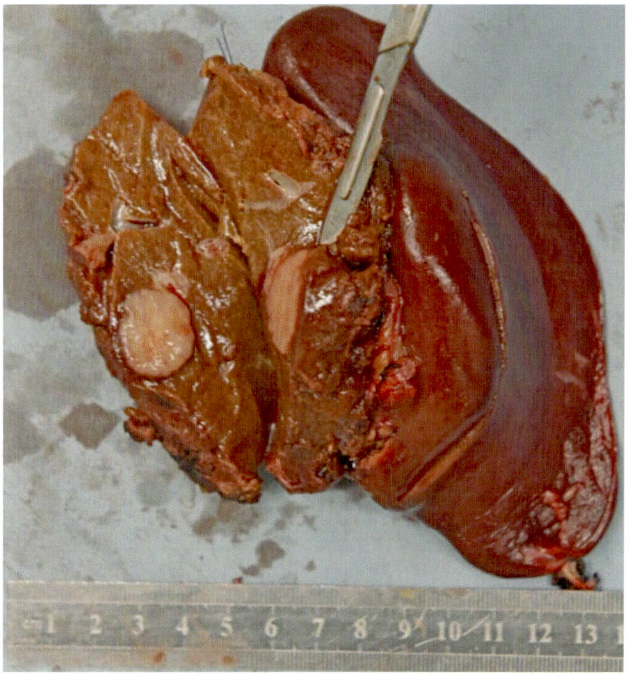

Fig. 79 The cross-section of the tumor

Anatomic Right Anterior Sectionectomy Using Glissonean Pedicle Transection Method

Jixiong Hu, Shengfu Huang, and Ning Zhou

Right anterior sectionectomy (RAS) of the liver, which is first described in 1956 [33], consists of resecting segment V and VIII, which are the liver central segments comprised between the right hepatic vein (RHV) and the middle hepatic vein (MHV). From a technical point of view, RAS remains a technically difficult procedure as it requires two transection planes [34]. In addition, there are a great number of hepatic veins and Glissonean pedicle branches that demand a division as compared to other anatomical hepatic resections [35, 36].

Surgical Indications

For patients with HCCs located within right anterior sector (segment V+ segment VIII), RAS was considered. In terms of liver function, Child-Pugh A and ICGR15 < 20% was thought to be essential for the safety of the planned operation [37]. Because cirrhosis is present in more than 80% of patients with HCC, preserving adequate functional hepatic parenchyma during hepatic resection is extremely important for postoperative patient survival [38]. From the perspective of clinical practice, RAS is preferred over the right hepatectomy or the mesohepatectomy (resection of segment V + VIII + IV). The surgical procedures included the right anterior pedicle isolation and division, mobilization of the liver, hepatic parenchymal transection, and management of the cut surface.

Operative Procedures	Technical Details
Laparotomy	◄ A right subcostal incision was made.
Mobilization of the right hemiliver	◄ The perihepatic ligaments were divided with electrocautery and the right adrenal gland was dissected away from the liver, and the retrohepatic short veins were divided and ligated individually up to the root of the right hepatic vein (RHV). The RHV was extrahepatically isolated, looped in order to be clamped if required. Occasimly, it is difficult to isolate the RHV, if so, the supra-and infra-hepatic inferior vena cava (IVC) was isolated and looped with a tourniquet, respectively.
Perihilar dissection	◄ Using perihilar Glissonean approach, the right hepatic pedicle and the right anterior pedicle was isolated and encircled with a vascular tape, respectively. The right anterior pedicle was clamped, divided and suture-ligated. The ischemic demarcation line between the right anterior sector and posterior sector, and the right anterior sector and segment IV was marked on the liver surface with electrocautery.
Parenchymal transection	◄ Hepatic parenchymal dissection was performed from the anterior and inferior liver surface posteriorly towards the IVC and superiorly towards the hepatocaval confluence along the demarcation line by a clamp crushing method. Left parenchymal transection was first carried out. After completion of the left transection plane, attention is then turned to the right-side transection. All large branches of the RHV and MHV were divided and ligated individually. The complete course of the RHV and MHV was fully exposedand tiny holes or lacerations on them were repaired.
Drainage and closure of the peritoneal cavity	◄ A tube was placed below the right subphrenic space and secured with silk-suture.

Intraoperative Key Points

1. RAS may require a longer liver parenchymal transection time, result in doubled area of cut surface and leave the right and middle hepatic veins exposed along the resection surface. Hemorrhage control remains the main problem in this surgical procedure [34, 35]. It is well known that low central venous pressure can reduce blood loss during hepatic parenchymal transection. In our major hepatectomies, we always ask anesthesiologists to decrease central venous pressure by reducing fluid volume and airway pressure to <15 mmHg (see section "Control of the Inflow and Outflow system during Liver Resection" in chapter "Basic Techniques for Hepatic Resection by the Glissonean Approach"). Left-sided hepatic parenchymal transection was performed under an intermittent Pringle maneuver (15 min of clamping and 5 min unclamping) to control inflow blood flow. Right-sided liver parenchymal transection was undertaken by clamping the right hepatic pedicle to obtain the right hemiliver blood inflow occlusion and reduce ischemic time of the left-sided remnant liver. Usually, severe bleeding during right anterior sectionectomy is caused by injuries to the exposed middle hepatic vein (MHV) and right hepatic vein (RHV) on the cut surfaces, especially for a large or deeply situated tumor that compresses or impinges on the RHV and/or MHV; such a massive venous backflow bleeding may occur at any time and may even lead to operative mortality. Therefore, we often preplace a vascular tape around the suprahepatic and infrahepatic IVC, respectively, or preliminary isolation and looping of the root of the RHV and MHV were performed prior to liver parenchymal transection. In case of severe venous backflow bleeding, clamping of the RHV and MHV or the common trunk of the MHV and LHV without caval clamping, associated with total or hemiliver blood inflow occlusion, or Pringle maneuver plus supra- and infrahepatic vena cava clamping (total hepatic blood exclusion), allows total control of backflow and inflow bleeding and unhurried and accurate repair of the injured vascular structures in a bloodless surgical field [39, 40]. Reports of RAP based on an open approach are very rare. RAP is the most highest technically demanding hepatic resection. Having performed RAP with complete exposure of the RHV and MHV on the cut surface and without blood transfusion, the true essence of hepatectomy may be obtained [41, 42].
2. Variations in anatomy of the portal vein branches in the hilar area are uncommon. Variations of the portal vein division were observed in 20–35% of the persons [43–45]. The commonest variant types is the portal trifurcation in which the main portal veins is divided into right anterior and posterior portal veins and the left portal branch, all arising from a common place. This type variant was observed in 10.9–15.0% of the persons [45, 46]. Encountering such an anatomical variant of the portal vein branches in the hilar area, in order to escape subsequent stricture occurring in the main portal vein that results from transection of the RAP, a safety margin of over 1 cm distal to its origin should be kept while dividing this pedicle. Another rare but potentially ravaging anomaly is the absence of the left portal vein. The left hemiliver was supplied by branches from the right anterior portal vein, and transection of the RAP can lead to the ischemia of the left hemiliver [47, 48]. The use of 3D reconstruction obtained from preoperative CT images seems to be the most valuable technique in recognizing the above-mentioned anomalies [45, 46, 49, 50].
3. In most patients (around 83–89%), the right posterior bile duct runs superiorly, dorsally, and inferiorly (Hjiorsjo crook) to the right main trunk of the portal vein and takes hold of the origin of the right anterior pedicle (RAP); transection of the RAP can cause injury to the right posterior bile duct if the transection is performed too close to the origin of the RAP [35, 51]. It is advisable to transect this pedicle about 1 cm distal to its origin and carefully check up the completeness of the right posterior pedicle (Fig. 80).

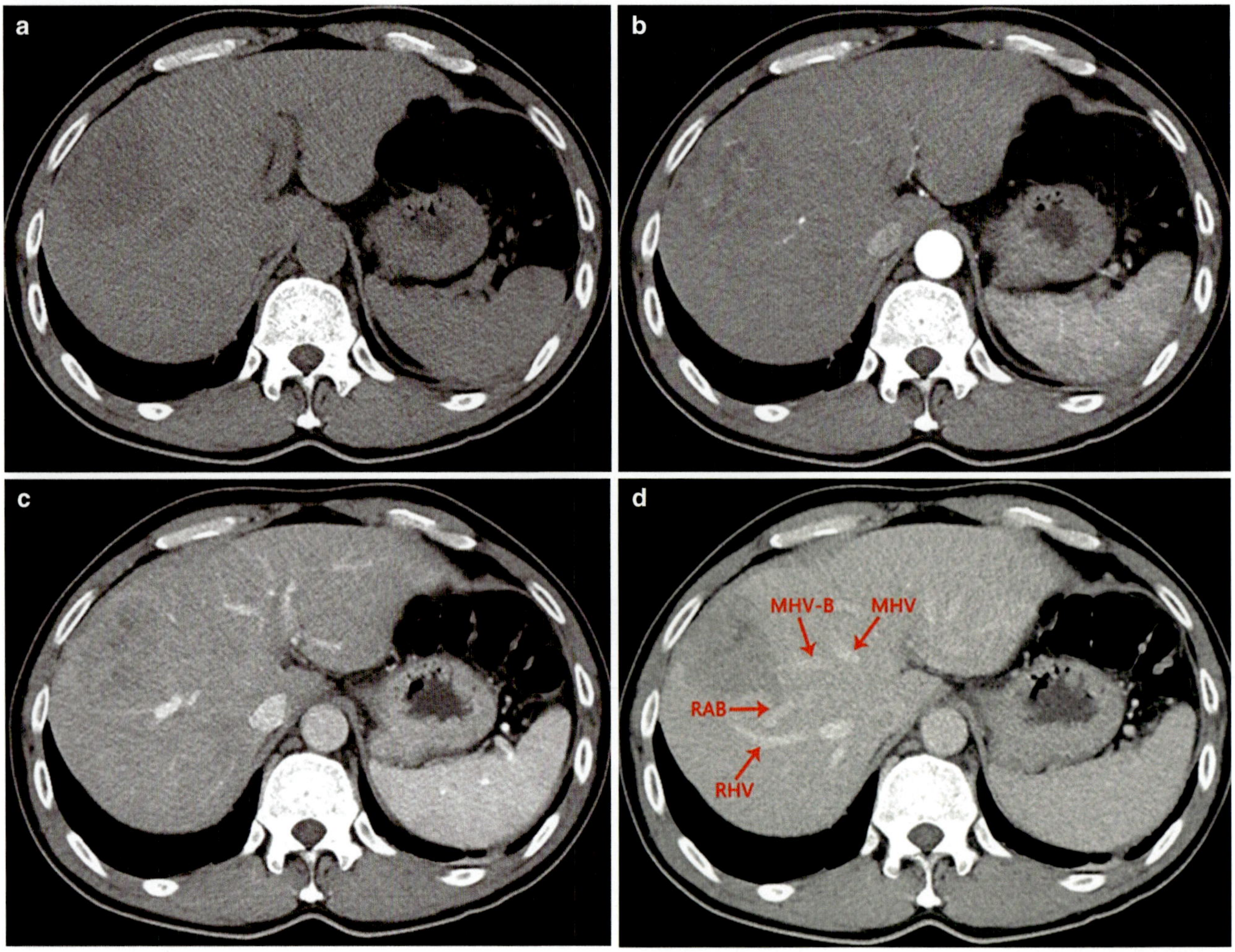

Fig. 80 (**a**) Preoperative CT (precontrast). The tumor, which appears slightly hypodense compared to the liver, is located in the right anterior sector. (**b**) Preoperative CT (hepatic arterial phase). The tumor shows heterogeneous enhancement. (**c**) CT (hepatic venous phase). The tumor shows enhancement fades and slight capsular enhancement. (**d**) Preoperative CT (interstitial phase). The tumor appears markedly hypodense due to washout. The tumor and its relationship with the hepatic veins. *RHV* right hepatic vein, *RAB* right anterior branch, *MHV-B* branch of MHV, *MHV* middle hepatic vein

Abdominal Incision and Mobilization of the Liver
(Figs. 81, 82, 83, 84, 85, 86, 87, 88, 89, and 90)

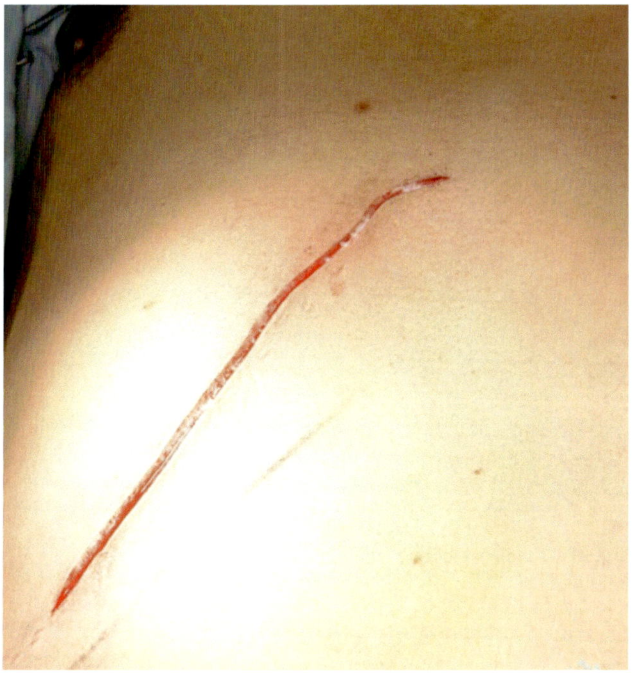

Fig. 81 A right subcostal incision was selected and made

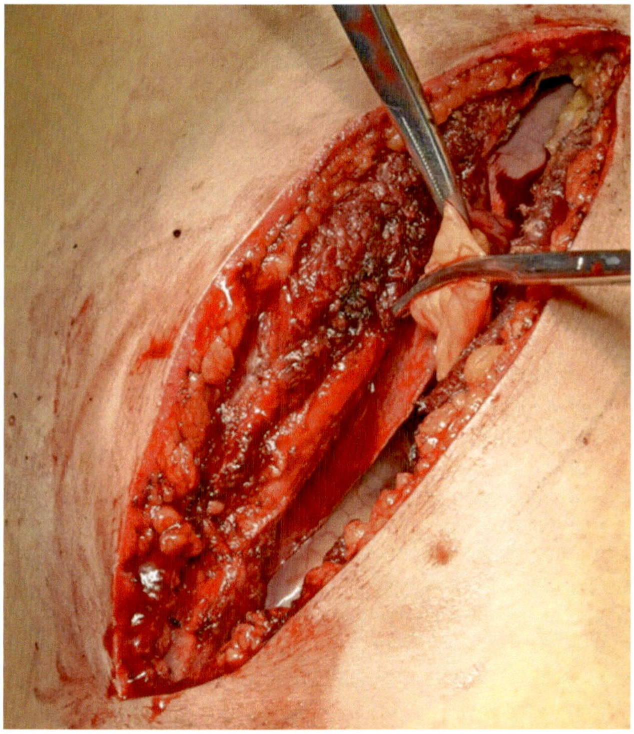

Fig. 82 Having entered into the abdominal cavity, the round ligament was divided and ligated

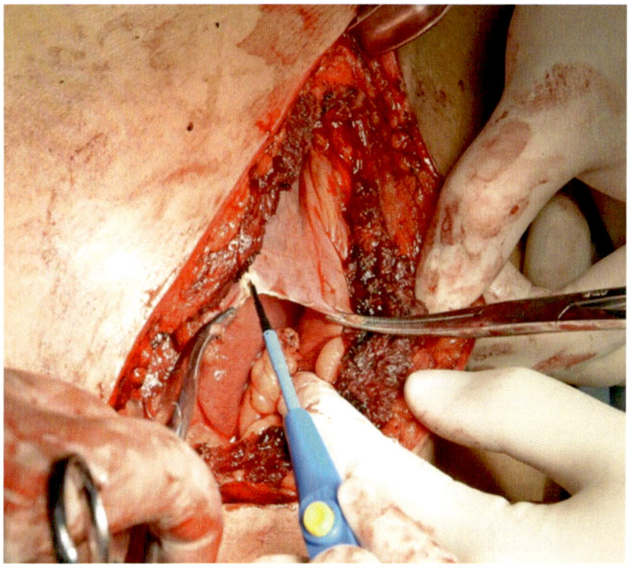

Fig. 83 The falciform ligament was electrocauterized

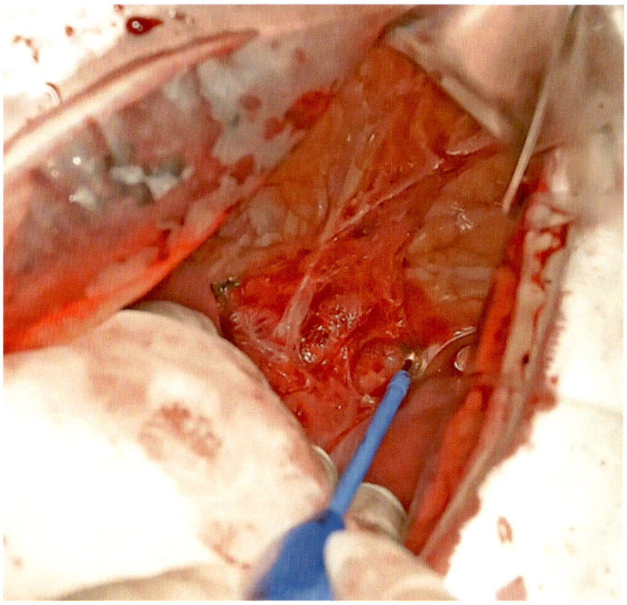

Fig. 84 Hepatocaval confluence was dissected

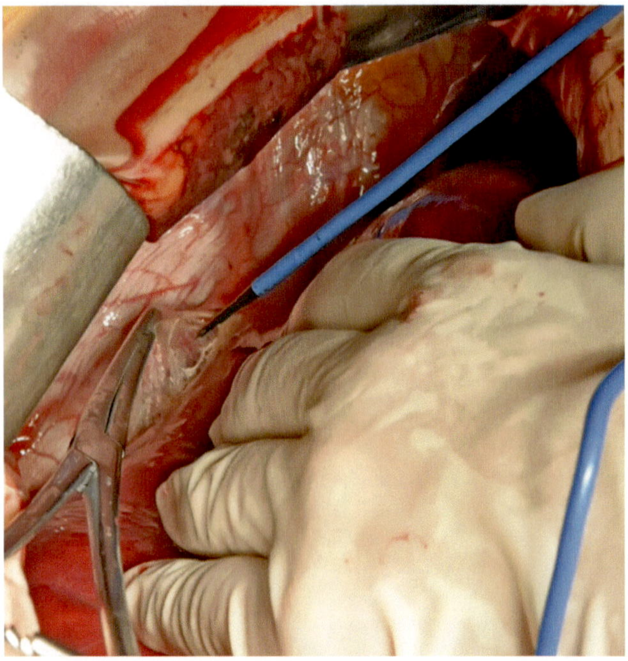

Fig. 85 The right coronary ligament was divided with electrocautery

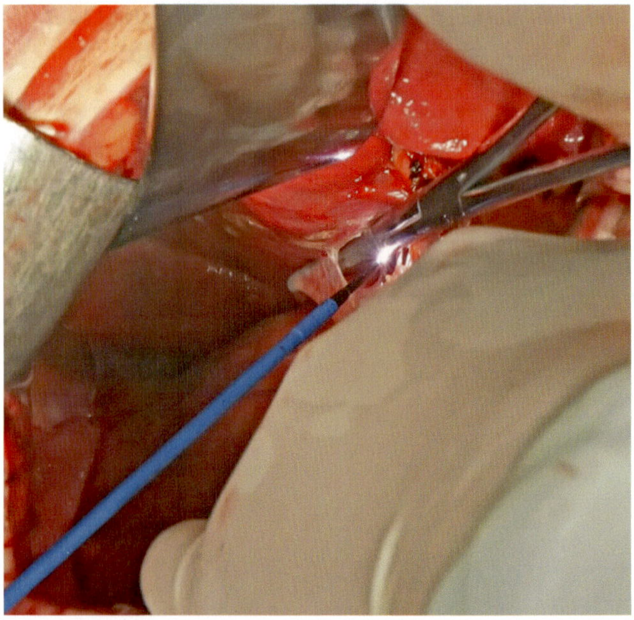

Fig. 87 The hepatocolic ligament was divided with electrocautery

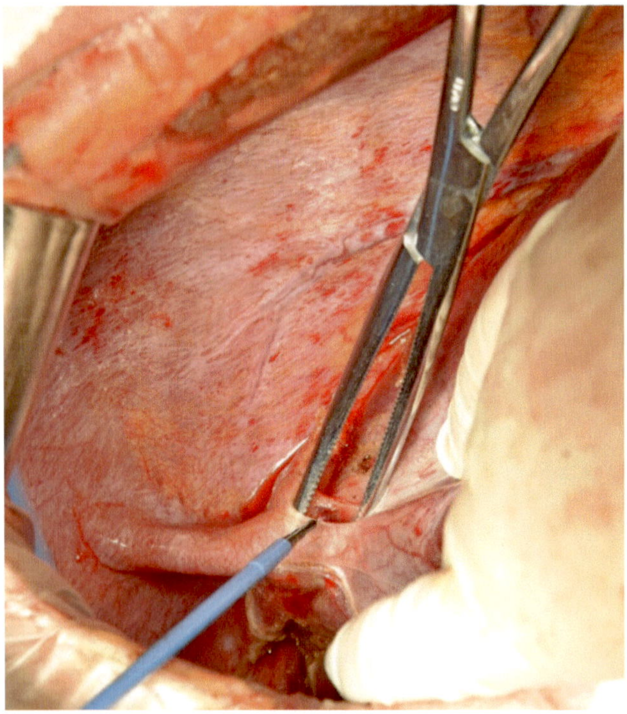

Fig. 86 The right triangular ligament was dissected

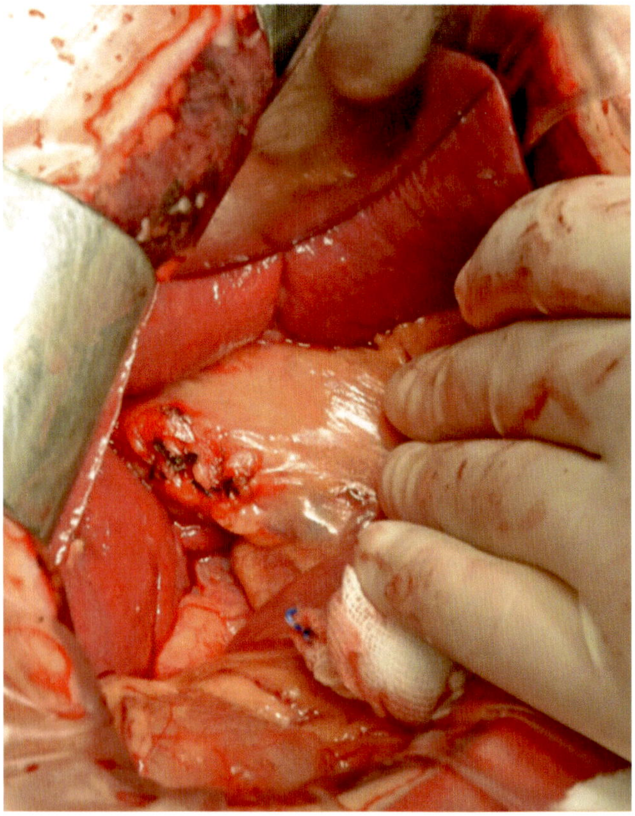

Fig. 88 Cholecystectomy was performed

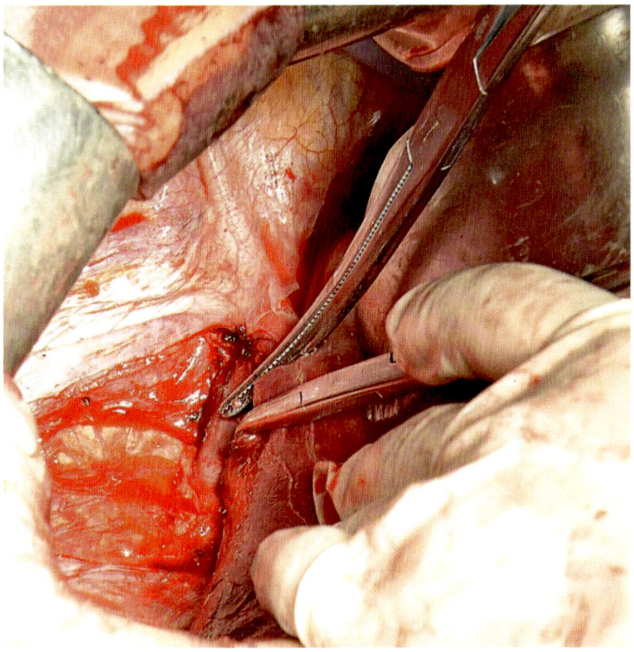

Fig. 89 Having dissected the right adrenal gland away from the liver, the right hemiliver was lifted upward and medially, and then the right-sided retrohepatic short veins were divided and ligated individually

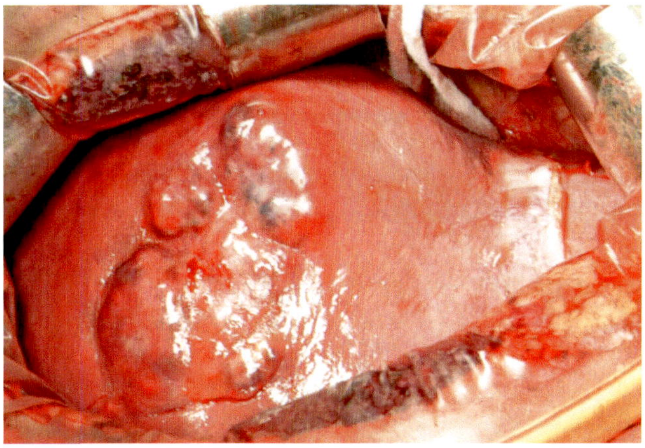

Fig. 90 The tumor was located within segments V and VIII, and a loop was pre-placed around the suprahepatic inferior vena cava (IVC) and infrahepatic IVC (see Fig. 93), respectively

Isolation of the Right Hepatic Pedicle
(Figs. 91, 92, and 93)

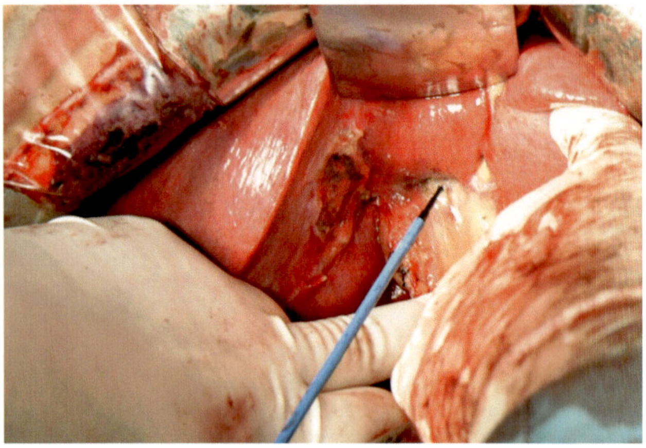

Fig. 91 One about 2.5 cm traverse incision was made in front of the hilar plate, and then using a large curved clamp, hepatic parenchyma above this incision was pushed upward, and the hilar plate was pulled down to expose the anterior and superior surface of the right hepatic Glissonean pedicle

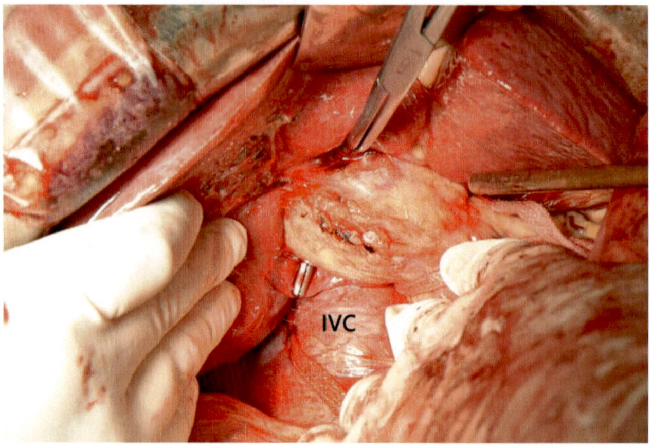

Fig. 93 Thus, the right hepatic Glissonean pedicle was isolated, and a loop was encircled with it. The infrahepatic inferior vena cava (IVC) and hepatic pedicle has been encircled with a tape, respectively

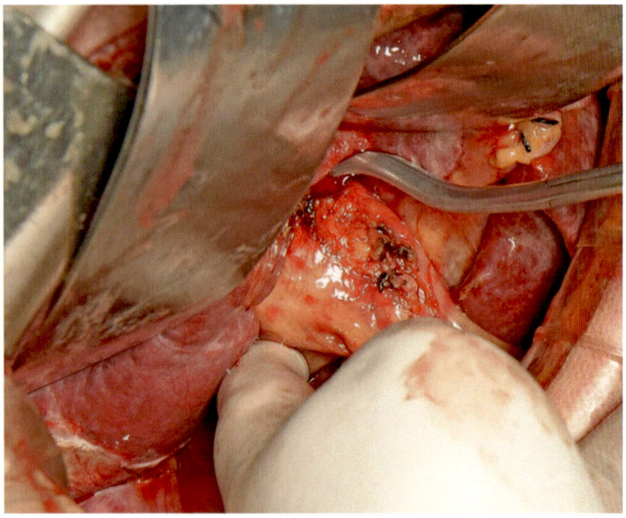

Fig. 92 The operator's left index finger was placed between the undersurface of the hilar plate and the anterior wall of the retrohepatic IVC, and then, a large curved clamp was inserting vertically into this incision and directly reached down to the tip of the index finger, using the index finger as a guide. The clamp was inserted furtherly to puncture the undersurface membrane of the hilar plate

Isolation of the Right Anterior Pedicle
(Figs. 94, 95, 96, and 97)

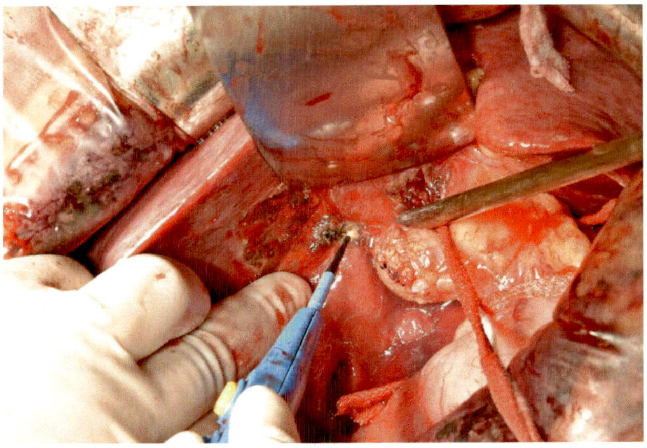

Fig. 94 Another small incision was made on the right edge of the gallbladder bed

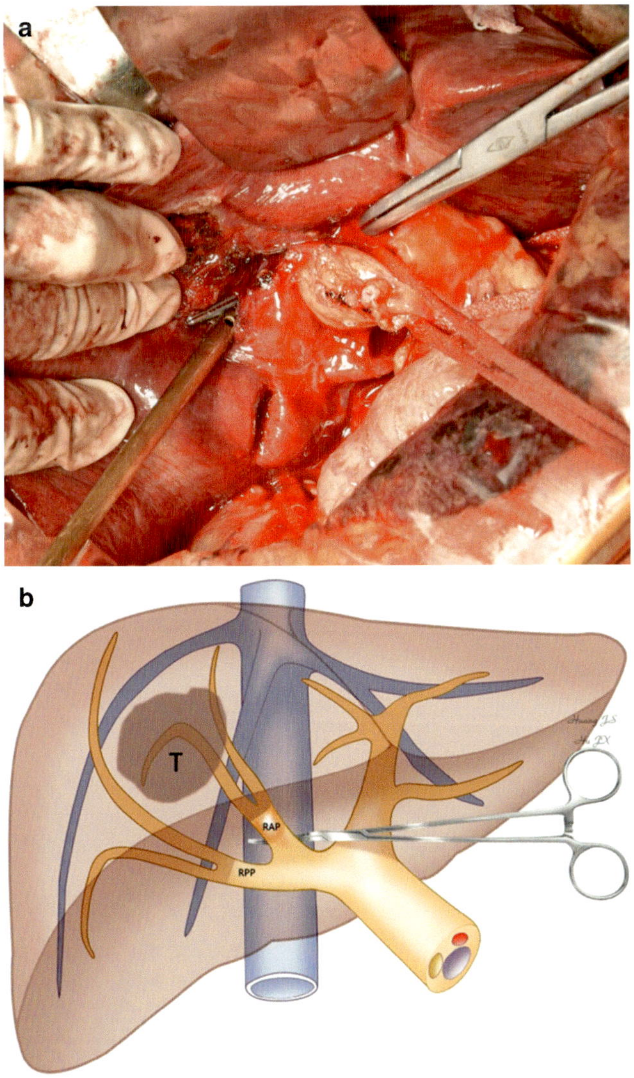

Fig. 95 (**a**) A large curved clamp was inserted into this incision in front of the hilus and passed out of this incision on the right edge of the gallbladder bed. (**b**) Schematic illustration of this procedure

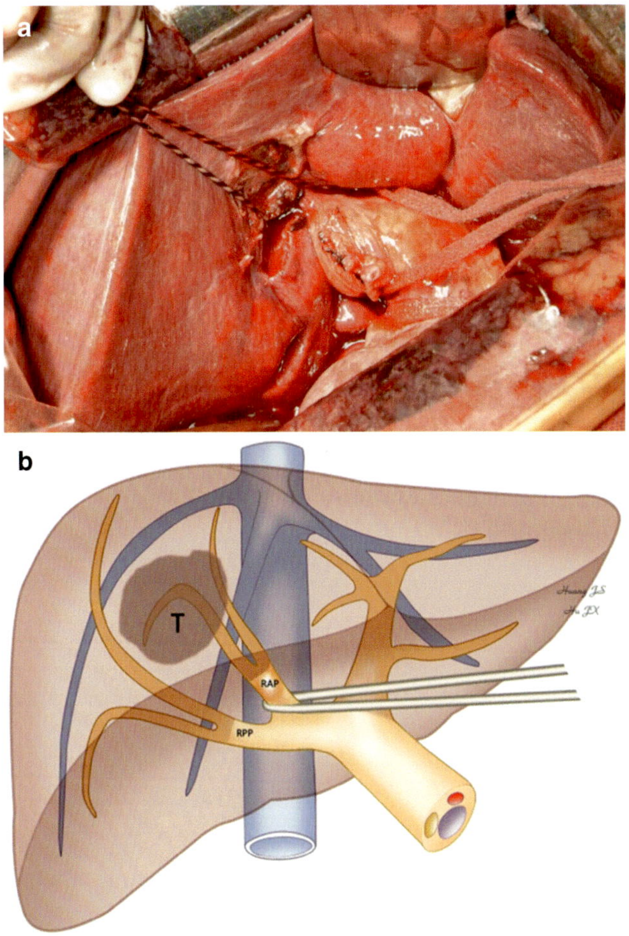

Fig. 96 (**a**) Schematic illustration of this procedure. Thus, the right anterior sectional Glissonean pedicle (RAP) was isolated and looped with a vascular tape. (**b**) Schematic illustration of this procedure. *RPP* right posterior sectional pedicle

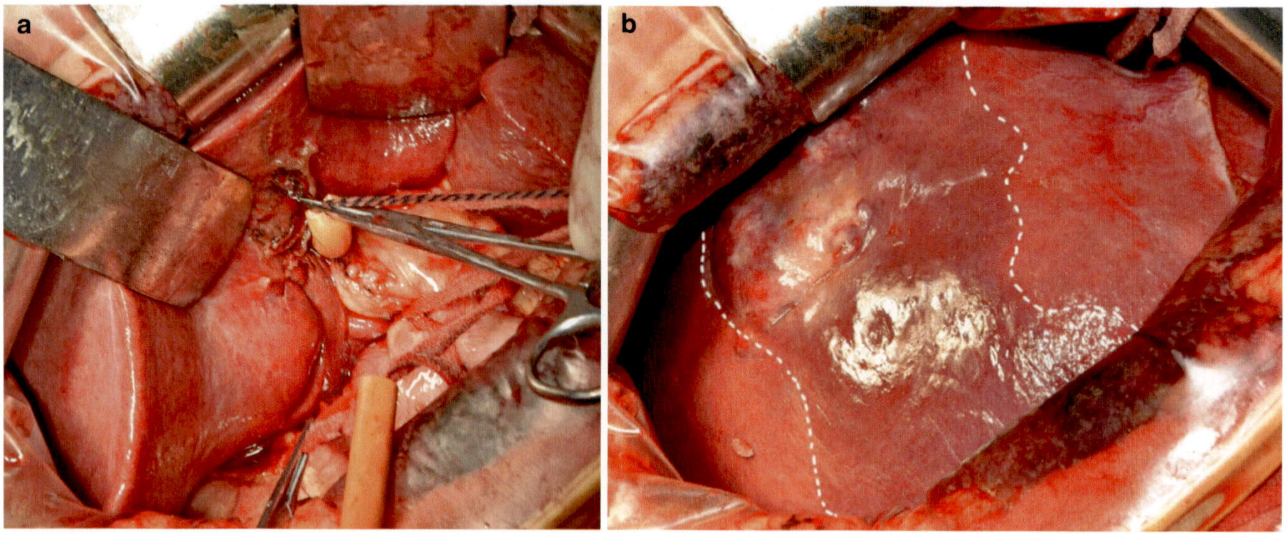

Fig. 97 (**a**) To identify the target section, having temporarily test-clamped the right anterior sectional Glissonean pedicle. (**b**) Obvious ischemic demarcation line appeared on the liver surface

Division of the Right Anterior Pedicle (Fig. 98)

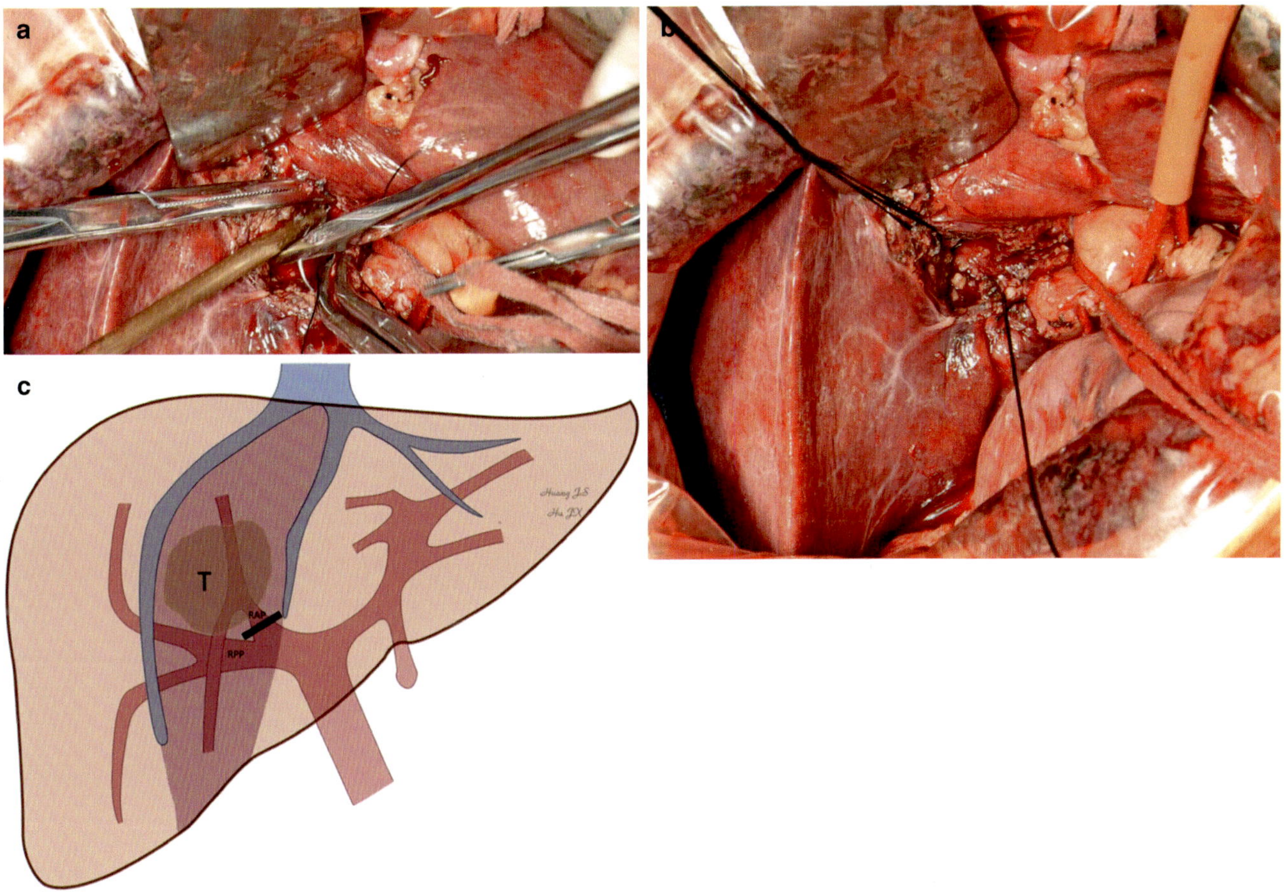

Fig. 98 (**a**, **b**) The right anterior sectional Glissonean pedicle was clamped, divided, and suture-ligated. (**c**) Schematic illustration of this procedure. *RPP* right posterior sectional pedicle, *RAP* right anterior sectional pedicle

Marking the Cut Line (Fig. 99)

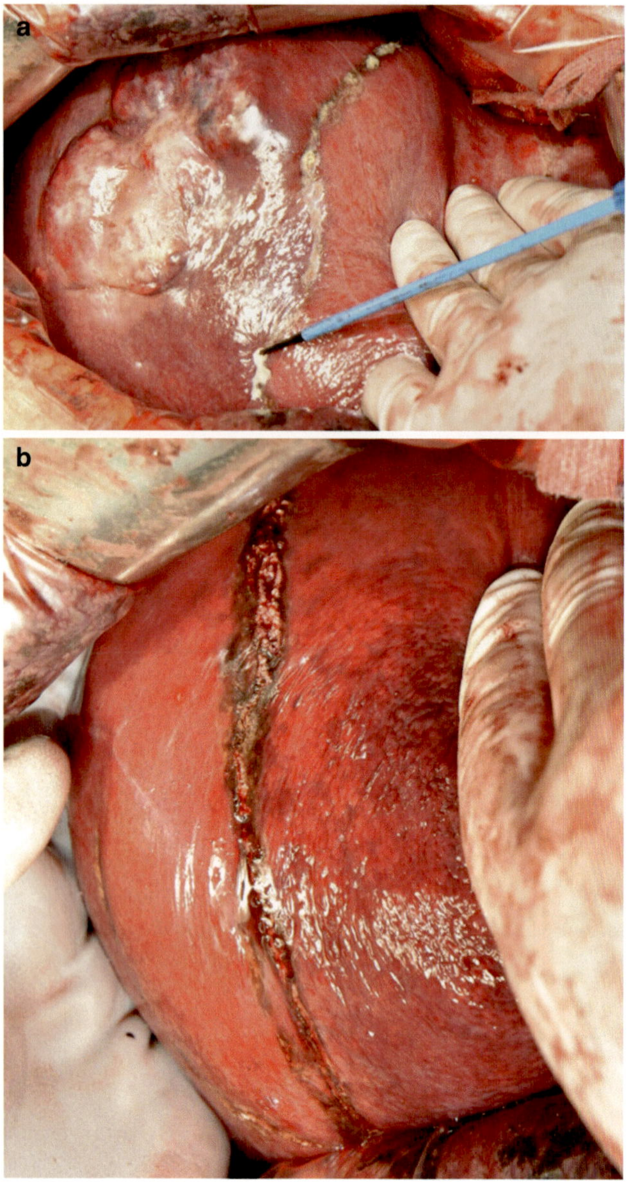

Fig. 99 (**a**, **b**) Left-sided (**a**) and right-sided (**b**) ischemic demarcation line was marked on the liver surface with electrocautery

Hepatic Parenchymal Transection (Left-Sided)

(Figs. 100, 101, 102, and 103)

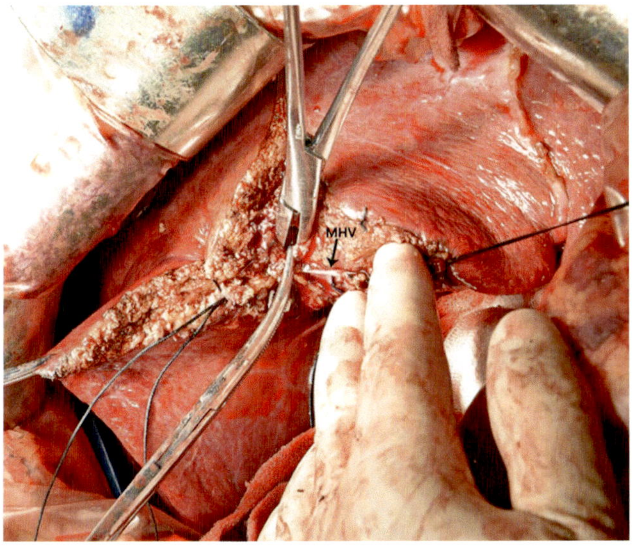

Fig. 100 Having clamped the infrahepatic inferior vena cava (IVC), and using Pringle maneuver (15 min of clamping and 5 min unclamping), left-sided hepatic parenchymal transection was carried out caudo-cranially

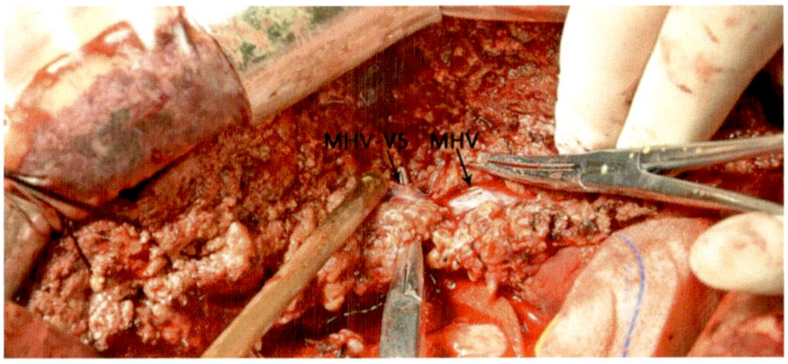

Fig. 101 Branch of the middle hepatic veins (MHV) draining the ventral portion of segment V was dissected

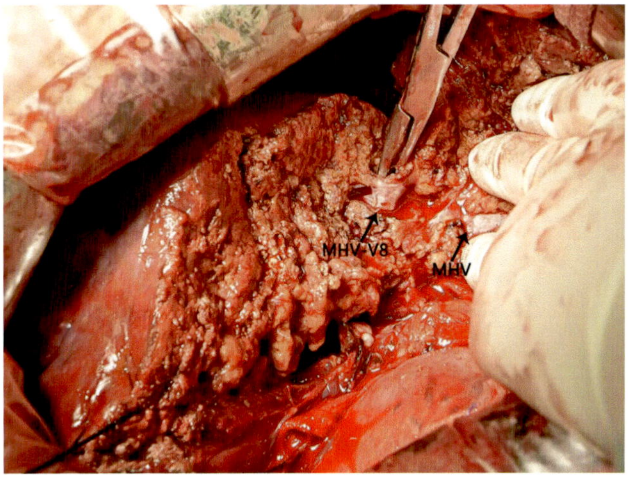

Fig. 102 Branch of the middle hepatic veins (MHV) draining the ventral portion of segment VIII was isolated, divided, and ligated

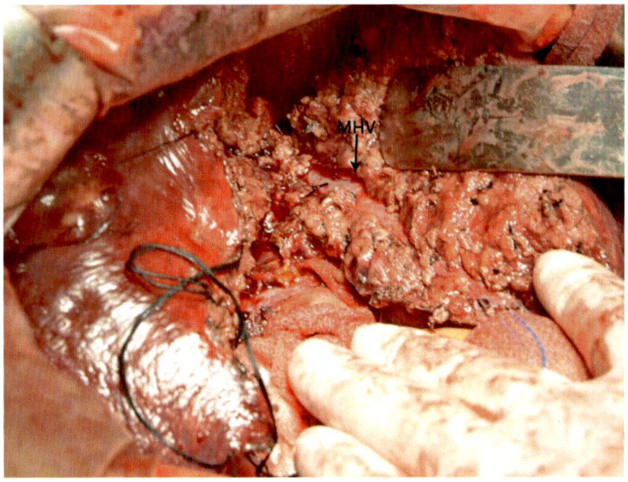

Fig. 103 Hepatic parenchyma around the root of the middle hepatic vein (MHV) was dissected, and the entry of the MHV into the suprahepatic inferior vena cava was exposed

Hepatic Parenchymal Transection (Right-Sided)
(Figs. 104, 105, 106, and 107)

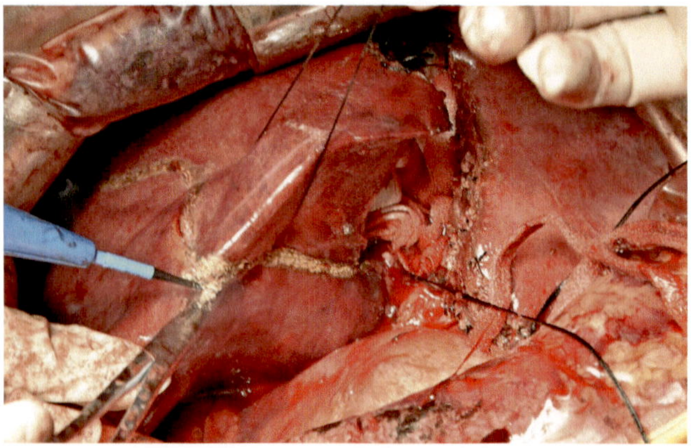

Fig. 104 Having clamped the infrahepatic vena cava and the right hepatic Glissonean pedicle, the right-sided hepatic parenchymal transection was carried out caudo-cranially, using the clamp-crushing method

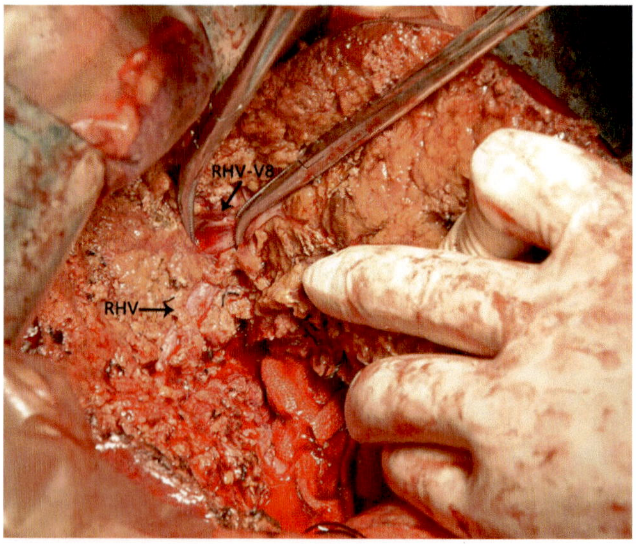

Fig. 106 Branch of the right hepatic veins (RHV) draining the dorsal portion of segment VIII was dissected

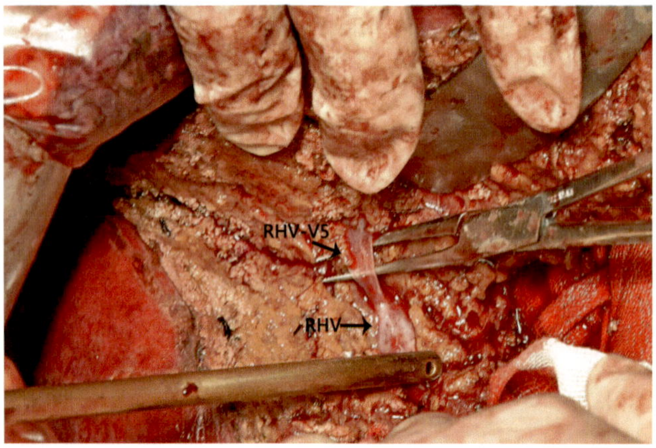

Fig. 105 Branch of the right hepatic veins (RHV) draining the dorsal portion of segment V was isolated, divided, and ligated

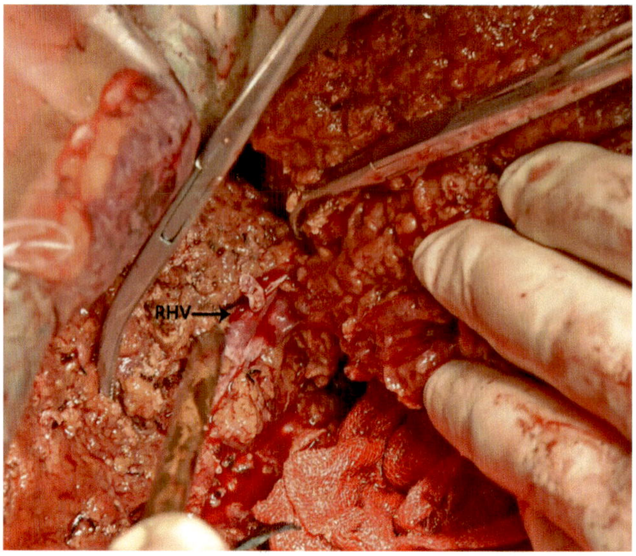

Fig. 107 Hepatic parenchyma around the root of the right hepatic vein (RHV) was dissected, and the entry of the RHV into the suprahepatic inferior vena cava (IVC) was exposed

Raw Area of the Residue Liver

(Figs. 108, 109, 110, and 111)

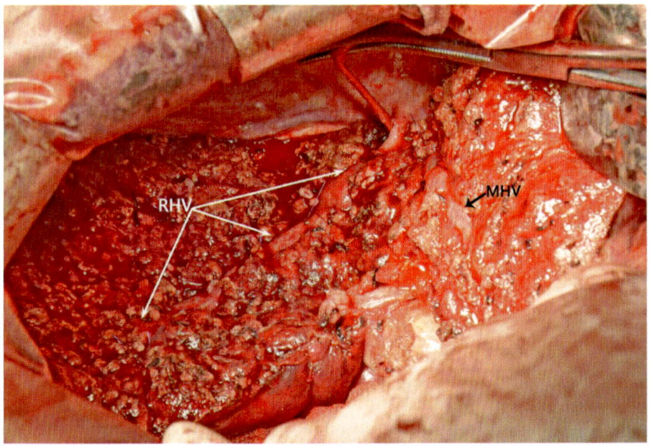

Fig. 108 Having removed the specimen, the whole course of the right hepatic vein (RHV) was obviously exposed on the right-sided cut surface. *MHV* middle hepatic vein

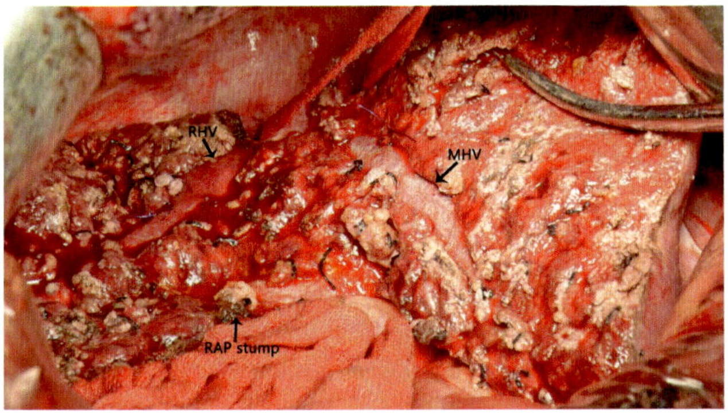

Fig. 109 The whole course of the middle hepatic vein (MHV) was also exposed on the left-sided raw area. Vascular and biliary ramifications on the both sided cut surface were carefully electrocauterized or suture-ligated. At last, the cut surface was covered with fibrin glue and gelatin sponge, and a tube was placed below the right subphrenic space and into the Winslow hole, respectively. *RHV* right hepatic vein, *RAP stump* stump of right anterior pedicle

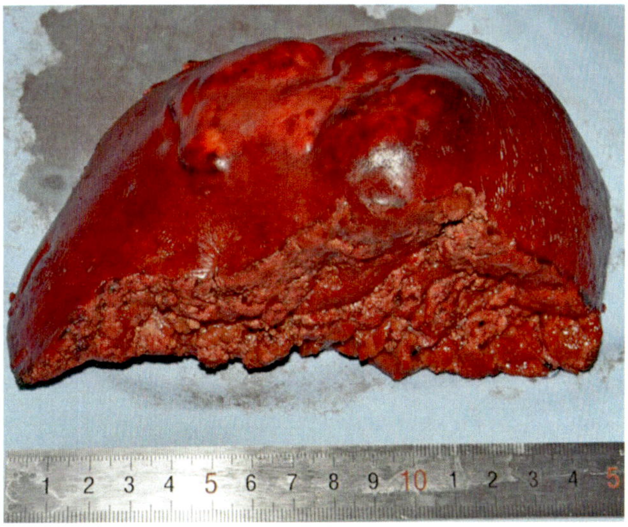

Fig. 110 Anterior view of the specimen

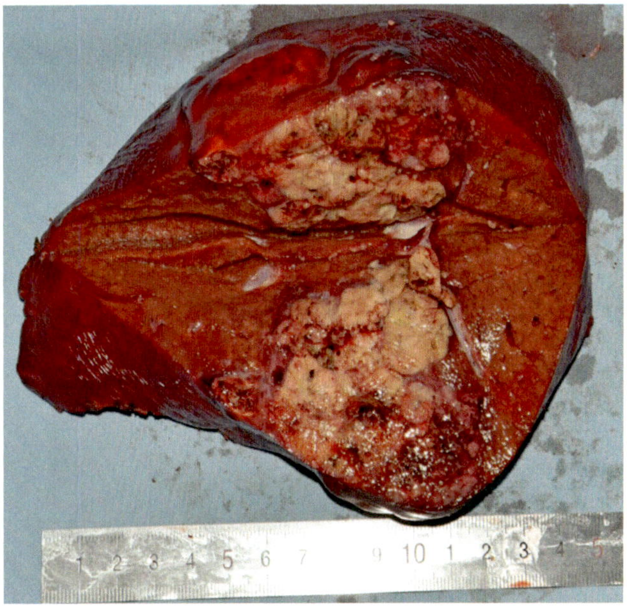

Fig. 111 Middle split surface of the specimen. The tumor occupied a part of both segments V and VIII

Right Posterior Sectionectomy (S6 + S7 Resection)

Jixiong Hu, Yinhuai Wang, and Jilong Wang

Right posterior sectionectomy (RPS) (anatomical resection of segments VI and VII) consists of removing segments VI and VII, which lie behind the right hepatic vein (RHV) and account for about 1/3 of the total liver volume. Right hepatectomy would traditionally be the treatment of choice for tumor located adjacent to the RHV in order to optimize tumor resection margin [52]. It has been generally accepted that posthepatectomy liver failure (PHLF) is the most severe complication occurring after hepatic resection due to poor liver reserves [53]. The sacrifice of non-cancerous segments V and VIII in RH could possibly reduce about 15–20% of the total liver volume [54]; theoretically, RPS is more preferred over RH with reference to reducing postoperative liver failure [55].

Surgical Indications

Patients were excluded if (A) the tumor was just only located in segment VI or VII; (B) the tumor was not a solitary lesion, and (C) the tumor had previous rupture. The surgical indications and procedures for resection of right posterior sector lesions were determined on the basis of the tumor-vasculature relationship and future remnant liver reserve. Generally, in terms of the location of the tumor, patients with tumor occupying both segments VI and VII or tumor infiltrating the Glissonean sheath proximal to the bifurcation of segment VI or VII branch were potential candidates for RPS.

Routine preoperative assessment includes cardiopulmonary evaluation, anesthetic evaluation, and review of the general condition of the patient. Imaging evaluation included abdominal ultrasound, high-resolution and contrast-enhanced computed tomography (CT), and/or magnetic resonance imaging. Hepatic function was evaluated by Child-Pugh scoring [56] and the indocyanine green retention rate at 15 min (ICGR 15) [5]. RPS was considered in patients with a left lobe ESLV (estimated liver volume) smaller than 30% and ICGR 15 smaller than 20%. The relationship between the tumor and the right hepatic vein should be discreetly evaluated preoperatively and must be kept intact. The surgical procedures included the right posterior pedicle isolation and division, mobilization of the right hemiliver, looping and hanging of the right hepatic vein, parenchymal transection, and management of the cut surface.

Indications for Methylene Blue Staining

Methylene blue injection was indicated when the tumor was not associated with macroscope portal vein thrombosis that is identified in the preoperative CT [57, 58]. When the right posterior pedicle was clamped, the boundary of ischemic demarcation too only appeared on the liver surface. It is well known that the morphology of hepatic segment is not regular and that the intersegmental plane of the liver has an uneven or curved surface [59, 60]; therefore, based only along the ischemic demarcation line on the liver surface, it is difficult to perform appropriate and precise anatomical hepatic transection. By injecting methylene blue through the feeding portal vein to achieve continuous methylene blue staining within the target segment(s), this method can achieve an obvious target segment boundary within hepatic parenchyma. Thus, the hepatic parenchyma transectional plane can be identified according to the range of staining within the liver parenchyma to improve the precision of anatomical hepatic resection.

Operative Procedures	Technical Details
Laparotomy ↓	◂A right subcostal incision.
Mobilization of the right hemiliver ↓	◂The perihepatic ligaments were divided and the right adrenal gland was dissected away from the right hemiliver, and the retrohepatic short veins were divided and ligated individually up to the root of the right hepatic vein (RHV). The RHV was extrahepatically isolated, looped and handed.
Perihilar dissection and dye injection ↓	◂Using perihilarGlissonean approach, the right posterior pedicle was isolated and looped, and then, Methylene blue was injected into the right posterior pedicle, and thereafter, this pedicle was divided and suture-ligated. The demarcation line between the colorized area and normal color area was marked on the liver surface with electrocautery to decide the limit of hepatic parenchymal dissection.
Hepatic parenchymal transection ↓	◂Hepatic parenchymal dissection was undertaken from the anterior and inferior liver surface posteriorly towards the IVC and superiorly towards the hepatocaval confluence along the demarcation line by a clamp crushing method. All large branches of the RHV were divided and ligated individually. The whole course of the RHV was fully exposed.
Drainage and closure of the abdominal cavity	◂A tube was placed below the right subphrenic space and secured with silk-suture.

Intraoperative Key Points

1. Right posterior sectionectomy is a technically demanding hepatectomy for which the demarcation of the liver territory to be resected is advocated. Theoretically, having transecting the right posterior pedicle, an ischemic demarcation area for the posterior section can be obtained on the liver surface, and this ischemic demarcating line corresponds to the right portal scissura. However, having clamped the right hepatic pedicle, the ischemic demarcation boundary disappeared between the right anterior and posterior sections within the liver parenchyma because the whole right hemiliver is under ischemic condition. The advantage of staining the target segment(s) by injecting methylene blue into the feeding portal vein can improve the precision of anatomical resection based on the range of liver tissue staining within the hepatic parenchyma.
2. Attention should be paid to the variations in anatomy of the portal vein branches in the hilar area. The main portal vein is divided into right anterior and posterior portal veins and the left portal branch at the same level. This type variant is the commonest type [44, 45]. Under such a variant type, in order to escape subsequent stricture occurring in the main portal vein that results from transection of the right posterior pedicle, it is recommended to transect the RSP distal to its origin. In addition, we also should take care of anther variant type of the right posterior portal vein. This variant type is that the right posterior vein arises directly from the main portal vein as its first branch below the hepatic hilum [44, 45]. While transecting the RSP, caution should be taken to prevent causing injury to the main trunk of the portal vein.
3. Long clamping time could be considered potential cause of postoperative complications [61–63]. To reduce ischemic-reperfusion injury, Pringle maneuver should be avoided in performing RPS. Transection of the RSP and/or clamping of the right hepatic pedicle is an effective measure to control bleeding during parenchymal proceedings. In case of severe venous backflow bleeding from the RHV, the root of the RHV can be clamped, especially while performing parenchymal transection near to the hepatocaval confluence (Fig. 112).

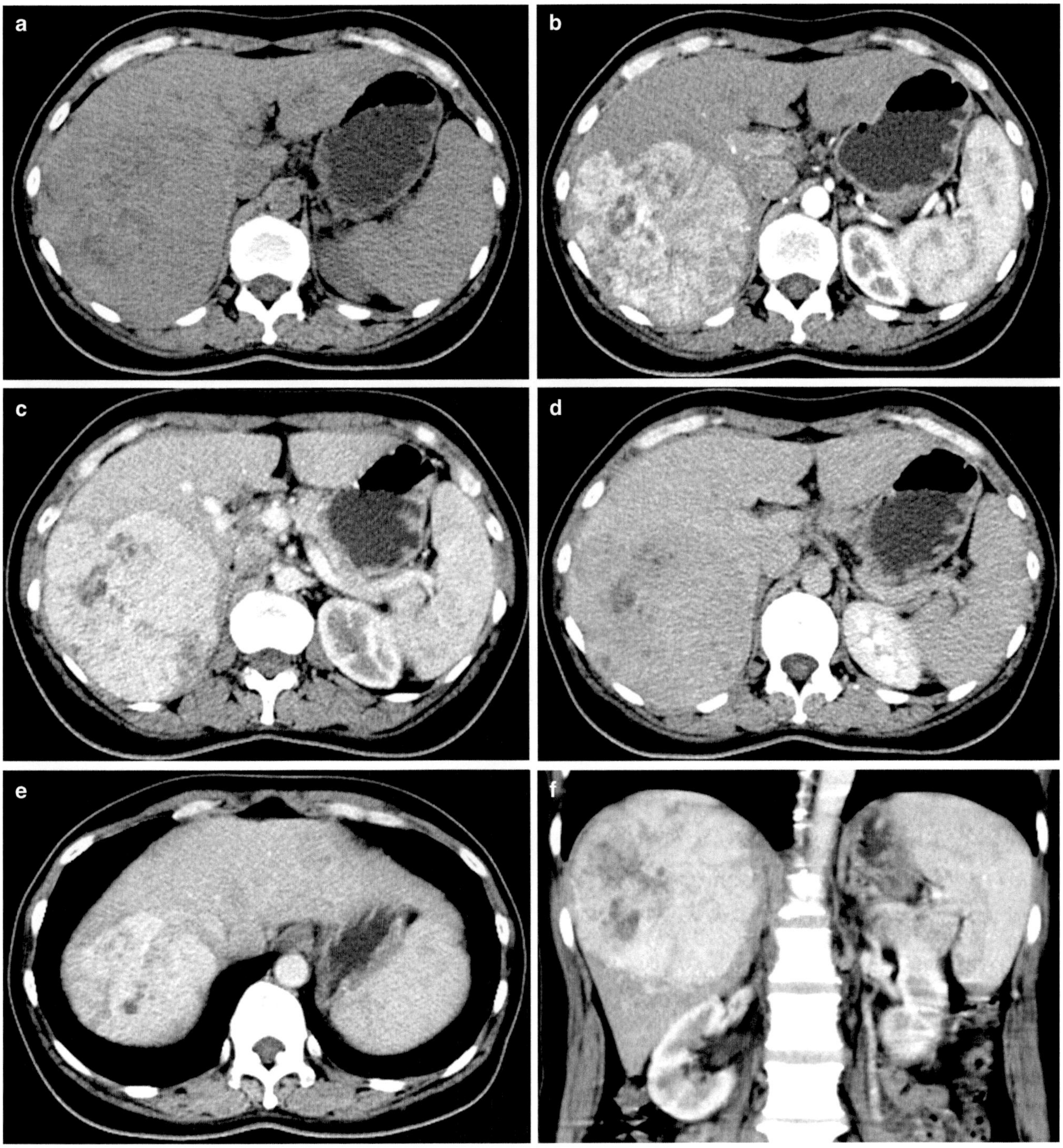

Fig. 112 (**a**) Preoperative CT (precontrast). The tumor, which appears isodense or slightly hypodense compared to the liver, is located at segments VI and VII. (**b**) Preoperative CT (hepatic arterial phase). The tumor shows heterogeneous enhancement. (**c**) Preoperative CT (hepatic venous phase). The tumor shows enhancement fades. (**d**) Preoperative CT (interstitial phase). The tumor shows markedly hypodense due to washout. (**e**) Preoperative CT. Right hepatic vein (RHV) is adjacent to the tumor but not infiltrated by the tumor. (**f**) Preoperative CT (coronal section of the tumor)

Abdominal Incision and Mobilization of the Liver
(Figs. 113, 114, 115, 116, 117, 118, 119, 120, and 121)

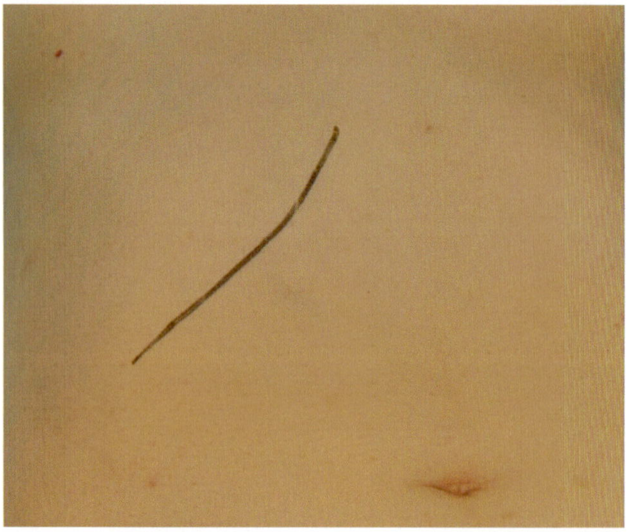

Fig. 113 A right subcostal incision was selected and made

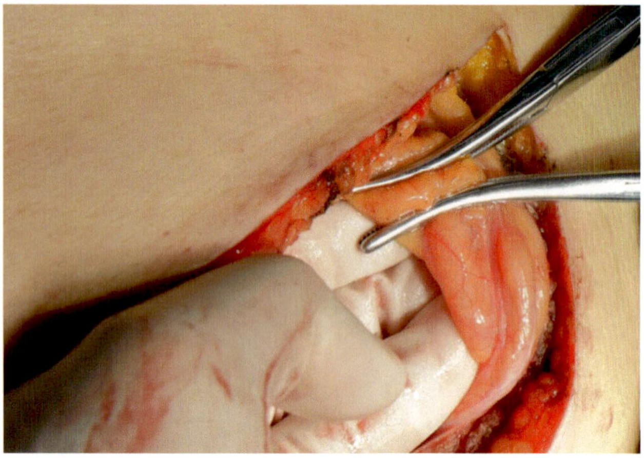

Fig. 114 Having entered into the abdominal cavity, the round ligament was divided and ligated

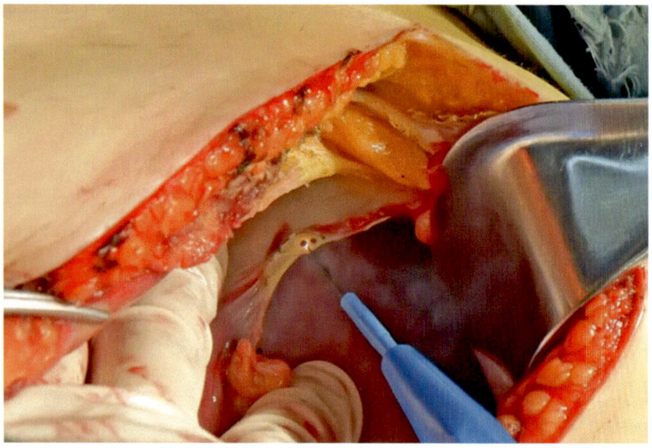

Fig. 115 The falciform ligament was electrocauterized near to the liver surface

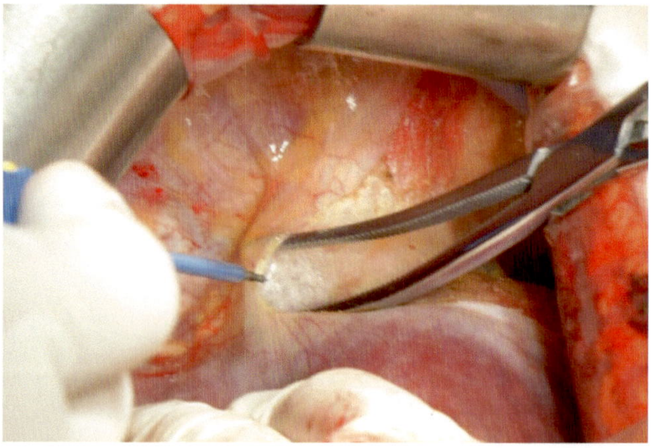

Fig. 116 Hepatocaval confluence was dissected to expose the entry site of the hepatic veins into the suprahepatic inferior vena cava (IVC)

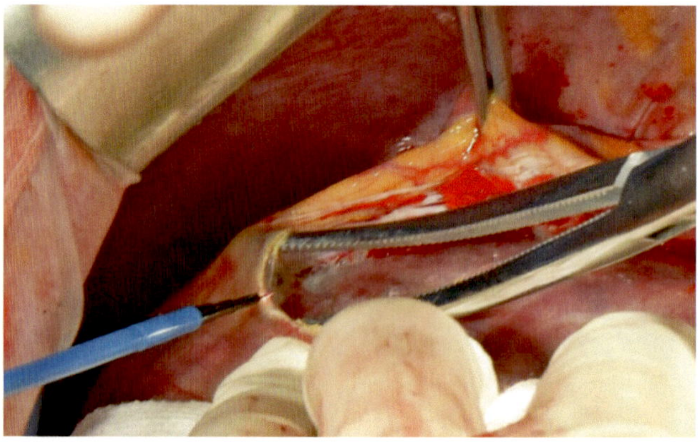

Fig. 117 The right coronary ligament was divided with electrocautery

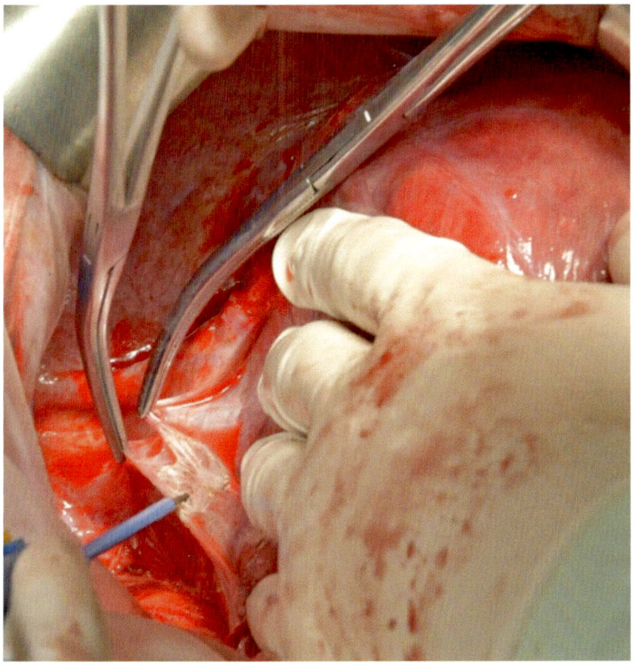

Fig. 118 The anterior layer of the right triangular ligament was dissected

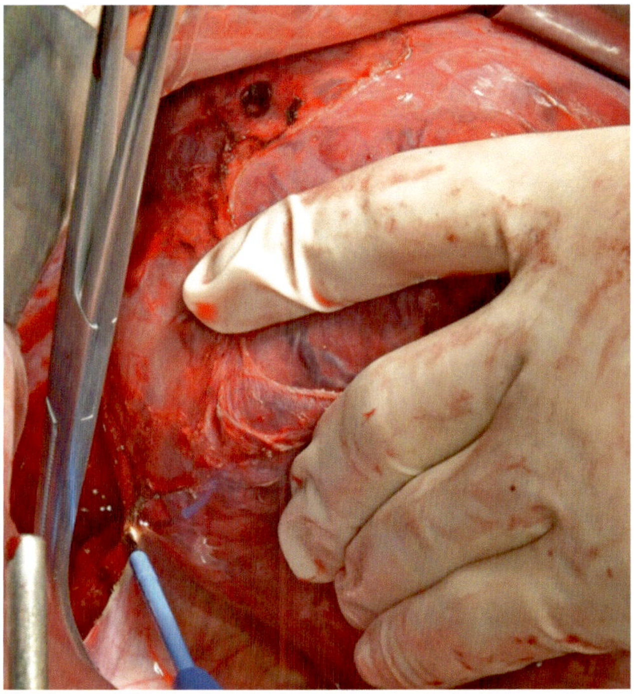

Fig. 119 The posterior layer of the right triangular ligament was electrocauterized

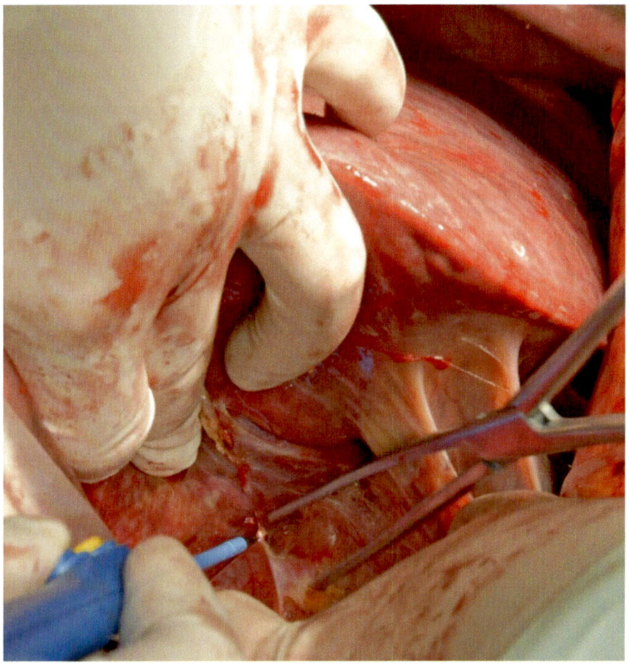

Fig. 120 Hepatocolic ligament was divided

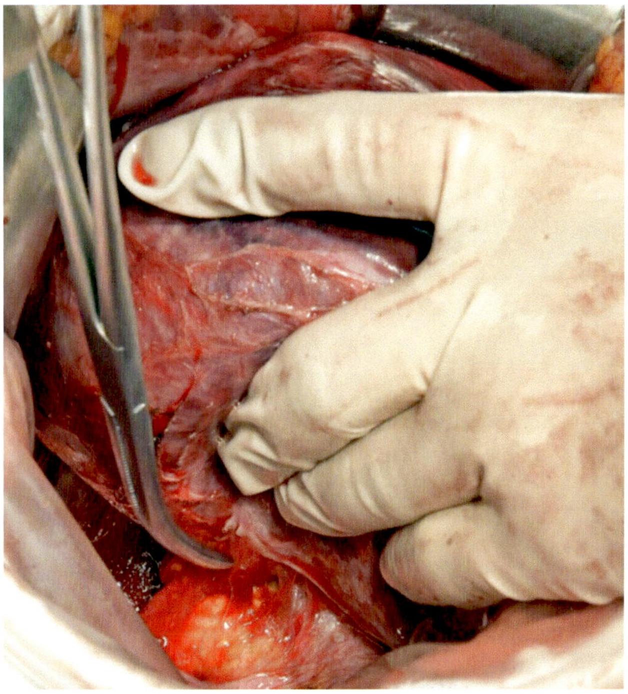

Fig. 121 The right adrenal gland was dissected away from the right hemiliver

Isolation of the RHV and IVC

(Figs. 122, 123, 124, 125, and 126)

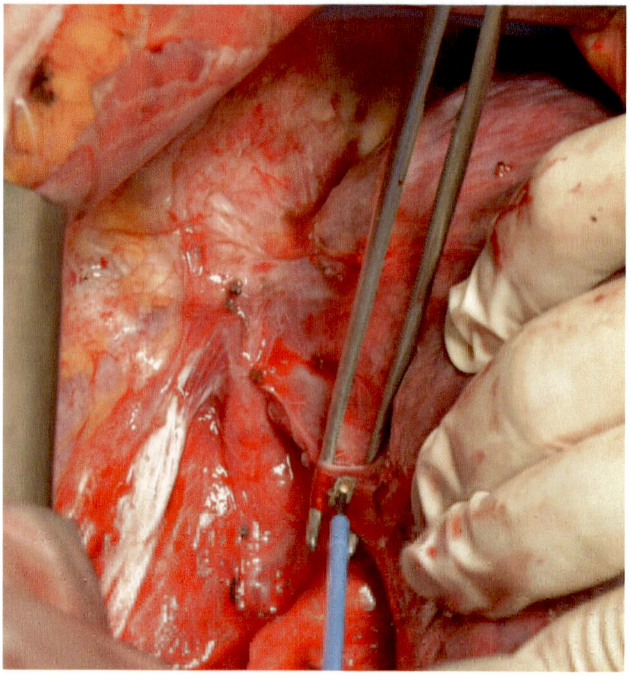

Fig. 122 The hepatocaval ligament was isolated and electrocauterized

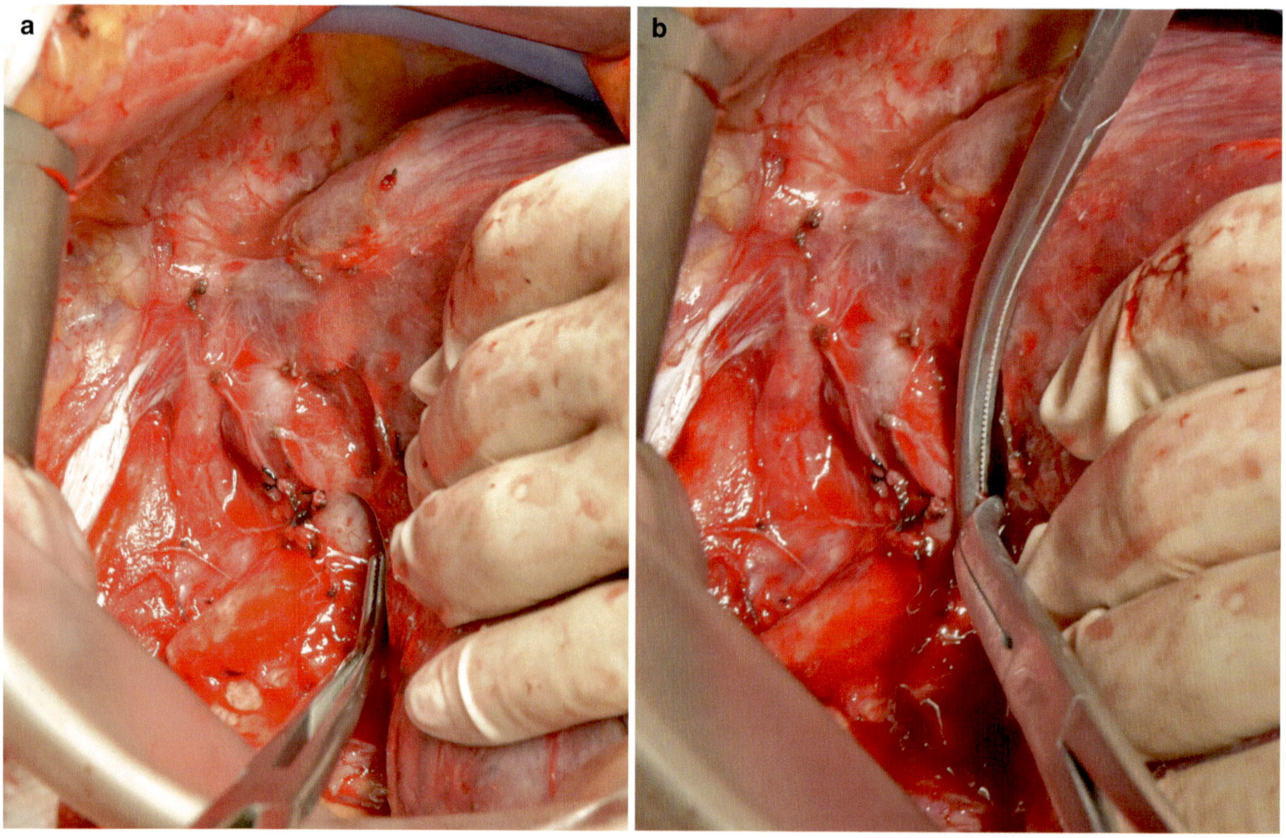

Fig. 123 (**a**, **b**) The retrohepatic short veins were divided and ligated individually

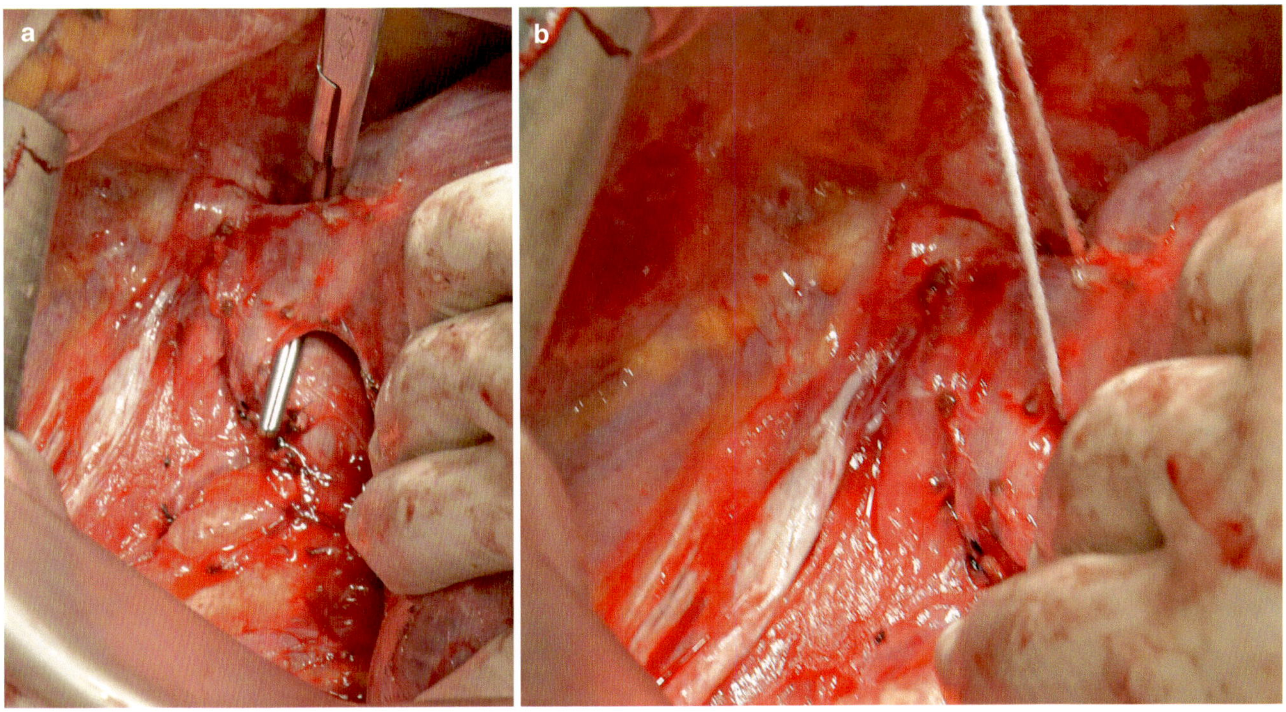

Fig. 124 (**a**, **b**) The right hepatic vein (RHV) was isolated and encircled with a tourniquet

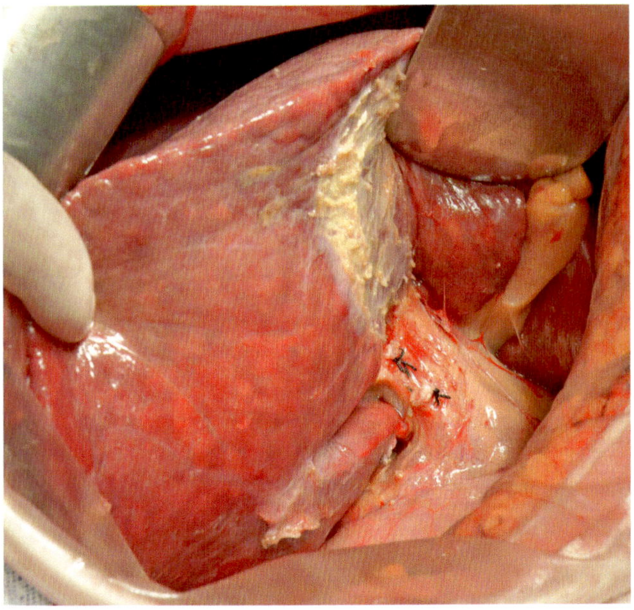

Fig. 125 Cholecystectomy was performed

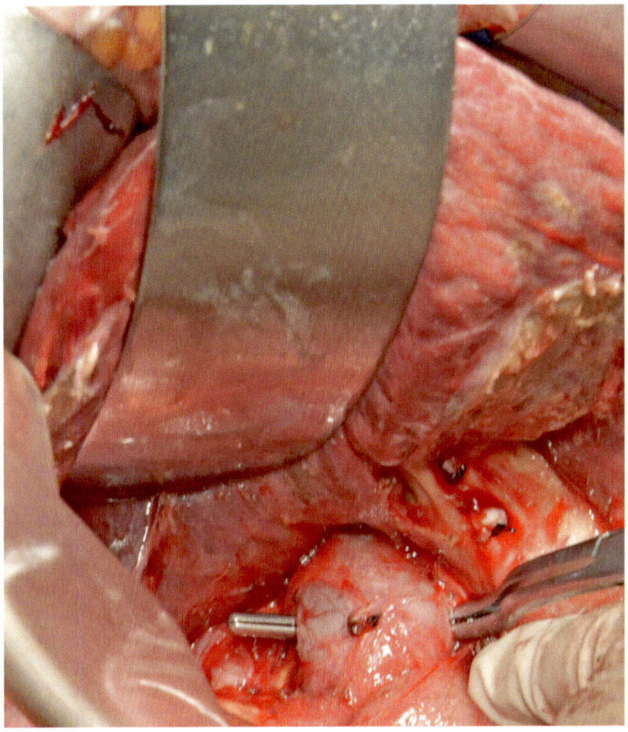

Fig. 126 The infrahepatic inferior vena cava was isolated and pre-placed with a loop

Isolation of the Right Hepatic Pedicle (RHP)
(Figs. 127, 128, and 129)

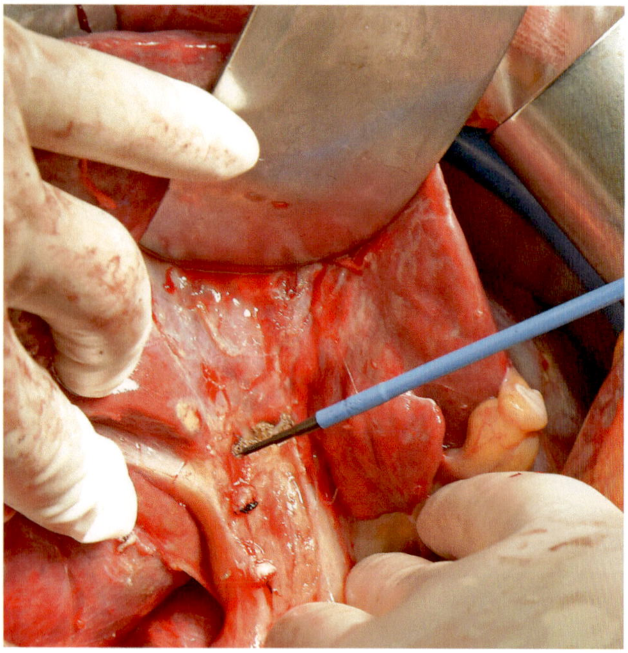

Fig. 127 One small incision was made in front of the hilus

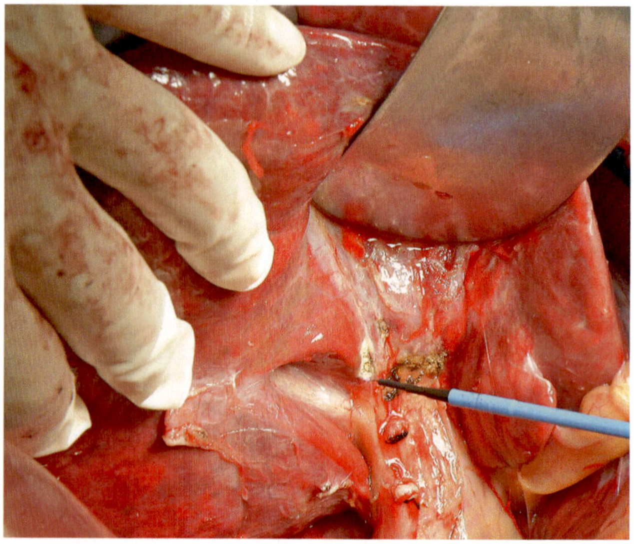

Fig. 128 Another incision was made at the right edge of the gallbladder bed

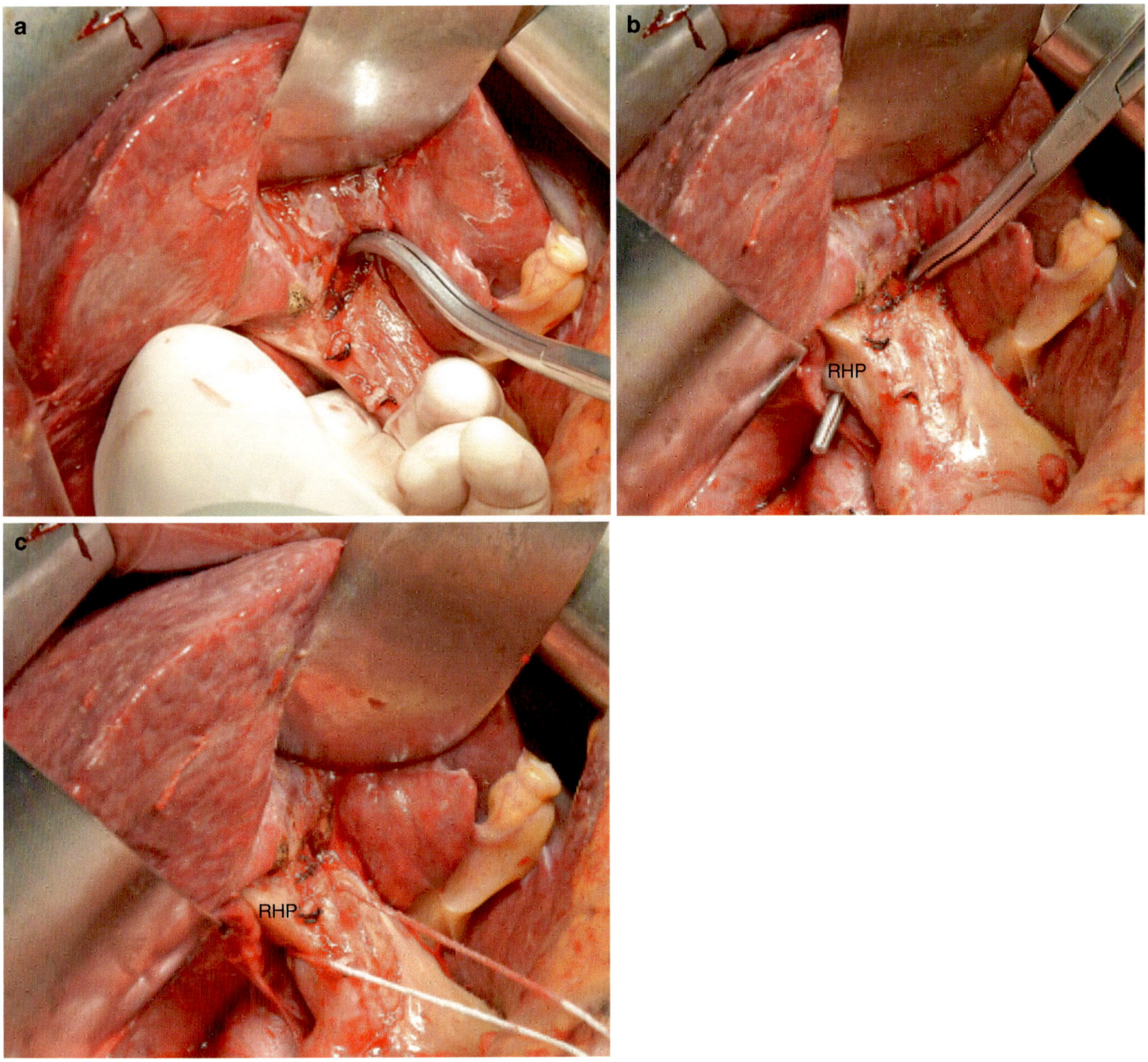

Fig. 129 (**a**) A large curved clamp was inserted into this incision in front of the hilus, and the operator's left index finger was put between the undersurface of the hilar plate and the anterior wall of the retrohepatic inferior vena cava, and then, using the index finger as a guide, (**b**) the clamp was inserted furtherly and directly reached to the tip of the finger and punctured through the undersurface membrane and passed out of the right edge of the right hepatic pedicle. (**c**) Thus, the right hepatic Glissonean pedicle was isolated and encircled with a loop

Isolation of the Right Posterior Pedicle (RPP)
(Fig. 130)

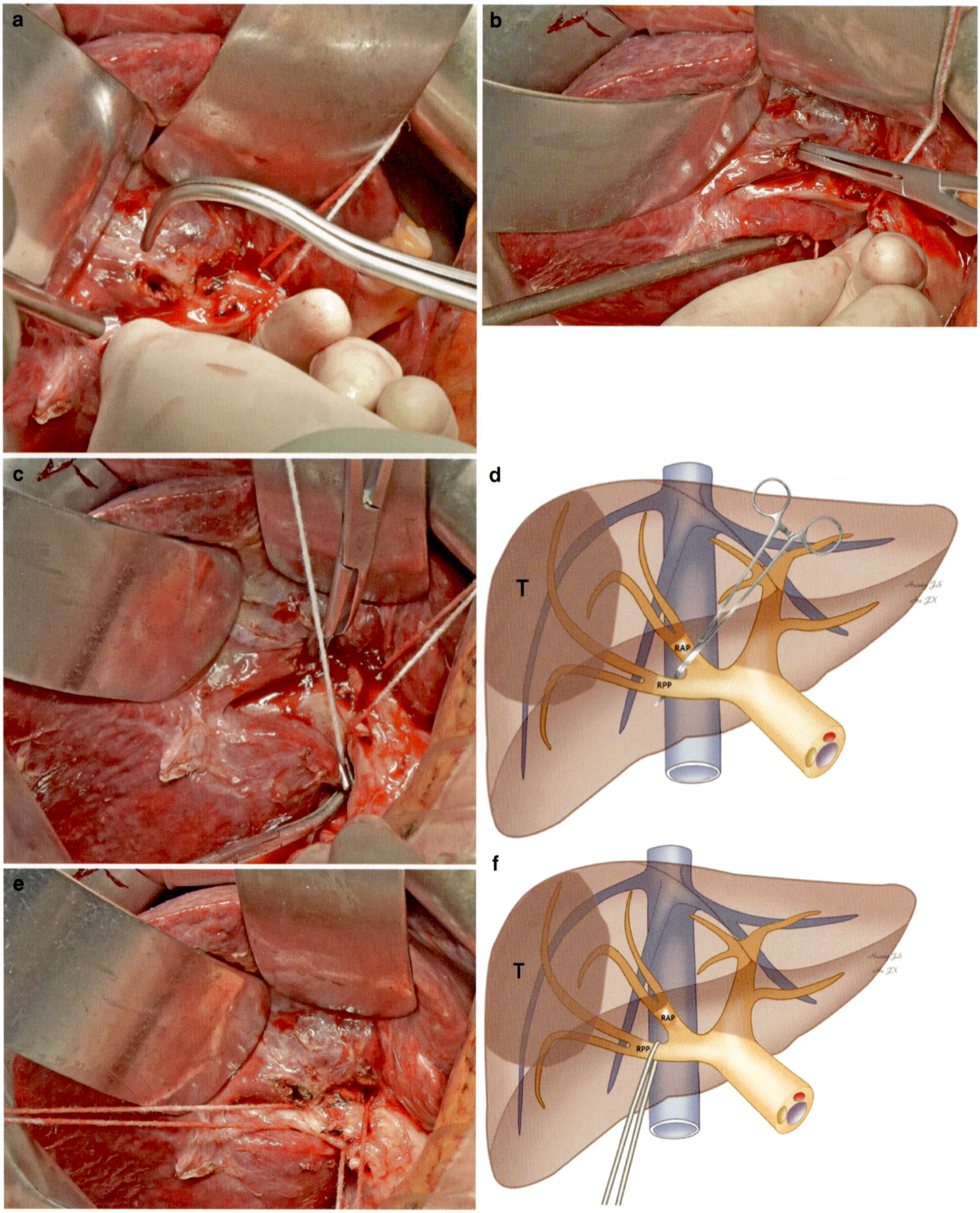

Fig. 130 (**a**) A large curved clamp was inserted into the incision at the right edge of the gallbladder, and meanwhile, the operator's left index finger was placed below the undersurface of the right hepatic pedicle. (**b**) Using the finger as a guide, the clamp was inserted downward and directly reached down to the fingertip and passed out of the right edge of the right hepatic pedicle. (**c**, **e**) Thus, the right posterior Glissonean pedicle was isolated and encircled with a tourniquet. (**d** and **f**) Schematic illustration of this procedure. *RPP* right posterior sectional pedicle, *RAP* right anterior sectional pedicle

Staining of the Right Posterior Sector
(Figs. 131 and 132)

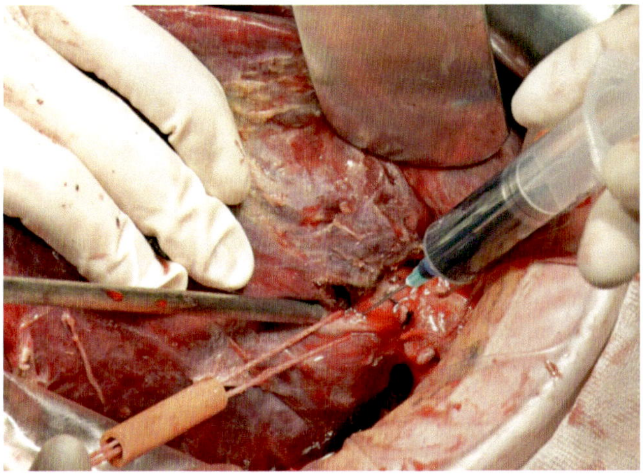

Fig. 131 Methylene blue was injected into the portal trunk of the right posterior sector

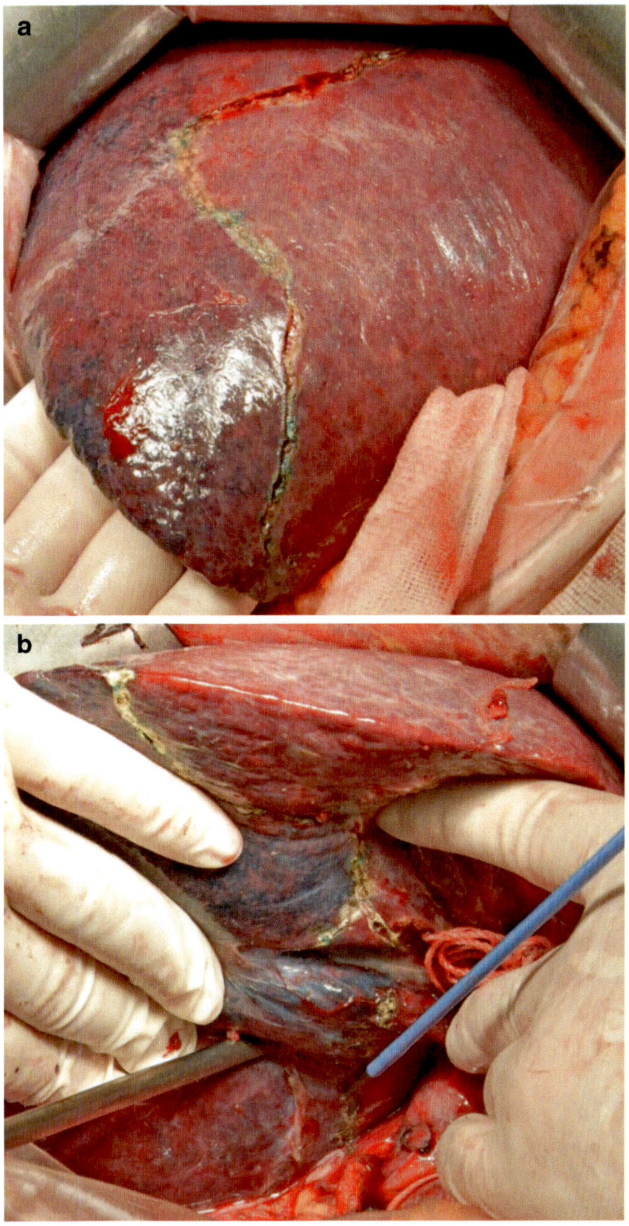

Fig. 132 (**a**, **b**) The right posterior sector was colorized. Along the demarcation line, the parenchymal transection line was marked on the liver surface with electrocautery

Division of the Right Posterior Pedicle (Fig. 133)

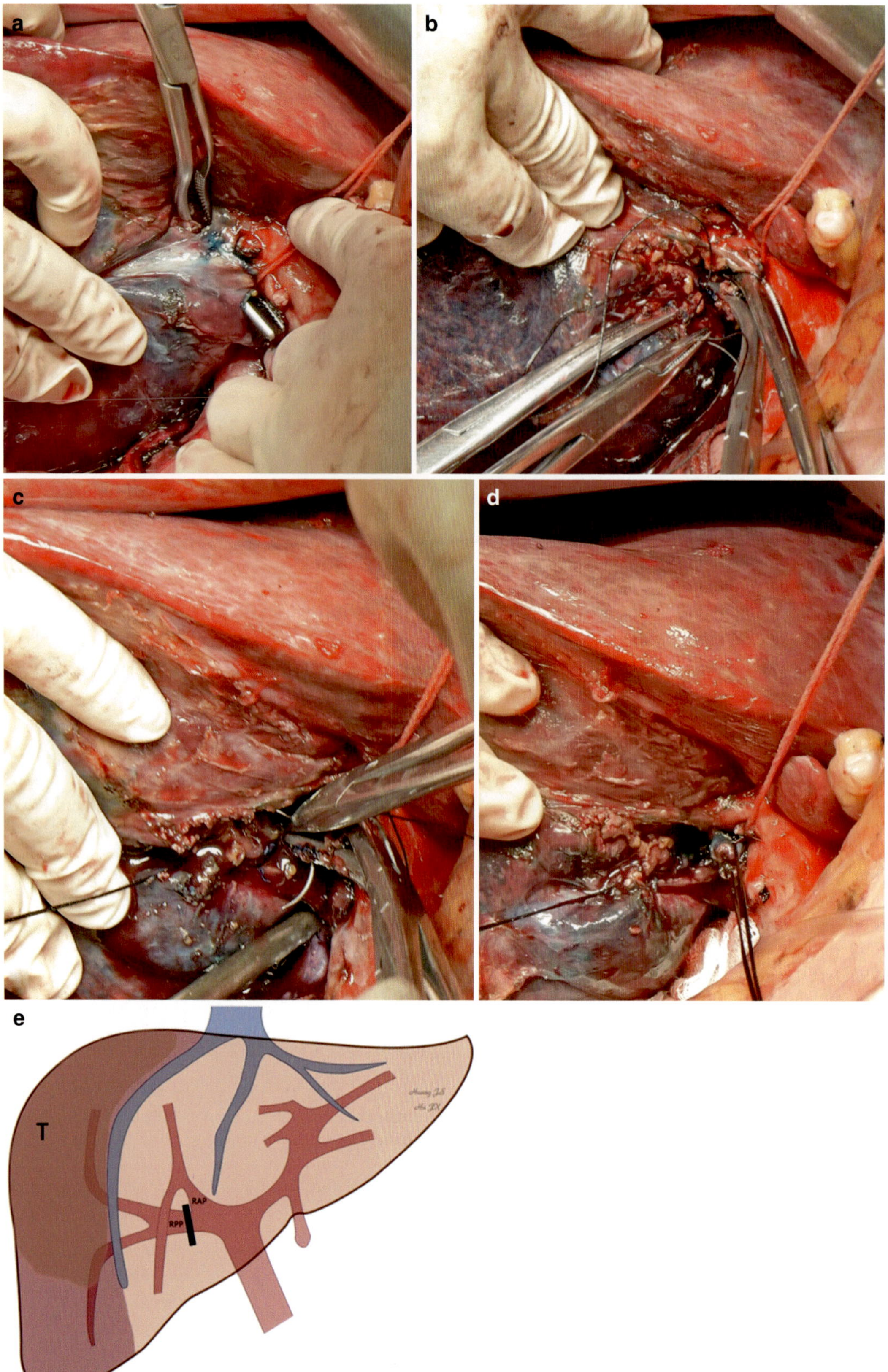

Fig. 133 (**a**–**d**) The right posterior Glissonean pedicle was isolated (**a**), clamped (**b**), divided, and suture-ligated (**c**, **d**). (**e**) Schematic illustration of this procedure. *RPP* right posterior sectional pedicle, *RAP* right anterior sectional pedicle

Hepatic Parenchymal Transection
(Figs. 134, 135, 136, 137, and 138)

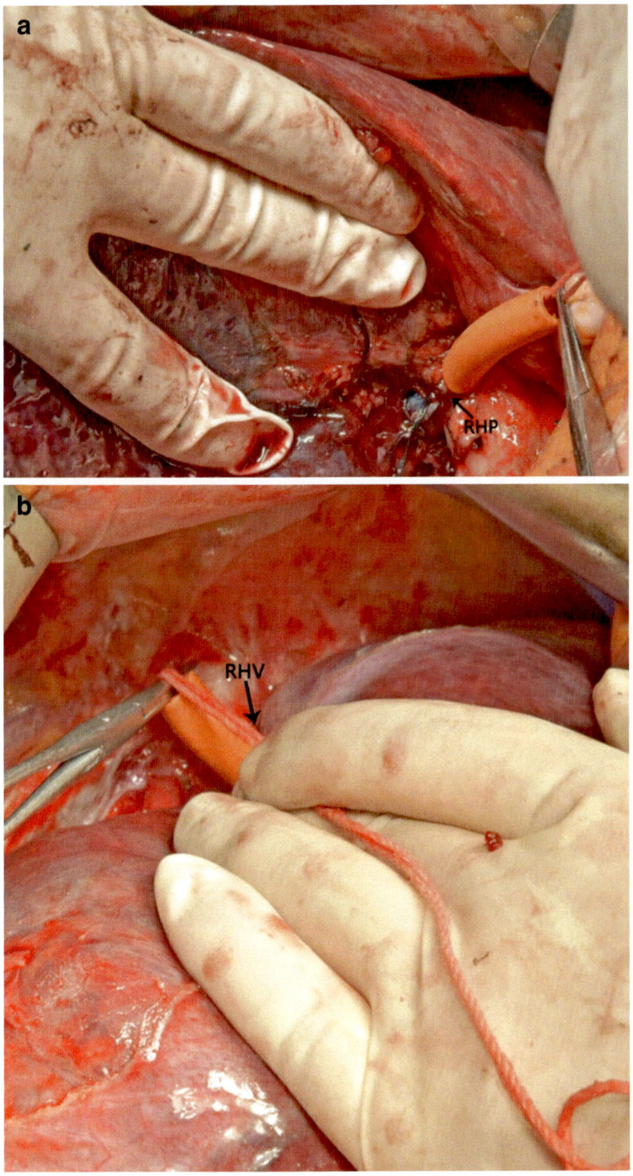

Fig. 134 (**a**, **b**) Prior to hepatic parenchymal dissection, the right hepatic pedicle (RHP) (**a**) and the right hepatic vein (RHV) (**b**) were clamped, respectively, to reduce bleeding during transecting proceedings

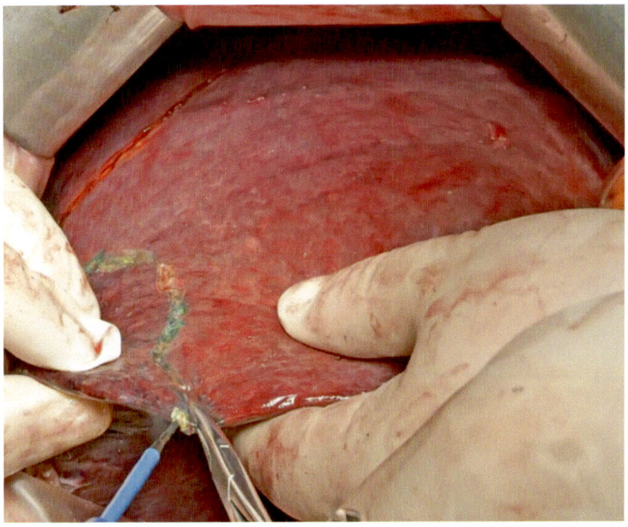

Fig. 135 Parenchymal transection was carried out caudo-cranially along the ischemic line, using the clamp-crushing method

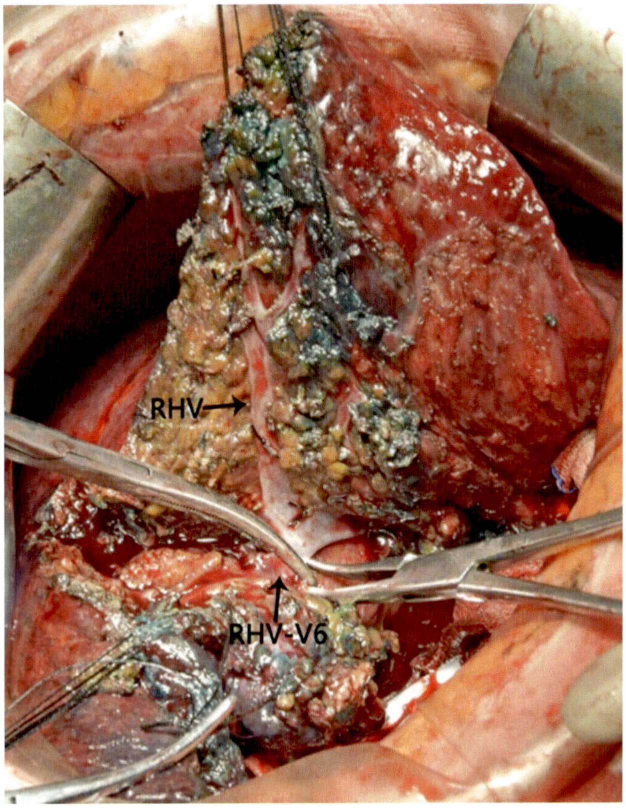

Fig. 136 Branch of the right hepatic vein (RHV) draining segment VI was isolated, divided, and ligated

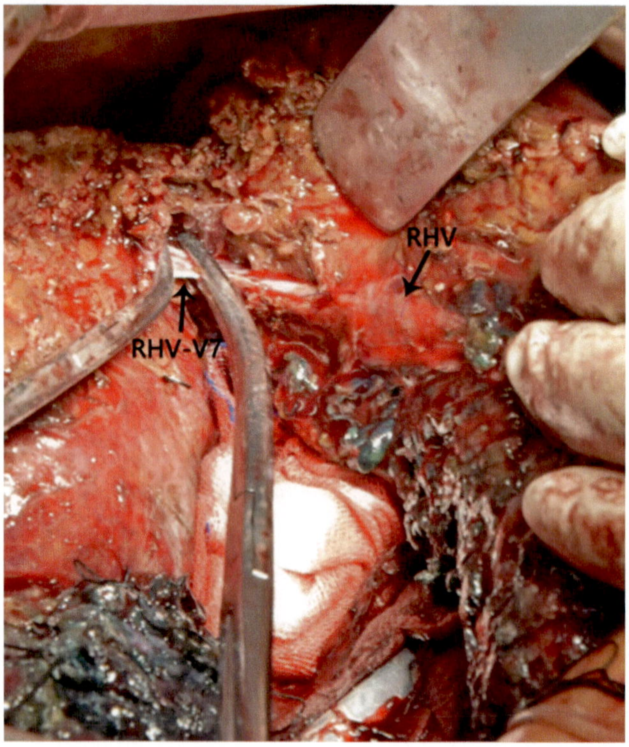

Fig. 137 Branch of the right hepatic vein (RHV) draining segment VII was dissected

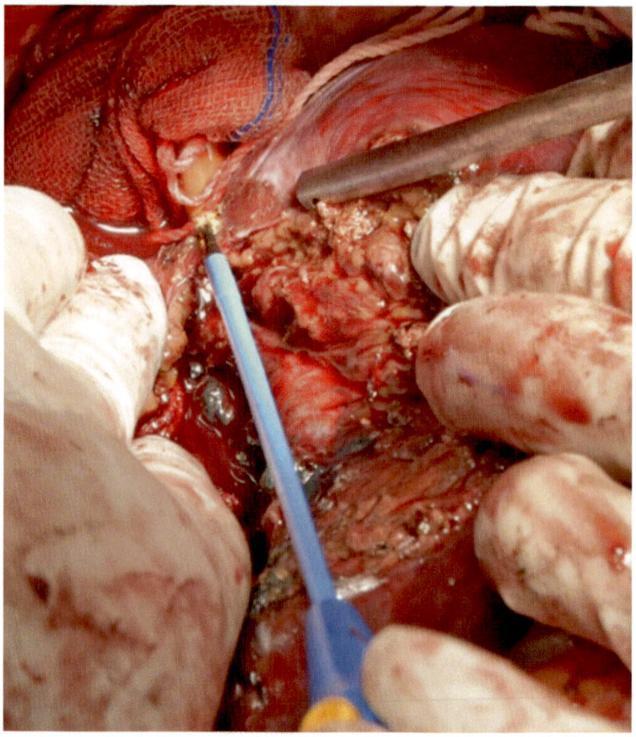

Fig. 138 The hepatic parenchyma around the root of the right hepatic vein (RHV) was dissected to remove the specimen and expose the entry of the RHV into the suprahepatic inferior vena cava (IVC)

Raw Area of the Residue Liver and Specimen
(Figs. 139, 140, 141, and 142)

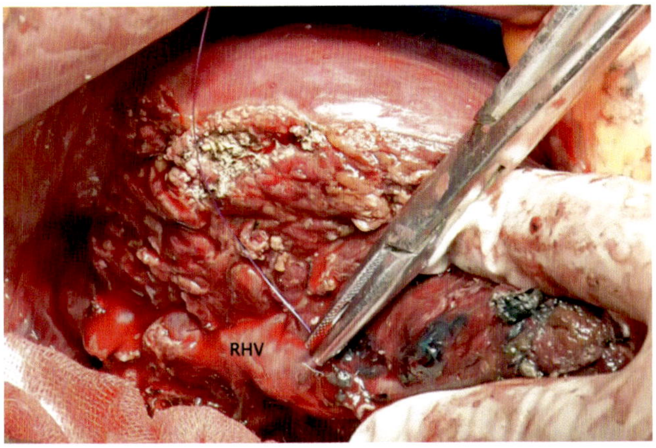

Fig. 139 Having removed the specimen and unclamped the right hepatic pedicle and the right hepatic vein (RHV), the vascular and biliary ramifications on the resectional surface of the residual liver were sutured with silk thread and/or polypropylene 1–0 and/or 2–0, and the tiny holes on the right hepatic vein were repaired with 4–0 and 5–0 polypropylene. *IVC* inferior vena cava

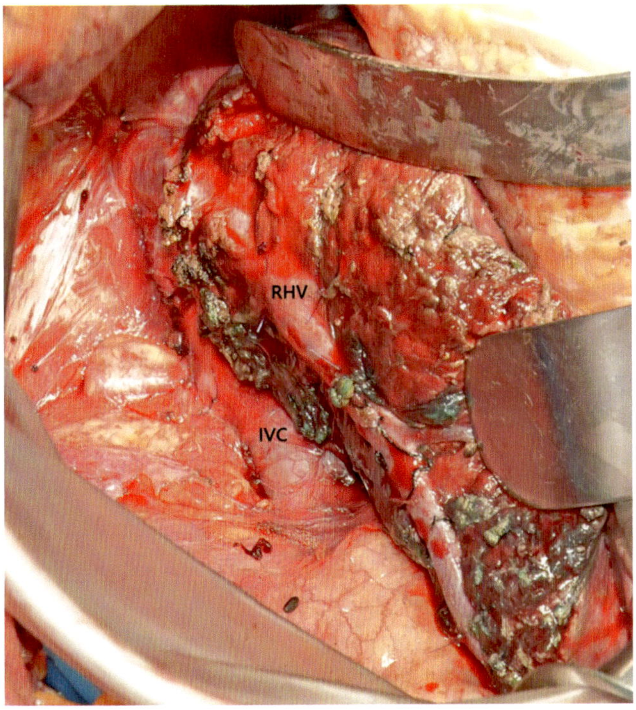

Fig. 140 The whole course of the right hepatic vein was shown on the cut surface

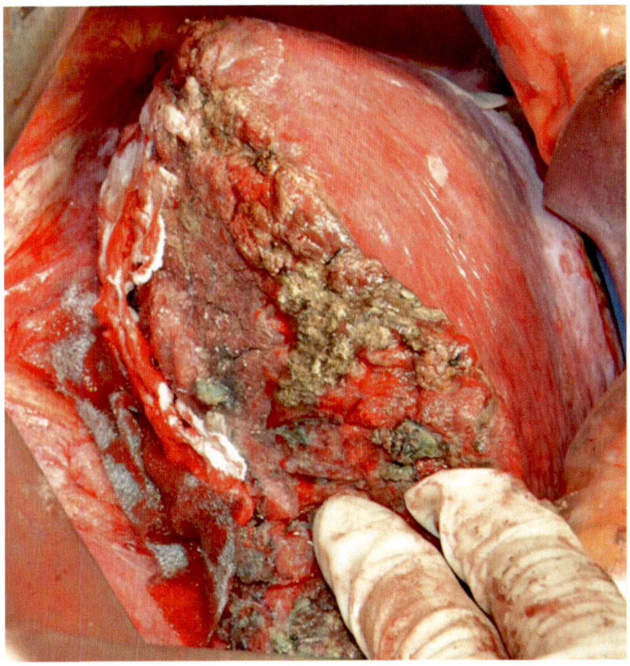

Fig. 141 The transection surface was covered with fibrin glue and other hemostatic agents. Always, a drain close to the liver section surface was used

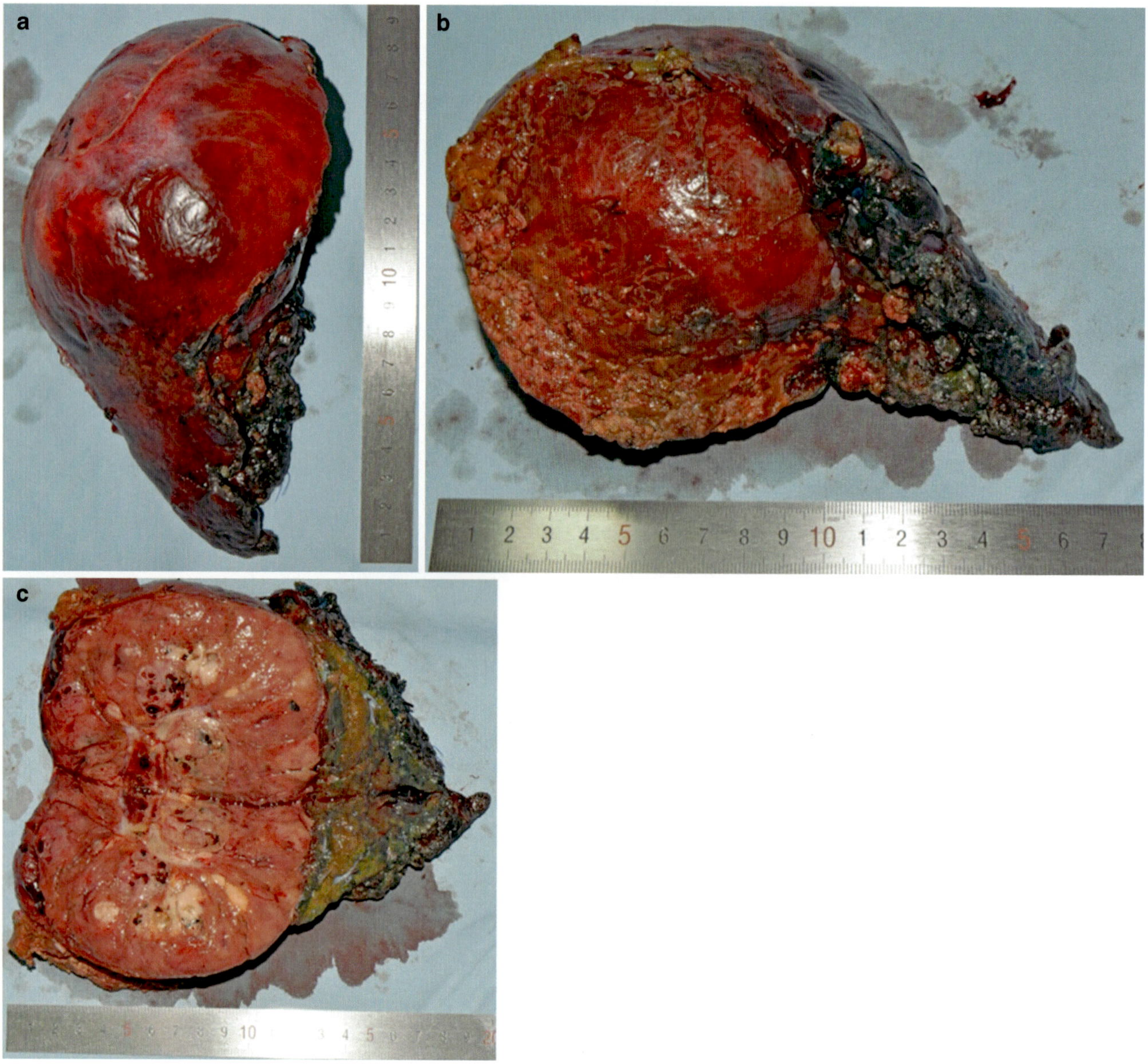

Fig. 142 The specimen. (**a**) Anterior surface. (**b**) Cut surface. (**c**) Split surface

Left Lateral Sectionectomy (S2 + S3 Resection)

Jixiong Hu, Xundi Xu, and Zhongkun Zuo

Surgical Indications for Left Lateral Sectionectomy

According to the Brisbane 2000 Terminology of Liver Anatomy and Resection [64], left lateral section corresponds to Couinaud segments II and III. Therefore, left lateral sectionectomy is referred to resection of segments II and III. Each of segments II and III accounted for <10% of total liver volume (TLV) in most persons [4]. The portal branches of segments II and III are small in number and have little anatomical variations [6]. The branching patterns of portal vein supplying segment II (P_2) and segment III (P_3) are as follows: P_2 arises from the cross of the left portal vein and Rex's recessus, and P_3 arises from the left angle of the cul-de-sac. Uncommon anatomical variations include a branch originating from the trunk of the umbilical portion of the portal vein or a common trunk formed by infusion of the two branches. Based on the relatively simple anatomical characteristics of segments II and III, a left lateral sectionectomy is a comparatively clear resection that is quite easily performed by transecting inflow and outflow structures intrahepatically or extrahepatically [27]. For tumors confined to segments II and III, left lateral sectionectomy is indicated for patients with preoperative serum total bilirubin level less than 1.0 mg/dl and ICGR15 less than 20% [65].

Hepatocellular carcinoma (HCC) is distinguished by its early venous invasion, which leads to form microscopic and then macroscopic portal vein tumor thrombus (PVTT) [66]. PVTT is a very important prognostic factor and predictor for postoperative early recurrence [67, 68]. According to the Barcelona Clinic Liver Cancer (BCLC) staging classification, sorafenib is the appropriate treatment modality for patients with HCC associated with macroscopic portal vein tumor thrombus (BCLC stage C) [69]. Liver resection is contraindicatated in HCC patients with Vp3 (tumor thrombus extension to the right or left portal vein) and Vp4 (tumor thrombus extension to the trunk of the portal vein or to the contralateral branch of the portal vein) and should be selected only for patients with small single tumors without portal hypertension or hyperbilirubinemia [30]. Nevertheless, liver resection for HCC with Vp1 (tumor thrombus confined to the segmental branch of the portal vein) and Vp2 (tumor thrombus confined to the sectional branch of the portal vein), combined with transarterial chemoembolization (TACE), was proposed in Japan Society of Hepatology (JSH) algorithm [70]. Up to now, many studies have reported that many patients inflicted by HCC with macroscopic PVTT have satisfactory prognosis following hepatectomy, in combination with either preoperative TACE or postoperative arterial infusion therapy [66, 71, 72]. In China, the treatment of choice for HCC with macroscopic PVTT is similar to the Japanese standard. For tumors located within the left lateral section and with macroscopic PVTT, the surgical indications are similar to that for the same located tumors without PVTT.

Isolated Left Lateral Sectionectomy (Fig. 143)

Operative Procedures	Technical Details
Laparotomy	◀ A right subcostal incision was made.
Mobilization of the left hemiliver	◀ The left hemiliver was freed off of its surrounding structures.
Isolation and division of the left hepatic vein	◀ The left hepatic vein was extrahepatically isolated, clamped, divided and suture-ligated.
Division of the pedicle of segment 3(S_3-P)	◀ The pedicle of segment 3 was extrahepatically isolated, clamped, divided and suture-ligated.
Parenchymal transection and Division of the the pedicle of segment 2(S_2-P)	◀ Parenchymal transection was carried out caudal-cranially along the cut line. The pedicle of segment 2 was intrahepatically isolated, clamped, divided and secured.

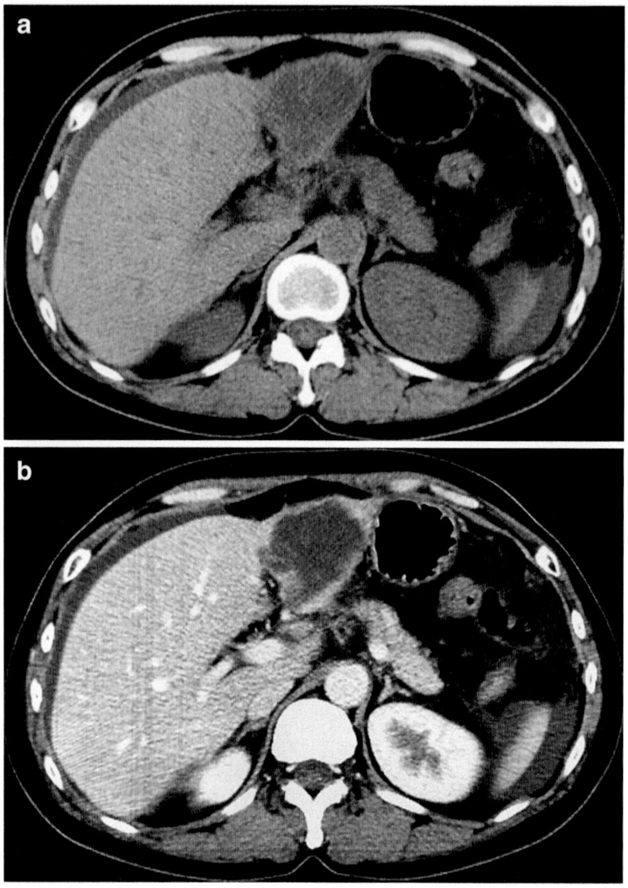

Fig. 143 (**a**) Preoperative CT (precontrast). The tumor, which appears hypodense, is located in the left lateral lobe. (**b**) Preoperative CT (hepatic venous phase). The tumor shows prominently hypodense due to less enhancement

A Right Subcostal Incision and Mobilization of the Left Hemiliver (Figs. 144, 145, 146, 147, 148, 149, 150, and 151)

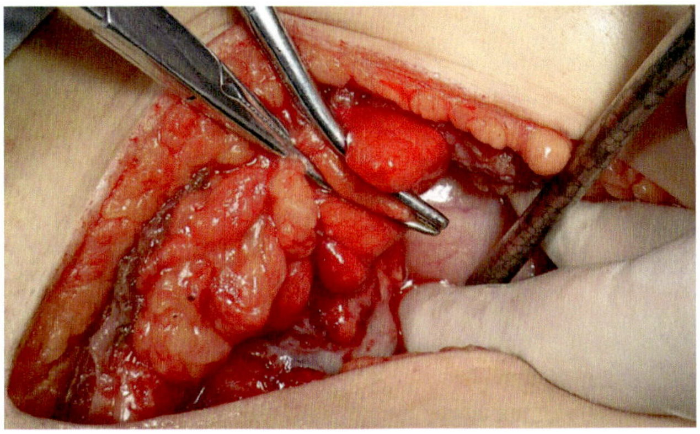

Fig. 144 The round ligament was divided

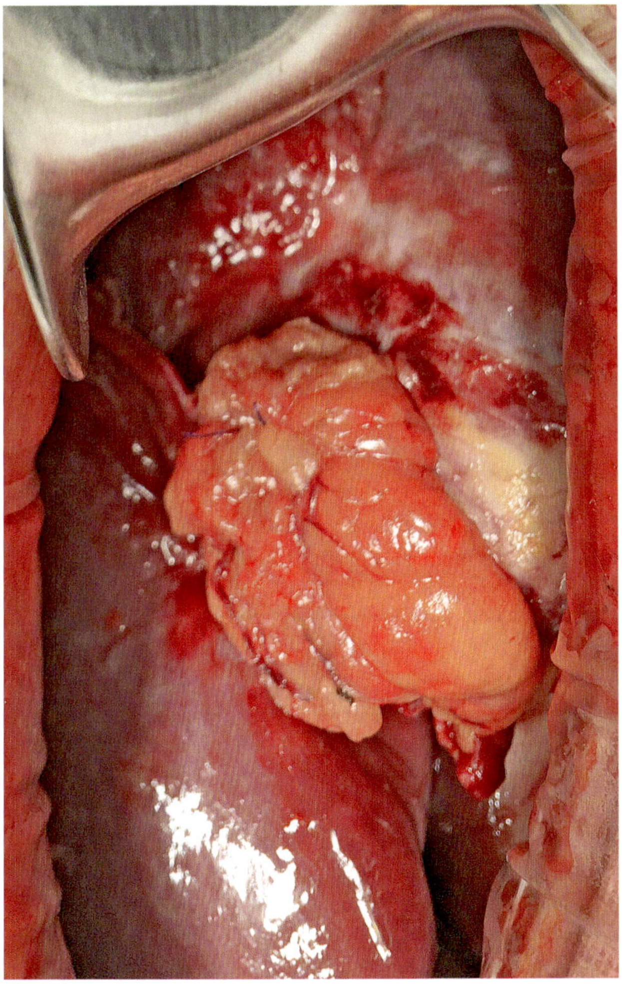

Fig. 145 The tumor was located within segments II and III

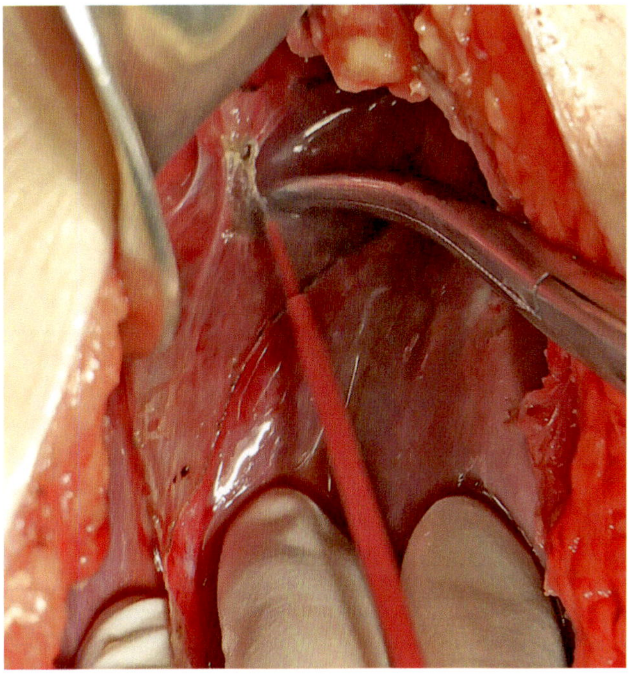

Fig. 146 The falciform was divided upward, and the dissection was continued to expose the anterior surface of the suprahepatic IVC and extrahepatic LHV. *IVC* inferior vena cava, *LHV* left hepatic vein

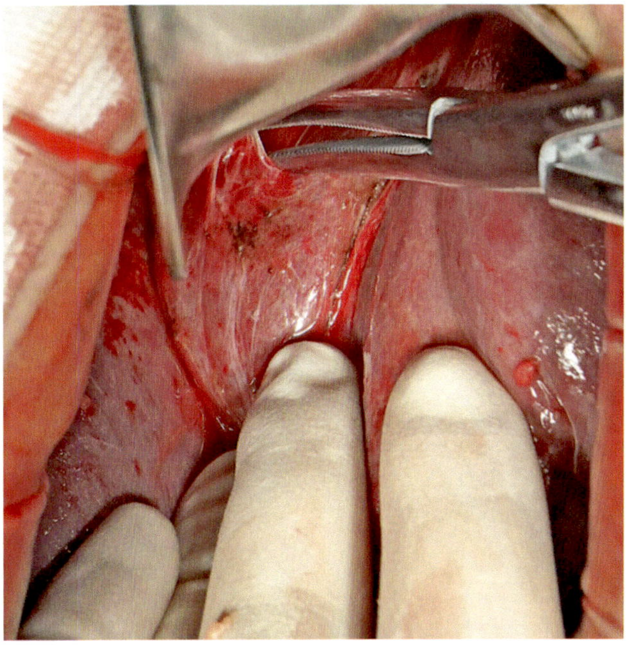

Fig. 147 The left coronary ligament was dissected

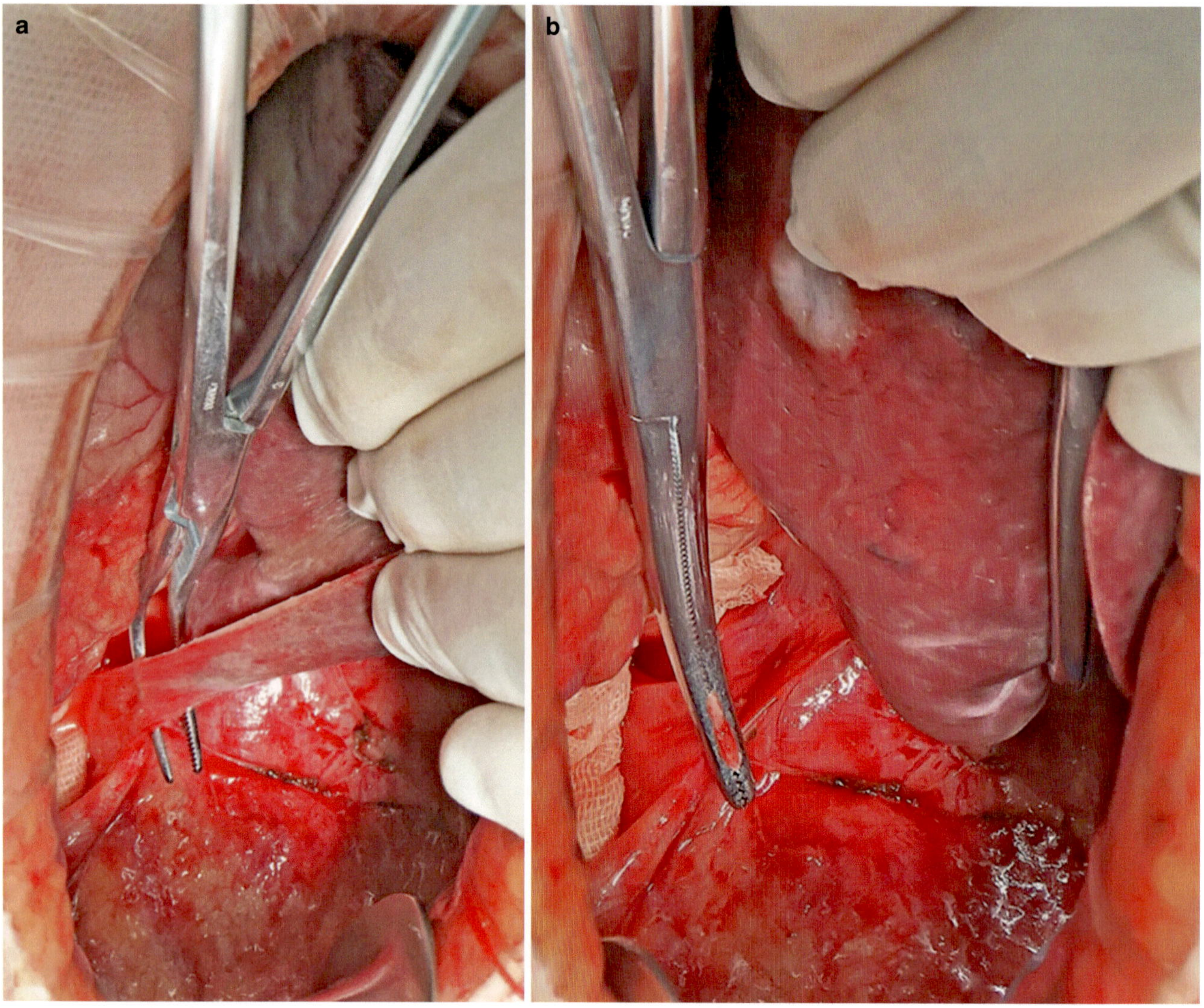

Fig. 148 (**a**, **b**) The left triangular was isolated, divided, and ligated

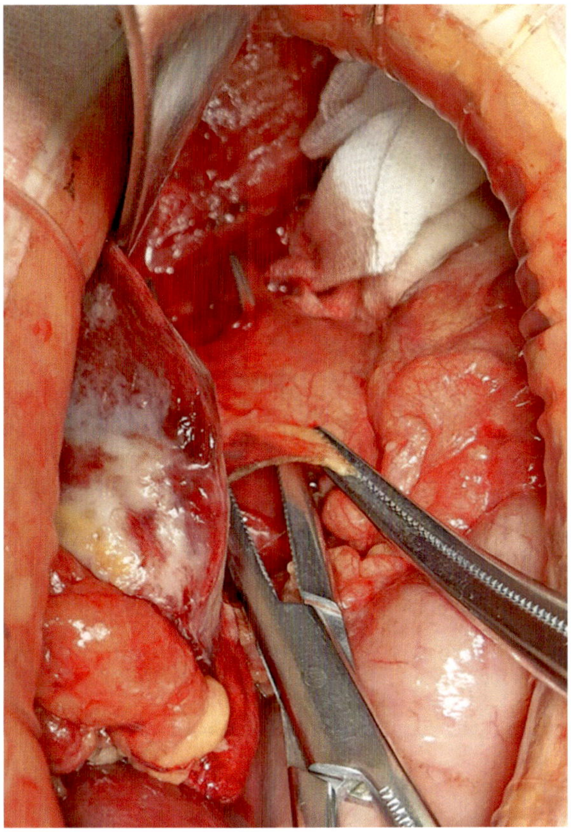

Fig. 149 The gastrohepatic ligament was divided

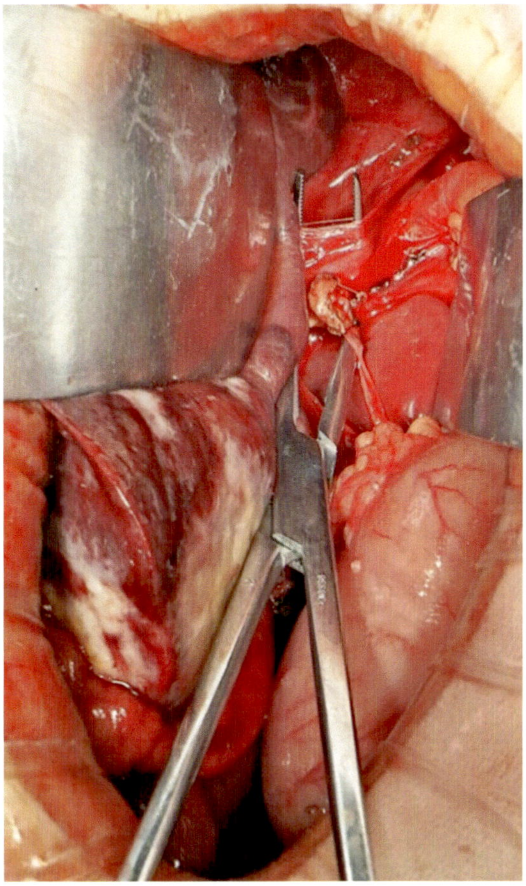

Fig. 150 The ligamentum venosum was divided

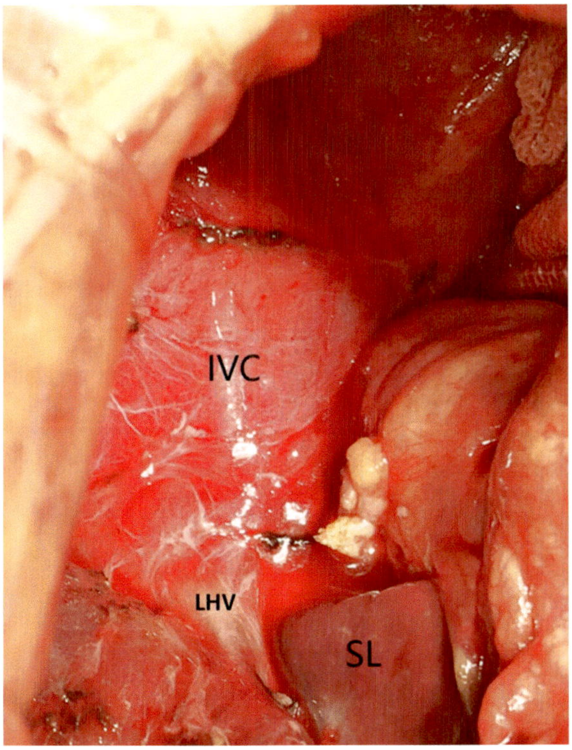

Fig. 151 The left-sided area of the hepatocaval confluence was exposed. *IVC* inferior vena cava, *LHV* left hepatic vein, *SL* Spiegel lobe

Isolation and Division of the Left Hepatic Vein (Fig. 152)

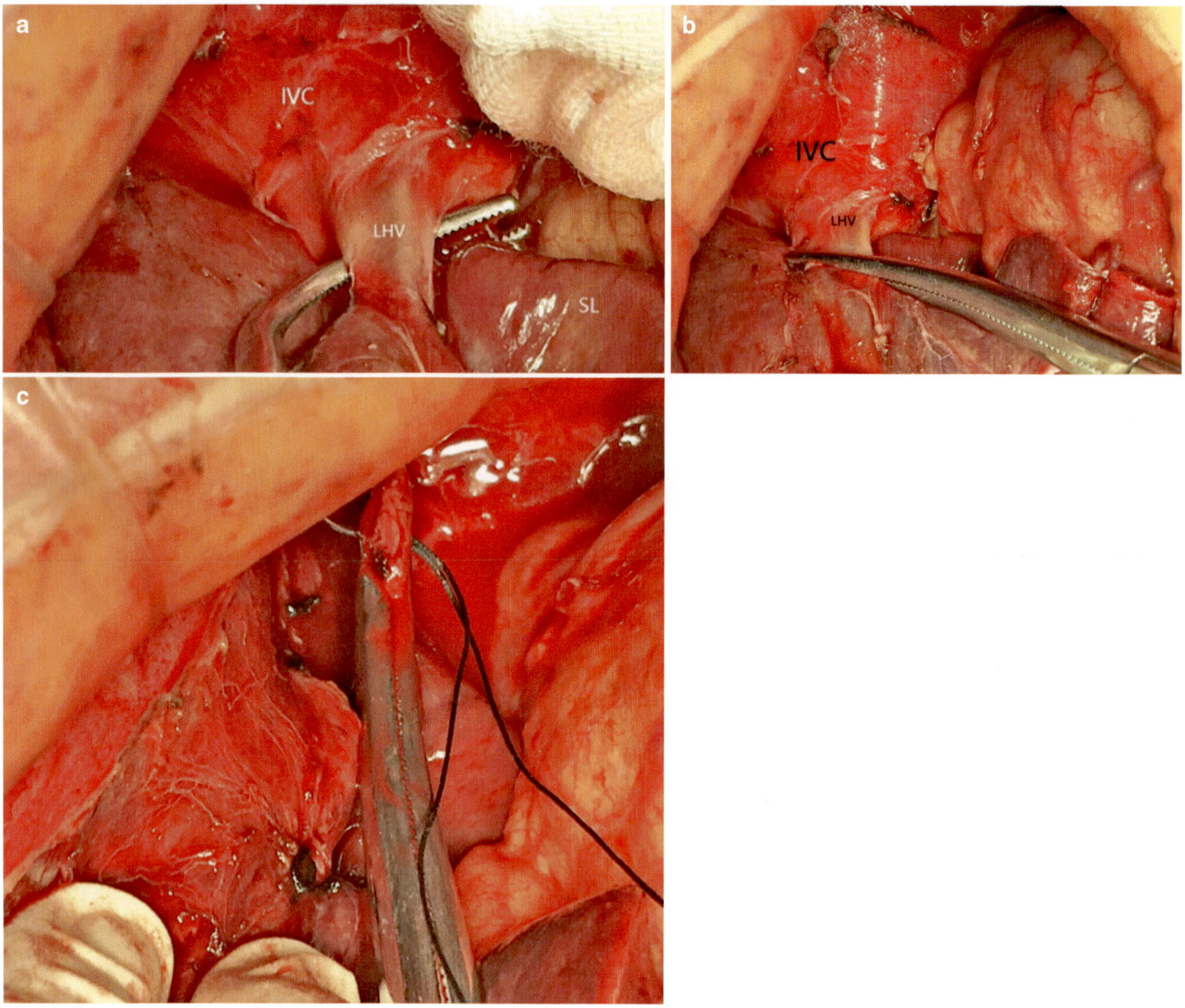

Fig. 152 (**a**–**c**) The left hepatic vein was extrahepatically isolated, divided, and suture-ligated. *IVC* inferior vena cava, *LHV* left hepatic vein, *SL* Spiegel lobe

Isolation and Division of the Pedicle of Segment III (Figs. 153 and 154)

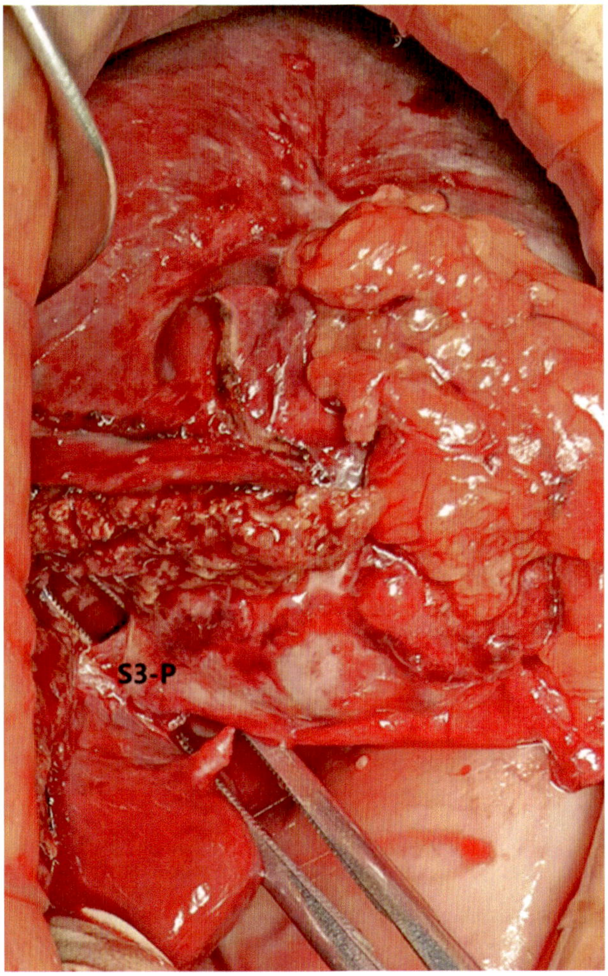

Fig. 153 The pedicle of segment III was isolated. S3-P, pedicle of segment III

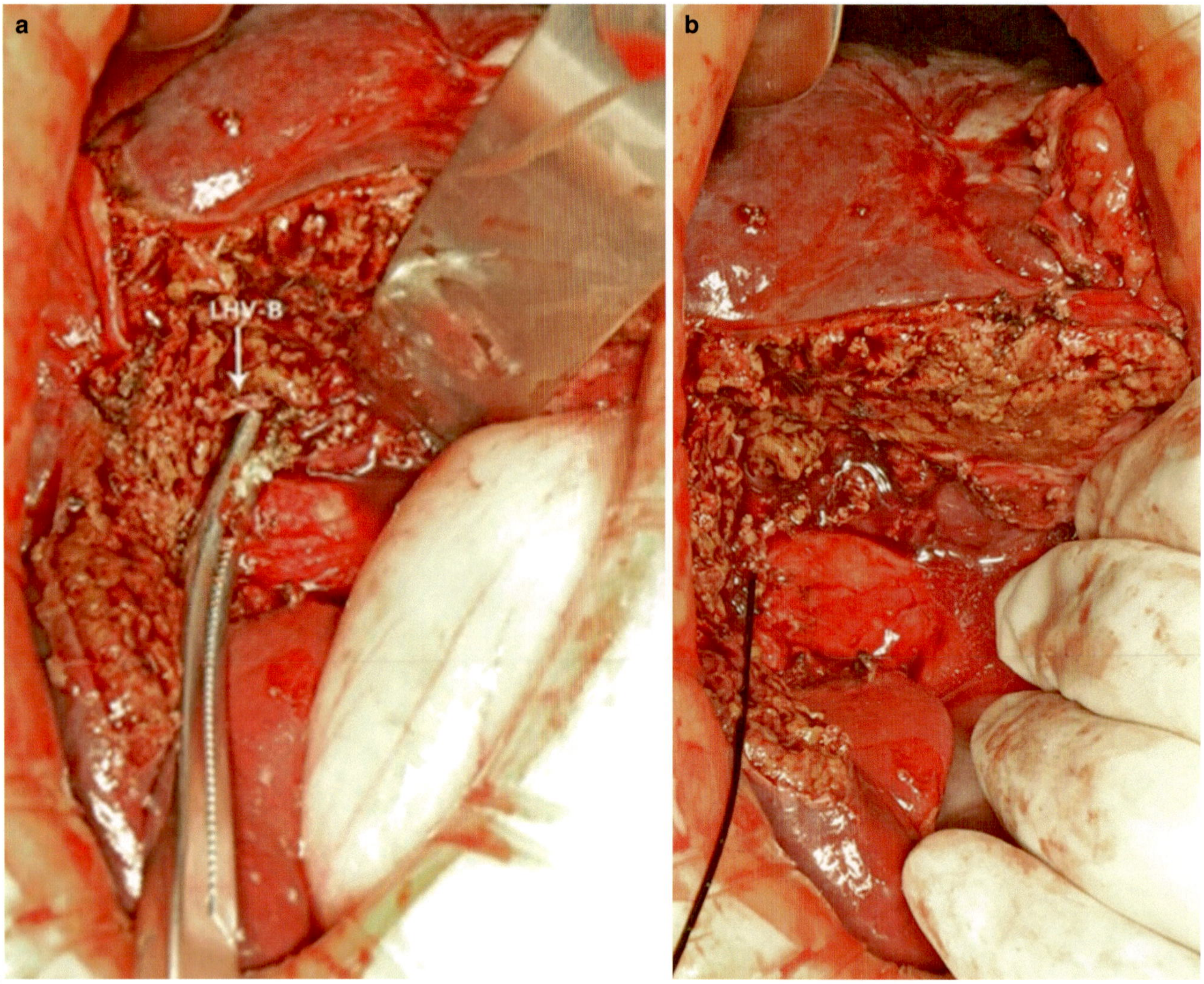

Fig. 154 (**a**, **b**) The pedicle of segment III was divided, and the proximal stump was suture-ligated. *LHV-B* branch of the left hepatic vein. Segment III was ischemic

Hepatic Parenchymal Transection and Management of S_2-P (Figs. 155, 156, and 157)

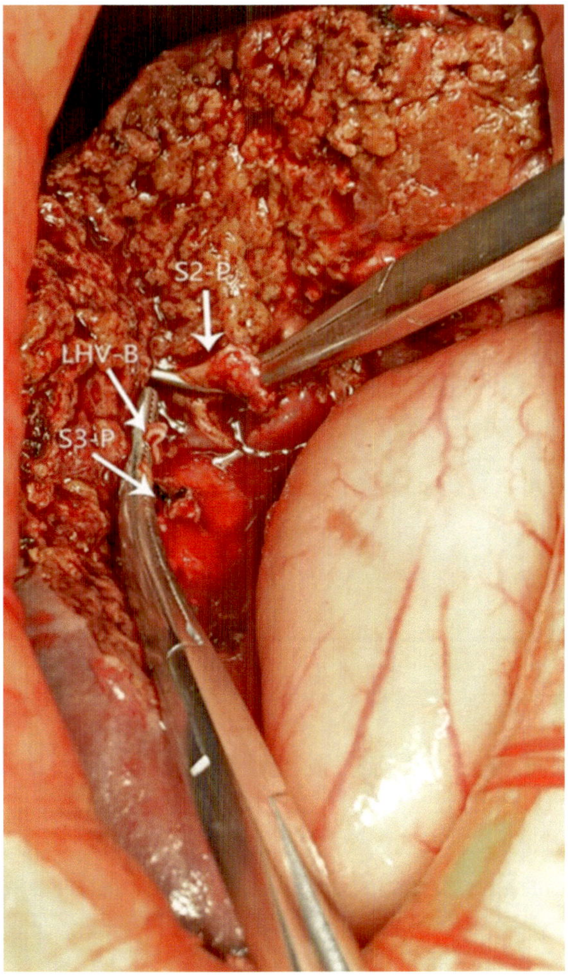

Fig. 155 The hepatic parenchymal transection line was corresponding to the left edge of the falciform ligament. The hepatic parenchymal transection was performed caudo-cranially, using clamp-crushing method. A large branch of the LHV was divided and ligated. The pedicle of segment II was isolated, divided, and ligated. *LHV* left hepatic vein, *S2-P* pedicle of segment II, *S3-P* pedicle of segment III

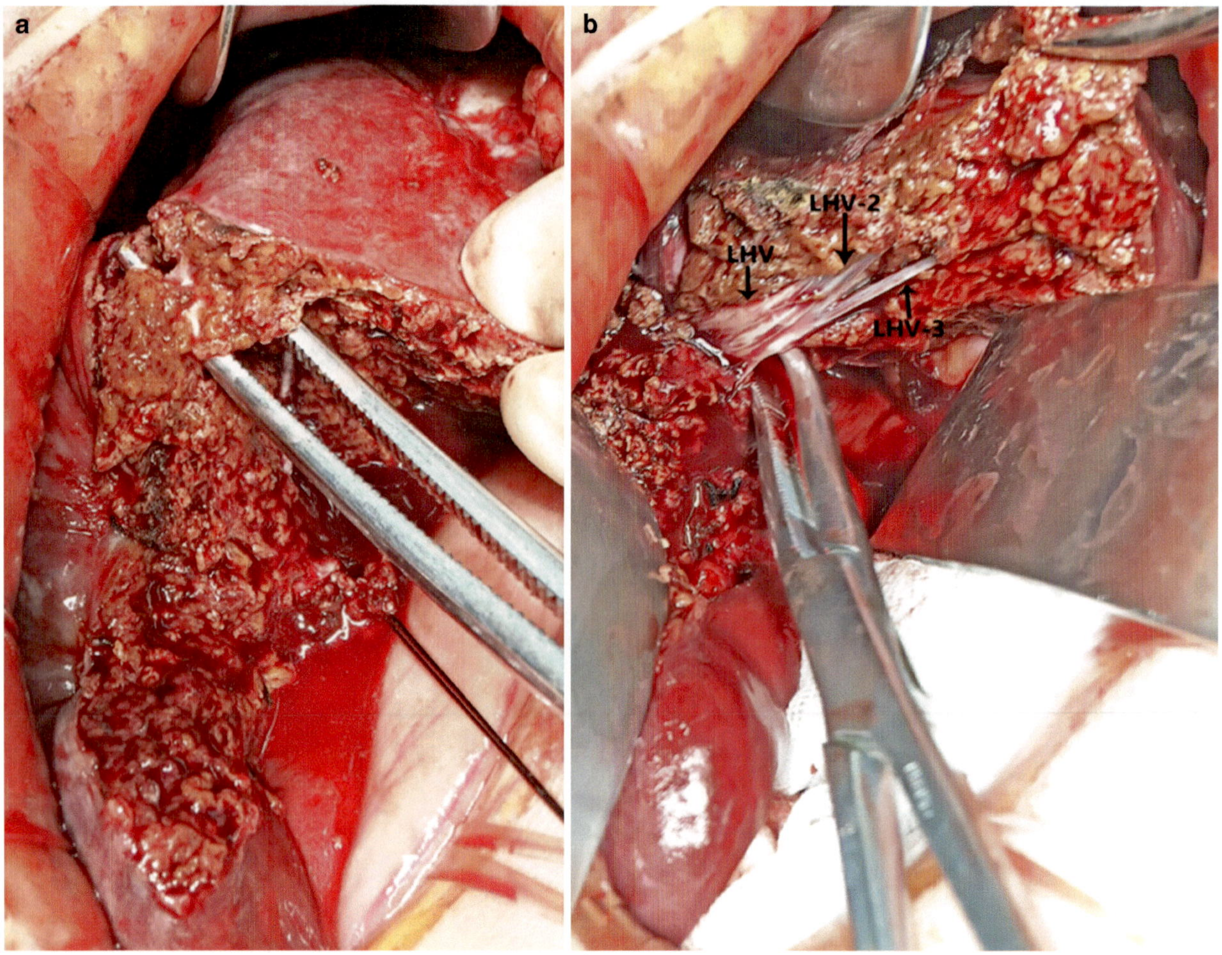

Fig. 156 (**a**, **b**) The parenchymal transection was continued upward to the root of the LHV. *LHV* left hepatic vein, *LHV-2* LHV draining segment II, *LHV-3* LHV draining segment III

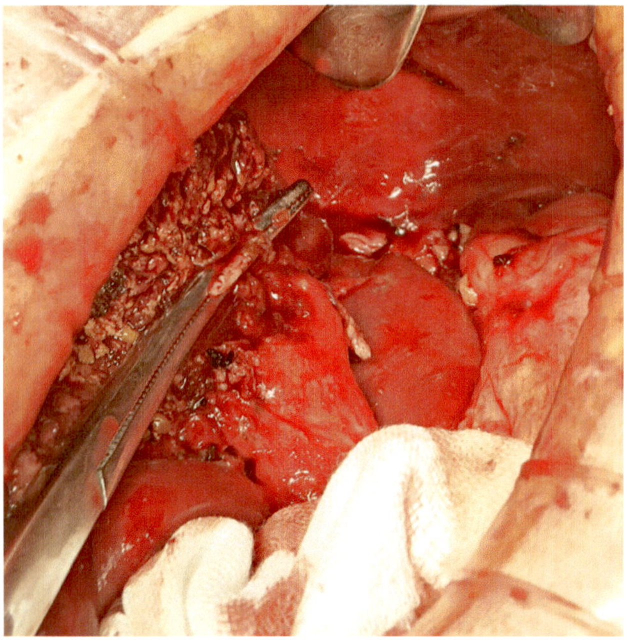

Fig. 157 The hepatic tissue surrounding the root of the LHV was crushed and ligated. *LHV* left hepatic vein

Raw Area of the Remnant Liver and the Specimen
(Figs. 158 and 159)

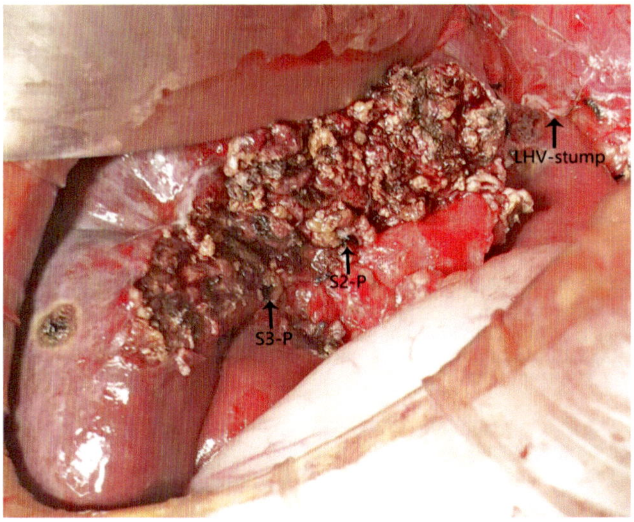

Fig. 158 The cut surface of the residual liver. *LHV-S* proximal stump of the left hepatic vein, *S2-P* pedicle of segment II, *S3-P* pedicle of segment III

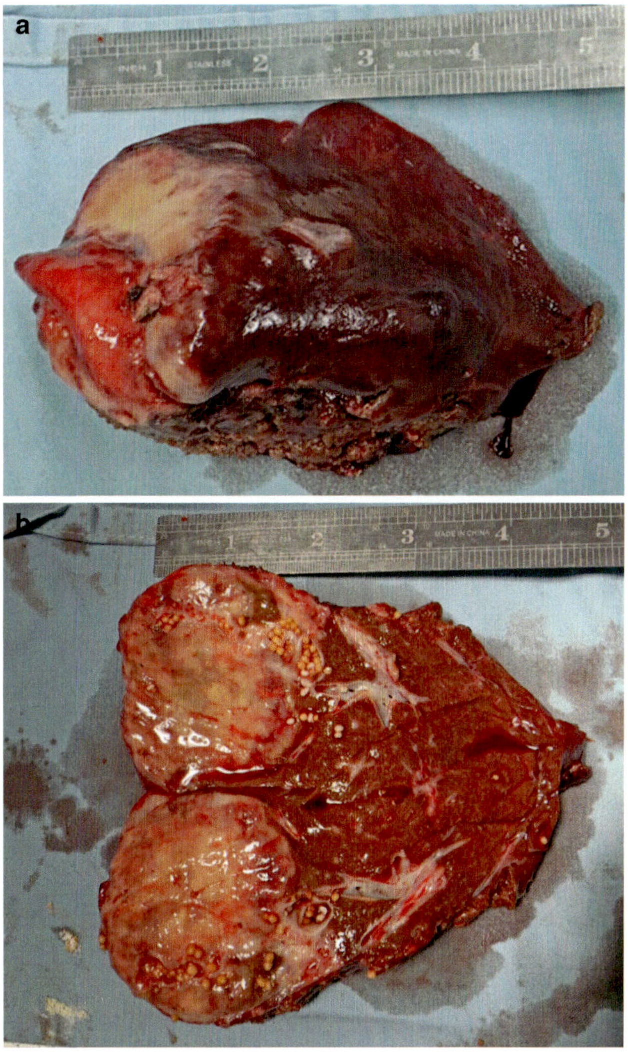

Fig. 159 (**a**, **b**) The specimen

Left Lateral Sectionectomy with Removal of the Portal Vein Tumor Thrombosis (PVTT) (Fig. 160)

Operative Procedures	Technical Details
Laparotomy ↓	◀ A right subcostal incision was made
Mobilization of the left hemiliver ↓	◀ The left hemiliver was dissected away from its surrounding structures.
Management of the pedicle of segment 3(S_3-P) ↓	◀ The pedicle of segment 3 was extrahepatically isolated, divided, the proximal stump of P_3 was opened and the tumor thrombus was removed from this stump. Then, the stump was transfix-sutured.
Transection of hepatic parenchymal and the pedicle of segment 2(S_2-P)	◀ Parenchyma was transected caudal-cranially along the cut line. S2-P was intrahepatically transected. The left hepatic vein was also intrahepatically transected.

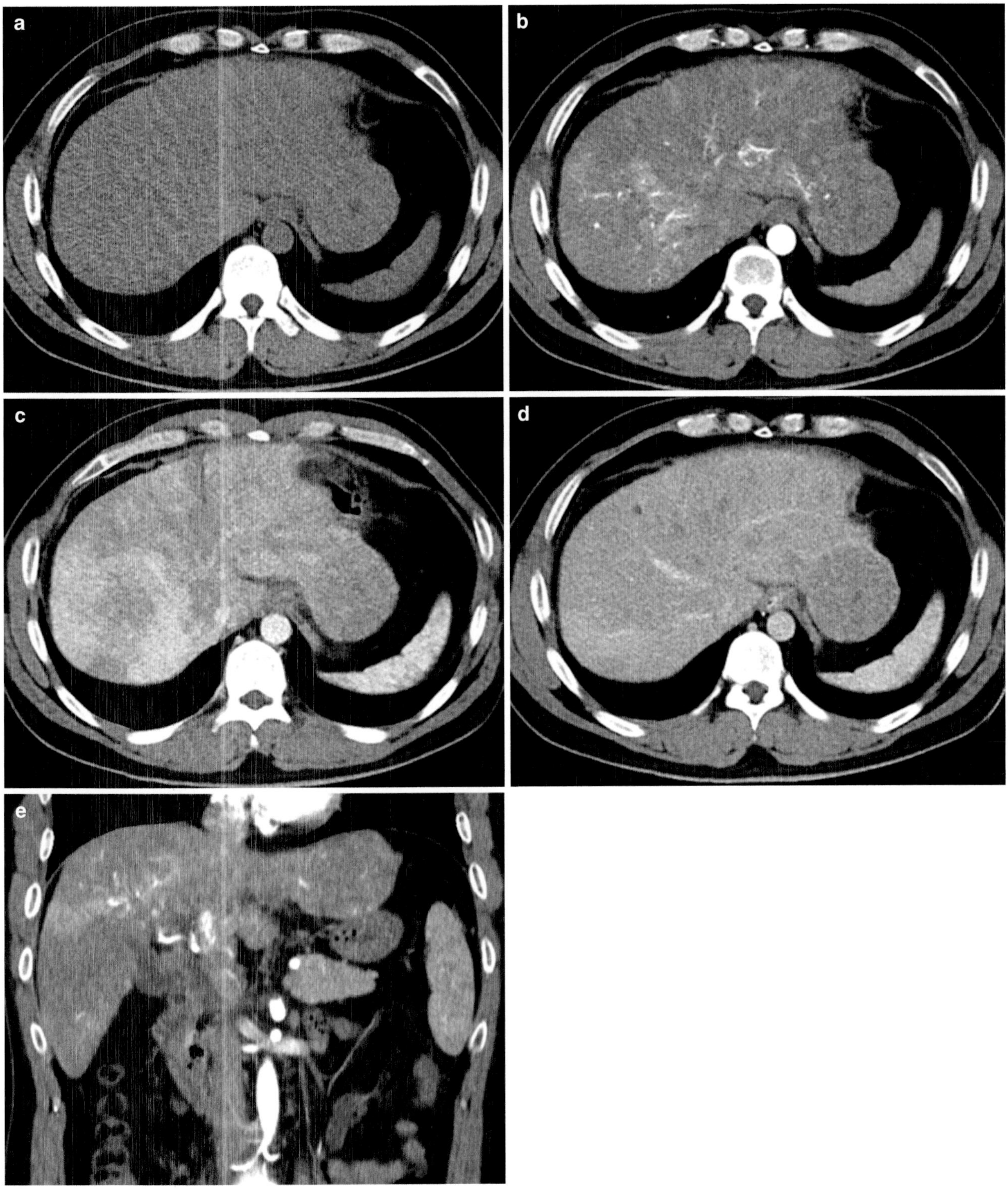

Fig. 160 (**a**) Preoperative CT (precontrast). The tumor, which appears mildly hyperdense, is located at margin of segments II and III. (**b**) Preoperative CT (early hepatic arterial phase). The tumor shows mildly homogeneous enhancement. (**c**) Preoperative CT (late hepatic arterial phase). The tumor shows mildly homogeneous enhancement. (**d**) Preoperative CT (hepatic venous phase). The tumor shows enhancement fades. (**e**) Preoperative CT (coronal section of the tumor)

Abdominal Incision and Mobilization of the Left Hemiliver (Figs. 161, 162, 163, 164, 165, and 166)

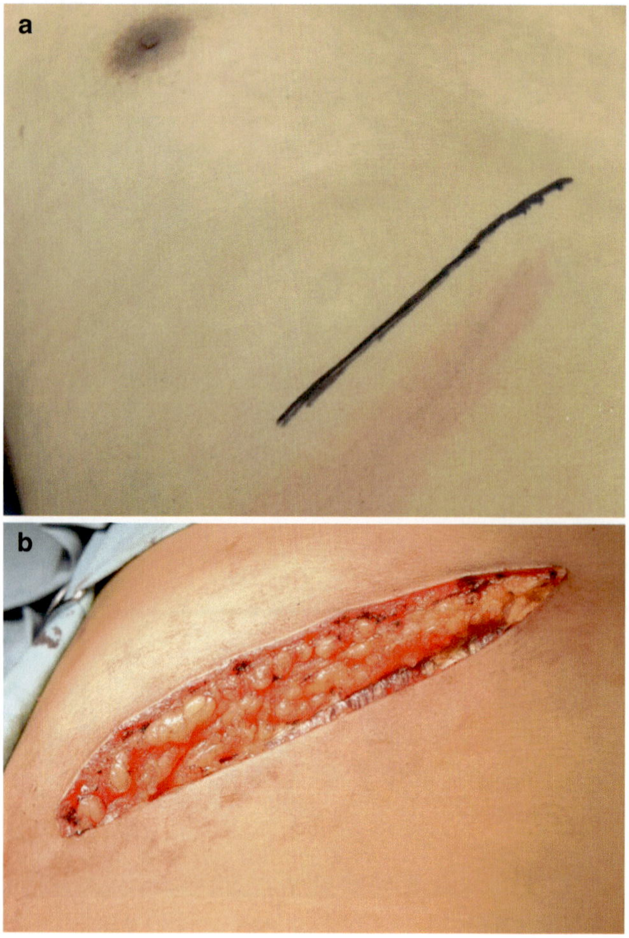

Fig. 161 (**a**, **b**) A right subcostal incision was selected and made

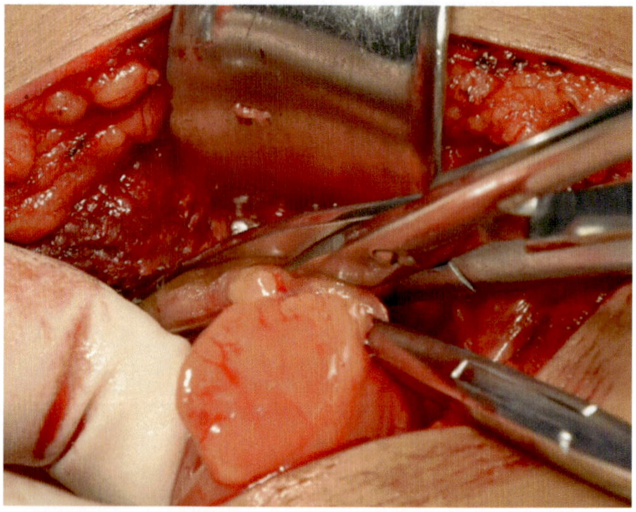

Fig. 162 The round ligament was divided and ligated

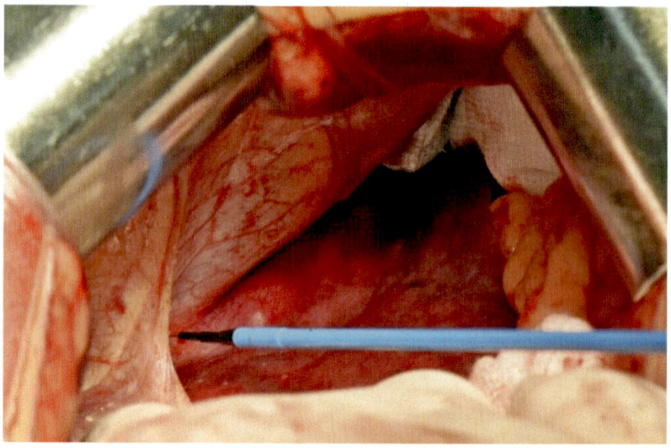

Fig. 163 Dissection of the falciform ligament

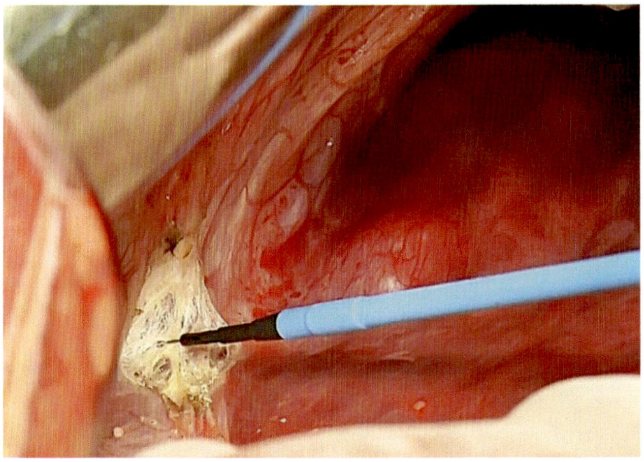

Fig. 164 Dissection of the hepatocaval confluence

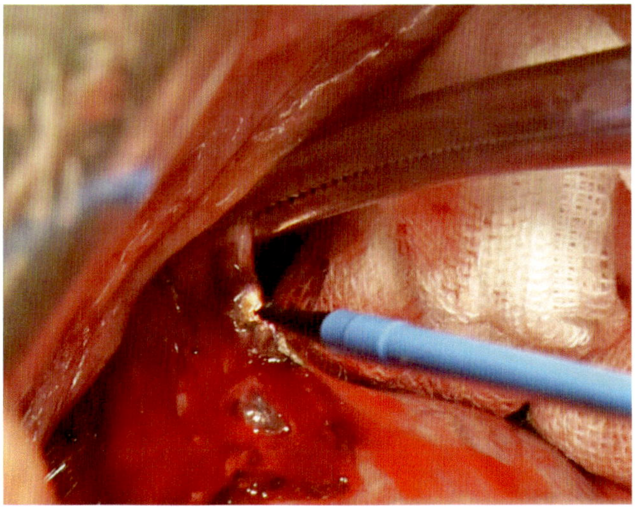

Fig. 165 The left coronary ligament was divided with electrocautery

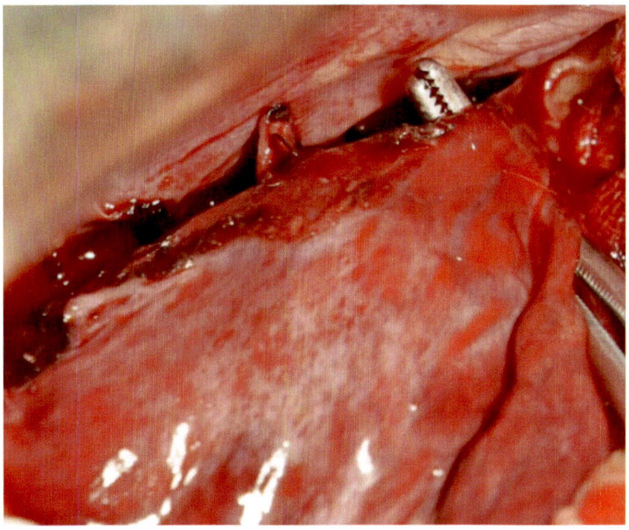

Fig. 166 The left triangular ligament was isolated, divided, and ligated

Management of the Pedicle of Segment III
(Figs. 167, 168, 169, 170, 171, 172, 173, and 174)

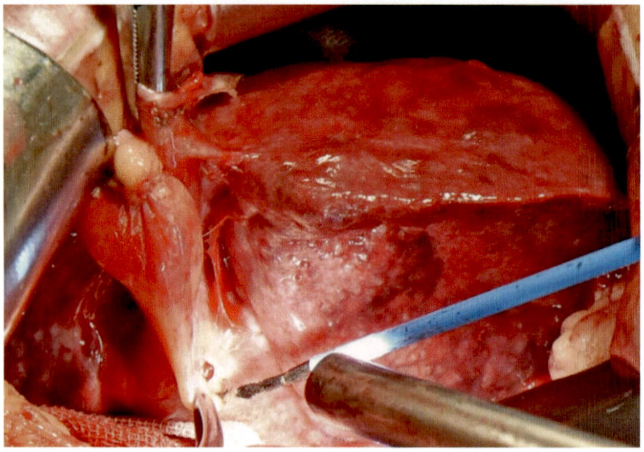

Fig. 167 Dissection in the plane just to the left of the umbilical fissure

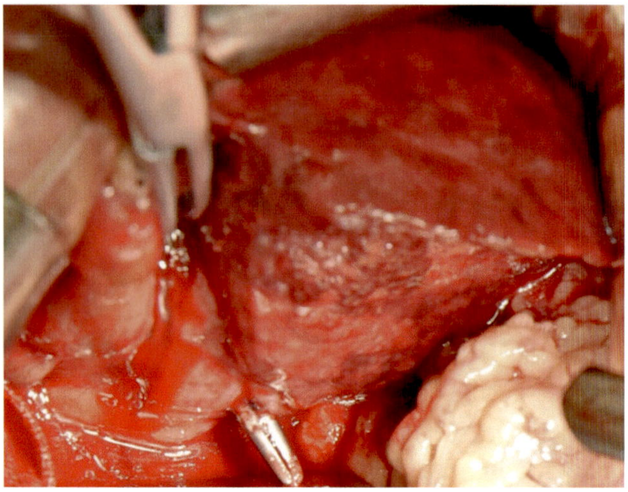

Fig. 168 A small incision was made at the left edge of the base of the round ligament. A large curved clamp was inserted into this incision and pushed vertically and downward and punctured out of the inferior edge of left hepatic pedicle. Thus, the pedicle of segment III was isolated

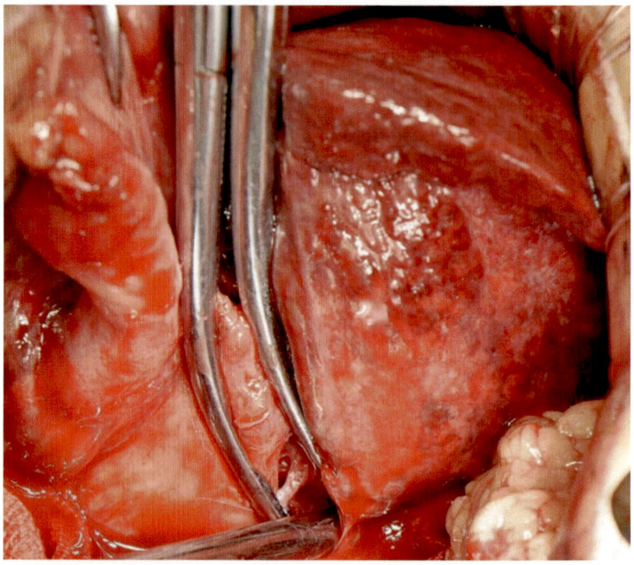

Fig. 169 The pedicle of segment III (S_3-P) was clamped with two large curved clamps and divided

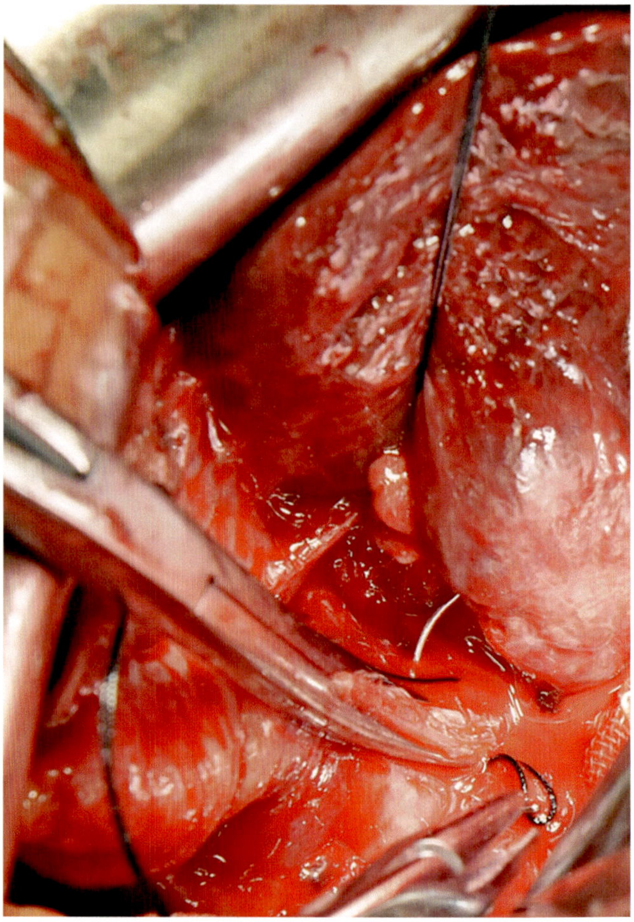

Fig. 170 The distal stump of S_3-P was ligated. The proximal stump was loosened, and the remaining proximal stump of S_3-P was re-clamped and suture-ligated

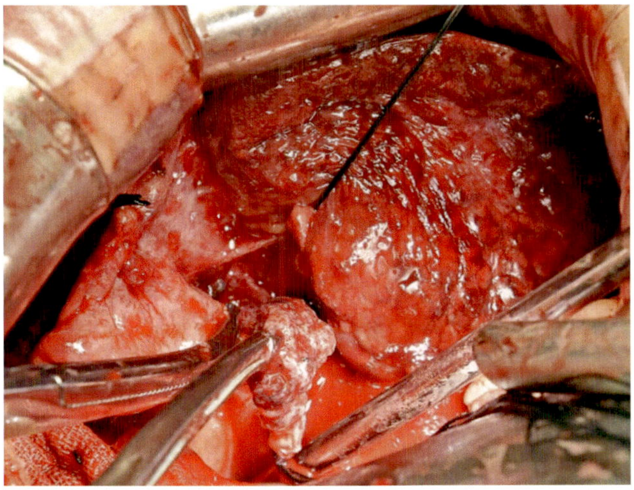

Fig. 171 The tumor thrombus were pulled out of the proximal stump of P_3

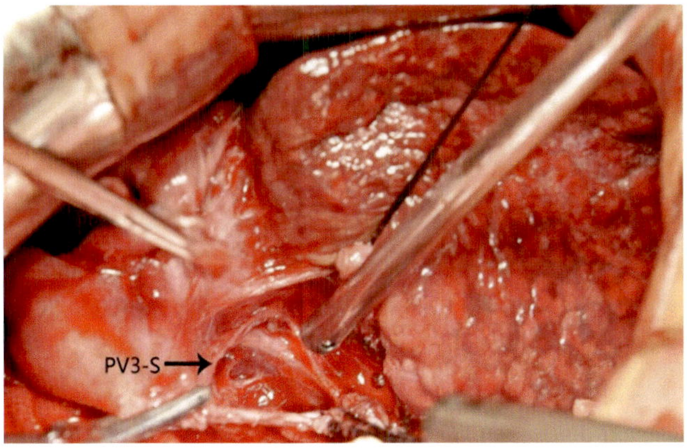

Fig. 172 The proximal stump of P_3 was shown. *P_3-S* stump of the portal vein supplying segment III

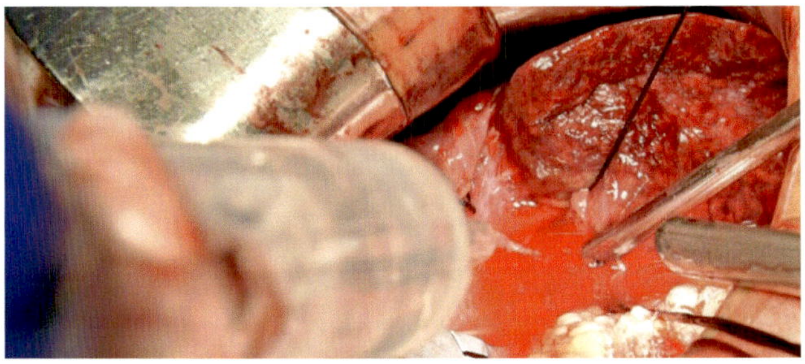

Fig. 173 A laveur was inserted into the proximal stump of the P_3, and the lumen of the P_3 was lavished, and then, the tape encircling around the hepatic pedicle was unloosened and let the portal vein blood stream wash away the possible residual tumor thrombus

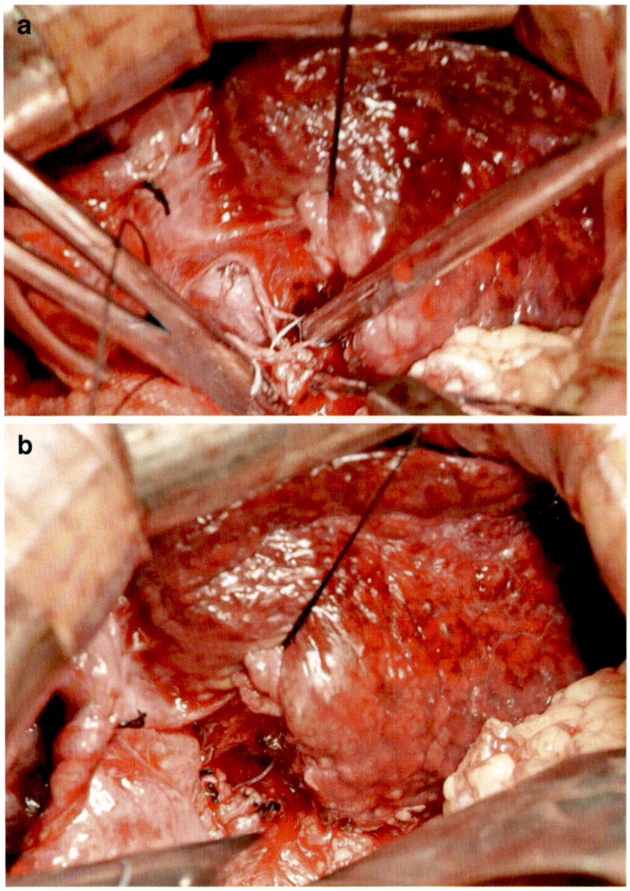

Fig. 174 (**a**, **b**) The proximal stump of P_3 was suture-ligated

Transection of Hepatic Parenchymal and S_2-P (Figs. 175, 176, 177, 178, 179, and 180)

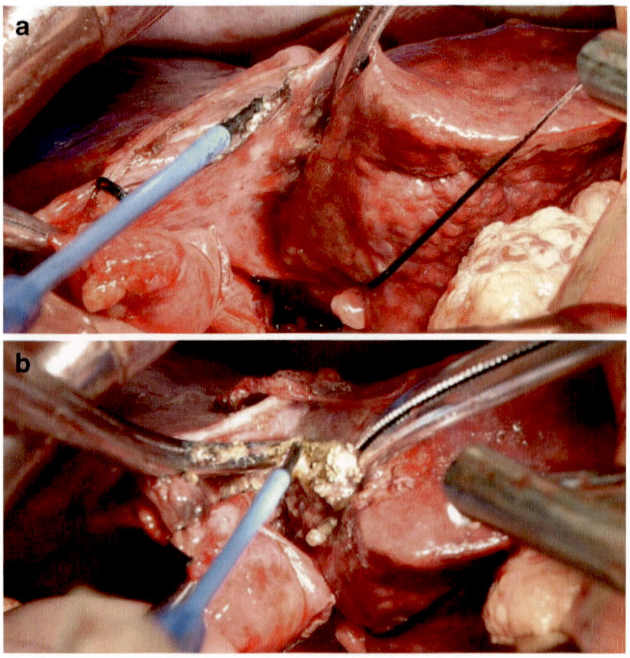

Fig. 175 (**a**, **b**) The hepatic parenchymal transection line was corresponding to the left edge of the falciform ligament. Parenchymal transection was performed caudo-cranially, using clamp-crushing method. All large vessels were ligated

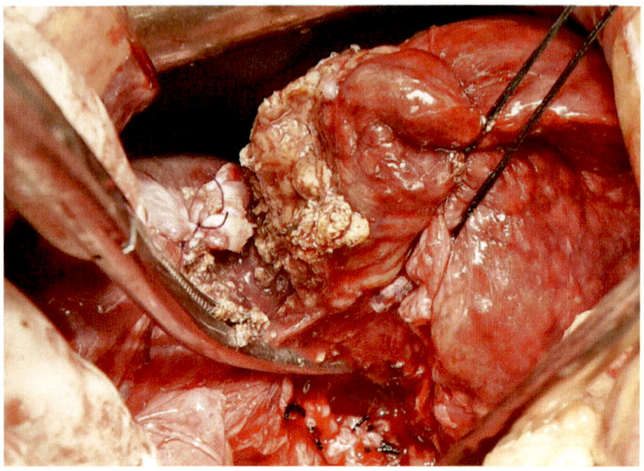

Fig. 176 The pedicle of segment II was isolated, divided, and ligated

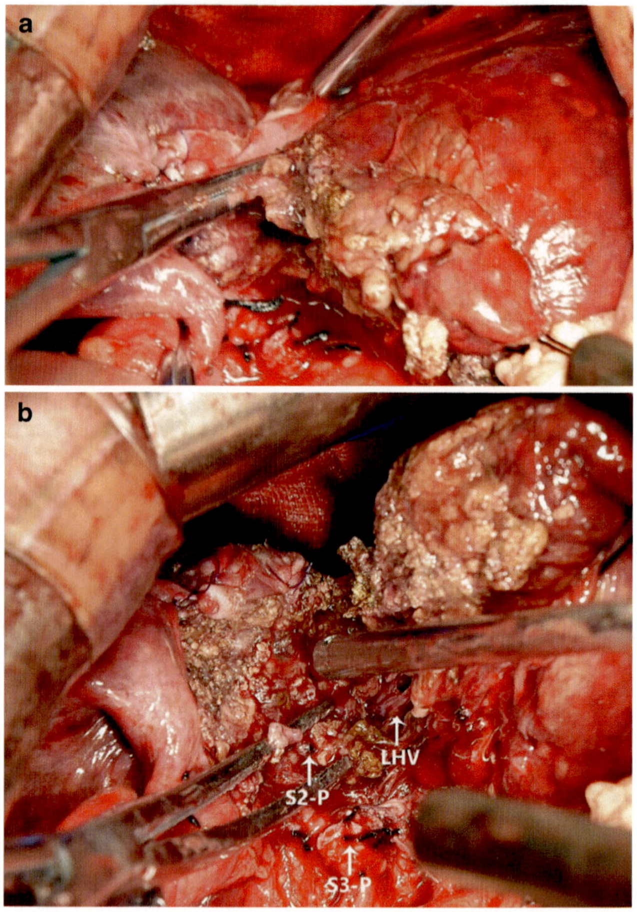

Fig. 177 (**a**, **b**) Parenchymal transection was continued upward to the root of the LHV. *LHV* left hepatic vein, *S_2-P* pedicle of segment II, *S_3-P* pedicle of segment III

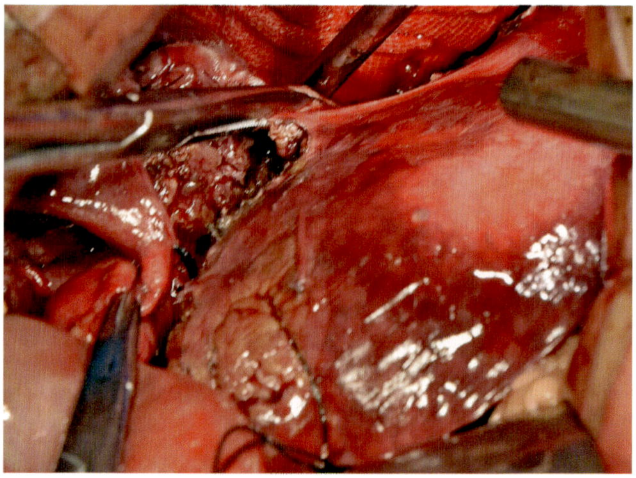

Fig. 178 The LHV was intrahepatically divided near its origin. *LHV* left hepatic vein

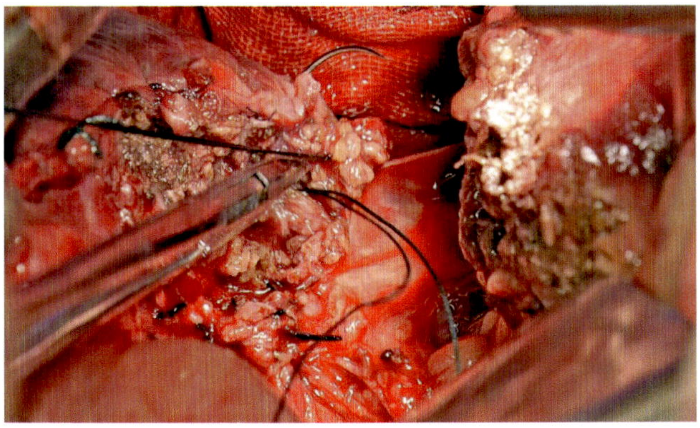

Fig. 179 The proximal stump of the LHV was suture-ligated. *LHV* left hepatic vein

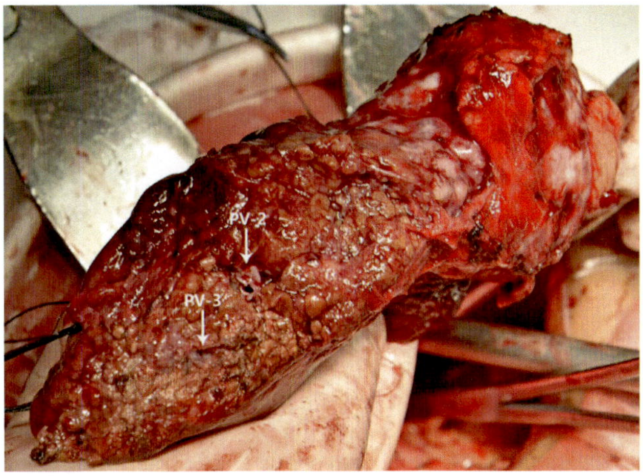

Fig. 180 Cut surface of the specimen. *PV-2* portal vein supplying segment II, *PV-3* portal vein supplying segment III

Raw Area of the Residual Liver and the Specimen
(Figs. 181 and 182)

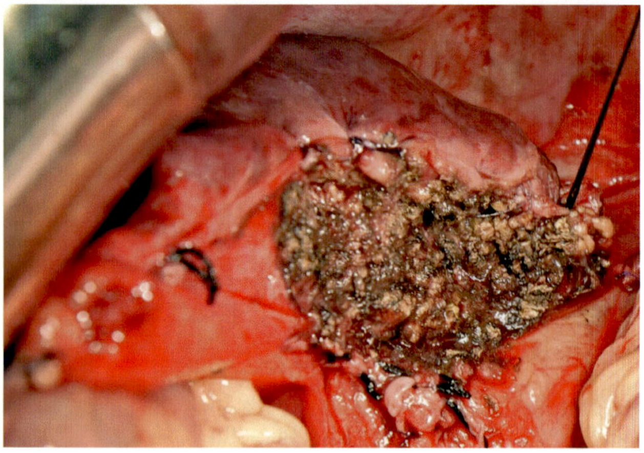

Fig. 181 Having removed the specimen, hemostasis in the cut surface of the residual liver was obtained by electrocautery, and >2 mm vascular and biliary branches were ligated

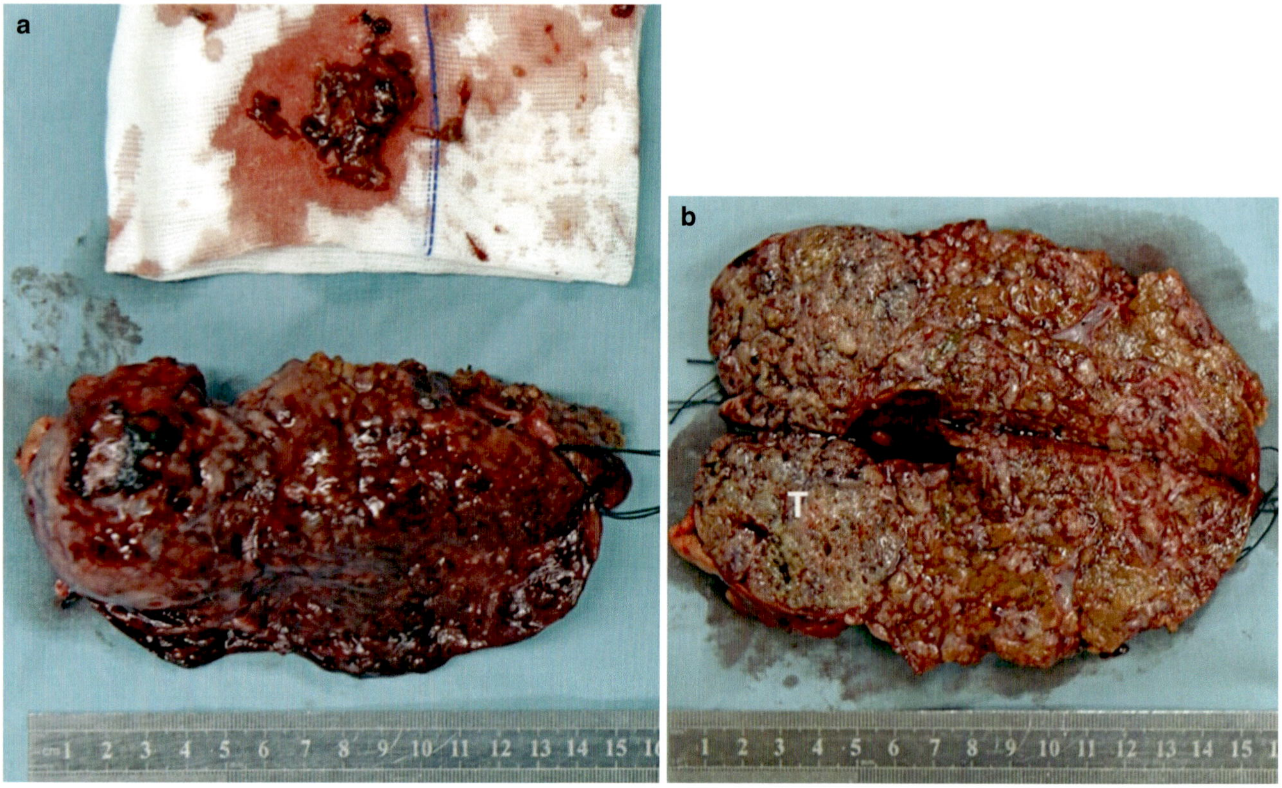

Fig. 182 (**a**, **b**) Tumor emboli and the tumor. *T* tumor

Intraoperative Key Points

1. The left hepatic vein classically inserts into the middle hepatic vein in a comparatively intrahepatic site. This anatomy results in that extrahepatic isolation and division of the left hepatic vein is technically difficult and may cause massive bleeding due to injuries to this vein in most individuals. Therefore, no need of this attempt is required (see section "Hepatic Vein" in chapter "Clinical Anatomy of the Liver").
2. The umbilical vein passes in the plane anterior to the umbilical fissure and usually inserts into the left hepatic vein. This vein lies in the plane of resection for a left lateral sectionectomy and can be transected or conserved. Injures to this vein leads to bleeding during parenchymal transection.
3. For tumors with portal vein tumor thrombus, it is vital to completely remove the tumor thrombus from the proximal stump of the involved portal vein. No residual macroscopic tumor thrombus within the portal vein can decrease postoperative early recurrence.

Segmentectomy IV

Jixiong Hu, Guohuang Hu, and Jiangbei Deng

Segment IV is located between the right plane determined by the main scissura (main fissure, or the midplane of the liver) and the left plane defined by the umbilical fissure, and its posterior boundary is the Spiegel lobe of the caudate lobe, including about 10% of the total liver volume. An isolated resection of segment IV (S4) is a technically difficult operative procedure due to two hepatic parenchymal transection planes along two fissures, which are the course of the main hepatic veins.

Surgical Indications

The surgical indications and types of hepatic resection of segment IV HCCs were determined by the tumor-related factors, remnant liver functional reserve, and the patient's general conditions. When a tumor is located in the superior part (S4a) or it is deeply located or in contact with the middle hepatic vein (MHV), it is well accepted that anatomical segmentectomy IV was preferred over nonanatomic partial resection (wedge resection or enucleation) [73, 74], because anatomical segmentectomy IV has the advantage of hepatic parenchymal sparing when compared with that of a left hemihepatectomy or a mesohepatectomy and especially in those patients with cirrhotic liver. However, when a tumor is located in the lower part of S4 (S4b), a wedge resection is a possible procedure [75]. In terms of the evaluation of the liver function, the Pugh-Child classification [56] and the indocyanine green retention rate at 15 min (ICGR 15) [5] were adopted. When a tumor was located within segment IV, and ICGR 15 was less than 30% and Pugh-Child classification was grade A or B, isolated segmentectomy is a feasible procedure.

Operative Procedures	Technical Details
Mobilization of the left liver	◀ A right subcostal incision was made. The perihepatic ligaments of the left liver were dissected and the hepato-caval confluence was exposed.
Isolation and division of the Glissonean pedicle of segment IV	◀ The Glissonean pedicle of segment IV was isolated, divided and silk-sutured, based on a perihilarGlissonean approach.
Hepatic parenchymal transection	◀ The ischemic demarcation line was marked on the liver surface with electrocautery. Parenchymal transection was undertaken according to the line using the clamp-crushing method. Because the tumor infiltrated the main trunk of the middle hepatic vein (MHV) near its origin, the main trunk was transected with the tumor close to its origin. Having delivered the specimen, the LHV and the proximal stump of the MHV was exposed.
Drainage and closure of the abdominal cavity	◀ A tube was placed at and Winslow hole and secured.

Intraoperative Key Points

1. When a tumor is strictly located within segment IVb, it is advisable to just perform subsegmentectomy IVB. Here are the several reasons why segment IVA is repeatedly not resected: (1) The most ravaging complication after hepatic resection is posthepatectomy liver failure. Thus, hepatic parenchyma-sparing policy is adopted to prevent postoperative liver failure [76]. (2) There are several small veins which run transversely through segment IVA and drain into the middle hepatic vein (MHV), and no obvious demarcation between segments I and IV exists. Removing segment IVA is technically demanding. (3) The Glissonean sheaths to segment IVA come from the main left Glissonean sheath and run transversely through the base of segment IV. Transecting these sheaths may cause injury to the sheaths to segments II and III [77].
2. The Glissonean pedicles of segment IV have more variations than other seven hepatic segments. The portal branches often are between three and ten in number, and the arterial and biliary branches are also variable. When these vasculatures and biliary tracts are traditionally dissected individually for isolated segmentectomy IV, the risk of causing injury to the Glissonean pedicles of segments II and III is considerably high. As shown in this chapter, the advantage of anatomical resection of segment IV based on an intrahepatic Glissonean approach is clearly demonstrated.
3. The MHV runs in the main portal scissura. It drains segment IV, and sometimes drains veins from segment V and/or VIII. When the tumor is within segment IV and infiltrates the main trunk of the main trunk of the MHV, the MHV must be resected to obtain an oncological clearance. The right hepatic vein (RHV) is located in the right portal scissura and receives venous branches from segments V, VI, VII, and VIII [78]. Just as demonstrated in this chapter, the MHV provides enough drainage to allow the segments V and VIII to survive (Fig. 183).

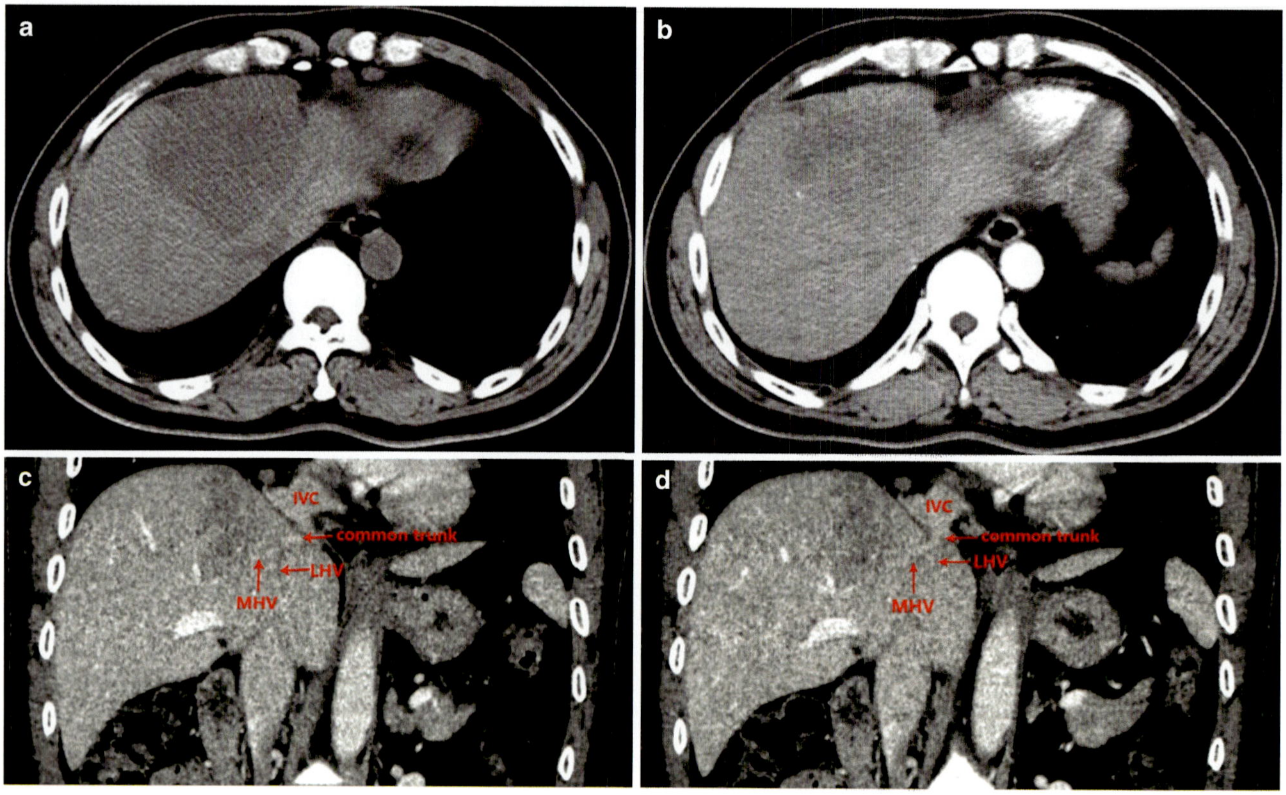

Fig. 183 (**a**, **b**) Preoperative CT. The tumor is located in segment IV and the paracaval portion of the caudate lobe near the hepatocaval confluence. The tumor shows mildly hypodense in precontrast (**a**) and heterogeneous enhancement in early hepatic arterial phase (**b**). (**c**, **d**) Preoperative hepatic vein reconstruction images show that the MHV is infiltrated by the tumor. *MHV* middle hepatic vein, *LHV* left hepatic vein, *IVC* inferior vena cava

Abdominal Incision and Exposure of Surgical Field (Fig. 184)

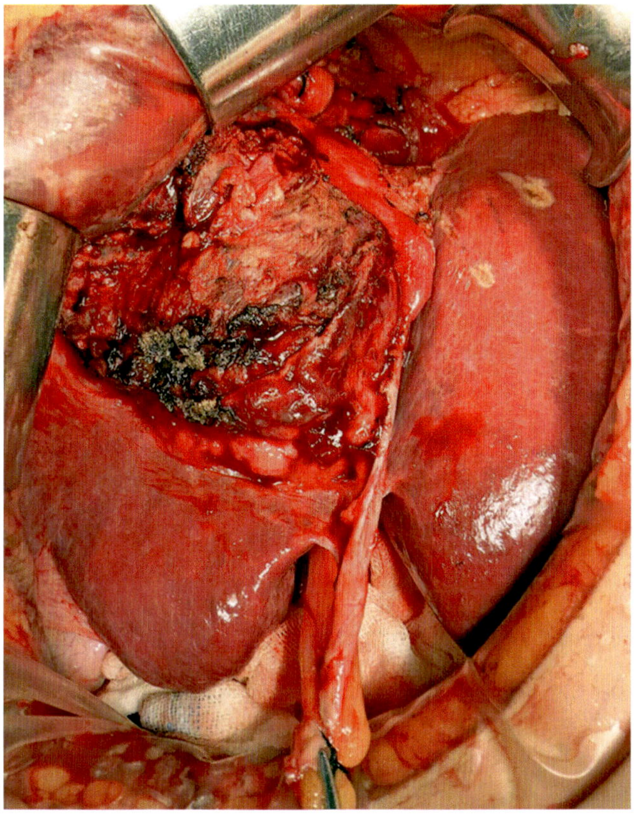

Fig. 184 The abdomen was opened via a right subcostal incision. The right costal arch was retracted cranially with two abdominal retractors. The tumor was located within segment IV, and a part of the tumor was above the liver surface

Isolation and Division of the Pedicle of Segment IV (Figs. 185, 186, 187, 188, 189, and 190)

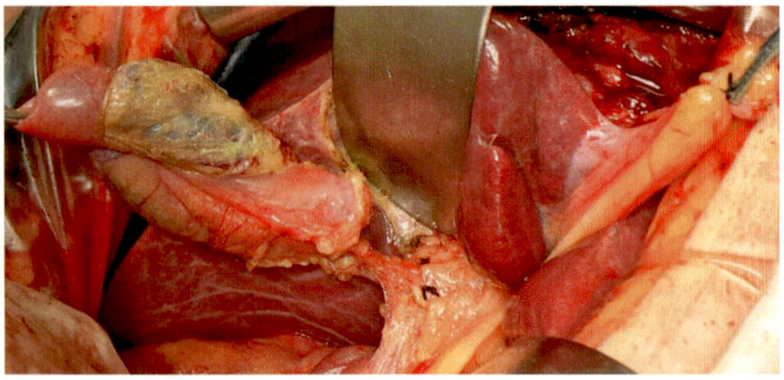

Fig. 185 The gallbladder cyst was being excised

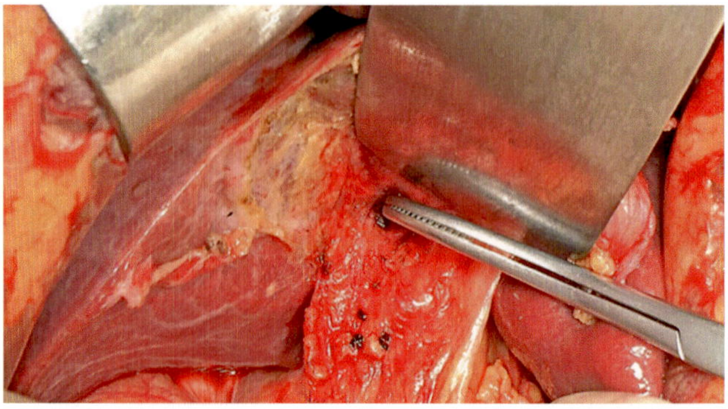

Fig. 186 A small anterior incision was made in front of the hilus, and the hepatic parenchyma around the small incision was divided with blunt dissection to expose the anterior surface of the left Glissonean pedicle and its course

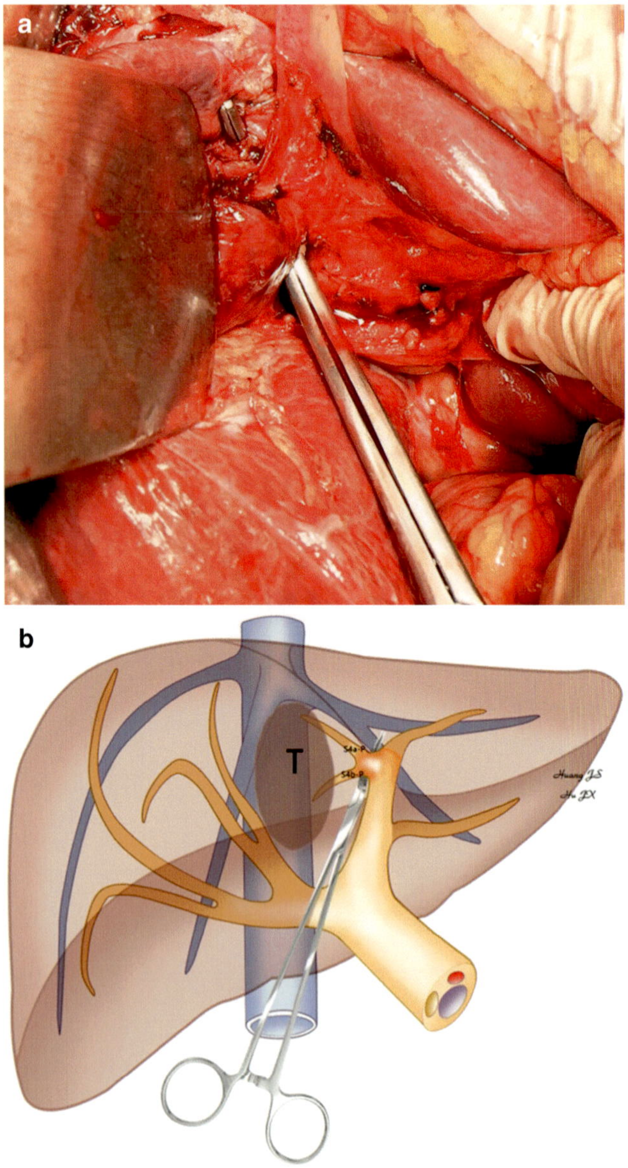

Fig. 187 (**a**) A second small incision was made in the right-sided margins of the basis of the round ligament, and a large curved clamp was inserted into the anterior incision in front of the hilus and passed out of the second incision. Thus, the Glissonean pedicle of segment IV was isolated. (**b**) Schematic illustration of this procedure

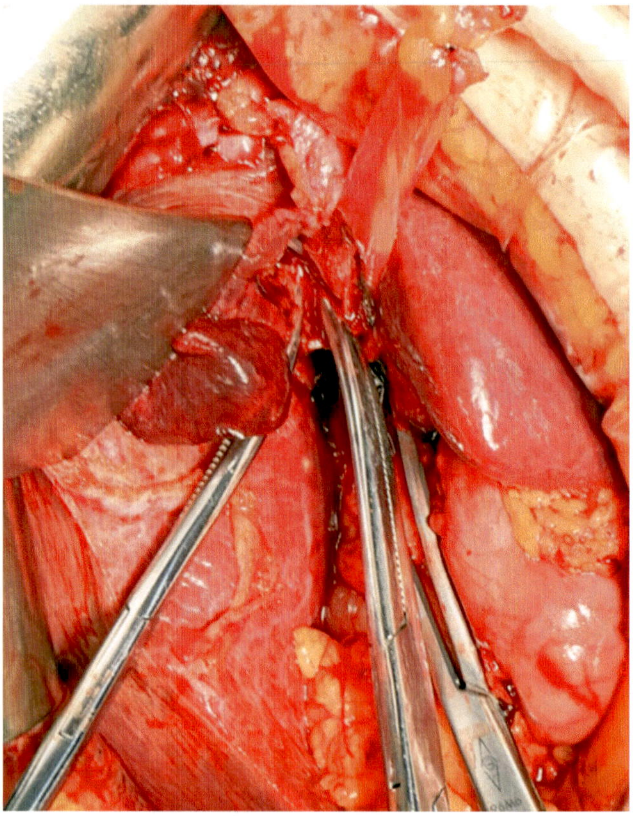

Fig. 188 The Glissonean pedicle of segment IV was clamped with two large curved clamps

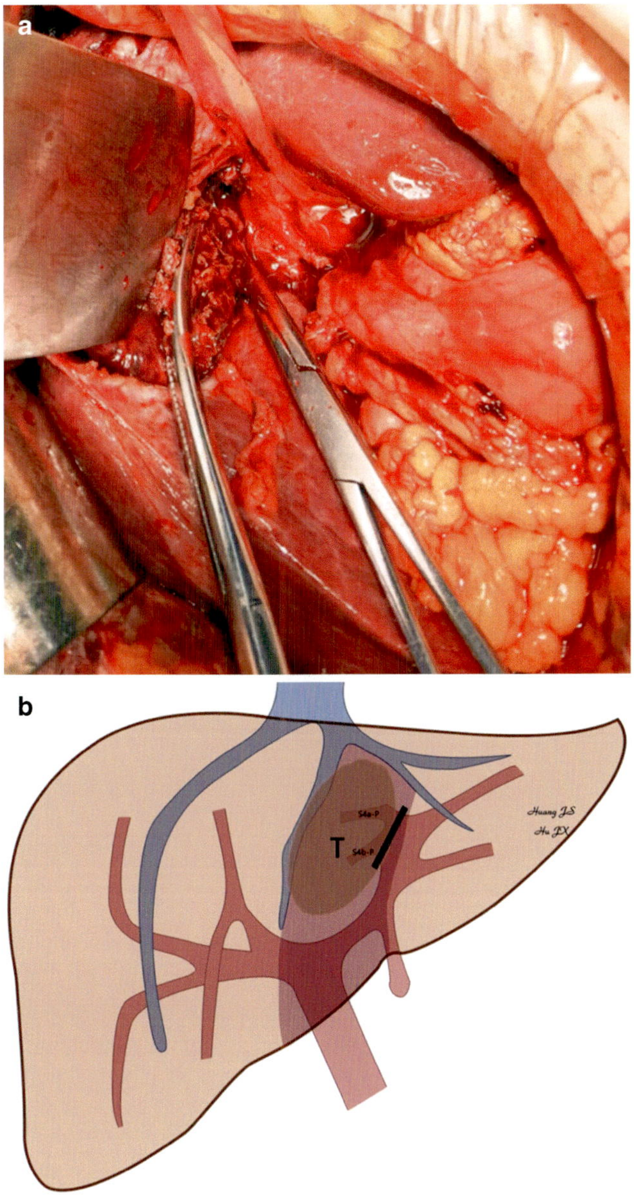

Fig. 189 (**a**) The Glissonean pedicle of segment IV was divided. The proximal stump was double silk-sutured; the distal stump was ligated. (**b**) Schematic illustration of this procedure

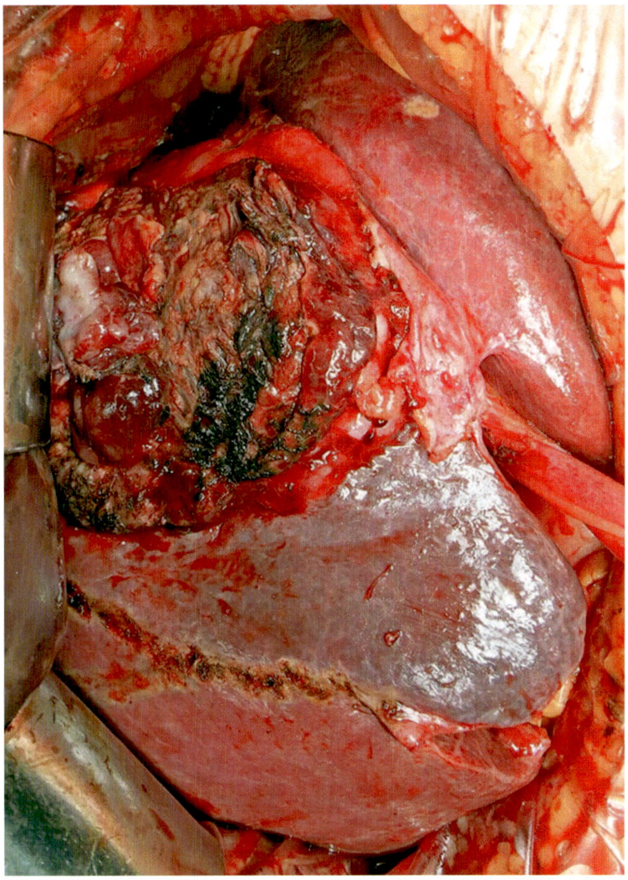

Fig. 190 Having divided the segment IV Glissonean sheath, inflow blood of the segment IV was completely occluded, and the whole segment IV was ischemic. On the liver surface, the right and left ischemic demarcation line of the segment IV was clearly obvious and was marked with electrocautery

Hepatic Parenchymal Transection (Fig. 191)

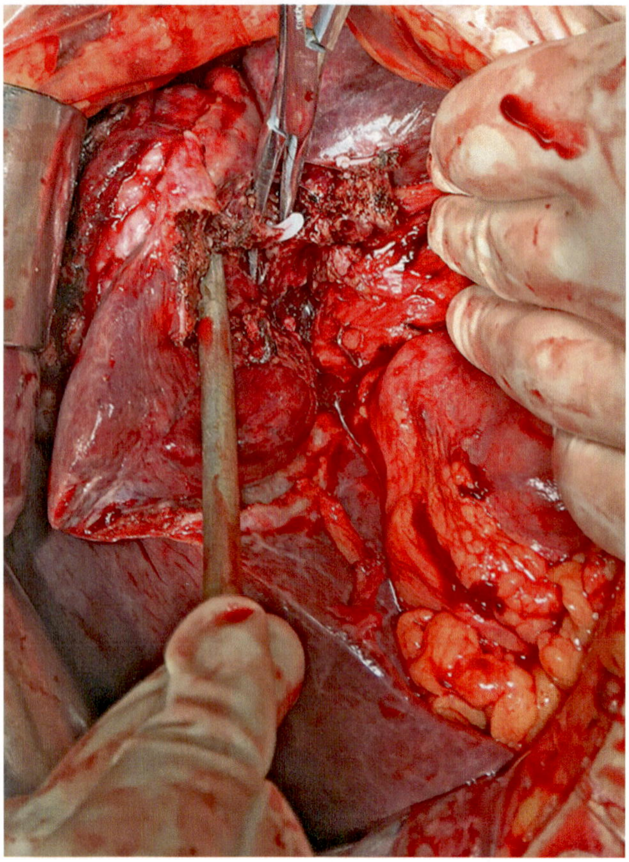

Fig. 191 Having fully mobilized the left liver, hepatic parenchymal transection was carried out along the ischemic demarcation line on the both sides using finger-fracture and/or clamp-crushing methods. The left-sided hepatic parenchyma transection proceeded near to the root of the left hepatic vein. It was found that the middle hepatic vein and the left hepatic vein comprise of the common trunk before entering into the suprahepatic IVC and the main trunk of the MHV was directed invaded by the tumor. The root of the MHV was isolated and divided. Its proximal stump was double sutured with silk thread. *IVC* inferior vena cava, *MHV* middle hepatic vein

Raw Area of the Residue Liver and the Specimen

(Figs. 192, 193, 194, 195, and 196)

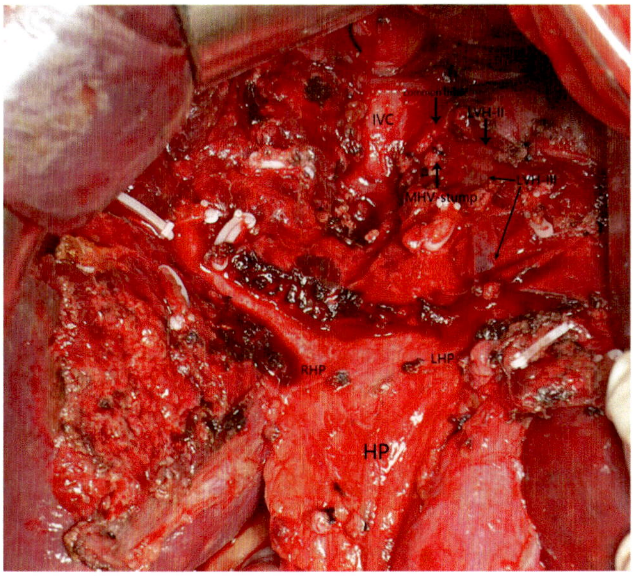

Fig. 192 Having performed hepatic parenchymal transection, the specimen was removed. The vascular and biliary ramification on the cut surface of the liver remnant were sutured with silk thread and/or polypropylene 3–0 and 4–0, and the tiny holes on the left hepatic vein and the anterior wall of retrohepatic inferior vena cava (IVC) were repaired with 5–0 and 6–0 polypropylene. *HP* hepatic pedicle, *RHP* right hepatic pedicle, *LHP* left hepatic pedicle, *MHV* middle hepatic vein, *LHV* left hepatic vein

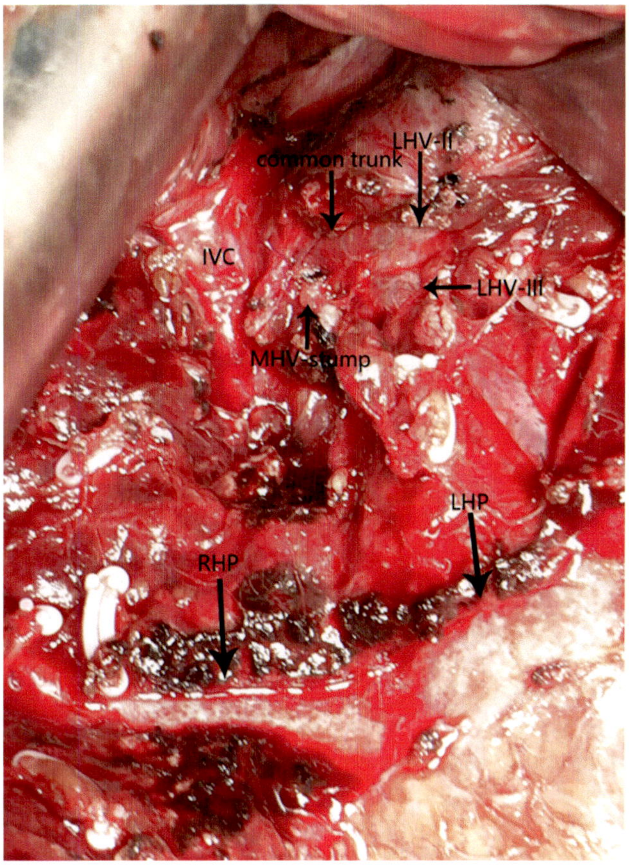

Fig. 193 The local and enlarged view of the cut surface. The paracaval portion of the caudate lobe was en bloc removed with the tumor. The common trunk of the MHV and the LHV, the proximal stump of the MHV, segment II and III branches of the LHV were clearly shown on the surface. *RHP* right hepatic pedicle, *LHP* left hepatic pedicle, *MHV* middle hepatic vein, *LHV* left hepatic vein, *IVC* inferior vena cava

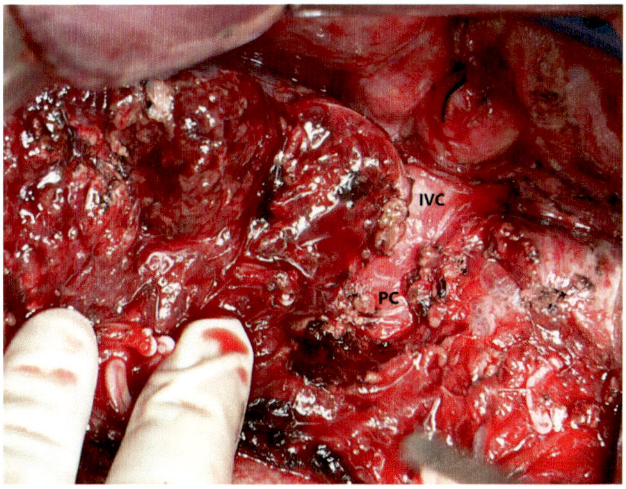

Fig. 194 The anterior wall of the retrohepatic IVC was longititudely exposed. The paracaval portion (PC) of the caudate lobe was also removed with the tumor. *IVC* inferior vena cava

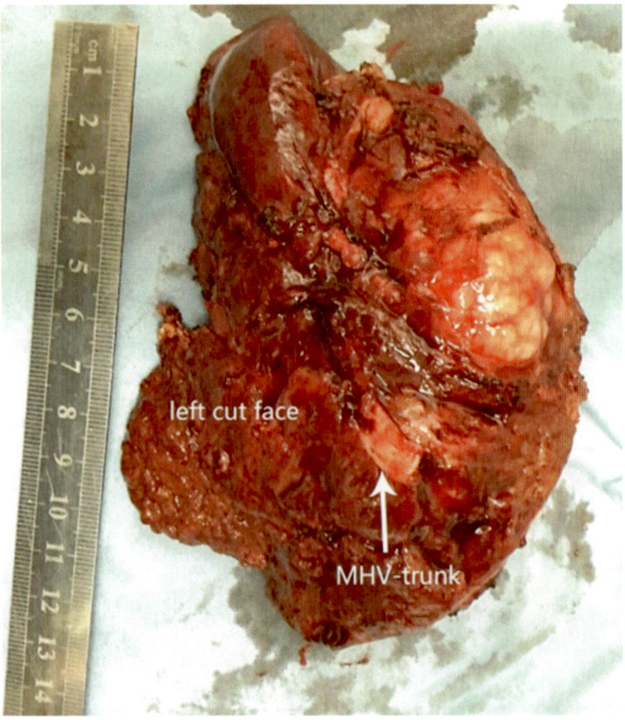

Fig. 195 The specimen contained a part of the main trunk of the MHV. *MHV* middle hepatic vein

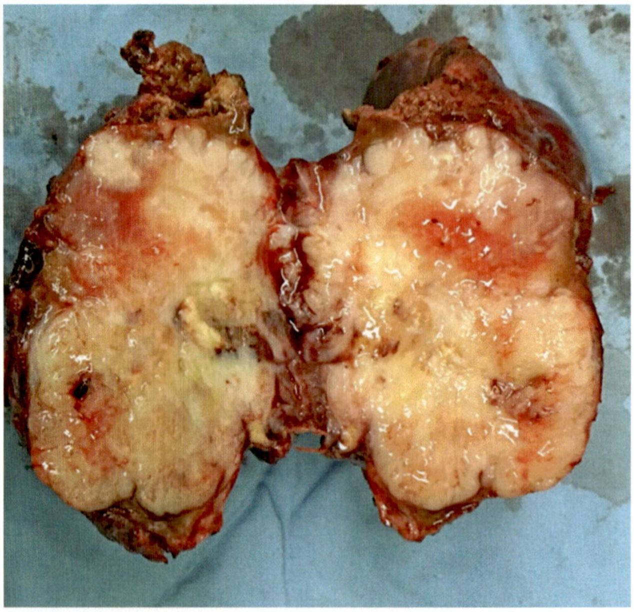

Fig. 196 The specimen was opened up. Pathology confirmed the diagnosis of HCC. *HCC* hepatocellular carcinoma

Mesohepatectomy (S4 + S5 + S8 Resection)

Jixiong Hu, Hongbo Xiao, and Zhongkun Zuo

For HCCs located centrally within the liver (Couinaud's [79] segments IV, V, and VIII), extended right or left trisectionectomy are usually recommended [80], which would unavoidably sacrifice the non-tumor right posterior or left lateral segments and may cause postoperative liver failure [81]. In contrast, mesohepatectomy removes tumor-bearing central liver segments and leaves the right posterior and left lateral segments in situ. Therefore, mesohepatectomy is performed over this more aggressive extended hepatectomy in terms of preserving more functional liver tissues [40, 82–85]. However, it is technically more demanding than traditional extended trisectionectomy. The complexity of this surgical procedure is based on two hepatic parenchymal transections, doubled area of cut surface, proximity to important vascular and biliary structures (such as the RHV and LHV and the right and left hepatic pedicle), and need of maintaining hepatic pedicles to the remaining posterior and lateral segments. Any compromise of these important structures may cause congestion, ischemia, and necrosis of the liver residual and may result in postoperative liver failure and even death [40, 84–86]. Mesohepatectomy was first performed for gallbladder cancer in 1972 by McBride and Wallace [87]. Though it is still a challenging surgical procedure, since then, it has been reported to be a safe and feasible alternative to extended hepatectomy [82, 87–94].

Surgical Indications

For HCCs located centrally within the liver (Couinaud's segments IV, V, and VIII), mesohepatectomy was carried out when the future liver residual volume was estimated to be adequate. Routine preoperative imaging assessment concluded abdominal ultrasound, high-resolution and contrast-enhanced computed tomography (CT) and/or magnetic resonance imaging (MRI) to ascertain the number, size and location of the tumor and its relationship with adjacent important vascular and biliary vessels. The future liver residual volume was evaluated by preoperative CT or MRI, and it should be >50% for patients with cirrhosis or >30% for patients with non-cirrhotic livers [95]. In terms of liver function evaluation, Child-Pugh classification [56] and the indocyanine green retention rate at 15 min (ICGR15) [5] were used. Mesohepatectomy for centrally located HCC was indicated only for patients with Child-Pugh class A and with an ICGR15<10%. The patients with Child-Pugh class B and C liver function, hyperbilirubinemia, encephalopathy, hypalbuminemia, and ascites were excluded from this procedure.

Operative Procedures	Technical Details
Laparotomy	◀ A right subcostal incision.
↓	
Mobilization of the liver	◀ Freeing the liver from its surrounding structure.
↓	
Isolation and division of the right anterior sectional and the left medial sectional pedicle	◀ The right anterior sectional Glissonean pedicle and the left medial sectional Glissonean pedicle was isolated, divided and silk-sutured, respectively, based on a Glissonean approach.
↓	
Hepatic parenchymal transection	◀ Having clamped the infrahepatic inferior vena cava (IVC), parenchymal transection was performed according to the cut line marked on the liver surface using the clamp-crushing and/or finger fracture method. Having removed the specimen, The right hepatic vein (RHV), the left hepatic vein (LHV) and the anterior wall of the retrohepatic IVC were exposed.
↓	
Drainage and closure of the abdominal cavity	◀ A double-lumen tube was placed close to the cut surface.

Intraoperative Key Points

1. It is conceivable that achieving an anatomical mesohepatectomy based on Glissonean approach may be difficult in some patients [84]. For instance, in patients with dilated venous collaterals caused by portal hypertension and/or previous right quadrant operation, the incisions made on the hilus were inclined to bleed, and the subsequent proceedings were difficult to continue. Under such a circumstance, it is advisable to abandon this method and use other methods to perform the proposed anatomical mesohepatectomy.
2. For large HCCs centrally located within the liver, control of the intraoperative bleeding is the key to the success of the surgical proceedings [40, 92]. In case of no highly selective inflow blood occlusion can be achieved, the Pringle maneuver and the infrahepatic and suprahepatic IVC should be pre-placed with a vascular tape, respectively, to prepare for inadvertent injuries to the RHV, LHV, the right portal vein, and the left portal vein. It should be kept in mind that the priority policy is the reasonable usage of various kinds of bleeding control technology.
3. For tumors located within the central segments of the liver, its proximity to the important vascular vessels was always a problem for an adequate resection margin. It is generally accepted that the resection margin length should be more than 10 mm; however, in most anatomical mesohepatectomies, it is impossible to achieve this length. It is our policy to prefer mesohepatectomy over traditional aggressive extended trisectionectomy when the resection margin can be kept negative [85]; especially in China, most patients (>85%) are associated with hepatitis B and cirrhotic liver, and the policy is appropriate and reasonable to reduce postoperative liver failure [95].
4. At this stage the right anterior pedicle is transected and suture-ligated, same attention is paid to prevent causing injury to the posterior bile duct (see section "Anatomic Right Anterior Sectionectomy Using Glissonean Pedicle Transection Method") [35, 49, 96, 97].
5. Anatomical mesohepatectomy is a technically complicated hepatic resection for which the demarcation of the liver area to be removed is advocated. Theoretically, having transecting the right anterior pedicle and the pedicle of segment IV, the right-sided ischemic demarcation line between the right anterior and posterior section and the left-sided ischemic demarcation line between segment IV and left lateral section can be obtained on the liver surface. However, having clamped the right or left hepatic pedicle, the ischemic demarcation boundary would disappear within the liver parenchyma. The advantage of staining the target section(segment) by injecting methylene blue into the feeding portal vein can facilitate to precisely and strictly resect the target section (segment) based on the range of liver tissue staining within the hepatic parenchyma [57] (Fig. 197).

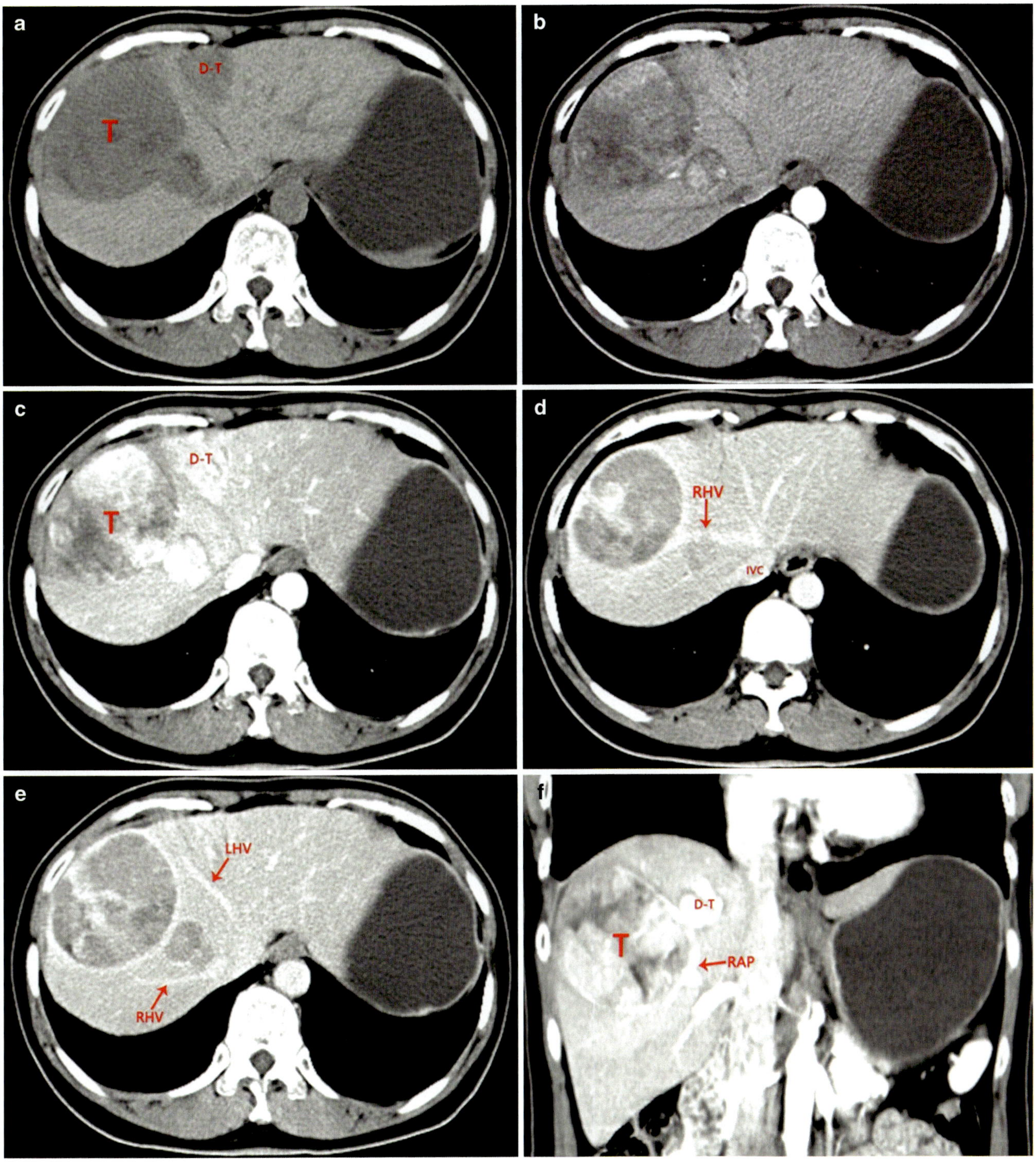

Fig. 197 (**a**) Preoperative CT (precontrast). The tumor, which appears hypodense, is located in segments IV, V, and VIII. (**b**) Preoperative CT (early hepatic arterial phase). The tumor shows heterogeneous enhancement. (**c**) Preoperative CT (late hepatic arterial phase). The tumor shows further enhancement. (**d**) Preoperative CT (hepatic venous phase). The tumor shows enhancement fades and prominent capsular enhancement. (**e**) Preoperative CT (hepatic venous phase). The tumor shows enhancement fades and prominent capsular enhancement. (**f**) Preoperative CT (coronal section of the tumor). *T* tumor, *D-T* daughter tumor, *RHV* right hepatic vein, *IVC* inferior vena cava, *MHV* middle hepatic vein, *RAP* right anterior sectional pedicle of portal vein

Abdominal Incision and Mobilization of the Liver
(Figs. 198, 199, 200, 201, 202, 203, 204, and 205)

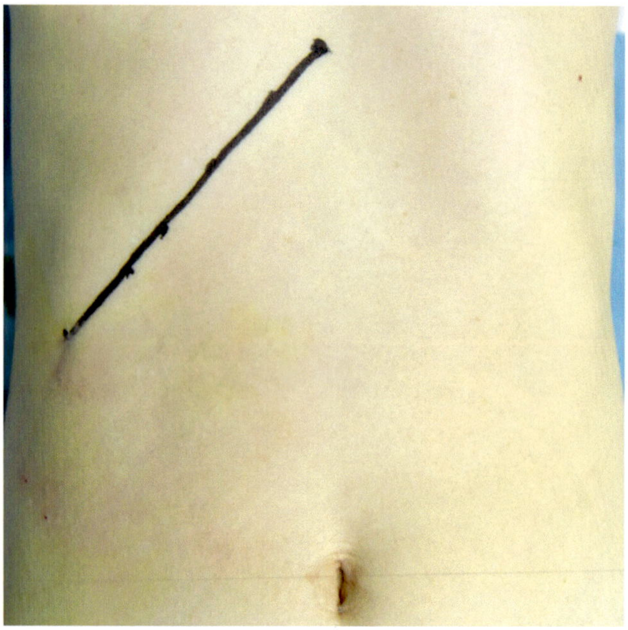

Fig. 198 A right subcostal incision was selected and made

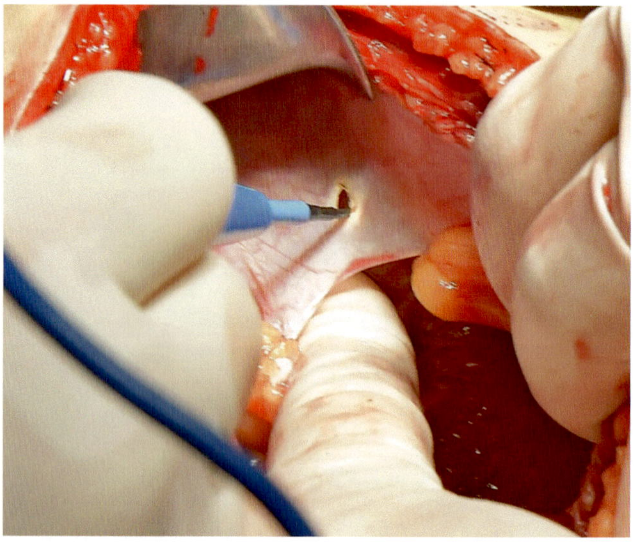

Fig. 200 The falciform was dissected away from the anterior abdominal wall

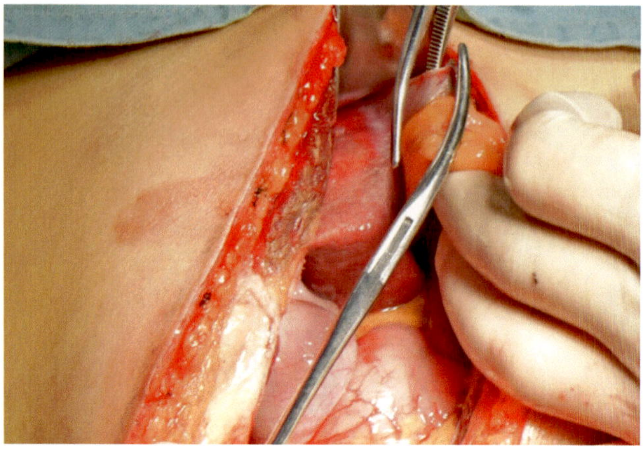

Fig. 199 Having entered into the abdominal cavity, the round ligament was divided and ligated

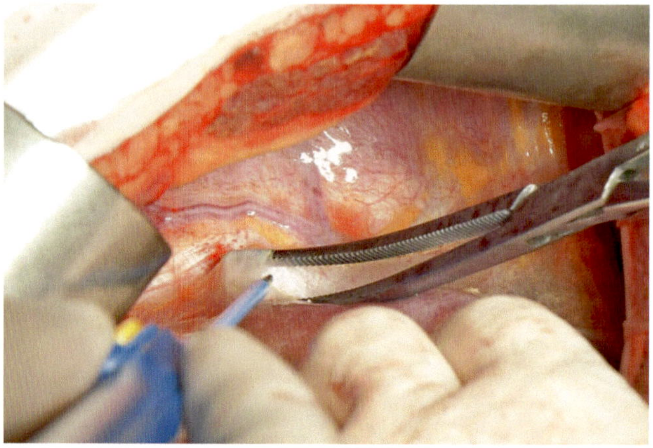

Fig. 201 Hepatocaval confluence and the right coronary ligament was dissected

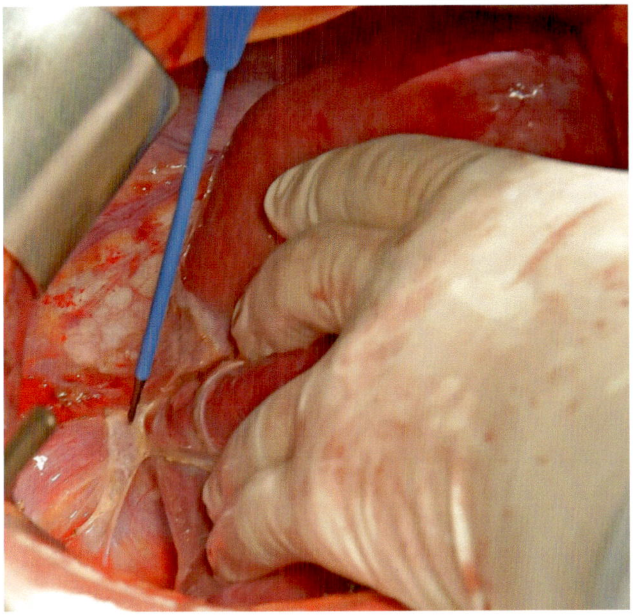

Fig. 202 The right triangular ligament was electrocauterized

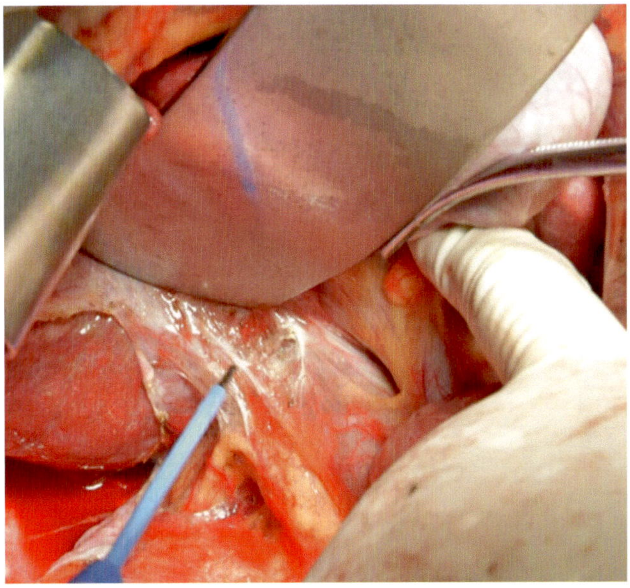

Fig. 204 The right adrenal gland was dissected away from the posterior portion of the right hemiliver

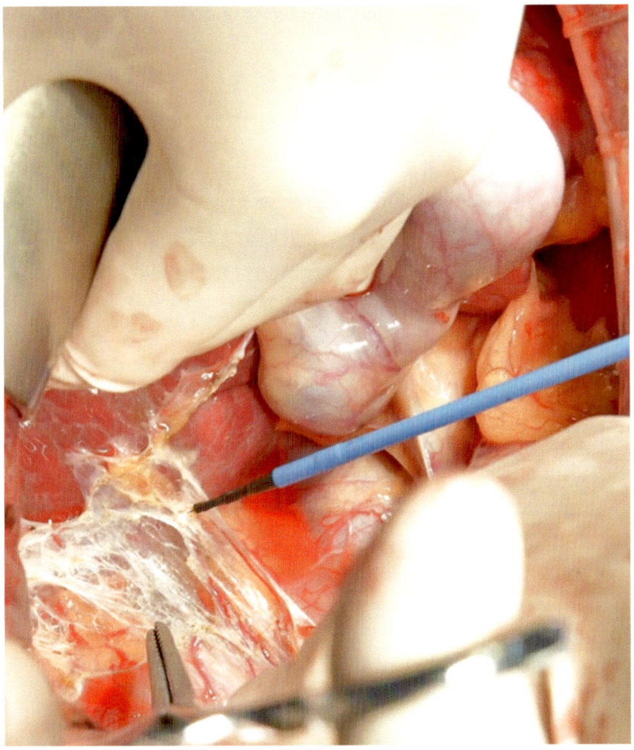

Fig. 203 The hepatocolic ligament was divided with electrocautery

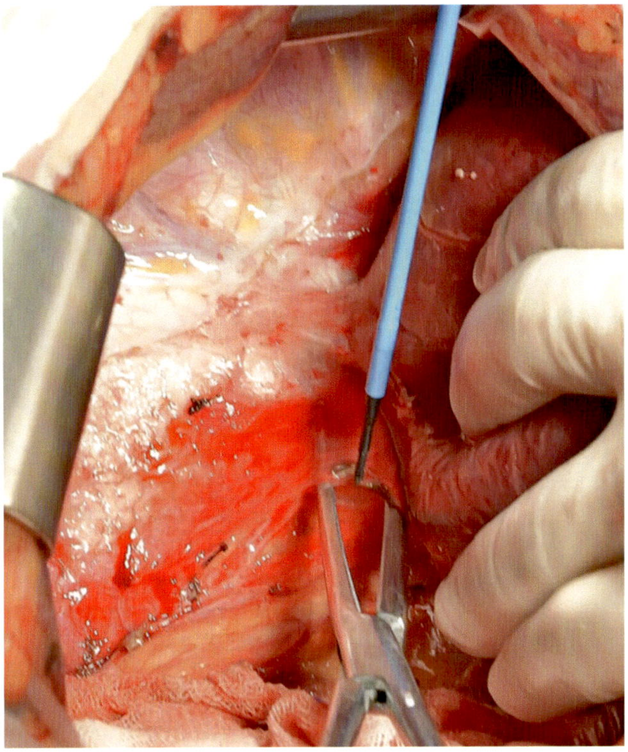

Fig. 205 The hepatocaval ligament was dissected to expose the right-sided and anterior wall of the retrohepatic inferior vena cava (IVC)

Preparation for Total Vascular Exclusion
(Figs. 206, 207, and 208)

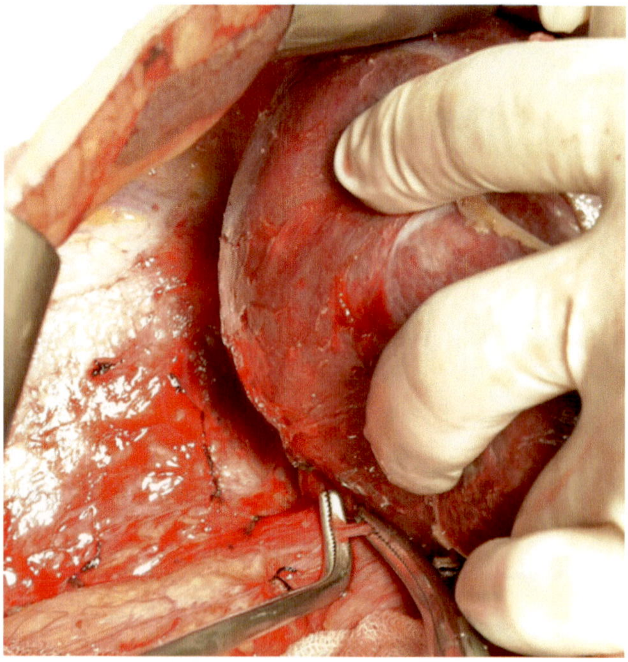

Fig. 206 The retrohepatic short veins were isolated, divided, and ligated individually caudo-cranially up to the root of the right hepatic veins (RHV)

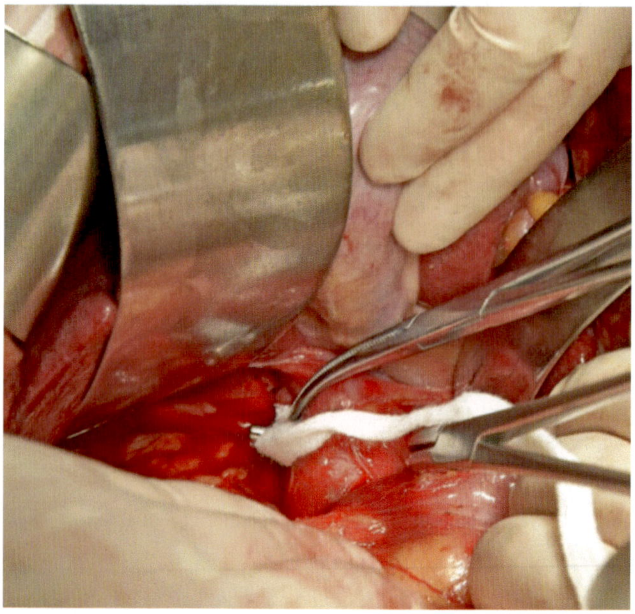

Fig. 208 The infrahepatic inferior vena cava (IVC) was also isolated and looped with a vascular tape

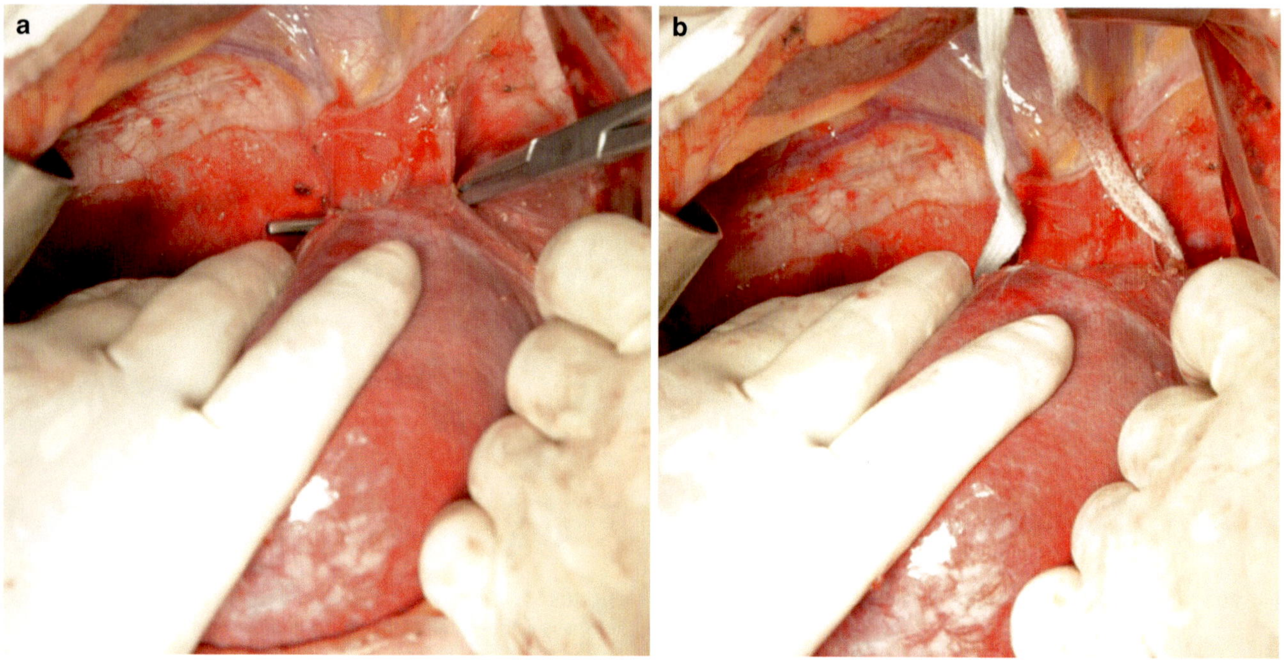

Fig. 207 (**a**, **b**) The suprahepatic inferior vena cava (IVC) was isolated and pre-placed with a tourniquet to control possible excessive bleeding in case of injuries to the main hepatic veins

Isolation of the Right Hepatic Pedicle

(Figs. 209, 210, and 211)

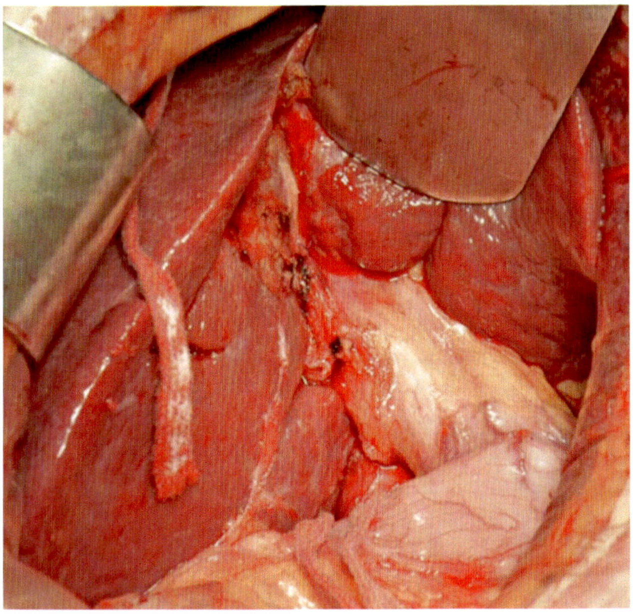

Fig. 209 Cholecystectomy have been performed

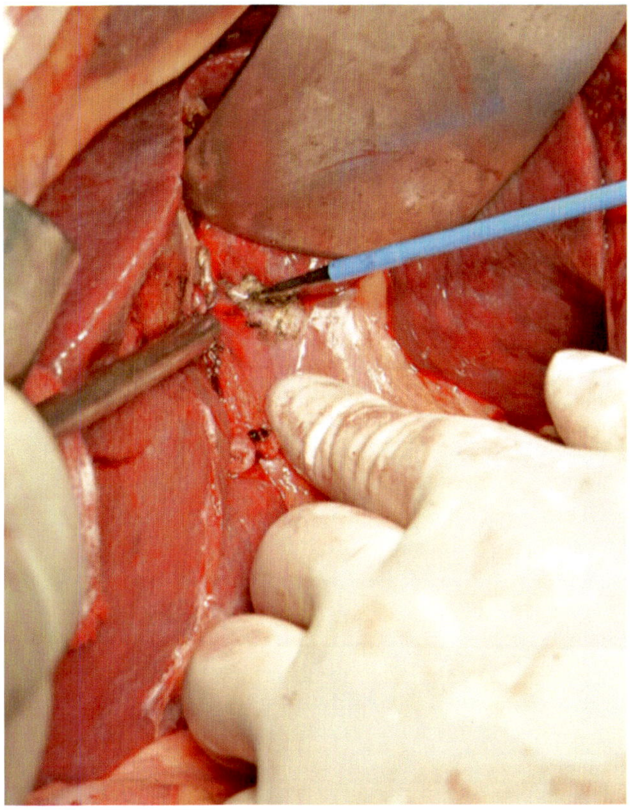

Fig. 210 A small anterior incision was made in front of the hilus, and the hepatic parenchyma around the small incision was divided with blunt dissection to expose the anterior surface of the right and the left Glissonean pedicle and its course

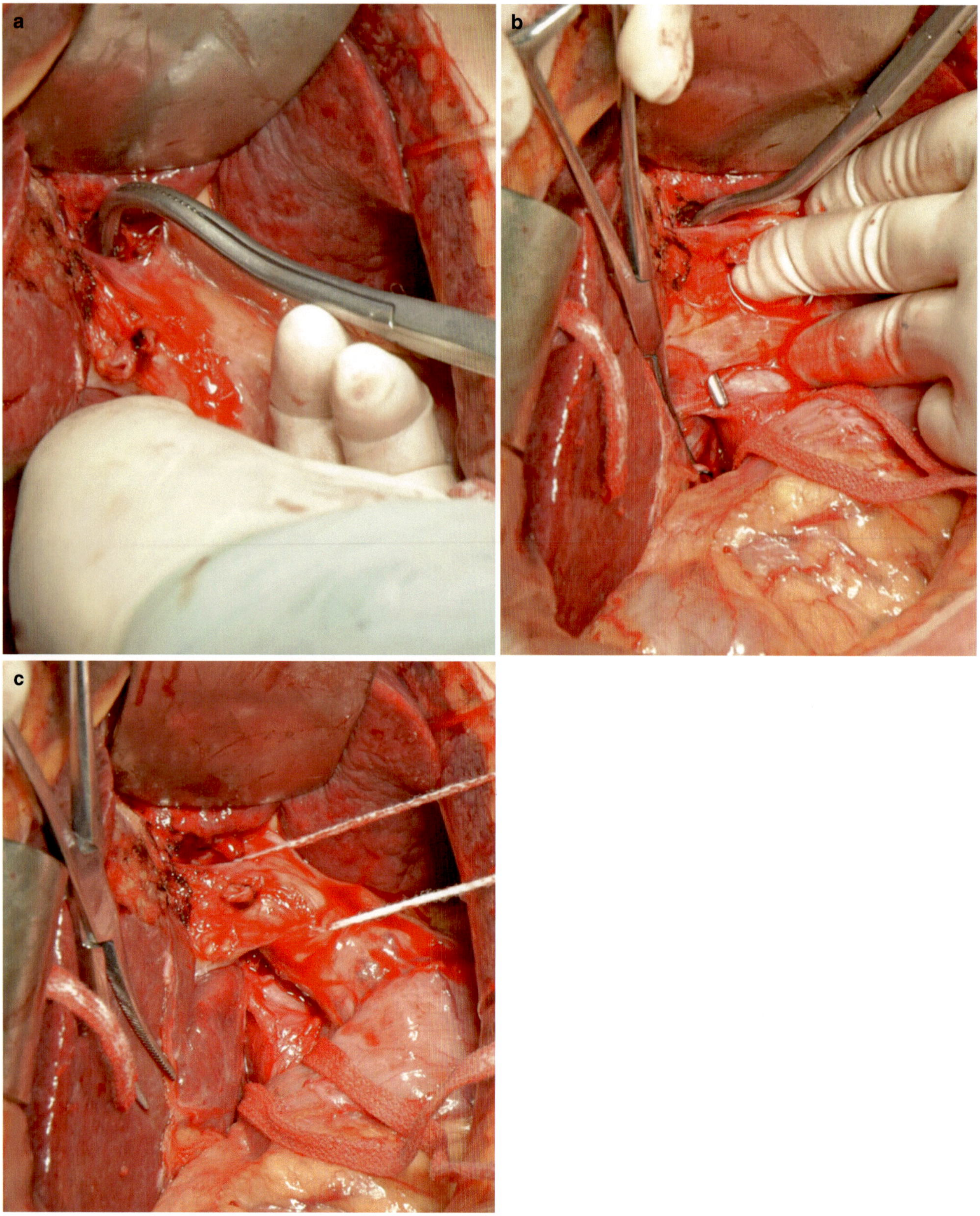

Fig. 211 (**a**) A large curved clamp was inserted vertically into this incision, and the operator's left index finger was put between the undersurface of the hilar plate and the anterior wall of the retrohepatic inferior vena cava (IVC). (**b**) The clamp was furtherly inserted to directly reach to the tip of the operator's left index finger, and using the finger as a guide, the clamp punctured through the undersurface membrane of the hilar plate and passed out of the right edge of the right hepatic pedicle. (**c**) Thus, the right hepatic pedicle was isolated and looped

Isolation of the Right Anterior Pedicle
(Figs. 212 and 213)

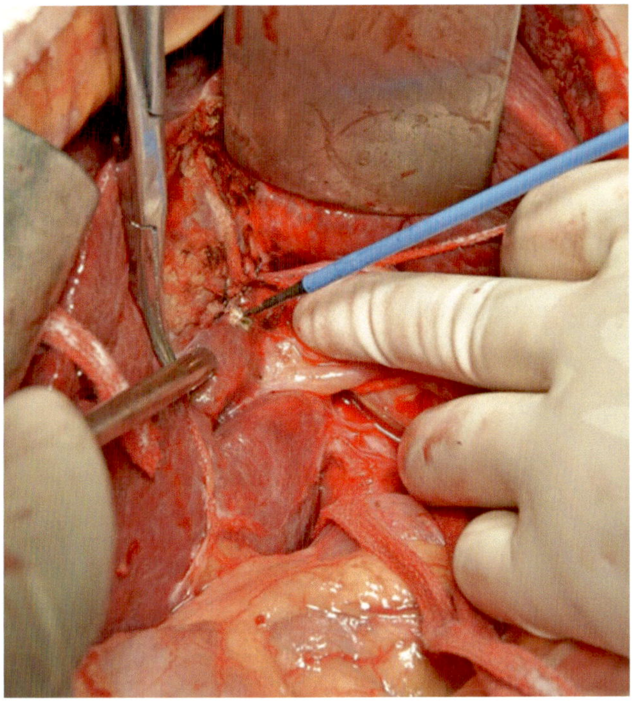

Fig. 212 Another small incision was made at the right edge of the gallbladder bed

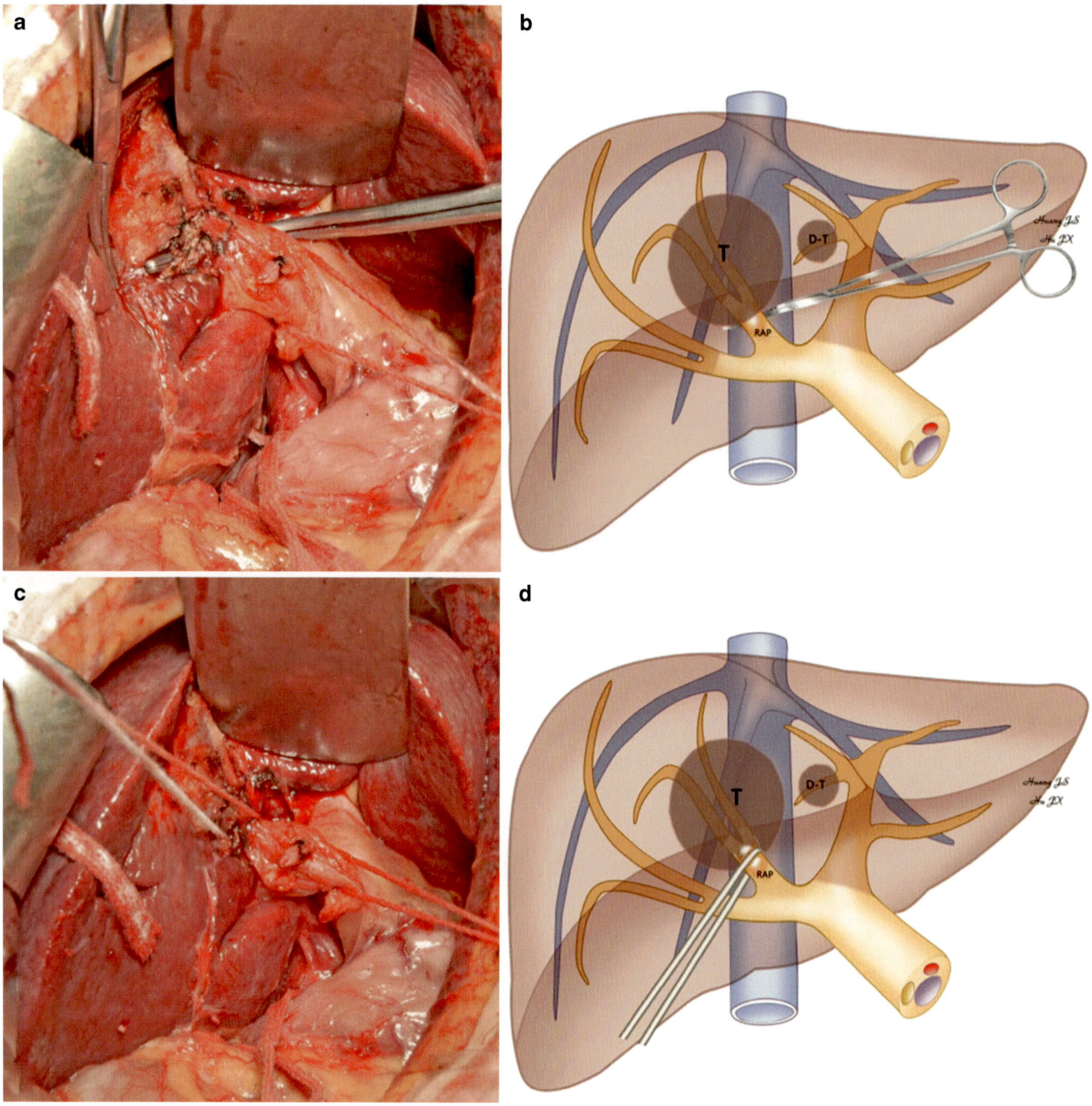

Fig. 213 (**a**) A large curved clamp was inserted into the incision in front of the hilar plate and pushed through out of the incision on the right edge of the gallbladder bed. (**b**) Schematic illustration of the maneuver. (**c**) Thus, the right anterior pedicle (RAP) was also isolated and encompassed by a vascular tape. (**d**) Schematic illustration of this procedure

Isolation of S4 Pedicle (Fig. 214)

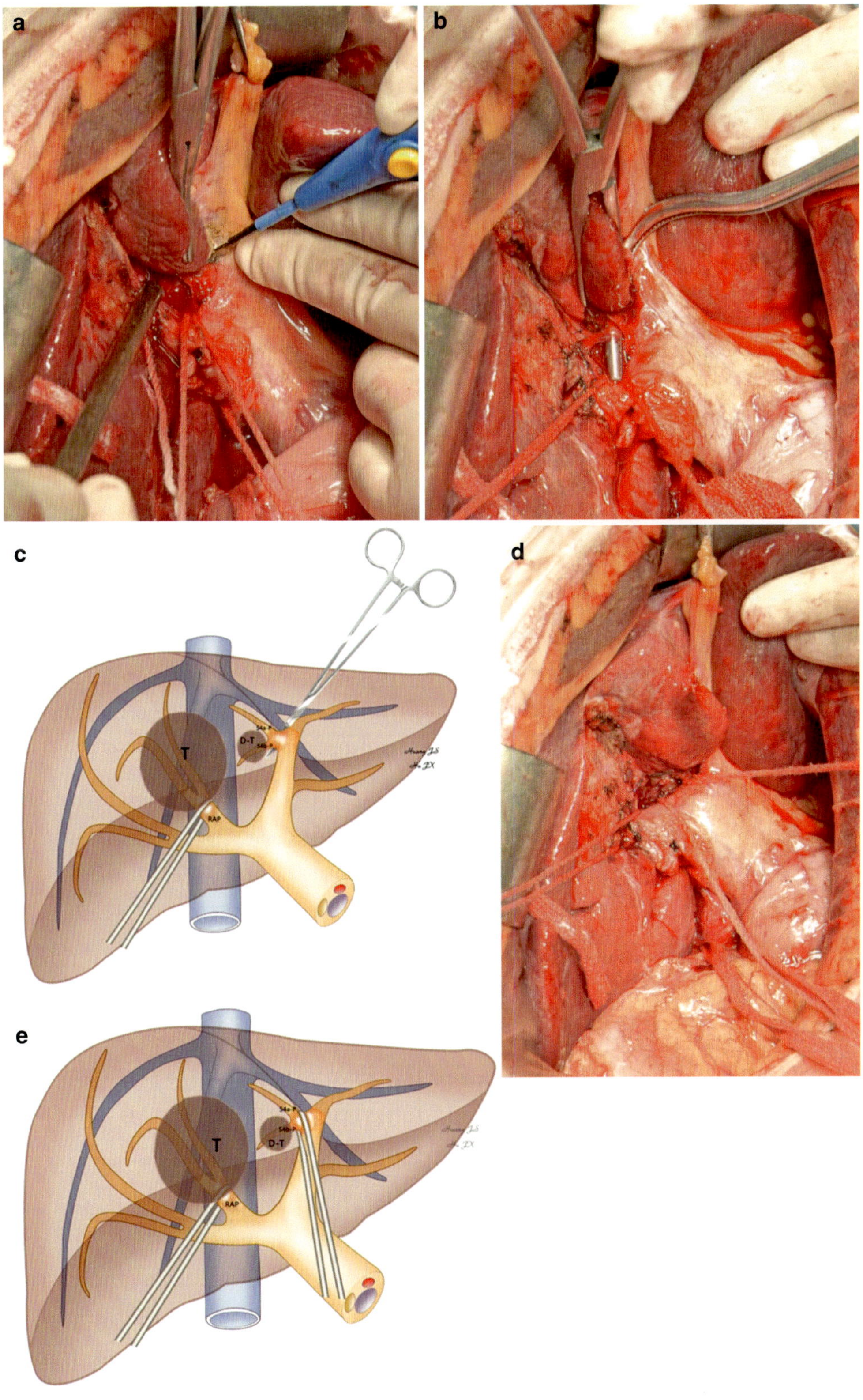

Fig. 214 (**a**) A third small incision was made in the right-sided margins of the basis of the round ligament. (**b**) A large curved clamp was inserted into this incision and passed out of the anterior incision in front of the hilus. (**c**) Schematic illustration of this maneuver. (**d**) Thus, the Glissonean pedicle of segment IV (S4) was isolated and then encircled with a vascular tape. (**e**) Schematic illustration of this procedure. *RAP* right anterior pedicle

Staining the Segments V, VIII, and IV and Marking the Cut Line (Figs. 215, 216, 217, 218, and 219)

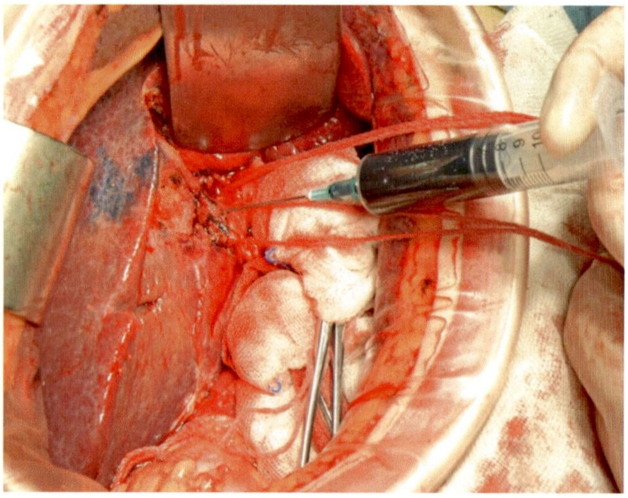

Fig. 215 Methylene blue was injected into the portal branch of the right anterior sector

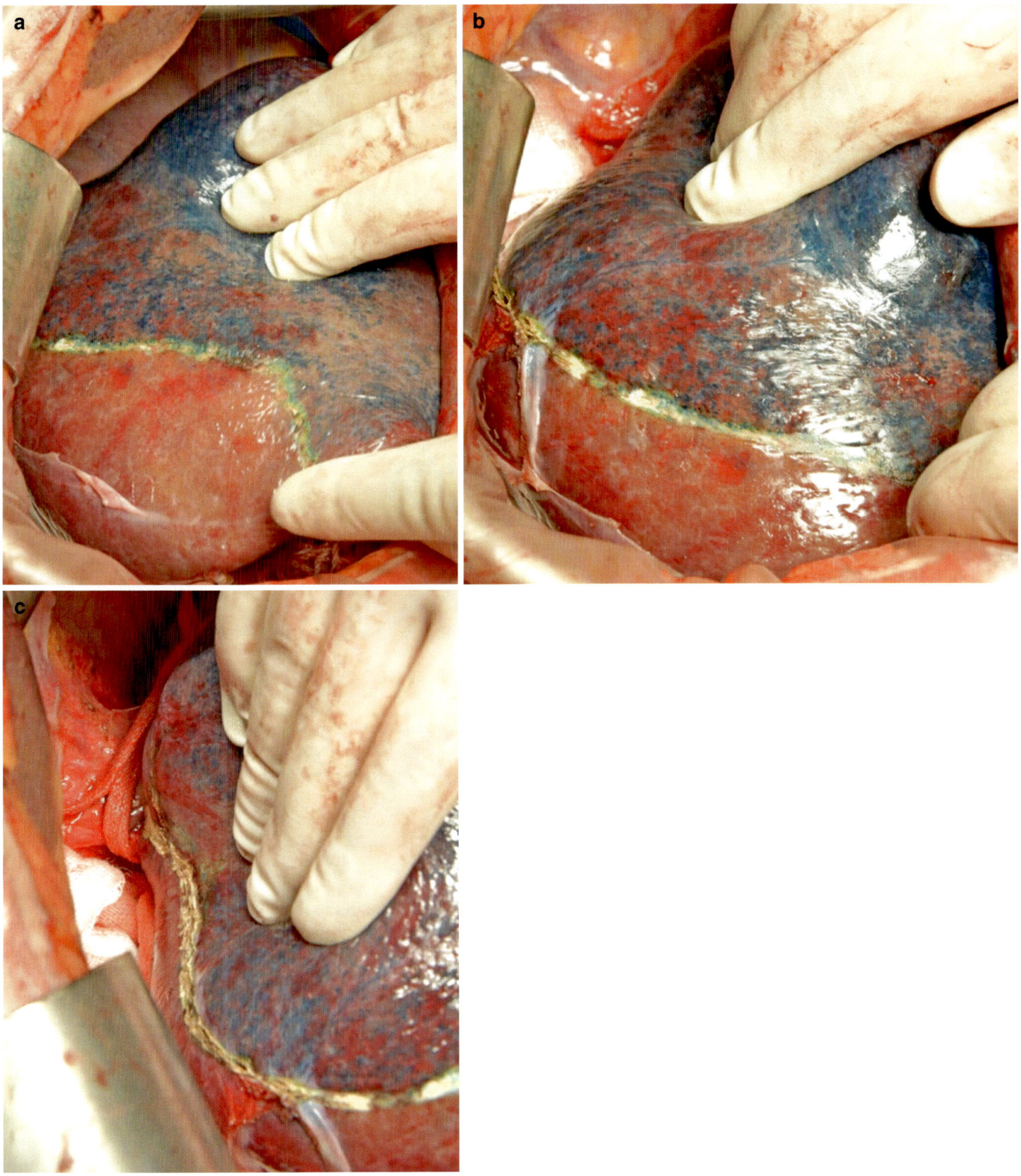

Fig. 216 (**a**–**c**) The right anterior sector was colorized. The demarcation line between the right anterior sector and posterior sector was marked on the liver surface with electrocautery

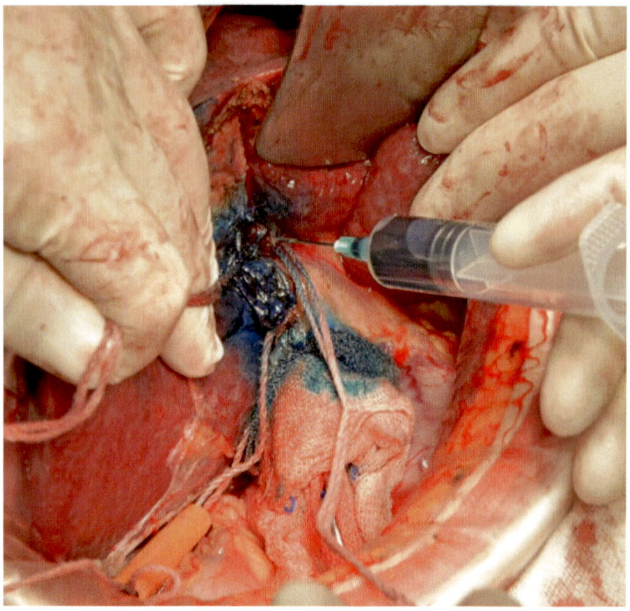

Fig. 217 Methylene blue was also injected into the portal branch of segment IV

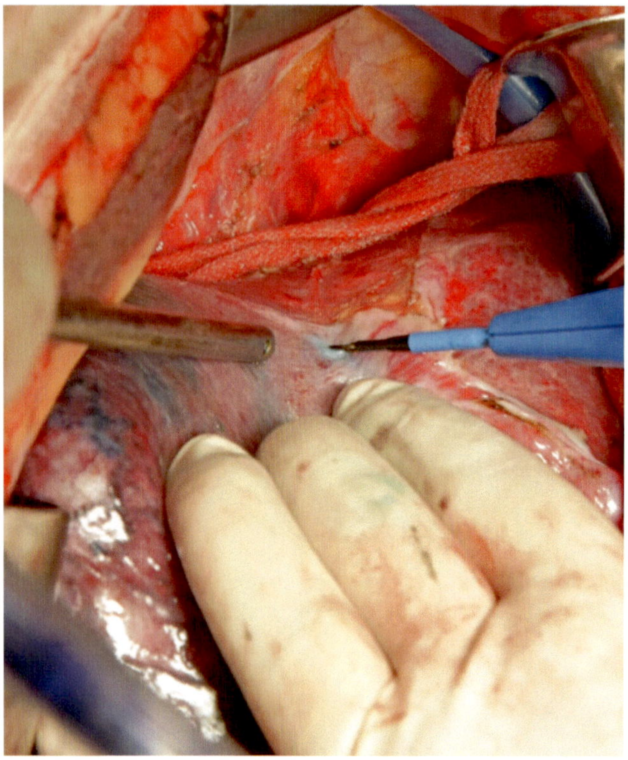

Fig. 218 Segment IV_A was colorized, and the demarcation line between this segment and segment II was marked on the liver surface with electrocautery

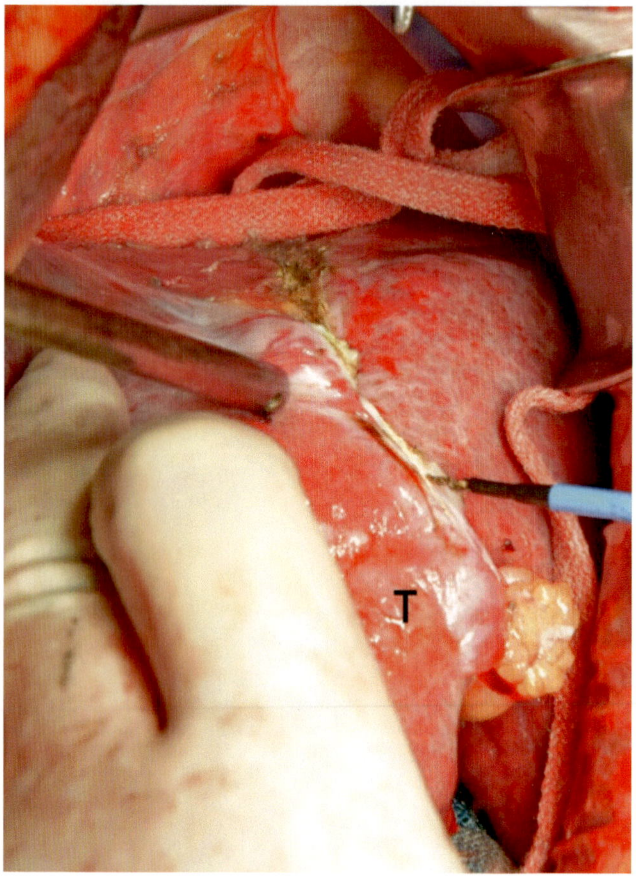

Fig. 219 Because the daughter tumor was located within segment IV_B, the transecting line between segment IV_B and segment III was marked on the left side of the falciform ligament

Division of the Right Anterior Pedicle

(Figs. 220, 221, 222, 223, and 224)

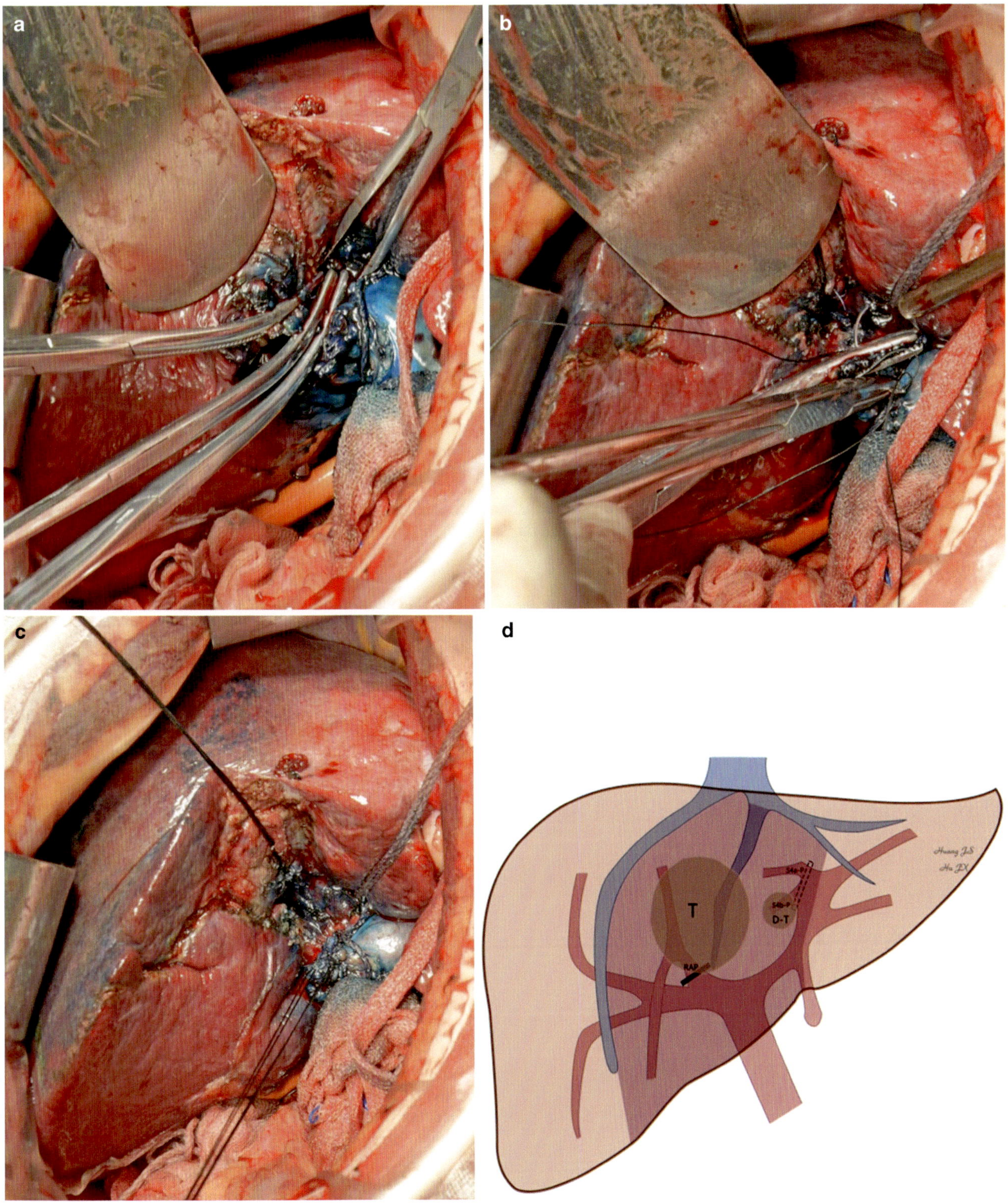

Fig. 220 (**a**) The right anterior Glissonean pedicle (RAP) was clamped. (**b**, **c**) The RAP was divided and suture-ligated. (**d**) Schematic illustration of this procedure

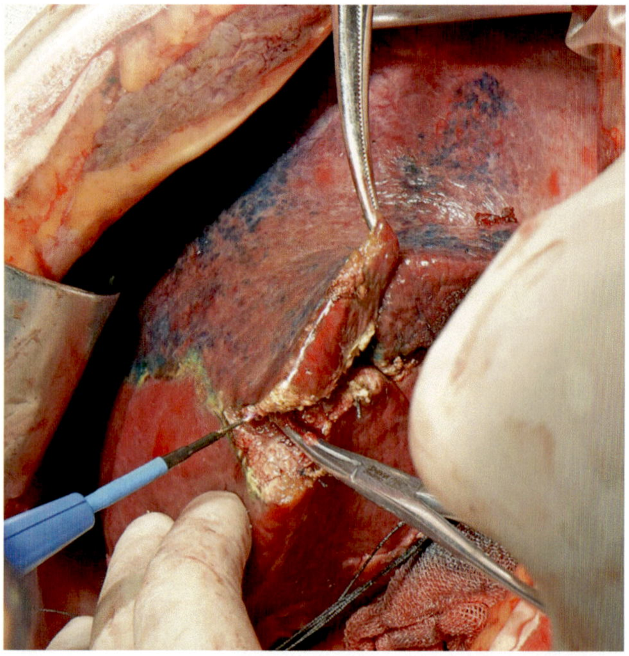

Fig. 221 Having clamped the right hepatic pedicle and infrahepatic IVC, hepatic parenchymal dissection was performed from the anterior and inferior liver surface posteriorly toward the retrohepatic IVC and superiorly toward the hepatocaval confluence along the demarcation line by a clamp-crushing method

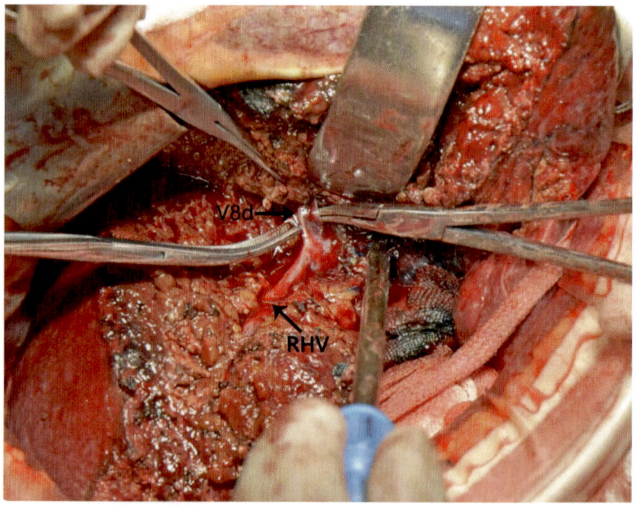

Fig. 223 Branch of the right hepatic vein (RHV) draining dorsal portion of segment VIII was isolated, divided, and ligated

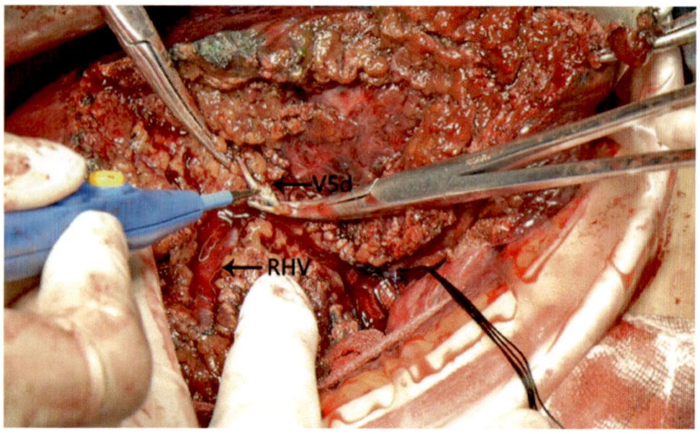

Fig. 222 Branch of the right hepatic vein (RHV) draining dorsal portion of segment V was dissected

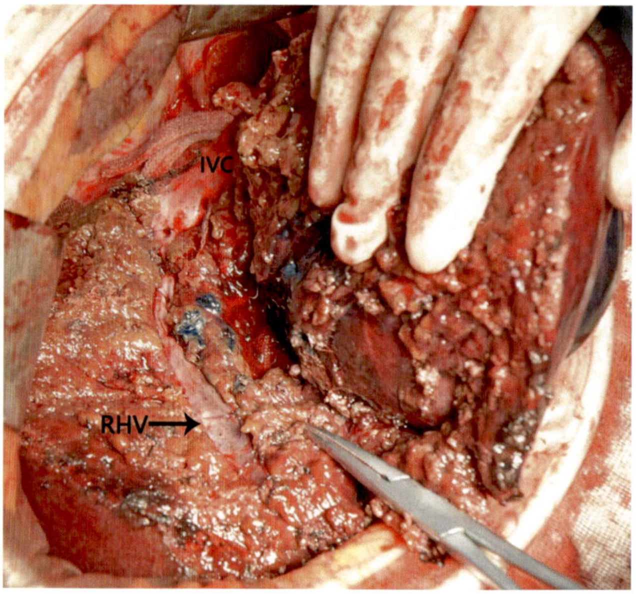

Fig. 224 The right-sided hepatic parenchymal transection has been performed, and complete exposure of the right hepatic vein (RHV) was shown on the raw surface of the residual liver

Division of the Pedicle of Segment IV (Fig. 225)

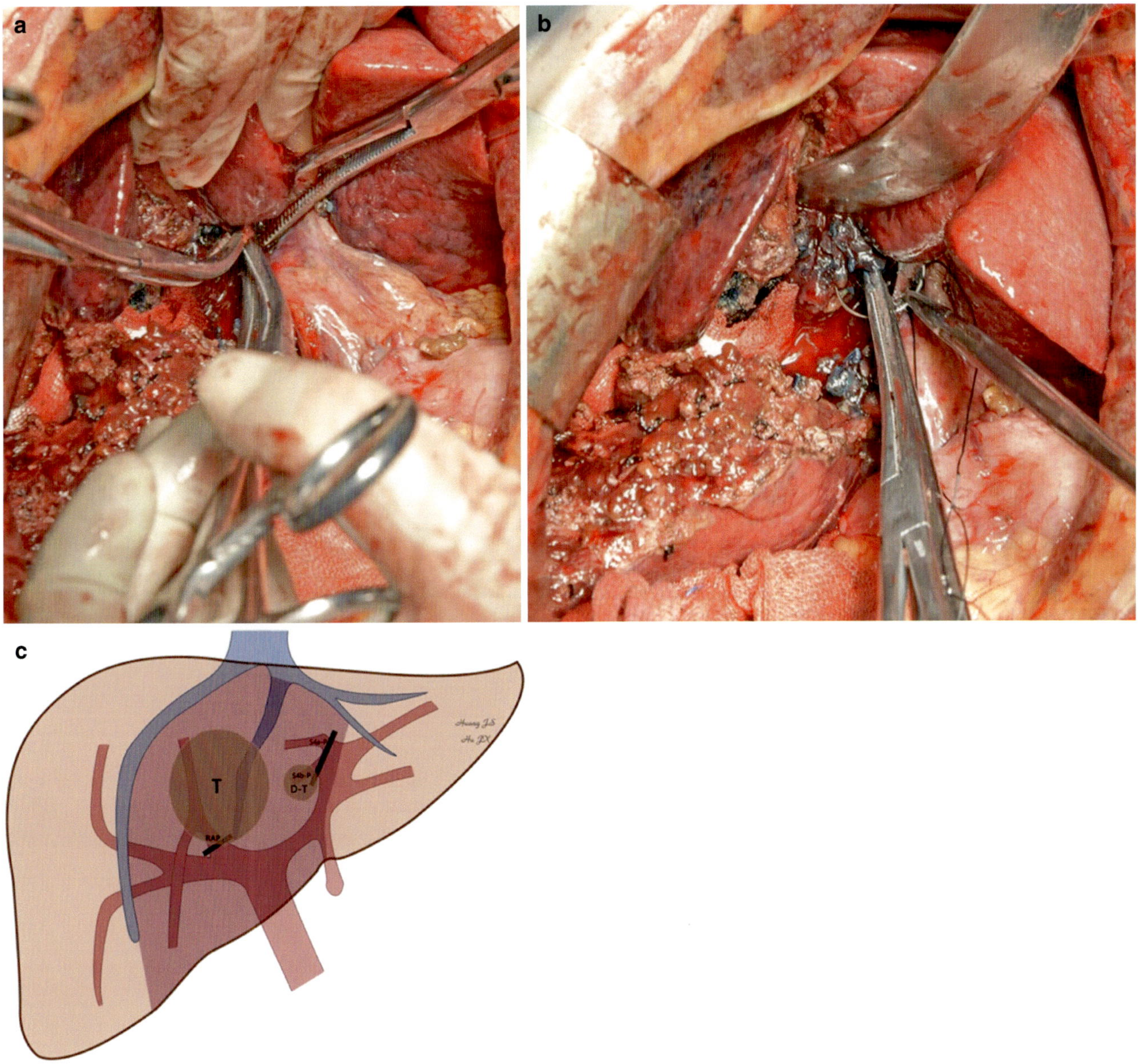

Fig. 225 (**a**, **b**) The segment IV Glissonean pedicle was clamped (**a**), divided, and suture-ligated (**b**). (**c**) Schematic illustration of this procedure

Hepatic Parenchymal Transection (Left-Sided)
(Figs. 226, 227, 228, and 229)

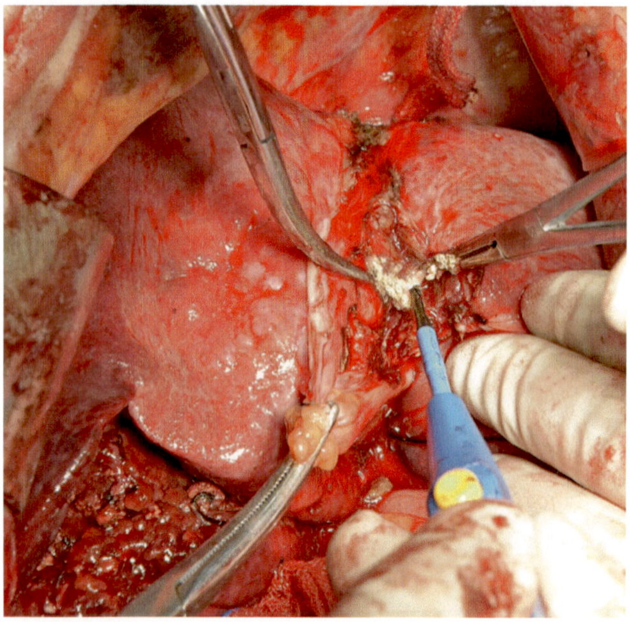

Fig. 226 Having clamped the left hepatic pedicle and the infrahepatic IVC, the left liver parenchyma transection was then performed using finger-fracture and clamp-crushing methods along the left cut line caudo-cranially

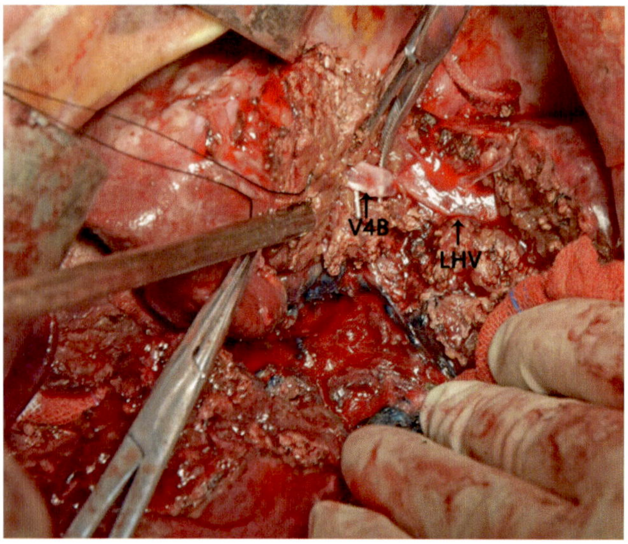

Fig. 227 Branch V_{4B} of the left hepatic vein (LHV) draining segment IVB was dissected

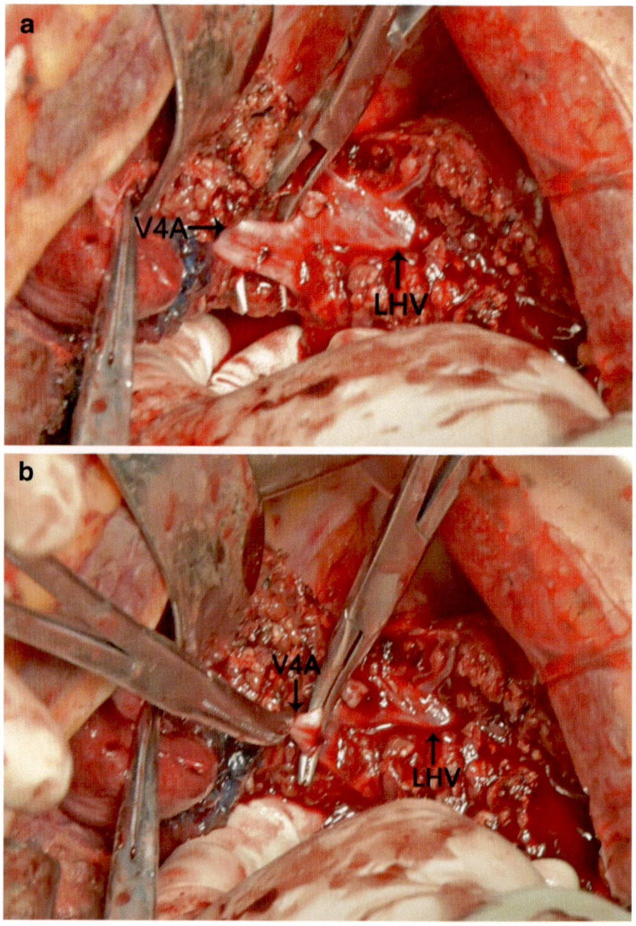

Fig. 228 (**a**, **b**) Branch V_{4A} of the left hepatic vein (LHV) draining segment IVA was isolated, divided, and ligated

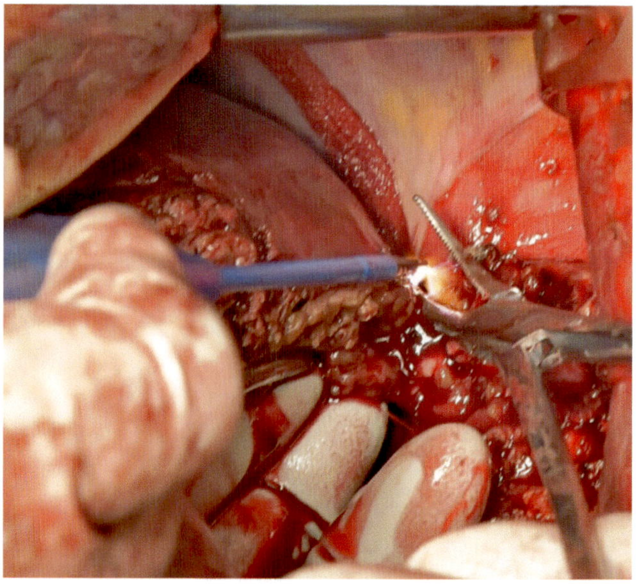

Fig. 229 The hepatic parenchyma around the root of the middle hepatic vein (MHV) and left hepatic vein (LHV) was dissected to expose their entry into the suprahepatic inferior vena cava (IVC)

Extrahepatic Management of the Middle Hepatic Vein (MHV) (Fig. 230)

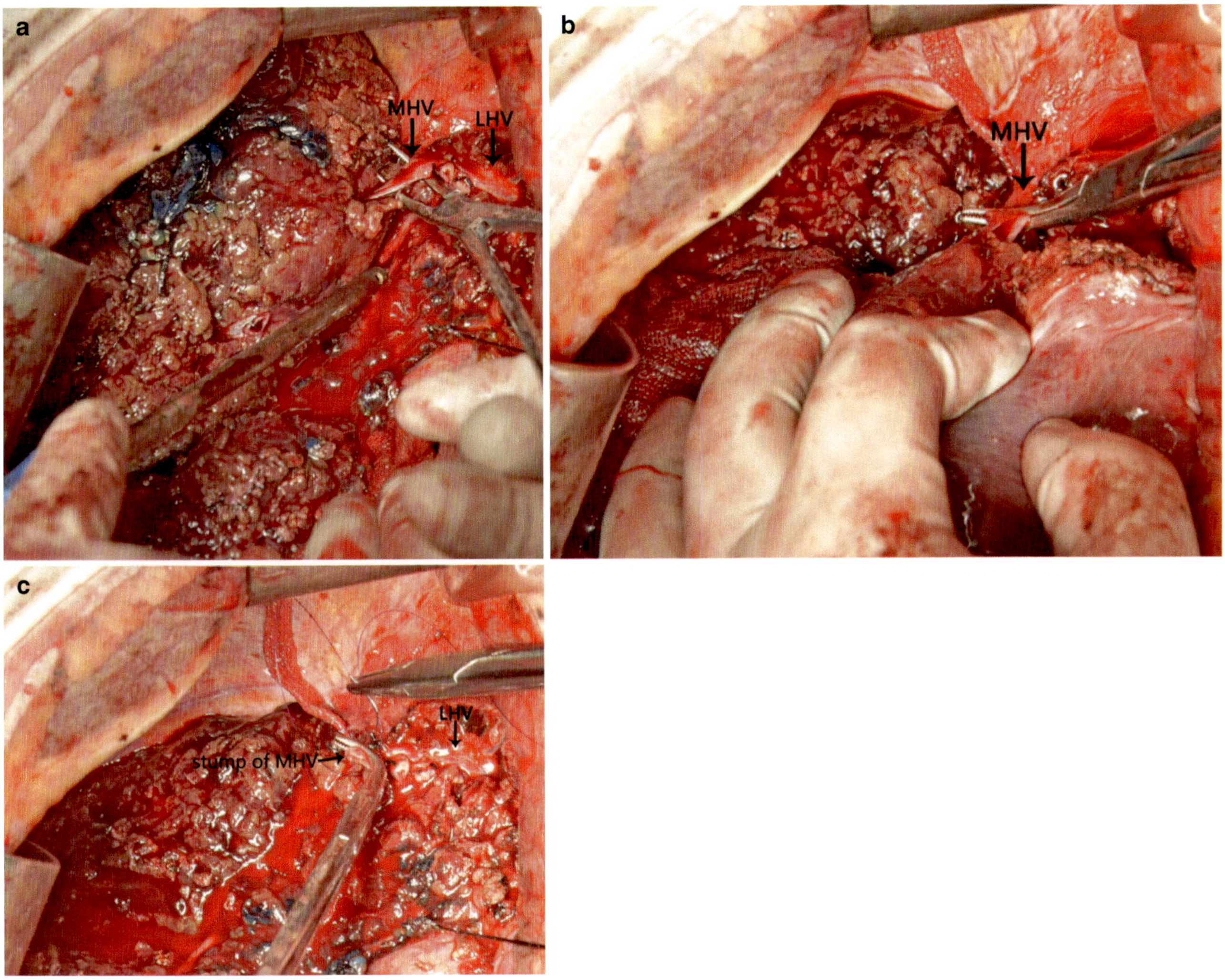

Fig. 230 (**a**–**c**) The middle hepatic vein (MHV) was extrahepatically isolated (**a**), clamped (**b**), divided, and suture-ligated (**c**). LHV, left hepatic vein

Hemostasis and Prevention of Bile Leak at the Raw Area (Fig. 231)

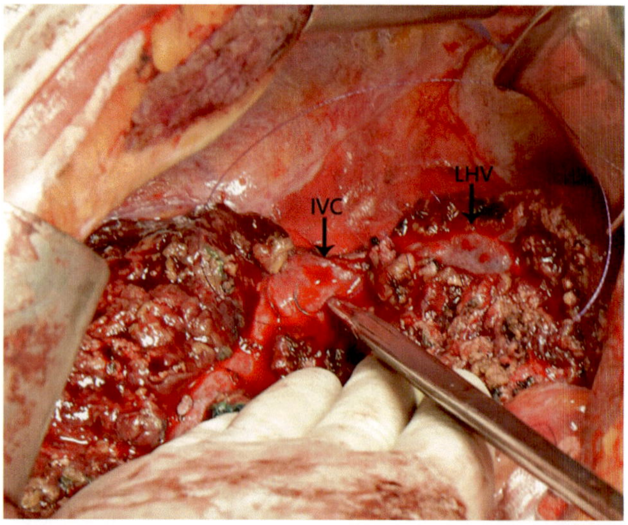

Fig. 231 Having removed the specimen, the tiny holes on the right hepatic vein (RHV) and left hepatic vein (LHV) were repaired with polypropylene 5-0. Other vascular and biliary ramifications on the raw surface were sutured with silk thread and/or polypropylene 3-0. *IVC* inferior vena cava

Raw Area of the Residue Liver and the Specimen
(Figs. 232, 233, and 234)

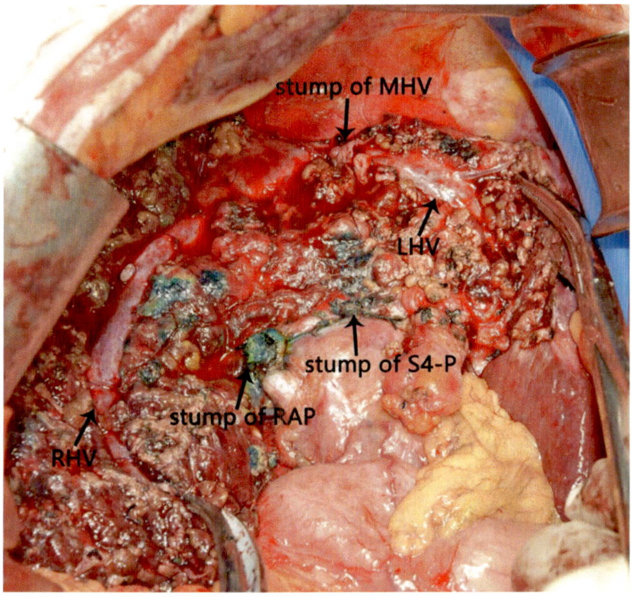

Fig. 232 Bird view of the raw area. At last, the raw area of the liver remnant was covered with fibrin glue or other hemostatic agents. In all cases, a drain close to the cut surface of the liver remnant was used. *RHV* right hepatic vein, *RAP* right anterior pedicle, *S4-P* segment IV pedicle, *MHV* middle hepatic vein, *LHV* left hepatic vein

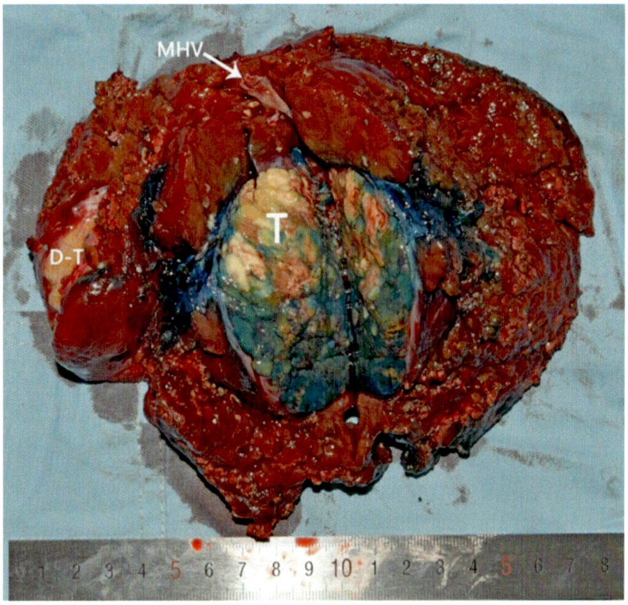

Fig. 234 The split surface of the tumor. *MHV* middle hepatic vein, *T* tumor, *D-T* daughter tumor

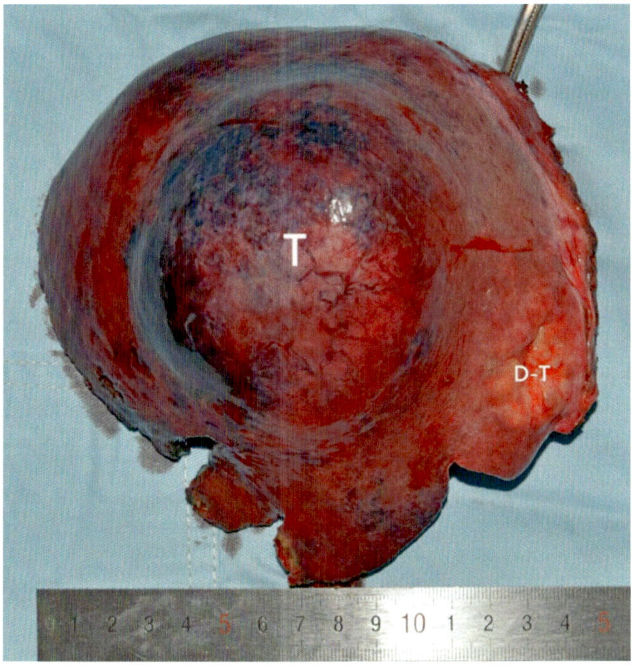

Fig. 233 The anterior surface of the specimen. *T* tumor, *D-T* daughter tumor

Segmentectomy VIII

Jixiong Hu, Weidong Dai, and Tenglong Tang

Segment VIII (SVIII) is the largest of the eight Couinaud segments [79], including 11–45 (median 24) percent of the total liver volume [60]. From a technical point of view, resection, isolated resection of single segment VIII, is technically challenging and complex [37, 98–101]. The pedicle(s) of segment VIII is(are) located deep inside hepatic parenchyma where it is sometimes difficult to isolate, loop, and transect it. SVIII is circumfused by the right hepatic vein (RHV) laterally, the middle hepatic vein (MHV) medially, and the retrohepatic inferior vena cava (IVC) posteriorly. Furthermore, it is difficult to decide the extent of resection due to no obvious anatomic landmarks on the liver surface. All these circumstances render a single resection of SVIII technically demanding.

Surgical Indications

The surgical indications and procedures for resection of SVIII HCCs were decided on the basis of the tumor-vessel relationships and future residual liver functional reserve. Generally, anatomical segmentectomy VIII was prioritized over wedge resection (WR), because anatomical resection of tumor-bearing hepatic segments has the advantage of reducing the risk of postoperative recurrence. Right anterior sectionectomy (RAS) or right hepatectomy was selected when the HCCs infiltrated the right anterior Glissonean pedicle or the right Glissonean pedicle (see sections "Right Hepatectomy (S5~S8 Resection)" and "Anatomic Right Anterior Sectionectomy Using Glissonean Pedicle Transection Method"). In terms of liver function, the acceptable ranges of sacrificed liver volumes were defined in detail on the basis of the indocyanine green retention rate at 15 min (ICGR 15). According to this criterion, anatomical segmentectomy VIII can be considered when the ICGR must be less than 30%.

Operative Procedures	Technical Details
Laparotomy ↓	◀ A right subcostal incision.
Isolation and division of the SVIII pedicle ↓	◀ The right hepatic Glissonean pedicle, the right anterior sectional Glissonean pedicle and the SVIII Glissonean pedicle was isolated and looped one by one.
Colorization ↓	◀ Methylene blue was injected into the pedicle of SVIII. Then, the pedicle of SVIII was divided. Color change appeared on the liver surface. According to color change and ischemic demarcation line, the cut line was marked on the liver surface with electrocautery.
Hepatic parenchymal transection ↓	◀ Having clamped the infrahepatic inferior vena cava and the right hepatic pedicle, parenchymal transection was performed using the clamp-crushing and/or finger fracture method. Having removed the specimen, The RHV, MHV, and the anterior wall of the retrohepatic IVC were exposed.
Drainage and closure of the abdominal cavity	◀ A double-lumen tube was placed close to the cut surface.

Intraoperative Key Points

1. It is conceivable that anatomic segmentectomy VIII may be difficult to achieve based on an intrahepatic Glissonean approach in some cirrhotic patients. For example, in case of portal hypertension or previous right upper quadrant abdominal surgery, it is sometimes very difficult to make incisions in front of the hilar plate because of severe bleeding. Under such circumstances, our policy is to perform anatomical segmentectomy VIII using other methods.
2. In most cases, the right anterior sectional Glissonean pedicle enters into hepatic parenchyma along a consistent course, and its divergence can be identified easily adjacent to the hilar plate. However, in few patients, the pedicles of segments V and VIII were lied deeply within the liver parenchyma, and it was technically demanding and time-consuming to identify them, respectively. For those patients, the right anterior pedicle was isolated and temporarily occluded, and then the left and right ischemic demarcation line was marked on the liver surface with electrocautery; meanwhile, the inferior parenchymal transection line, which corresponds to the traverse plane through the hilar hilum, was also marked on the liver surface. Along the boundary of segment VIII, hepatic parenchymal transection was carried out, and the pedicle of S8 was finally transected.
3. S_{VIII} is the most centrally located segment. HCCs confined to this segment usually are very adjacent to or adhere to the right hepatic vein and/or the middle hepatic vein. Therefore, a wide or an adequate resection margin (>10 mm) is usually impossible to obtain by single segmentectomy VIII. It is our policy that lesser operative margins are acceptable and an isolated anatomical resection of segment VIII should not be abandoned. Great care should be taken to guarantee a negative resection margin. Meanwhile, as aforementioned, during the hepatic parenchymal transectional proceedings, attention should be paid to prevent injury to the RHV and MHV. In case of severe backflow bleeding from the RHV and/or MHV, inflow and outflow blood occlusion should be employed to repair the injuries to the RHV and/or MHV. A bloodless operative field is essential for safely performing subsequent parenchymal transection.
4. Single anatomical Couinaud segment resection demands careful and precise isolation of the inflow pedicle(s), and knowledge of common anatomical variations of the target segment is necessary. Segment VIII classically has a single main pedicle that divides into a ventral and dorsal branch just before entering into segment VIII, just as seen in this resection. This is a noticeably consistent anatomic finding [27]. Another more important and common finding is that the pedicle of segment V (P5) may arise caudally from the extrasegmental trunk of the pedicle of segment VIII and supply the superior portion of segment V in as many as 69.2% of individuals [4, 6] (see Figs. 342, 344, 345, 347, and 349). Therefore, attention must be paid when transecting parenchyma toward the trunk of P8 because this surgical proceeding may inadvertently cause injury to P5 and result in ischemia of the superior portion of segment V (Figs. 235 and 236).

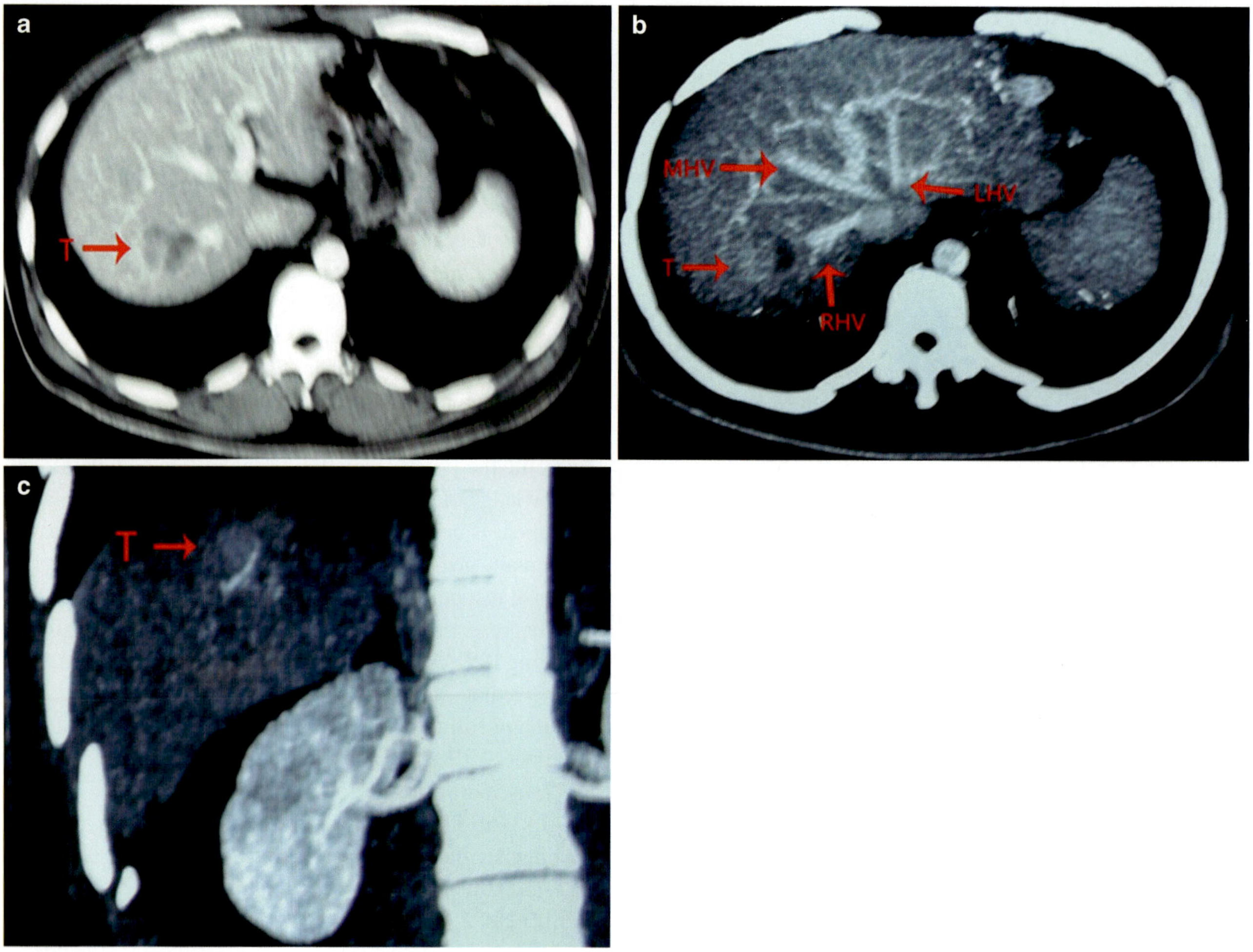

Fig. 235 (**a**, **b**) Preoperative CT shows the relationship between the tumor and the main vascular structure. The tumor shows heterogeneous enhancement in the hepatic arterial phase (**a**), further enhancing in the hepatic venous phase (**b**). (**c**) Coronary position. *T* tumor, *MHV* middle hepatic vein, *RHV* right hepatic vein, *LHV* left hepatic vein

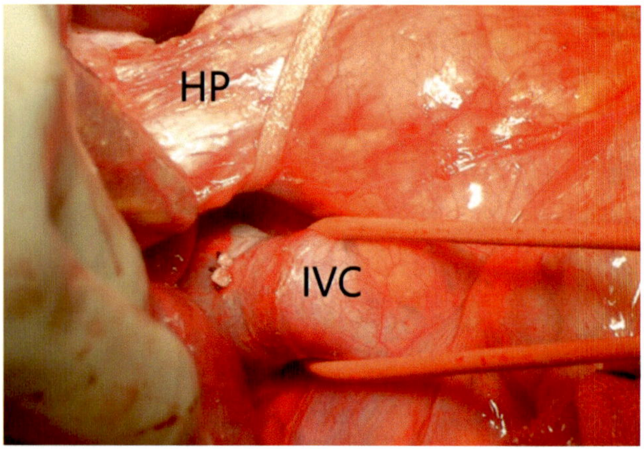

Fig. 236 A right subcostal incision was made. Having entered into the peritoneal cavity, the right hemiliver was mobilized. Then, a careful peritoneal exploration was made, and IOUS was made to ascertain in the relationship between the tumor and the main vasculature. In order to control intraoperative bleeding from the supplying vessels and backflow bleeding from the hepatic veins, hepatic pedicle (HP) and infrahepatic inferior vena cava (IVC) were encircled with a vascular tape, respectively

Isolation of the Right Hepatic Pedicle
(Figs. 237, 238, 239, and 240)

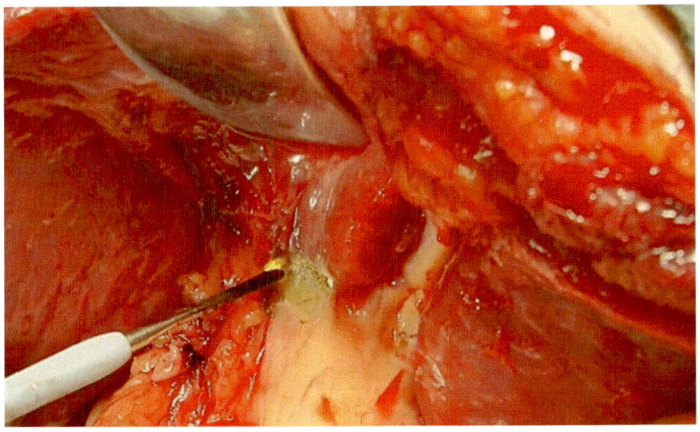

Fig. 237 An anterior small incision was made over the hepatic plate

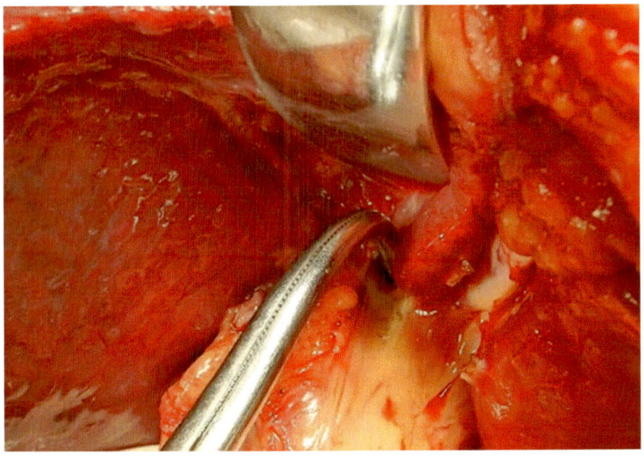

Fig. 238 A large right angle clamp was inserted into the incision

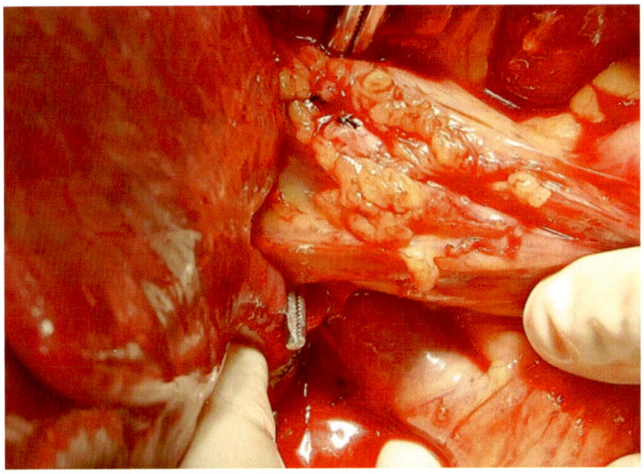

Fig. 239 A large curved clamp was inserted into this incision in front of the hilus, and the operator's left index finger was put between the undersurface of the hilar plate and the anterior wall of the retrohepatic inferior vena cava, and then, using the finger as a guide, the clamp was inserted furtherly and directly reached to the finger and punctured through the undersurface membrane and passed out of the right edge of the right hepatic pedicle. Thus, the right hepatic Glissonean pedicle was isolated and encircled with a vascular tape. The right hepatic pedicle was encompassed by a large right angle clamp

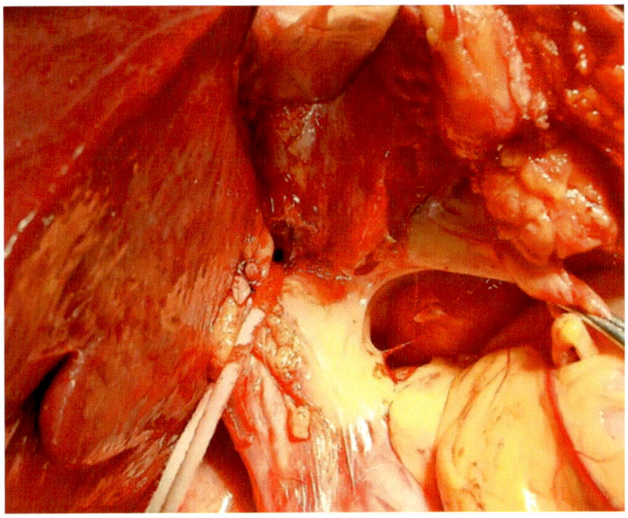

Fig. 240 The right hepatic pedicle was encircled with a vascular tape

Isolation of the Pedicle of Segment VIII (Figs. 241, 242, 243, 244, 245, 246, and 247)

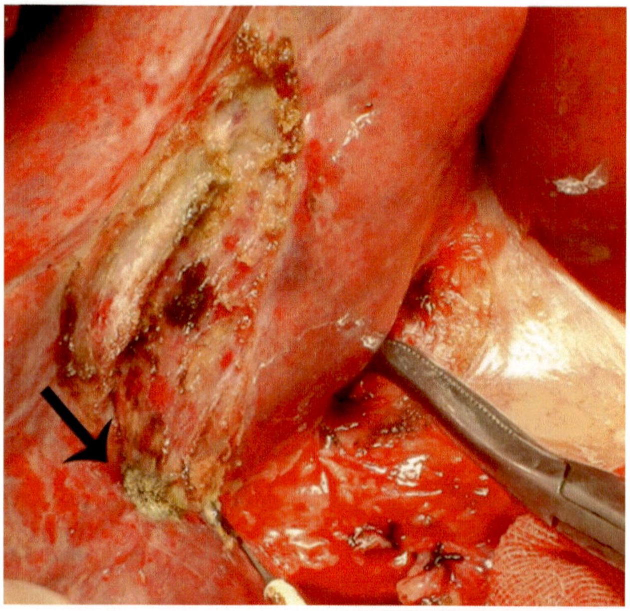

Fig. 241 Having performed cholecystectomy, another small incision was made on the right edge of the gallbladder bed (black arrow)

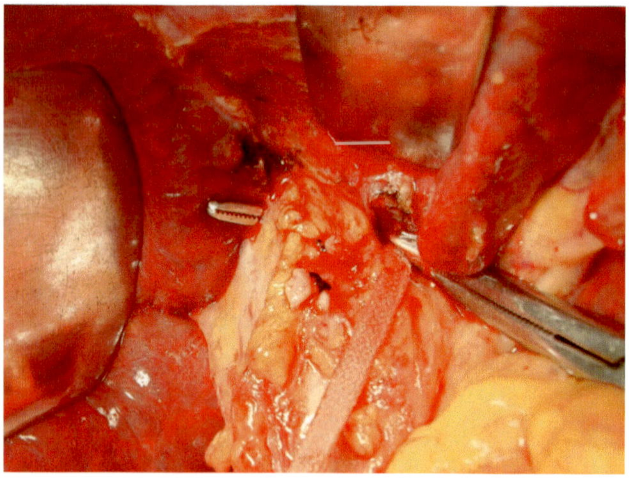

Fig. 242 A large right angle clamp was inserted into the incision over the hilar plate and pushed through out of the incision on the right edge of the gallbladder bed

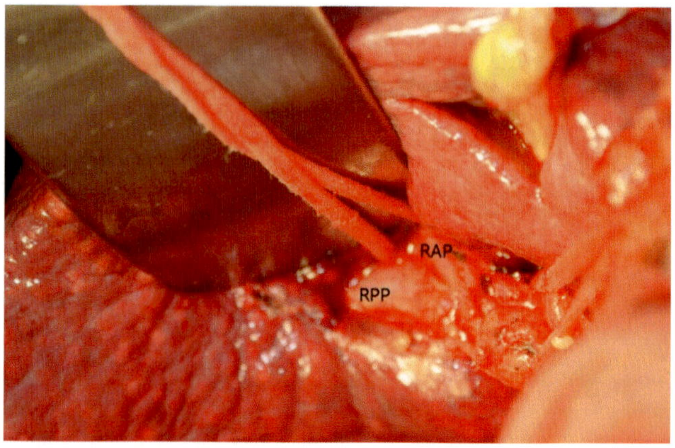

Fig. 243 The right anterior pedicle was also encompassed by a vascular tape. *RAP* right anterior pedicle, *RPP* right posterior pedicle

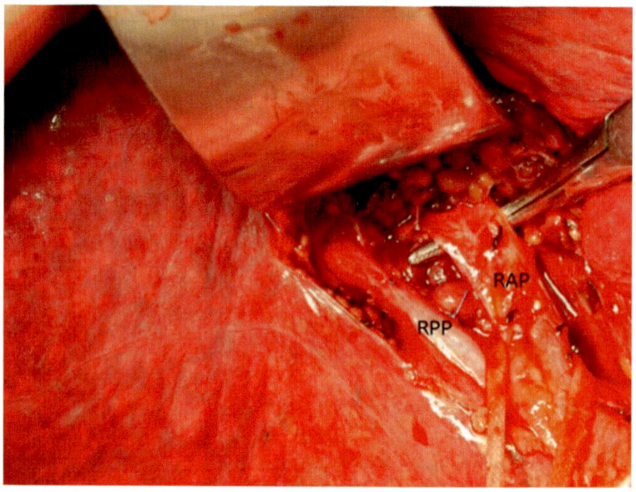

Fig. 244 The right anterior sectional pedicle was dissected on its superior and anterior surface for about 8–10 mm, where it was possible to ascertain bifurcation of segments V and VIII

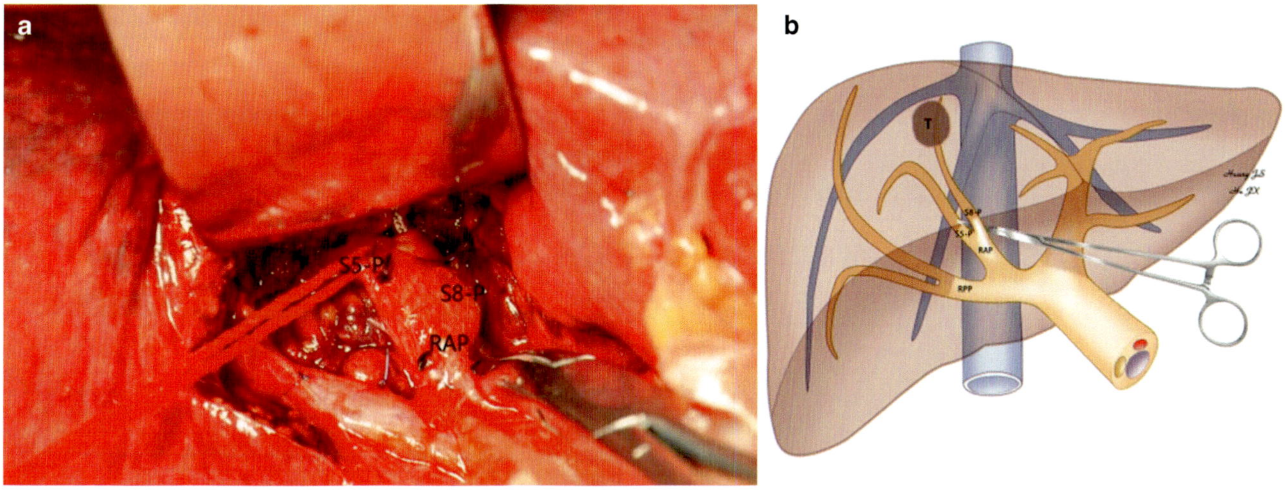

Fig. 245 (**a**) The pedicle of segment V was encircled with a vascular tape, and the pedicle of segment VIII was encompassed by a large right angle clamp alone (**a**). Schematic illustration of this procedure (**b**). *RAP* right anterior pedicle, *S5-P* pedicle of segment V, *S8-P* pedicle of segment VIII

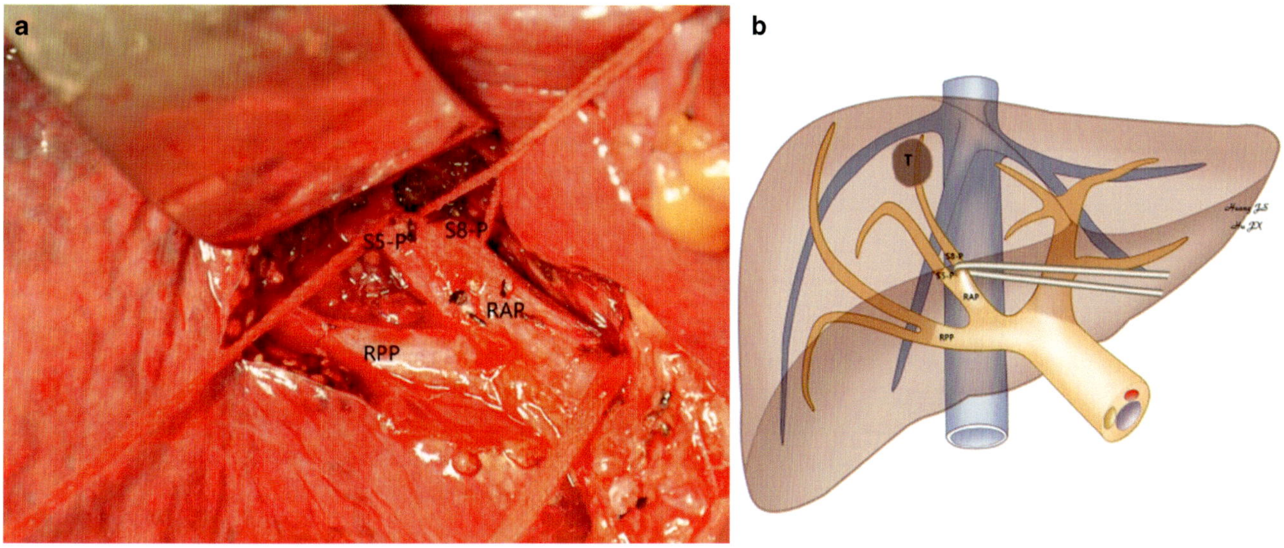

Fig. 246 (**a**) The pedicle of segment VIII was also looped by a vascular tape. (**b**) Schematic illustration of this procedure. *RAP* right anterior pedicle, *RPP* right posterior pedicle, *S5-P* pedicle of segment V, *S8-P* pedicle of segment VIII

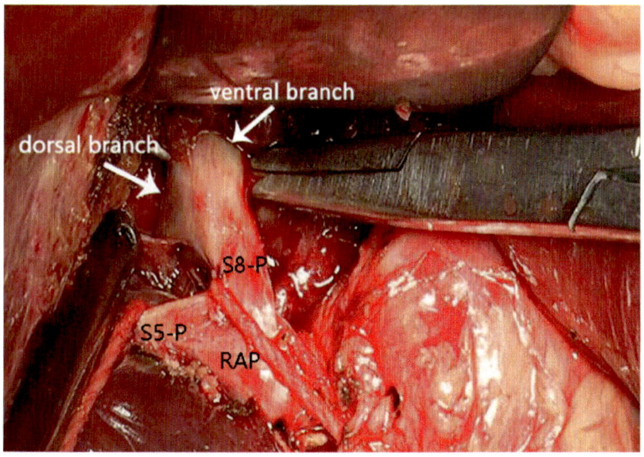

Fig. 247 To further trace the course of the pedicle of segment VIII, the ventral branch of the pedicle of segment VIII was encompassed by a right angle clamp. *RAP* right anterior pedicle, *S5-P* pedicle of segment V, *S8-P* pedicle of segment VIII

Staining Segment VIII and Marking the Boundary of S8 (Figs. 248, 249, and 250)

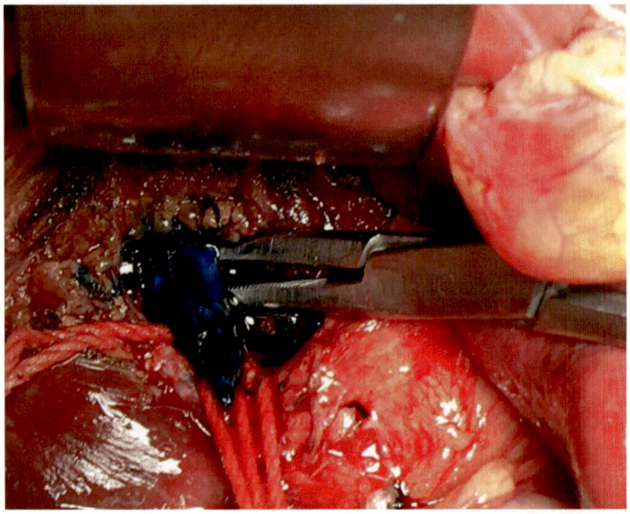

Fig. 248 Methylene blue was injected into the pedicle of segment VIII

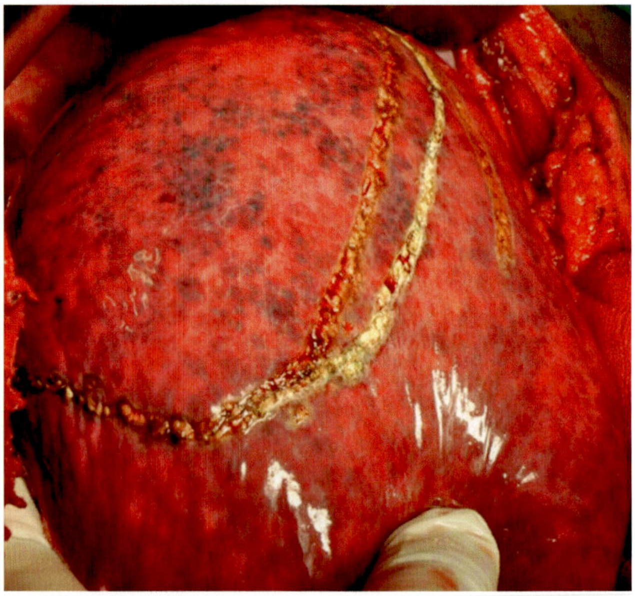

Fig. 250 The color of the surface of segment VIII was changed to blue. Along the edge of the blue area, the cut line was marked on the liver surface

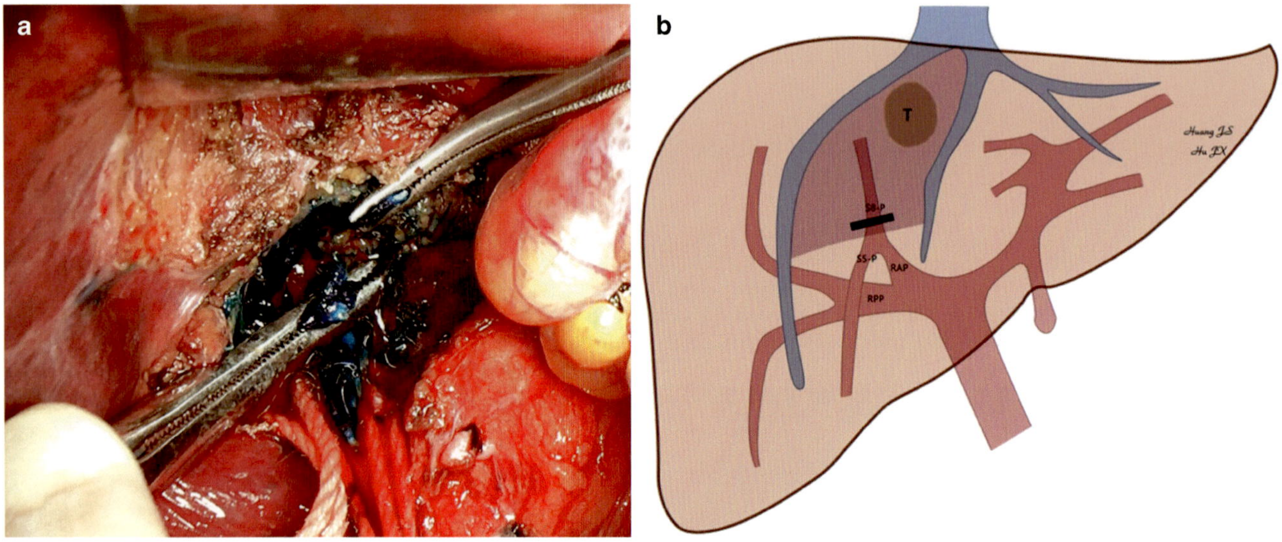

Fig. 249 (**a**) The pedicle of segment VIII was divided; the proximal stump was suture-ligated. (**b**) Schematic illustration of this procedure. *RAP* right anterior pedicle, *RPP* right posterior pedicle, *S5-P* pedicle of segment V, *S8-P* pedicle of segment VIII

Hepatic Parenchymal Transection of Segment VIII
(Figs. 251, 252, 253, and 254)

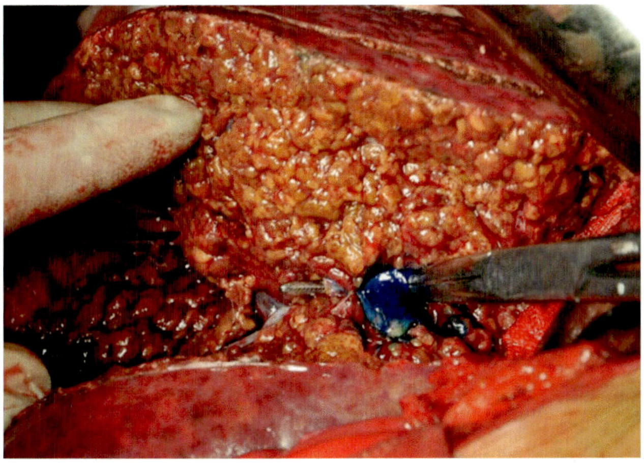

Fig. 251 Having clamped the hepatic pedicle (Pringle maneuver) and the infrahepatic inferior vena cava, hepatic parenchyma transection was started along the right-sided cut line. The dorsal branch of the pedicle of segment VIII was isolated and divided

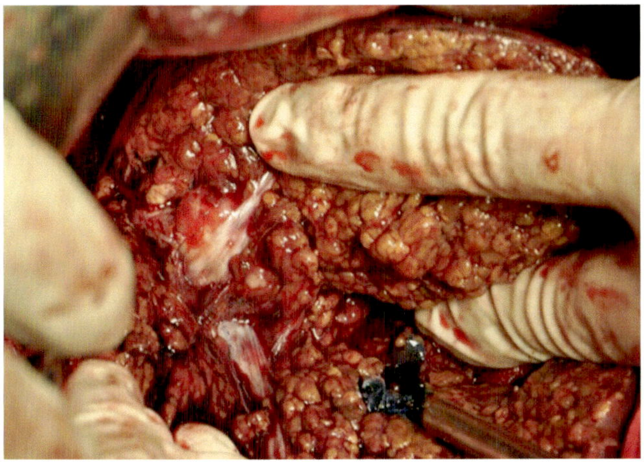

Fig. 252 The tumor was peeled away from the RHV. *RHV* right hepatic vein

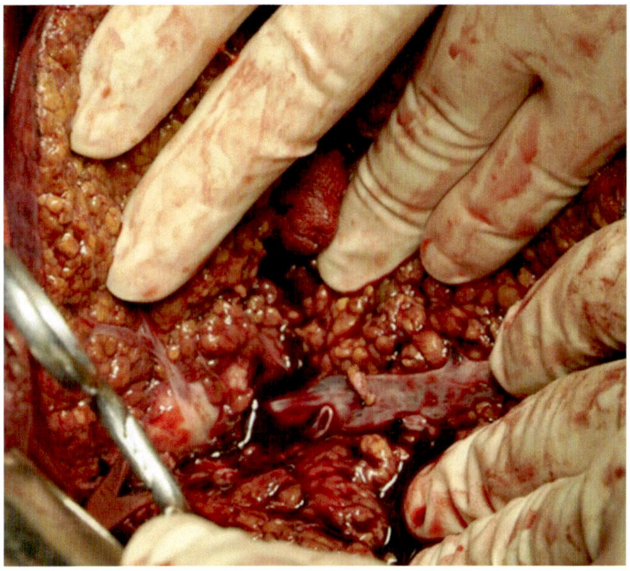

Fig. 253 Bleeding occurred from the holes on the RHV and the holes were sutured with silk thread and/or 4/0 and 5/0 polypropylene. *RHV* right hepatic vein

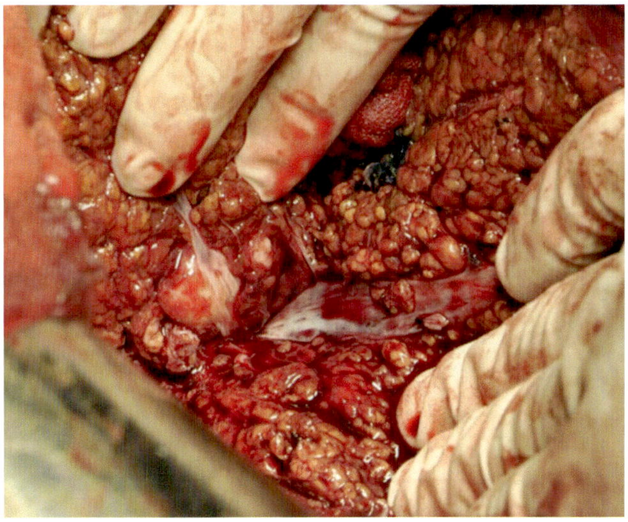

Fig. 254 Having repaired the RHV, bleeding has stopped. Then, the left-sided hepatic parenchyma was initiated. *RHV* right hepatic vein

Raw Area of the Residue Liver and the Specimen
(Figs. 255, 256, and 257)

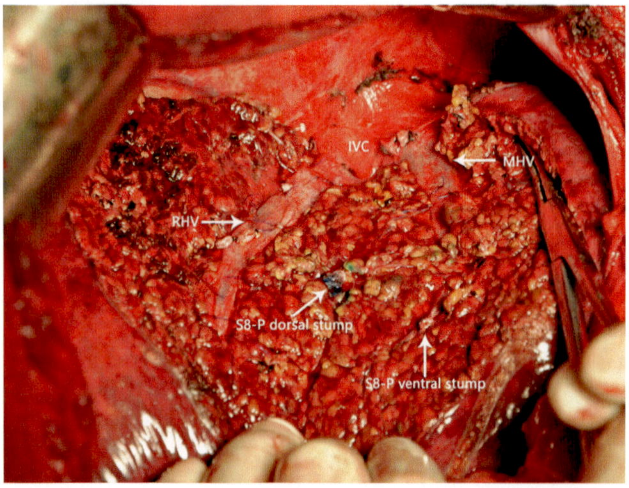

Fig. 255 Having removed the specimen, raw area after complete segment VIII resection. *IVC* inferior vena cava, *MHV* middle hepatic vein, *RHV* right hepatic vein, *S8-P* pedicle of segment VIII

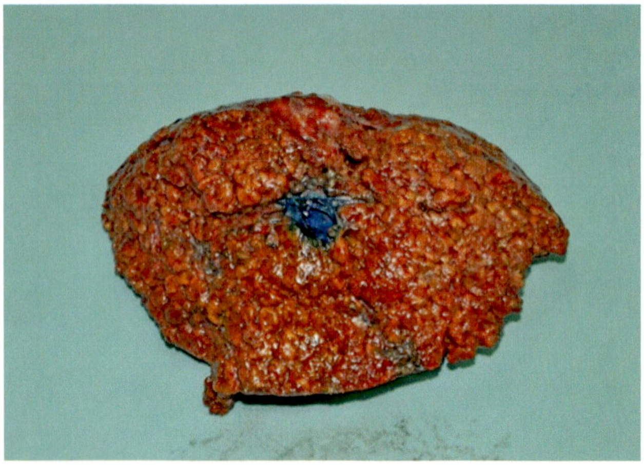

Fig. 256 The resection margin surface of the specimen

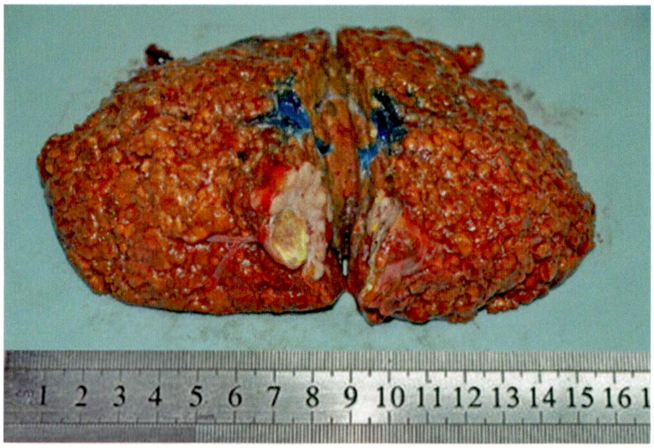

Fig. 257 The specimen was cut open, and the tumor was showed

Segmentectomy VII

Jixiong Hu, Xundi Xu, and Tenglong Tang

Despite great advances in hepatic resection techniques, resection of hepatocellular carcinomas (HCCs) located within Couinaud's segment VII still is technically demanding [55]. Segment VII is located between the plane determined by the vena cava and right hepatic vein (RHV) in situ and is sticked to the right diaphragm and the right posterior area without peritoneum (bare area) [6]. Therefore, segment VII always entails complete mobilization of the right hemiliver from the right diaphragm, right adrenal gland, and retrohepatic vena cava by dividing the perihepatic ligaments and the retrohepatic short veins. Meanwhile, the right posterior sector's pedicle and the bifurcation of the segment VII pedicle lie deep within the hepatic parenchyma, which makes it difficult to identify the boundary of segment VII before hepatic parenchymal transection using an intrahepatic Glissonean approach [12] and which makes further perihilar dissection necessary to access the segment VII pedicle [15, 16, 102, 103]. During hepatic transectional proceedings, the RHV branches draining segment VII should be divided and ligated individually in the deepest aspects of the liver. To our knowledge, reports of isolated anatomical segment VII are very rare. Makuuchi M [104] and Lim C [55] reported systematic segmentectomy VII using IOUS-guided dye injection method. Up to now, anatomical segmentectomy VII has not been reported based on an intrahepatic Glissonean approach.

Surgical Indications

The surgical indications and types of hepatic resection of segment VII HCCs were decided by the tumor-related factors, future remnant liver functional reserve, and the patient's general condition. Anatomical segmentectomy VII was preferred over nonanatomic partial resection (wedge resection or enucleation), because the en bloc removal of cancer-bearing hepatic segment has been generally accepted, at least theoretically, as the gold standard not only based on the portal vein branch but also because this systematic segmentectomy spares the remaining volume of the liver as much as possible, therefore reducing the risk of posthepatectomy liver failure (PHLF) [105–107]. Furthermore, systematic segmentectomy is reported associated with several benefits in terms of obtaining safe surgical margins and reducing intraoperative blood loss and blood transfusion and postoperative complications [108–110]. Right posterior sectionectomy (RPS) or right hepatectomy was adopted when the HCCs infiltrated the right posterior Glissonean pedicle or the right hepatic Glissonean pedicle, respectively; in terms of liver function, the acceptable ranges of sacrificed liver volumes were decided at great length on the basis of the Pugh-Child classification and the indocyanine green retention rate at 15 min (ICGR15). According to this criterion, anatomic segmentectomy VII can be considered when the total bilirubin was less than 1.0 mg/dl and the ICGR15 was less than 30%.

Operative Procedures	Technical Details
Laparotomy ↓	◀ A right subcostal incision was made. The perihepatic ligaments were dissected and the right adrenal gland was divided away from the right hemiliver, and the right-sided retrohepatic short veins were divided and ligated individually up to the root of the RHV.
Colorization ↓	◀ Using an intrahepatic Glissonean approach, the segment VII pedicle was isolated and looped, and then, Methylene blue was injected into this pedicle, and the pedicle was then divided and suture-ligated. The demarcation line between the area of color change and normal color area was marked on the liver surface with electrocautery to decide the limit of hepatic parenchymal transection.
Hepatic parenchymal transection ↓	◀ Having clamped the right hepatic pedicle and the right hepatic vein, hepatic dissection was carried out, using the clamp crushing method. The large branches of the RHV draining segment VII were divided and ligated, individually, and the pedicle was once more suture-ligated intrahepatically.
Drainage and closure of the abdominal cavity	◀ A tube was placed below the right subphrenic space and secured with silk-suture.

Intraoperative Key Points

1. The pedicle to the right posterior sector is the most deeply placed of the right pedicles [22, 62]. During the surgical proceedings of isolating and looping the right posterior pedicle, care must be taken to prevent injury to the portal pedicle originating from the right hepatic pedicle into the caudate process [5]. Further dissection is required to access to the pedicle of segment VI and segment VII. The right posterior pedicle (RPP) was dissected on its anterior, superior, and inferior surface for about 1–3 cm, where it was possible to ascertain the bifurcation of segment VI and VII. The number of the pedicle of segment VII is usually one, occasionally two. Having isolated the pedicle of segment VII, test clamping this pedicle should be attempted to ascertain this pedicle to supply the target segment. In addition, in order to precisely transect the deepest hepatic parenchyma, the target segment can be stained by injecting methylene blue into the supplying portal branch [111]. Having completed the parenchymal transection of segment VII, the proximal trunk of right hepatic vein (RHV) should be kept intact and exposed on the cut surface as a landmark of the segmental boundary.
2. In terms of the technical aspects of systematic segmentectomy VII for HCC confined to segment VII, complete mobilization of the right hemiliver to fully expose the hepatocaval confluence is a very important step in safely isolating and looping the root of the right hepatic vein (RHV), because venous bleeding from the RHV during transection of the deep hepatic parenchyma sometimes is very severe and may be lethal, and under such a circumstance, hemorrhage can stopped by clamping the root of the RHV. During freeing the right hemiliver off from its surrounding structures, attention should be paid to avoid bleeding from the right inferior phrenic vein, retrohepatic short veins, and the right adrenal gland.
3. Over the past 20 years, all hepatic resection (about 3000 cases) performed in our hospital have not undergone thoracophrenolaparotomy, no matter the tumors are located in any segment(s) or huge in diameter. Although thoracophrenolaparotomy provides good surgical field and working space for liver mobilization and hepatic parenchymal transection during segmentectomy VII for HCC confined to segment VII, this large incision may increase the risk of postoperative pulmonary complications, decrease postoperative patients' quality of life, and delay beginning of adjuvant chemotherapy after surgery. Based on our clinical experiences, no necessity for thoracotomy for segmentectomy VII for HCC confined to segment VII was needed (Fig. 258).

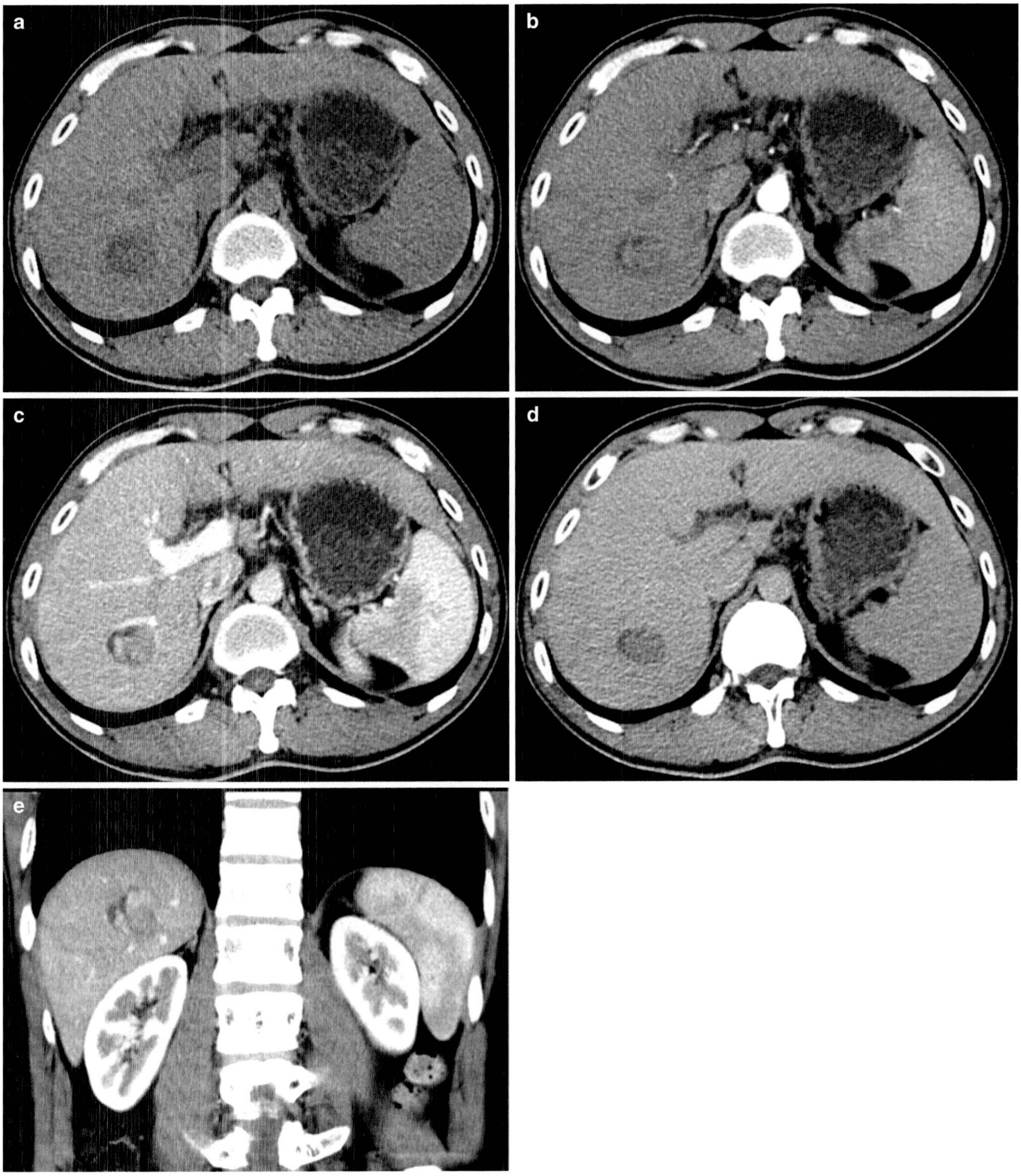

Fig. 258 (**a**) Preoperative CT (precontrast). The tumor, which appears mildly hypodense, is located in segment VII. (**b**) Preoperative CT (hepatic arterial phase). The tumor shows heterogeneous enhancement. (**c**) Preoperative CT (hepatic venous phase). The tumor shows enhancement fades. (**d**) Preoperative CT (interstitial phase). The tumor shows subtle washout. (**e**) Preoperative CT

Abdominal Incision and Mobilization of the Liver
(Figs. 259, 260, 261, 262, 263, 264, 265, and 266)

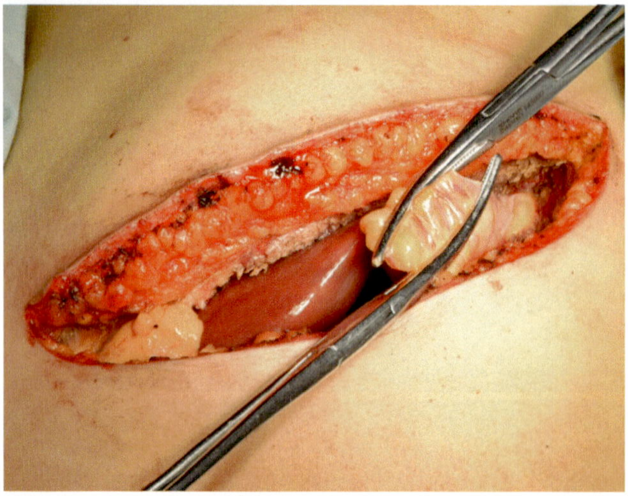

Fig. 259 A right subcostal incision was selected and made. Having entered into the abdominal cavity, the round ligament was divided and ligated

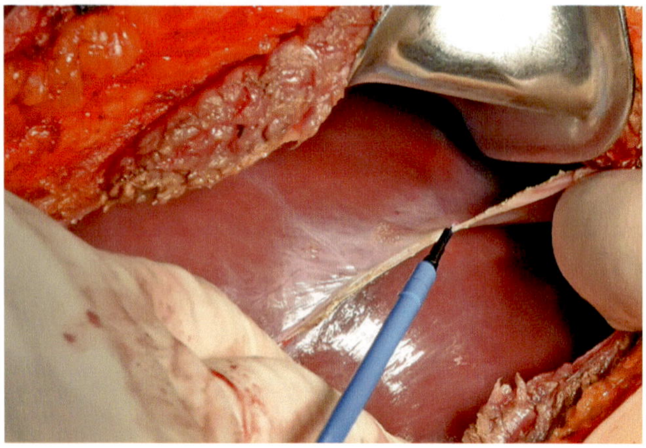

Fig. 260 The falciform ligament was divided with electrocautery

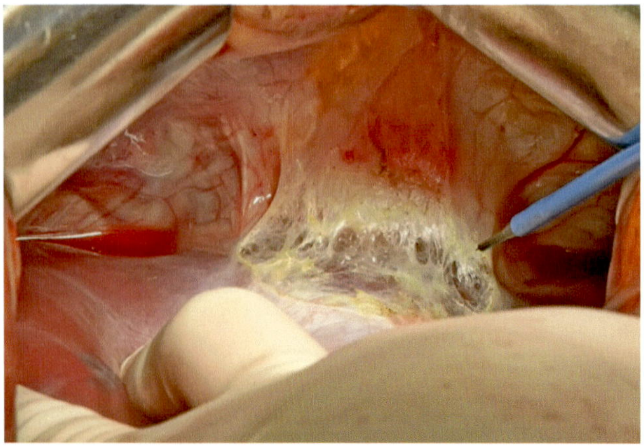

Fig. 261 Hepatocaval confluence was dissected

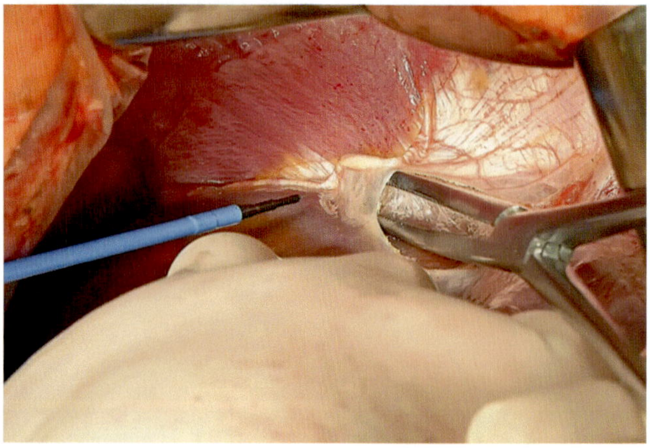

Fig. 262 The right coronary ligament was electrocauterized

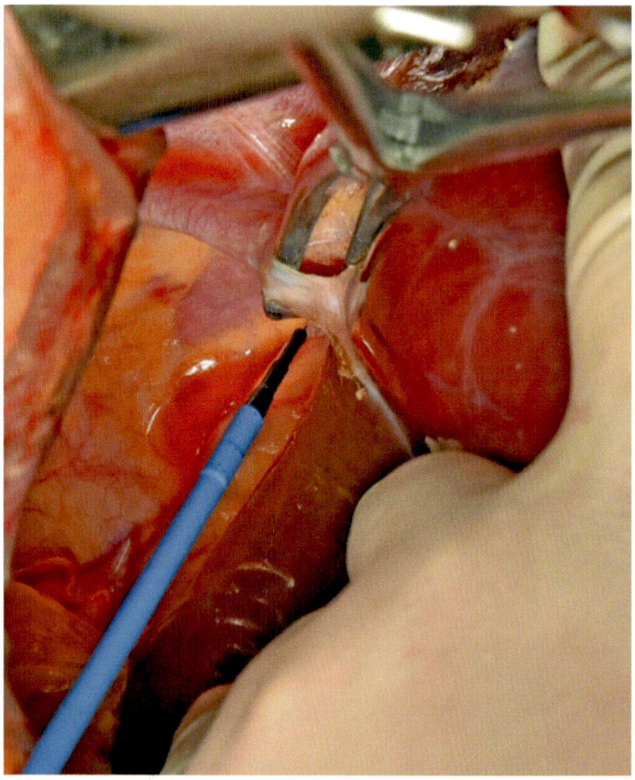

Fig. 263 The right triangular ligament was dissected

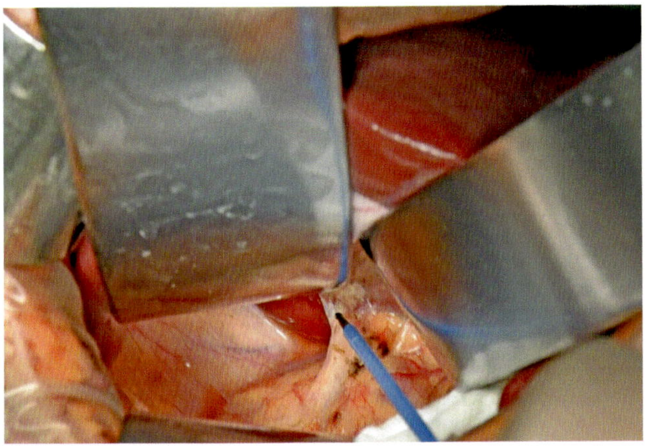

Fig. 264 The hepatocolic ligament was divided

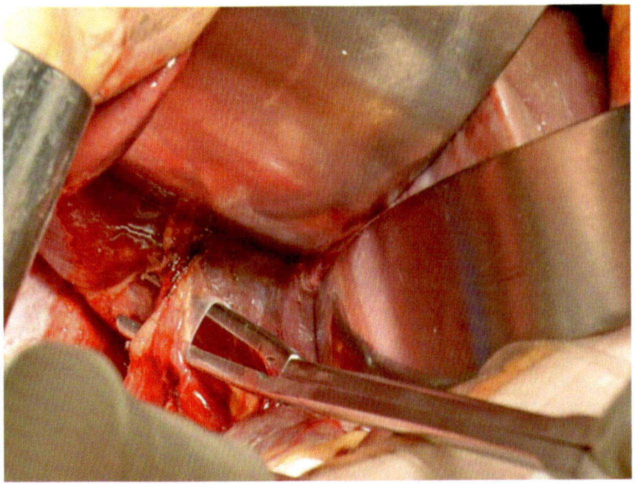

Fig. 265 The right adrenal gland was dissected away from the posterior sector of the right hemiliver

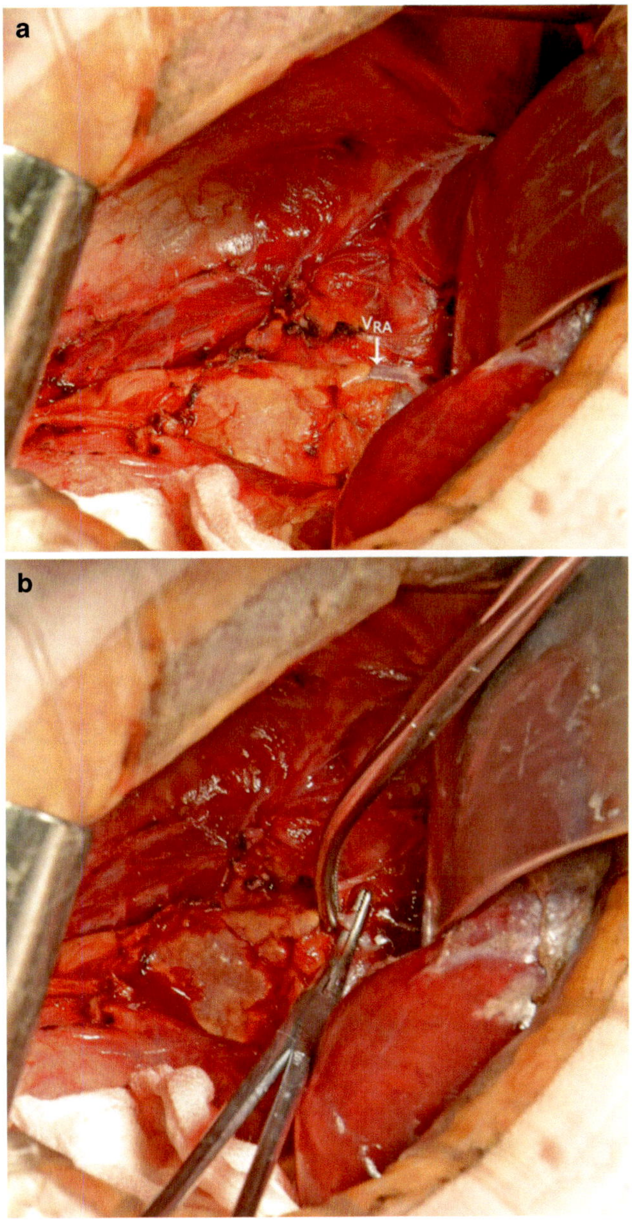

Fig. 266 (**a**, **b**) The vein draining the right adrenal gland (V_{RA}) was isolated, divided, and ligated

Isolation of the Right Hepatic Vein (RHV)
(Figs. 267, 268, and 269)

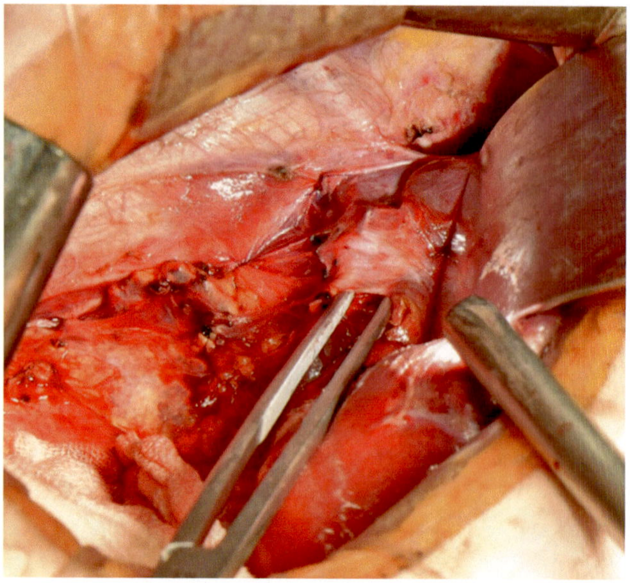

Fig. 267 The hepatocaval ligament was isolated and electrocauterized

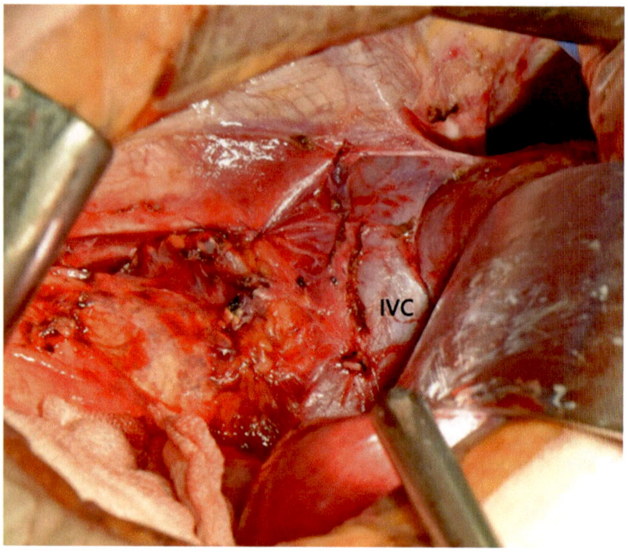

Fig. 268 The retrohepatic right-sided short veins were divided and ligated individually, and the retrohepatic inferior vena cava (IVC) was fully exposed

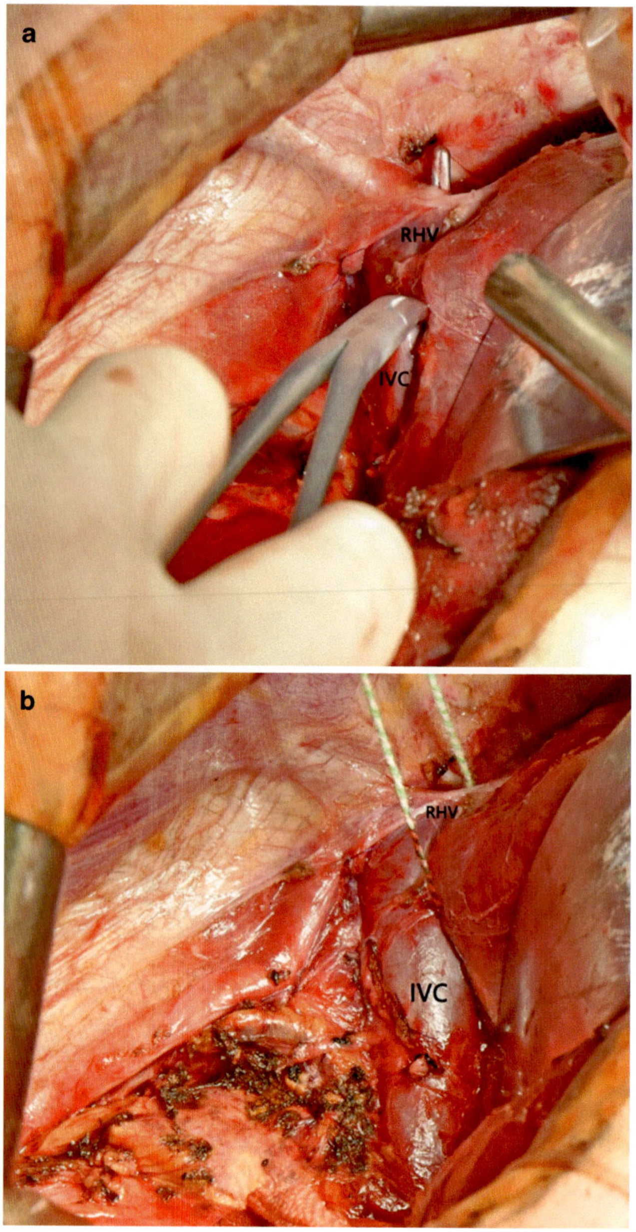

Fig. 269 (**a**, **b**) The right hepatic vein was isolated and pre-placed with a vessel loop

Isolation of the Right Hepatic Pedicle (RHP)
(Figs. 270, 271, and 272)

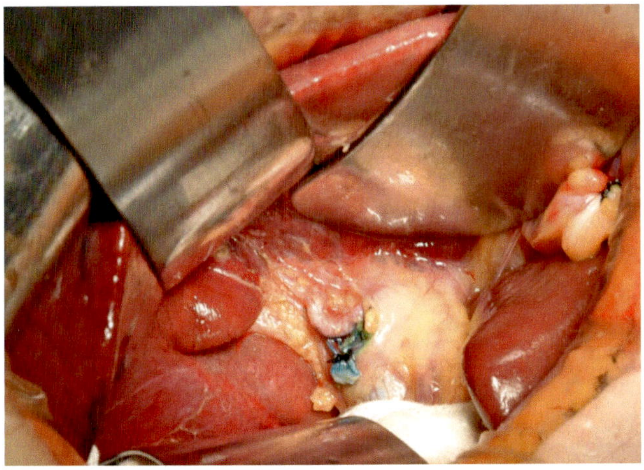

Fig. 270 Cholecystectomy was performed

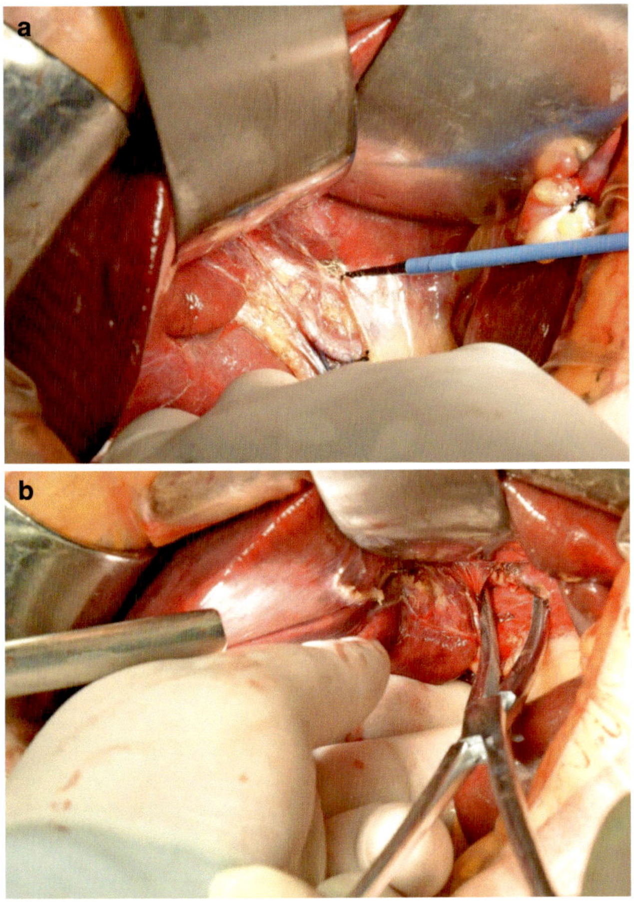

Fig. 271 (**a**, **b**) One small incision (about 2 cm) was made in front of the hilus. Hepatic parenchymal around this incision was pushed upward, and the hilar plate was pulled down

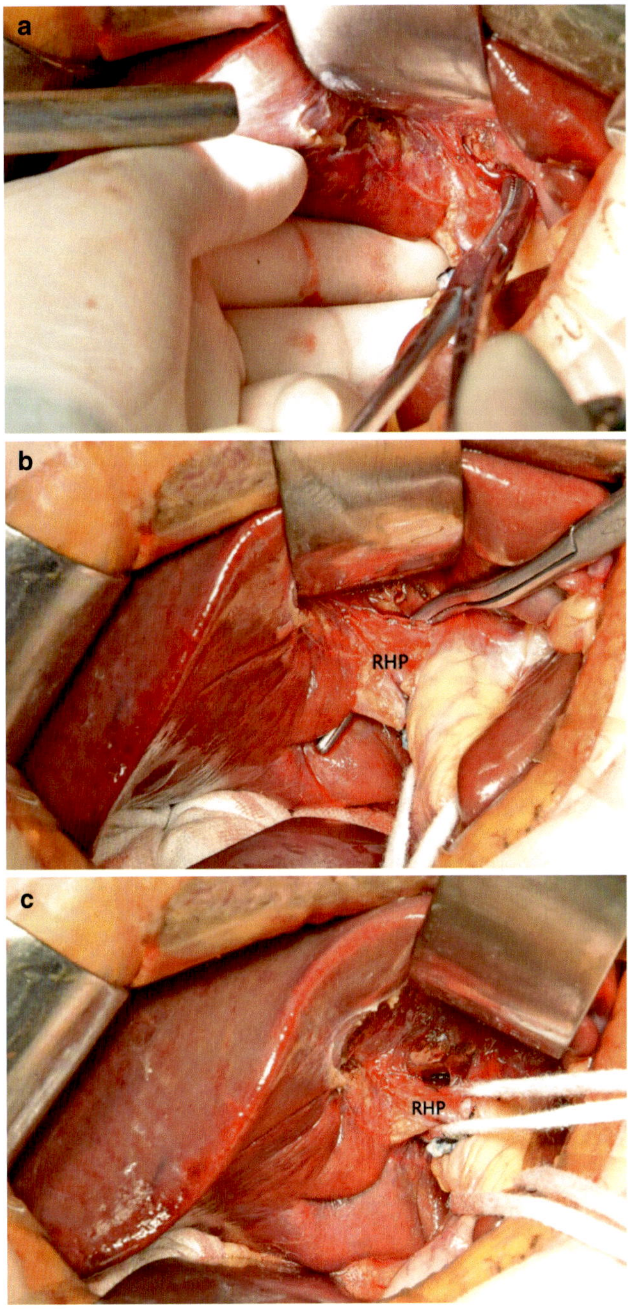

Fig. 272 (**a**–**c**) A large curved clamp was inserted into this incision, and the operator's left index finger was placed between the undersurface of the hilar plate and the anterior wall of the retrohepatic vena cava; using the index finger as a guide, the large clamp was pushed down to directly reach to the tip of the index finger and punctured through the undersurface membrane of the hilar plate and passed out of the right edge of the right hepatic pedicle. Thus, the right hepatic pedicle was isolated and encircled with a vascular tape

Isolation of the Right Posterior Pedicle (RPP)
(Figs. 273, 274, and 275)

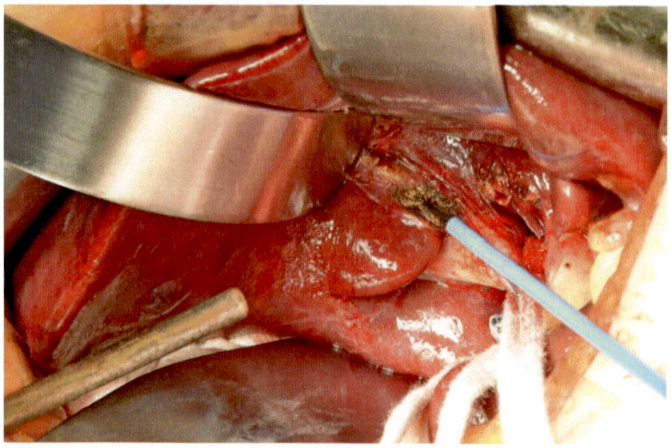

Fig. 273 Another small incision was made at the right edge of the gallbladder bed

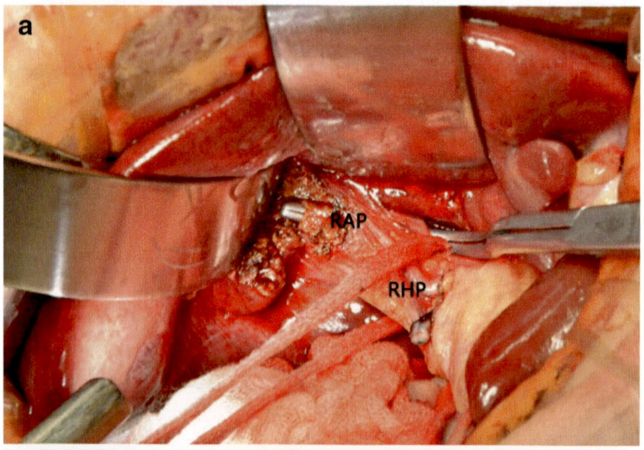

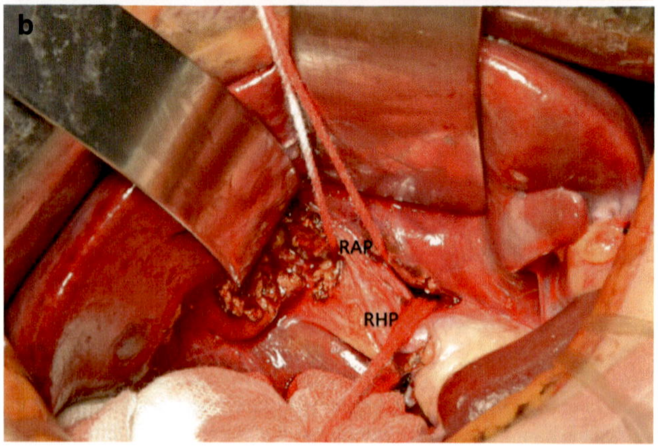

Fig. 274 (**a**, **b**) A large curved clamp was inserted into the incision in front of the hilum and passed out of this incision at the right edge of the gallbladder bed. Thus, the right anterior sector's pedicle (RAP) was isolated and looped

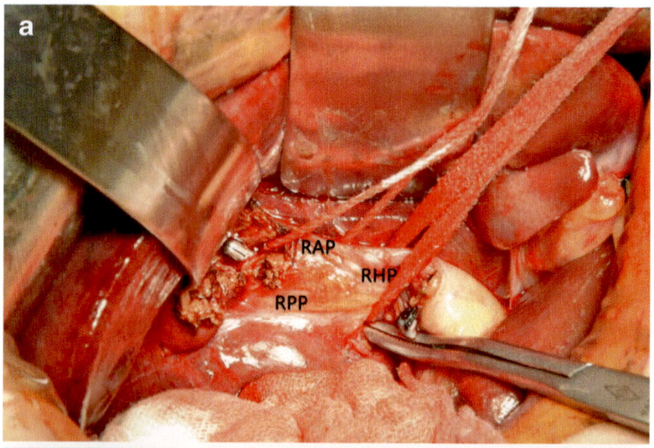

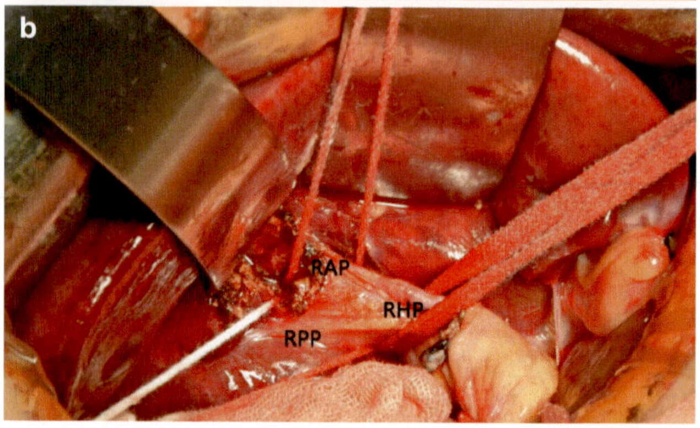

Fig. 275 (**a**, **b**) A large curved clamp was inserted upward from the inferior edge of the right hepatic pedicle and passed out of the incision at the right edge of the gallbladder bed. Thus, the right posterior pedicle (RPP) was isolated and encircled with a vessel loop

Isolation of Segment VII Pedicle (S_7-P)
(Figs. 276 and 277)

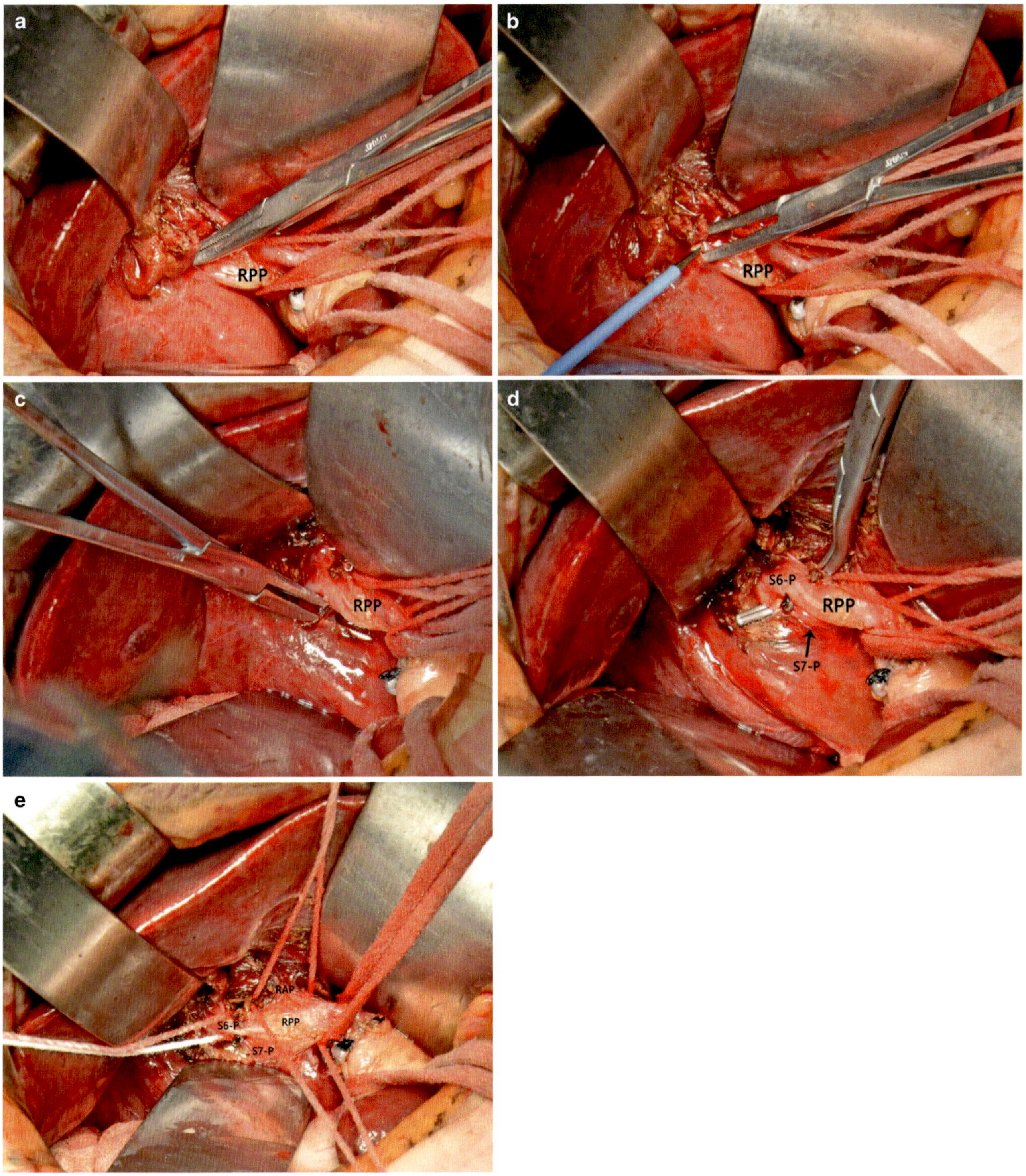

Fig. 276 (**a**–**e**) The right posterior sector's pedicle (RPP) and the bifurcation of the segment VII pedicle lies deep within the hepatic parenchyma, which makes further dissection necessary to access the segment VII pedicle. The right posterior pedicle was dissected on its superior, anterior and inferior surface for about 1–2 cm, where it was possible to ascertain bifurcation of segment VI and VII. The pedicle of segment VI was isolated and encircled alone. *S6-P* pedicle of segment VI, *S7-P* pedicle of segment VII, *RAP* right anterior sector's pedicle

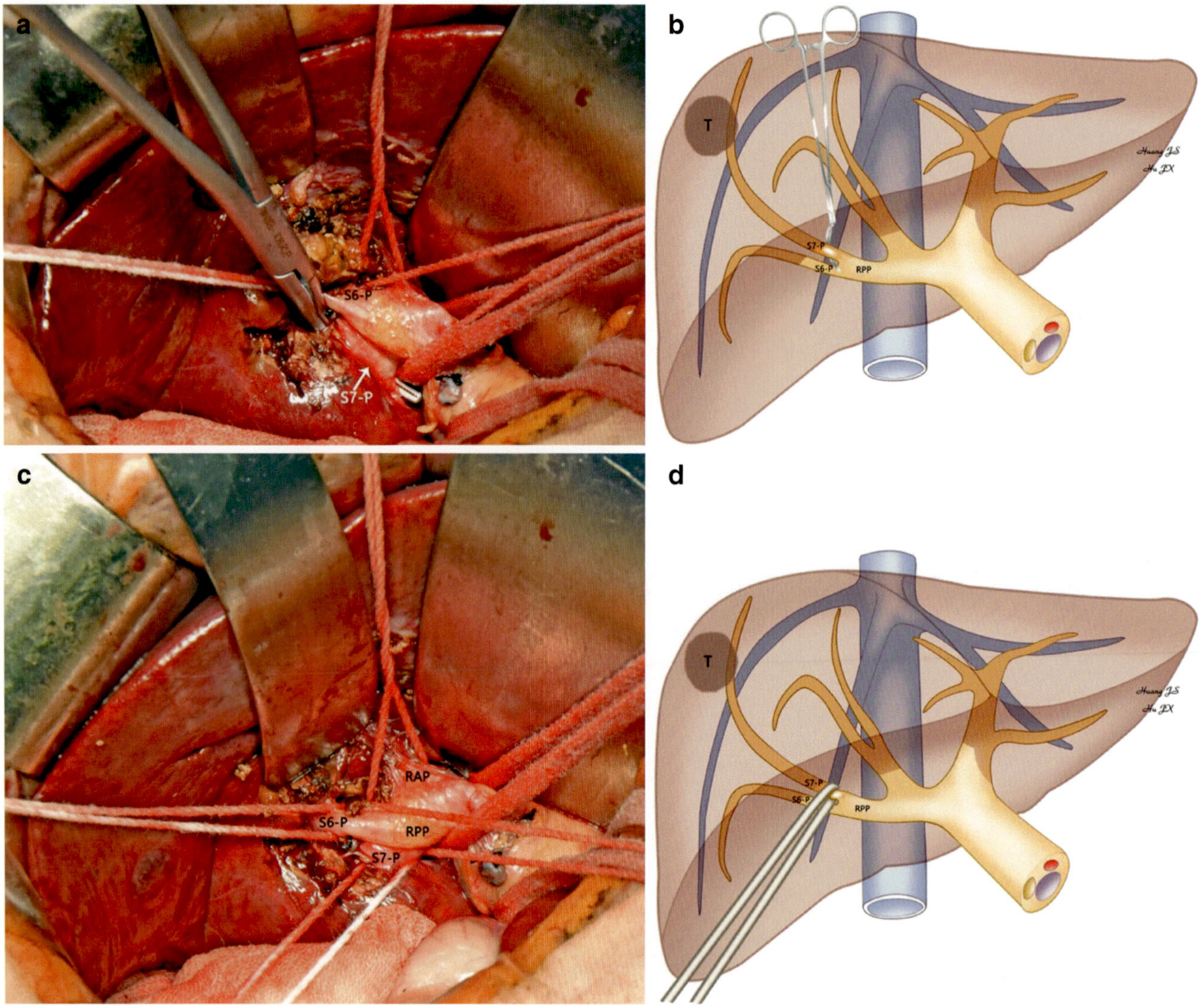

Fig. 277 (**a**, **c**) The segment VII pedicle was also isolated (**a**) and looped with a tourniquet alone (**c**). (**b** and **d**). Schematic illustration of this procedure. *S6-P* pedicle of segment VI, *S7-P* pedicle of segment VII, *RPP* right posterior sector's pedicle, *RAP* right anterior sector's pedicle

Staining Segment VII and Marking the Cut Line
(Figs. 278 and 279)

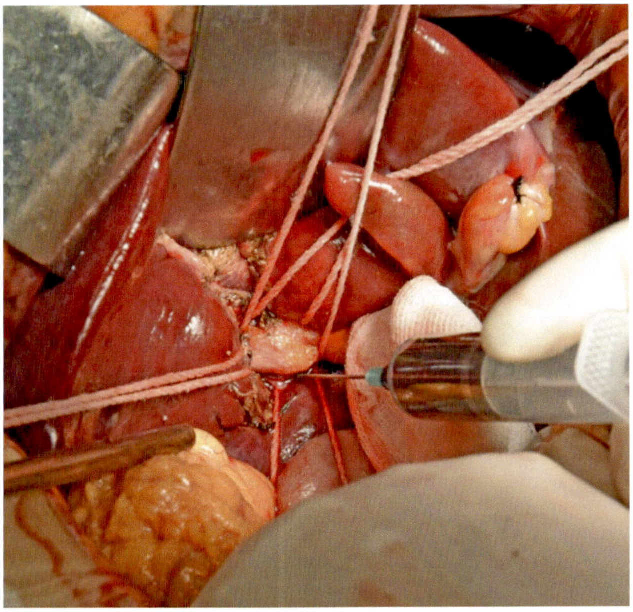

Fig. 278 Methylene was injected into the pedicle of segment VII

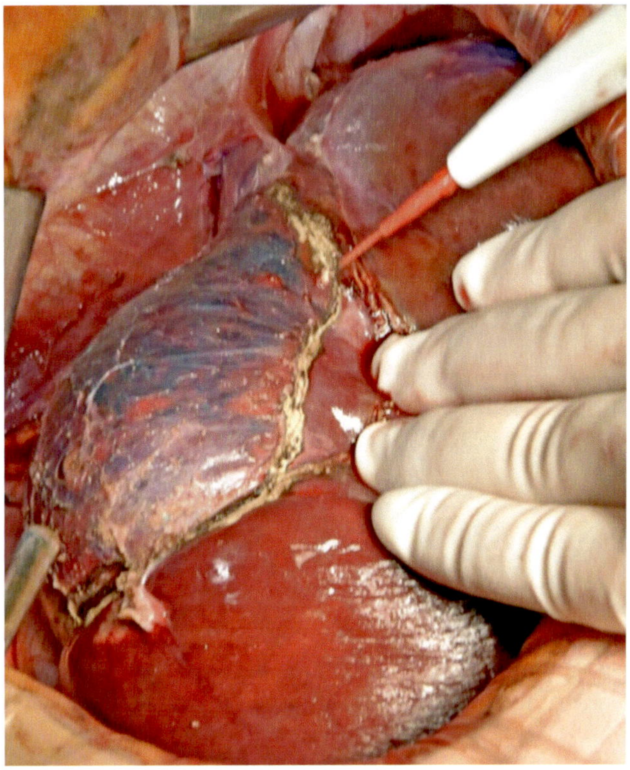

Fig. 279 Segment VII was colorized. The boundary of segment VII was marked with electrocautery

Division of Segment VII Pedicle (S_7-P)
(Figs. 280, 281, 282, 283, 284, and 285)

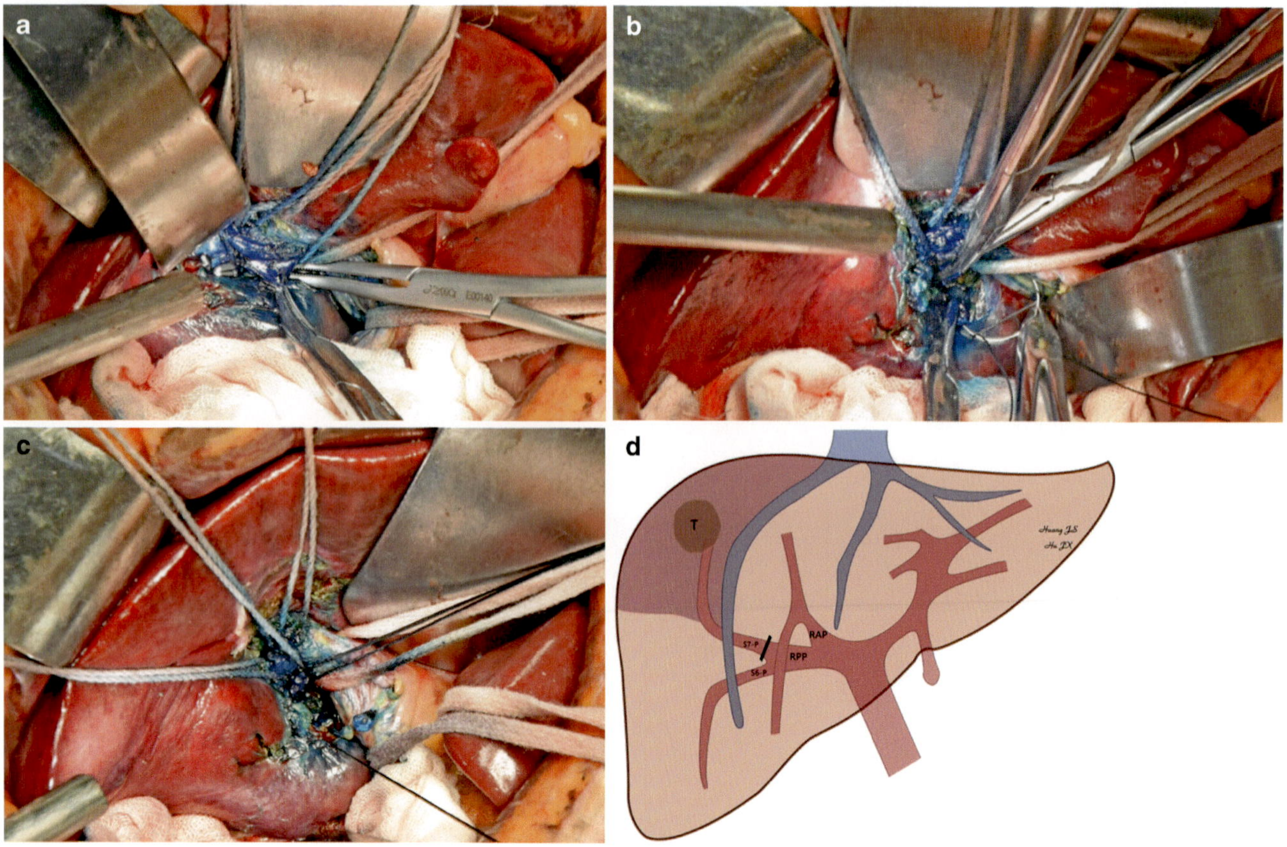

Fig. 280 (**a**–**c**) The pedicle of segment VII was clamped (**a**), divided, and suture-ligated. (**d**) Schematic illustration of this procedure. *S7-P* pedicle of segment VII, *S6-P* pedicle of segment VI, *RPP* right posterior sector's pedicle, *RAP* right anterior sector's pedicle

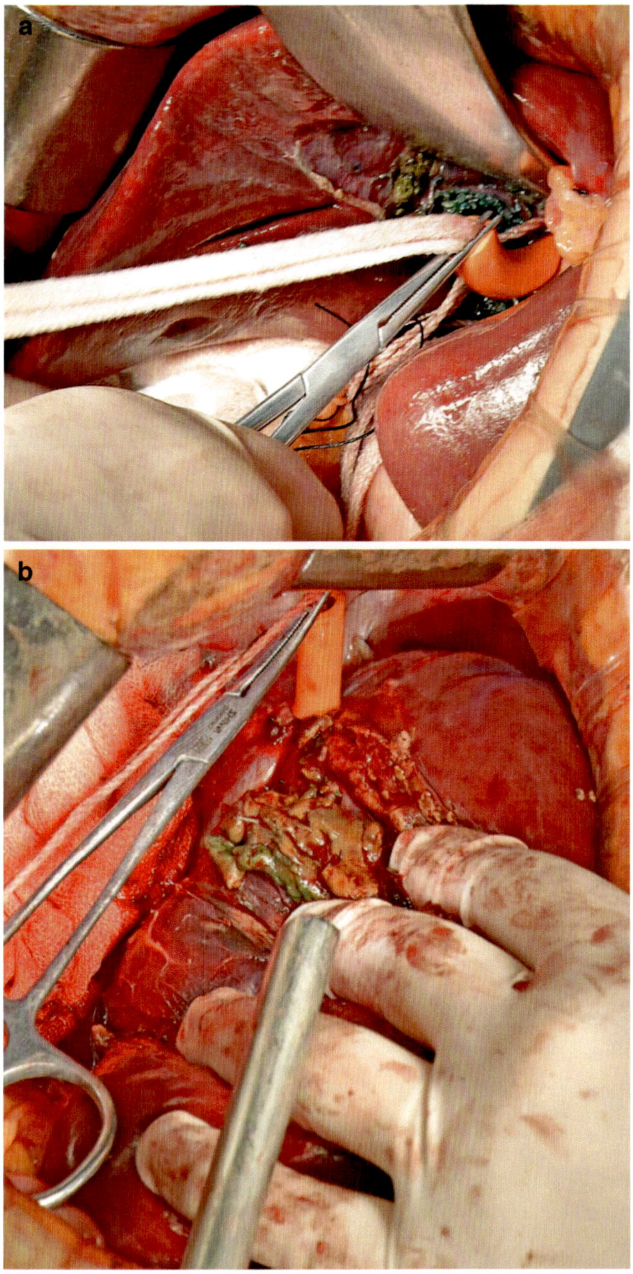

Fig. 281 (**a**, **b**) Before hepatic parenchymal transection, the right hepatic pedicle (**a**) and the right hepatic vein (RHV) (**b**) were clamped to occlude the right hemiliver inflow and outflow blood, respectively

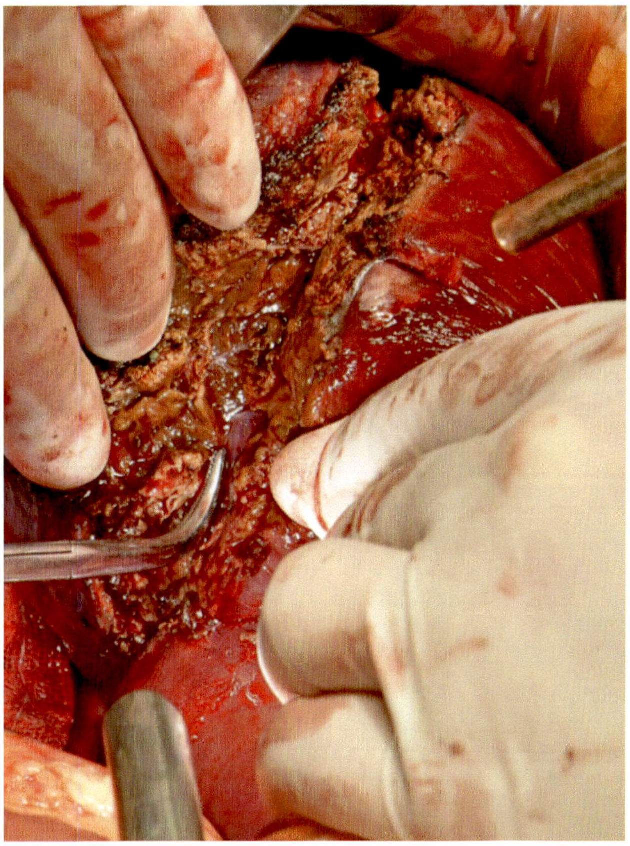

Fig. 282 Hepatic parenchymal transection was initiated between segment VI and segment VII along the stained boundary, using the clamp-crushing method. During the surgical proceedings, small vessels were electrocauterized, and large vessels were divided and ligated individually

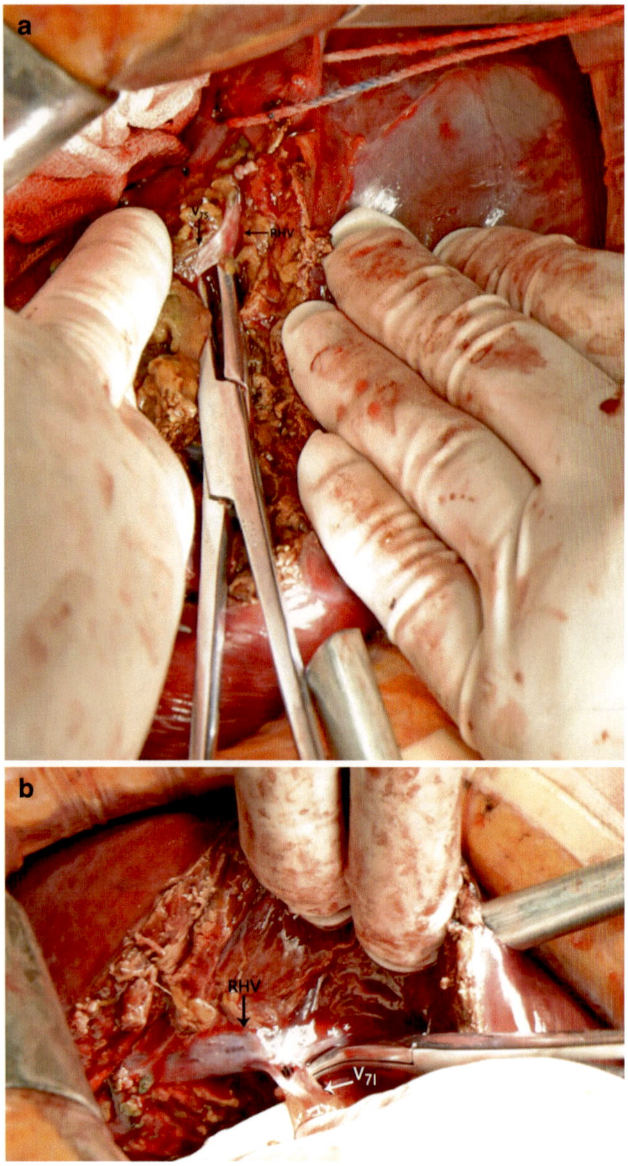

Fig. 283 (**a**, **b**) Hepatic parenchyma dissection was continued between segments VI and VII. The segment VII branches of the right hepatic vein (RHV) were divided and ligated individually if encountered. V_{7S} branch of the RHV draining the superior portion of segment VII, V_{7I} branch of the RHV draining the inferior portion of segment VII

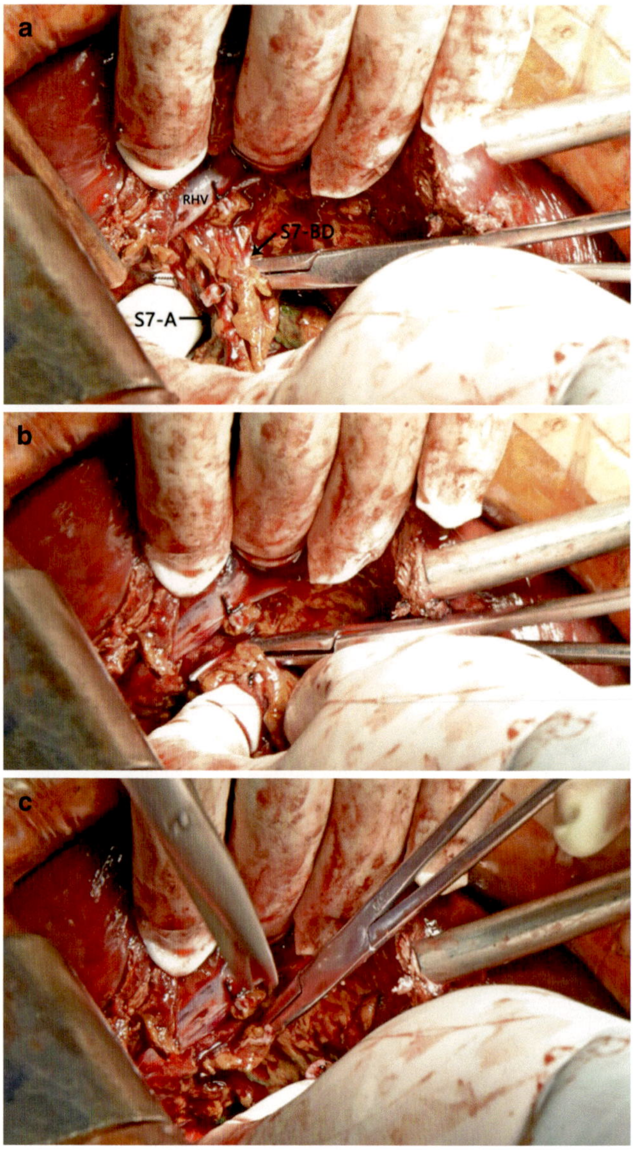

Fig. 284 (**a**–**c**) The artery and bile duct of segment VII was isolated, divided, and suture-ligated. *RHV* right hepatic vein

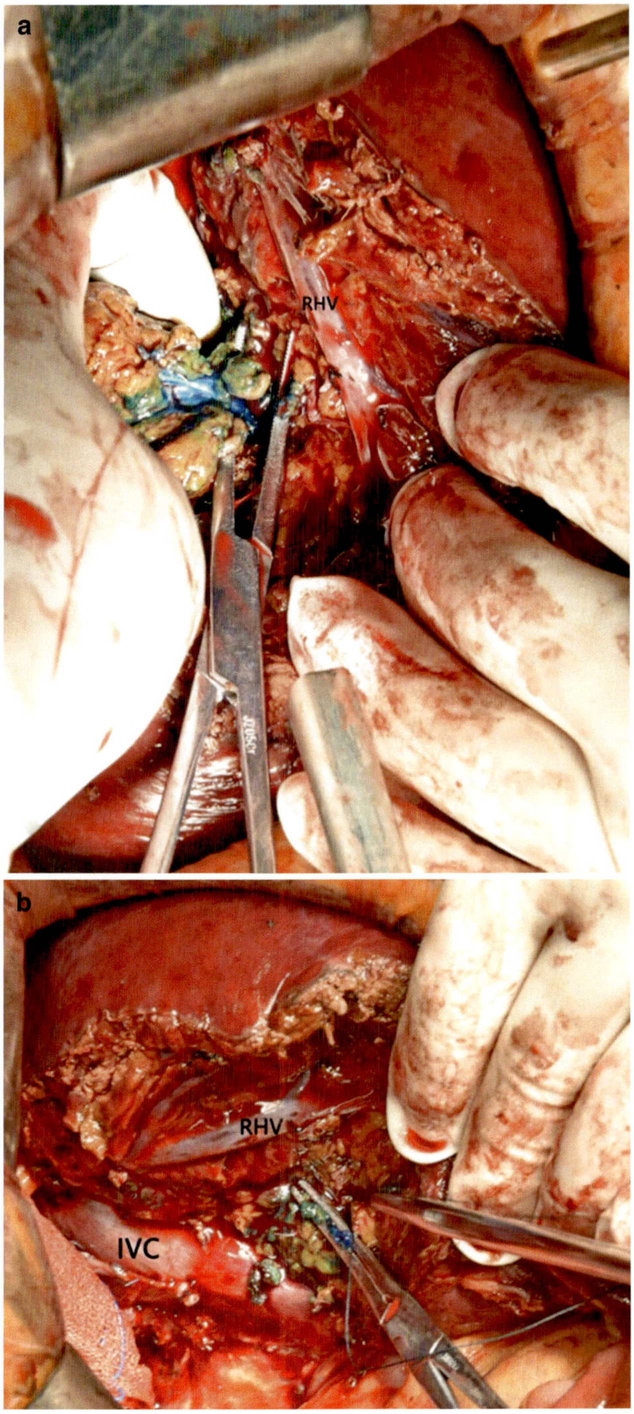

Fig. 285 (**a**, **b**) The branch of the portal vein supplying segment VII was isolated, divided, and suture-ligated. *RHV* right hepatic vein; *IVC* inferior vena cava

Hemostasis and Prevention of Bile Leak at the Cut Surface (Fig. 286)

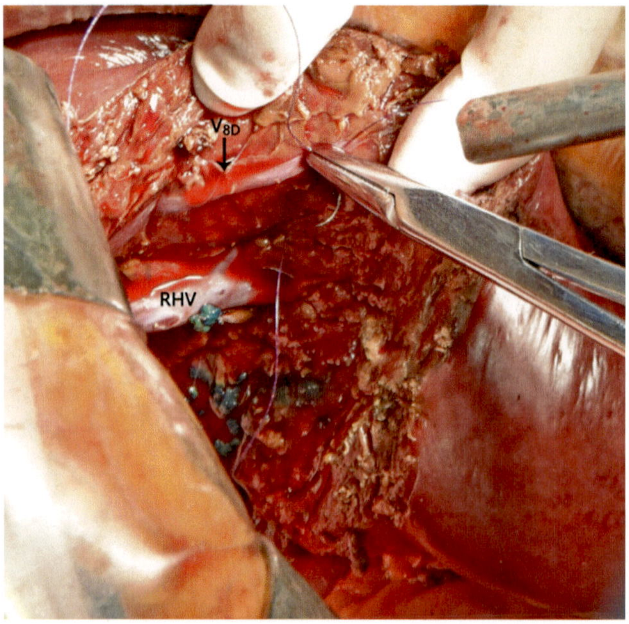

Fig. 286 Having unclamped the right hepatic vein (RHV) and the right hepatic pedicle, tiny holes on the RHV were repaired with 4–0 polypropylene individually. V_{8D} branch of the RHV draining the dorsal portion of segment VIII

Raw Area of the Residue Liver and the Specimen
(Figs. 287, 288, and 289)

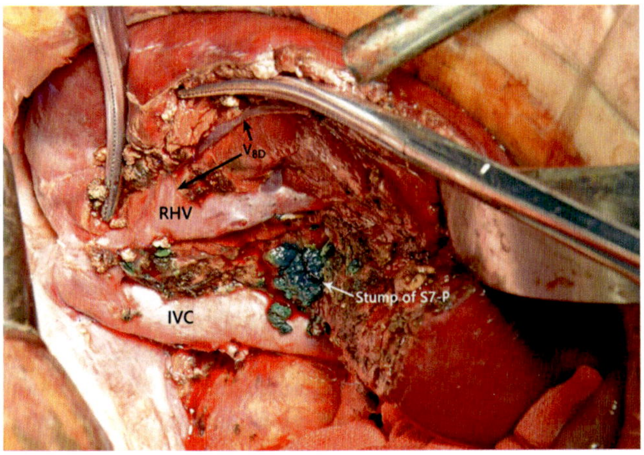

Fig. 287 The bird view of the cut surface. The main trunk of the right hepatic vein (RHV) draining segment VII was obviously shown. The stump of the pedicle of segment VII was colorized. *IVC* inferior vena cava, V_{8D} venous branch of the RHV draining the dorsal portion of segment VIII

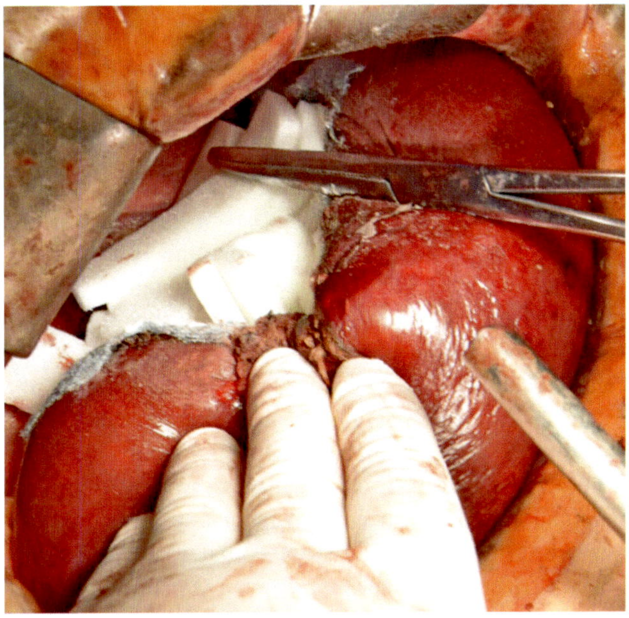

Fig. 288 The cut surface was covered with fibrin glue and gelatin sponge

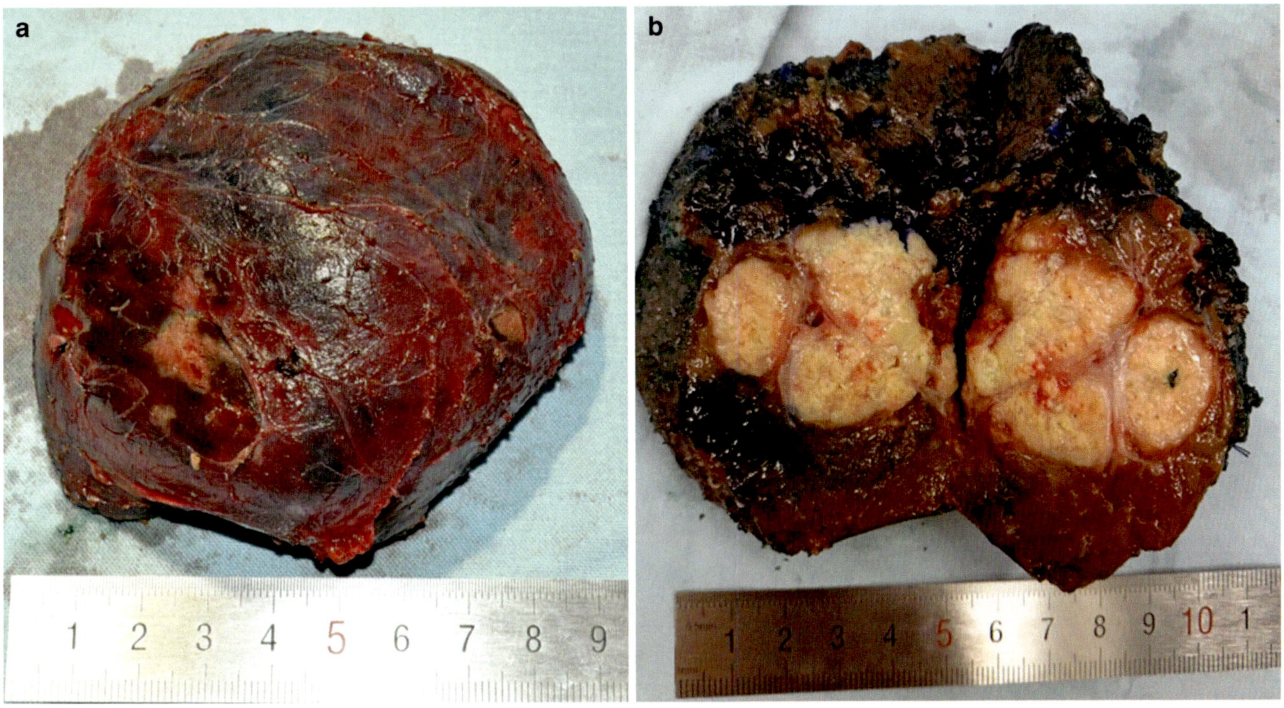

Fig. 289 (**a**, **b**) The specimen

Segmentectomy V

Jixiong Hu, Enxiang Zhou, and Zhongkun Zuo

Brief Description of the Anatomic Variations of Segment V

The boundary between segments V (caudal part of the right anterior sector) and VIII (cranial part of the right anterior sector) usually is obscure resulting from the lack of a clear anatomic landmark. To our knowledge, no reports on isolated anatomic segment V have been published in English literature. To perform an anatomic segmentectomy V, the right hepatic vein (RHV) is its right-sided landmark, and the middle hepatic vein (MHV) is its left-sided landmark.

A precise anatomical parenchymal transection along the border of each segment is very necessary to conserve the maximal functional hepatic parenchyma with minimal blood loss [104, 112–117]. However, the watershed of each segment does not pursue straight and consistent lines [4, 60]. The boundaries of segments vary among persons and frequently show a complex unpredictable branching of the Glissonean pedicles. The branching patterns of the right anterior section (sector) have been reported to vary most commonly among persons [118–121]. Segment V accounted for 12.6% (range, 4.4–20.0%) of total liver volume (TLV), and the number of P5s (P5 represents the branches of the portal vein feeding segment V) was usually from 1 to 6 [4, 77]. The branching types of P5 were categorized according to Couinaud's definition, which is based on the branching points of P5 [122]. The simple branching of P5 off the trunk of the portal vein supplying the right anterior section was encountered in only 30.8% of persons. In the remaining 69.2% of individuals, P5 deviated caudally from the trunk of P8 [4]. This fact that segment V classically does not have a dominant inflow pedicle and has numerous inflow branches makes single segment V resection technically demanding.

Surgical Indications for Segmentectomy V

The routine preoperative imaging studies included ultrasonography and high-resolution helical computed tomography (CT), CT angiography, MR, and, if necessary, PET-CT. For patients with HCCs within segment V, anatomical segmentectomy V was preferred over nonanatomic partial resection (wedge resection or enucleation). Right anterior sectionectomy (RAS) (see section "Anatomic Right Anterior Sectionectomy Using Glissonean Pedicle Transection Method") or right hepatectomy (see section "Right Hepatectomy (S5–S8 Resection)") was adopted when the HCCs infiltrated the right anterior Glissonean pedicle or the right hepatic Glissonean pedicle, respectively. In order to prevent postoperative hepatic dysfunction and failure, several criteria for safe liver resection have been proposed [123]. In China, the so-called Makuuchi criteria [5] are simple to apply and widely used to determine the extent of safe hepatic resection [124]. According to these criteria, the anatomical units to be resected (e.g., a hemiliver, section (sector), or segment) are chosen based on liver function estimated using preoperative serum total bilirubin level and ICGR15. Anatomic segmentectomy V can be considered when serum total bilirubin level is less than 1.0 mg/dl and the ICGR15 is less than 30% [125].

Isolated Segmentectomy V

Operative Procedures	Technical Details
Laparotomy ↓	◀ A right subcostal incision was made.
Isolation and division of the S5 pedicle ↓	◀ The right hepatic Glissonean pedicle, the right anterior sectional Glissonean pedicle and S5 Glissonean pedicle was isolated and encircled with a tourniquet successively.
Staining of S5 ↓	◀ Methylene blue was injected into the pedicle of S5. Then, the pedicle of S5 was divided and suture-ligated. Color change appeared on the liver surface. According to the color change and ischemic demarcation line, the cut line was marked on the liver surface with electrocautery.
Hepatic parenchymal transection ↓	◀ Having clamped the hepatic pedicle, parenchymal transection was undertaken using the clamp-crushing and/or finger fracture method. Having delivering the specimen, the right hepatic vein (RHV) and the middle hepatic vein (MHV) were exposed on the cut surface of the liver remnant.
Drainage and closure of the abdominal cavity	◀ A drain close to the liver cut surface was used.

Intraoperative Key Points

1. The aim of staining by injecting methylene blue into the branch of portal vein supplying the target segment is to precisely guide the deep parenchymal transection along the interface between the stained liver tissue and unstained liver tissue. However, if the methylene blue is quickly washed out, this aim cannot be obtained, such as occurred in these surgical proceedings. To prolong staining the tumor-bearing segment, two maneuvers should be done. First, inflow pedicle should be clamped immediately after injecting dye; second, the venous outflow system should be occluded (see section "Right Posterior Sectionectomy (S6+S7 Resection)").
2. Segmentectomy V is challenging in that it demands three lines of transection to contain segment V. Although the main inflow pedicles of segment V arise from the anterior sectional pedicle and also diverge caudally from the extrasegmental trunk of the inflow pedicle of segment VIII [4], occasionally segment V will have extra inflow pedicles from the posterior sectional pedicle or the central inflow pedicles at the main originating points in the hepatic porta [27]. It is important to appropriately take these extra inflow pedicles during parenchymal transection proceedings along the three lines of transection.
3. It is vital to preserve and expose the distal trunk of the right hepatic vein on the right-sided cut surface after ligating and dividing its terminal branches, since this is the venous drainage of segment VI. Although segment IVB can drain into the umbilical vein, the distal trunk of the middle hepatic vein should be preserved and exposed on the left-sided raw area after ligating and dividing its terminal branches, in case of no infiltration or invasion by the tumor. In addition, as the caudate lobe lies posteriorly and does not demand to be resected as part of segment V, the posterior extent of resection in segmentectomy V does not demand dissection down to the retrohepatic inferior vena cava (Fig. 290).

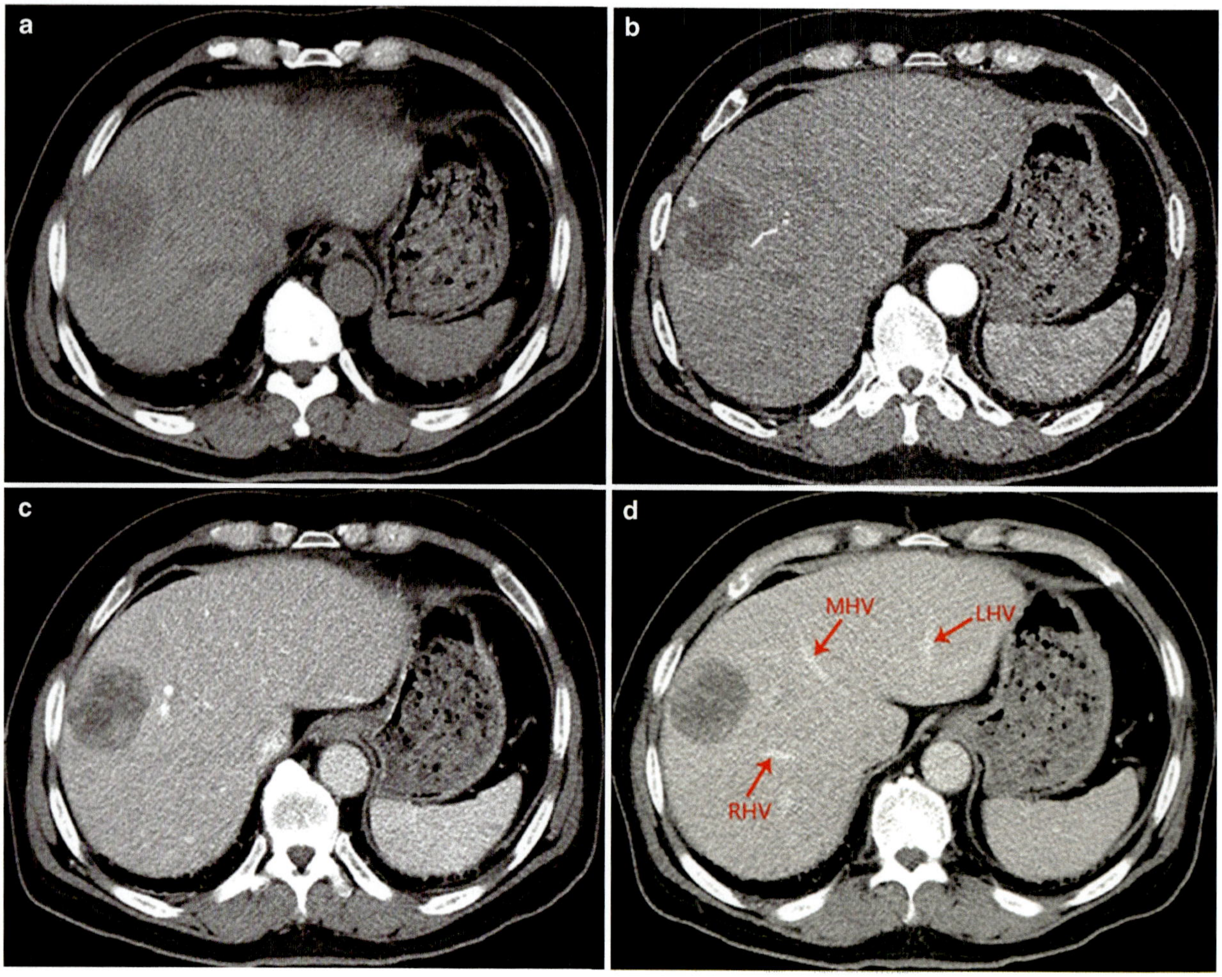

Fig. 290 (**a**) Preoperative CT (precontrast). The tumor, which appears mildly hypodense, is located in segment V. (**b**) Preoperative CT (hepatic arterial phase). The tumor shows mildly heterogeneous enhancement. (**c**) Preoperative CT (hepatic venous phase). The tumor shows enhancement fades. (**d**) Preoperative CT (interstitial phase). The tumor shows subtle washout. *RHV* right hepatic vein, *MHV* middle hepatic vein, *LHV* left hepatic vein

Abdominal Incision and Mobilization of the Right Hemiliver (Figs. 291, 292, 293, 294, 295, 296, and 297)

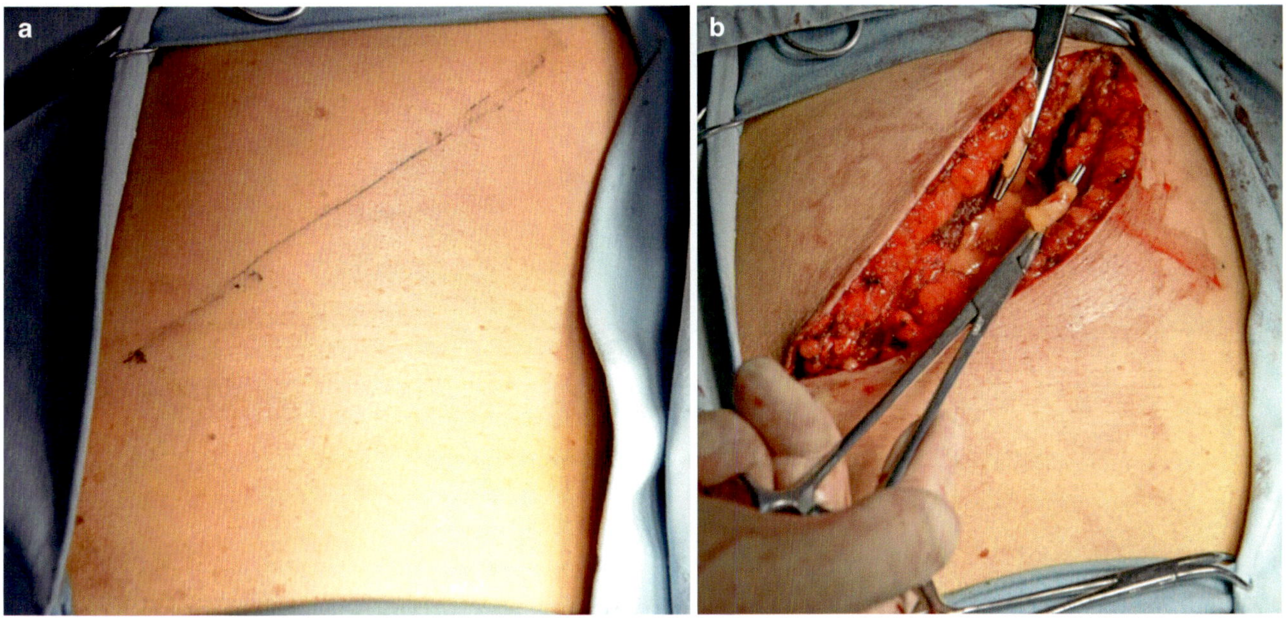

Fig. 291 (**a**, **b**) A right subcoastal incision was selected, and having entered into the peritoneal cavity, the round ligament was divided and ligated

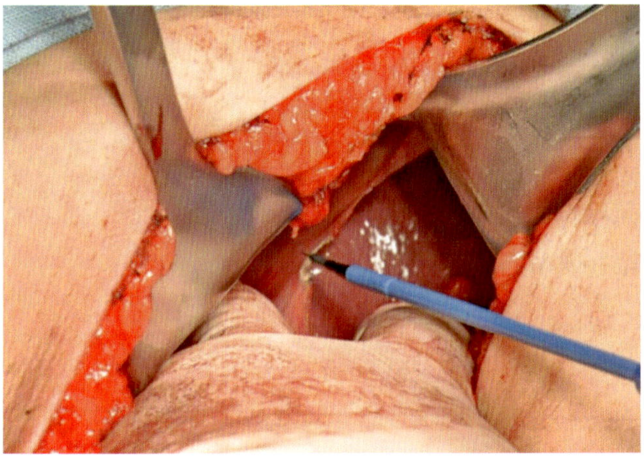

Fig. 292 The falciform ligament was electrocauterized

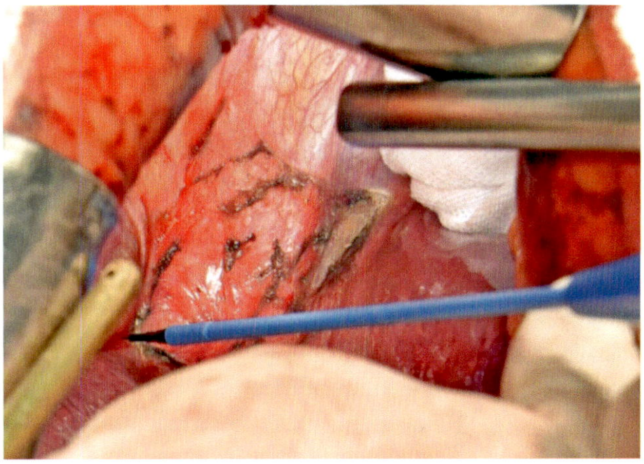

Fig. 293 Hepatocaval confluence was dissected and exposed

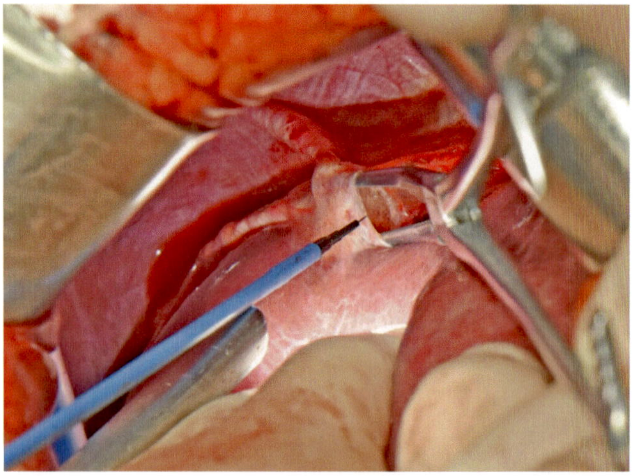

Fig. 294 The right coronary ligament was divided with electrocautery

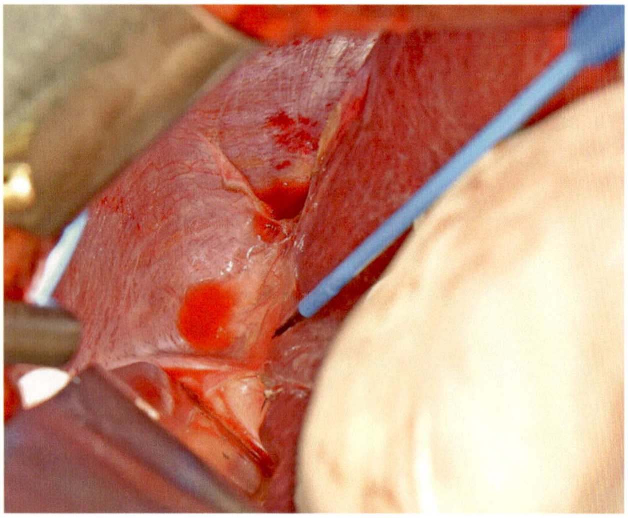

Fig. 295 The right triangular ligament was electrocauterized

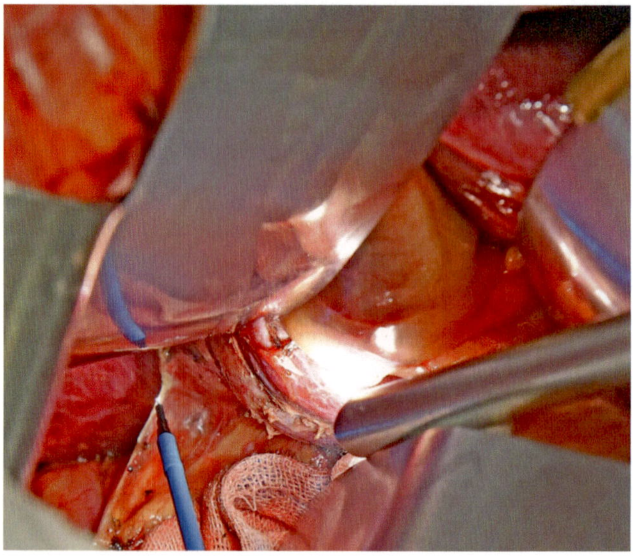

Fig. 296 The hepatocolic ligament was dissected

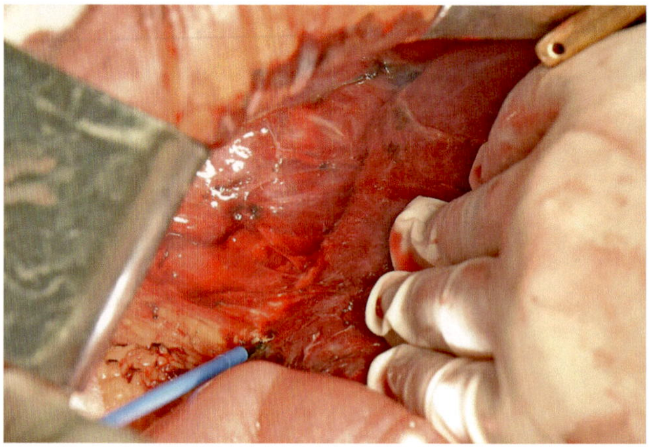

Fig. 297 The right adrenal gland was dissected off from the right posterior sector of the liver. At this time, the right hemiliver was fully mobilized

Isolation of the Pedicle of Segment V (S_5-P)
(Figs. 298, 299, 300, and 301)

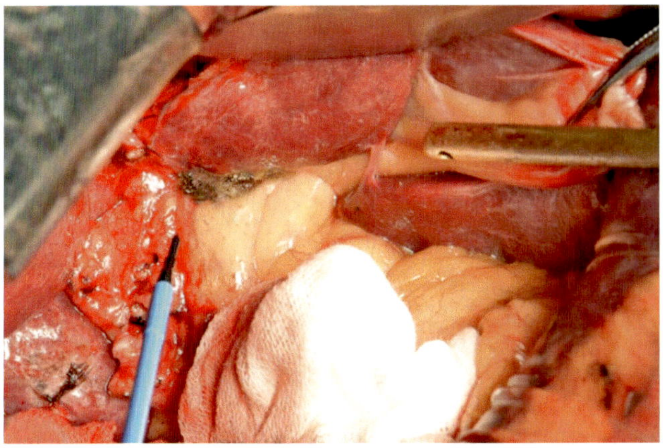

Fig. 298 A traverse small incision was made in front of the hilus with electrocautery, and the hepatic parenchyma around this incision was pushed upward to expose the anterior surface of the right hepatic Glissonean sheath

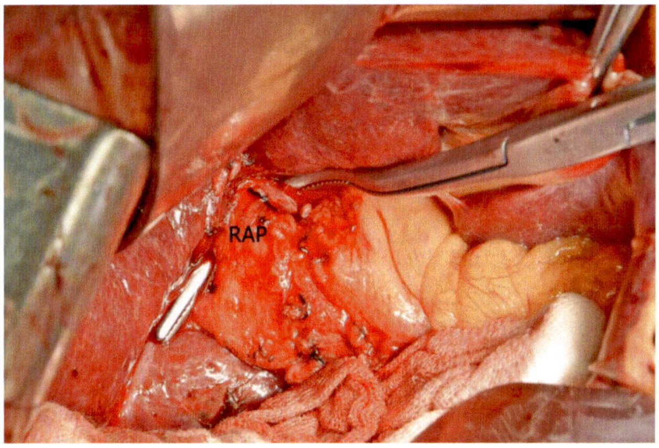

Fig. 299 A large curved clamp was inserted into this incision in the hilus and passed out of another small incision at the right edge of the gallbladder bed. Thus, the right anterior sectional Glissonean pedicle (RAP) was isolated

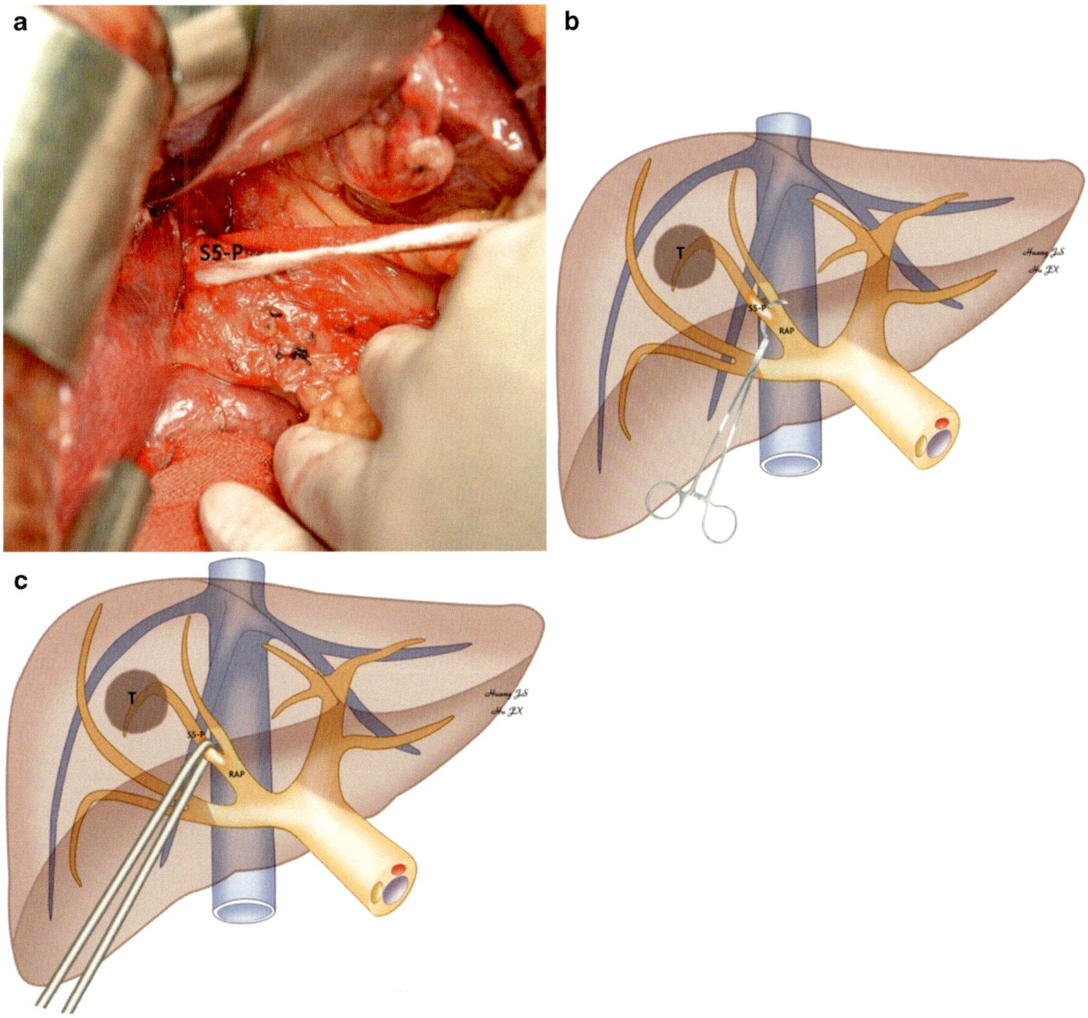

Fig. 300 (**a**) Having identified the right anterior sectional pedicle, further dissection was carried out to access the segment V pedicle. The right anterior sectional pedicle was dissected on its superior and anterior surface for about 10 mm, where the pedicle of the segment V was identified and encompassed by a vascular tape. (**b**, **c**) Schematic illustration of this procedure. *S5-P* pedicle of segment V

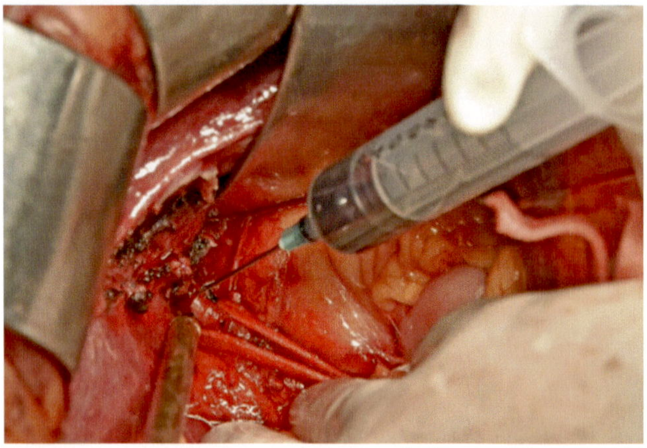

Fig. 301 Methylene blue was injected into the pedicle of the segment V, and the pedicle of segment V was temporarily clamped to prolong staining the liver tissue

Staining the Segment V and Marking the Cut Line (Figs. 302 and 303)

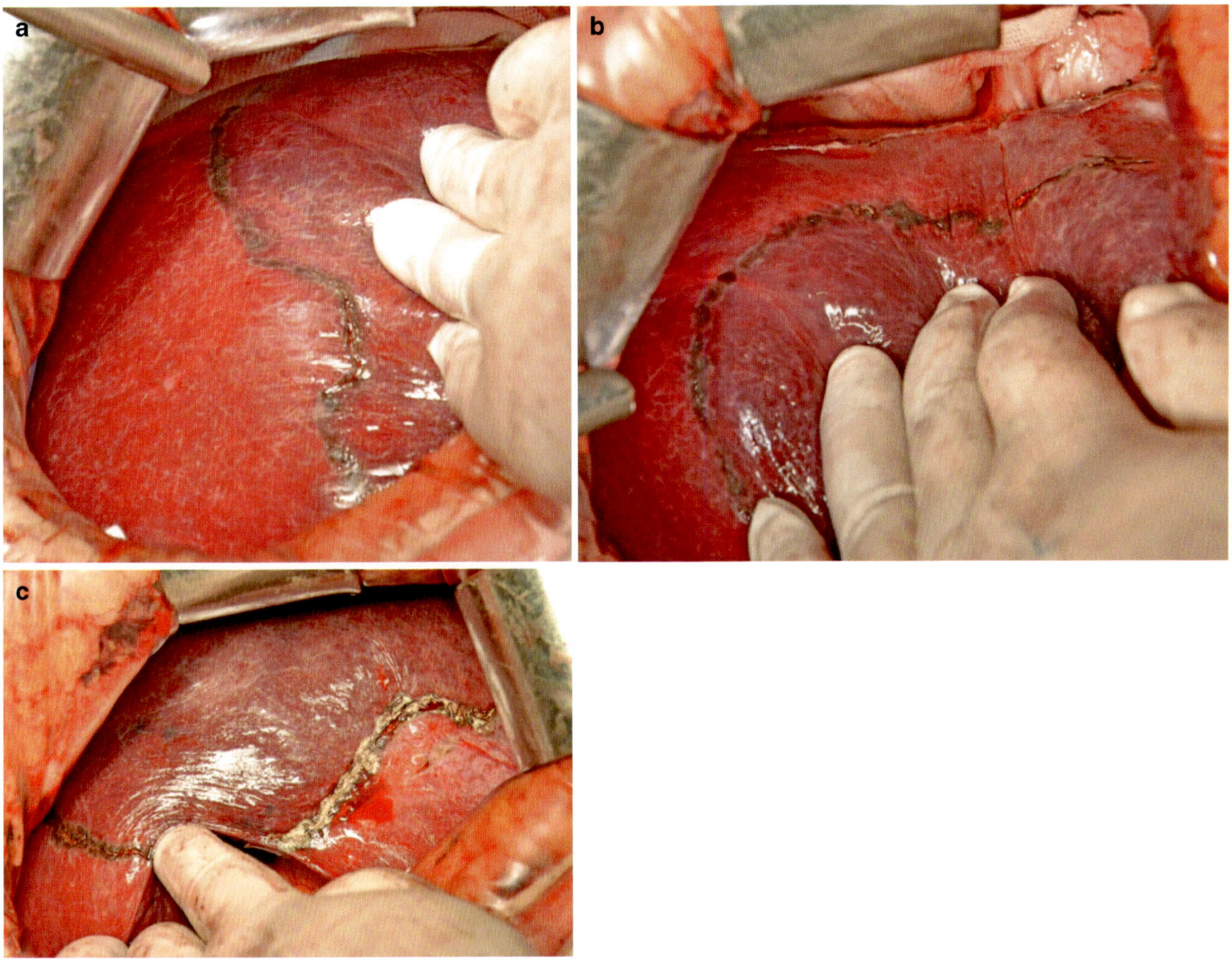

Fig. 302 (**a**–**c**) The ischemic and stained zone boundary was marked on the liver surface with electrocautery

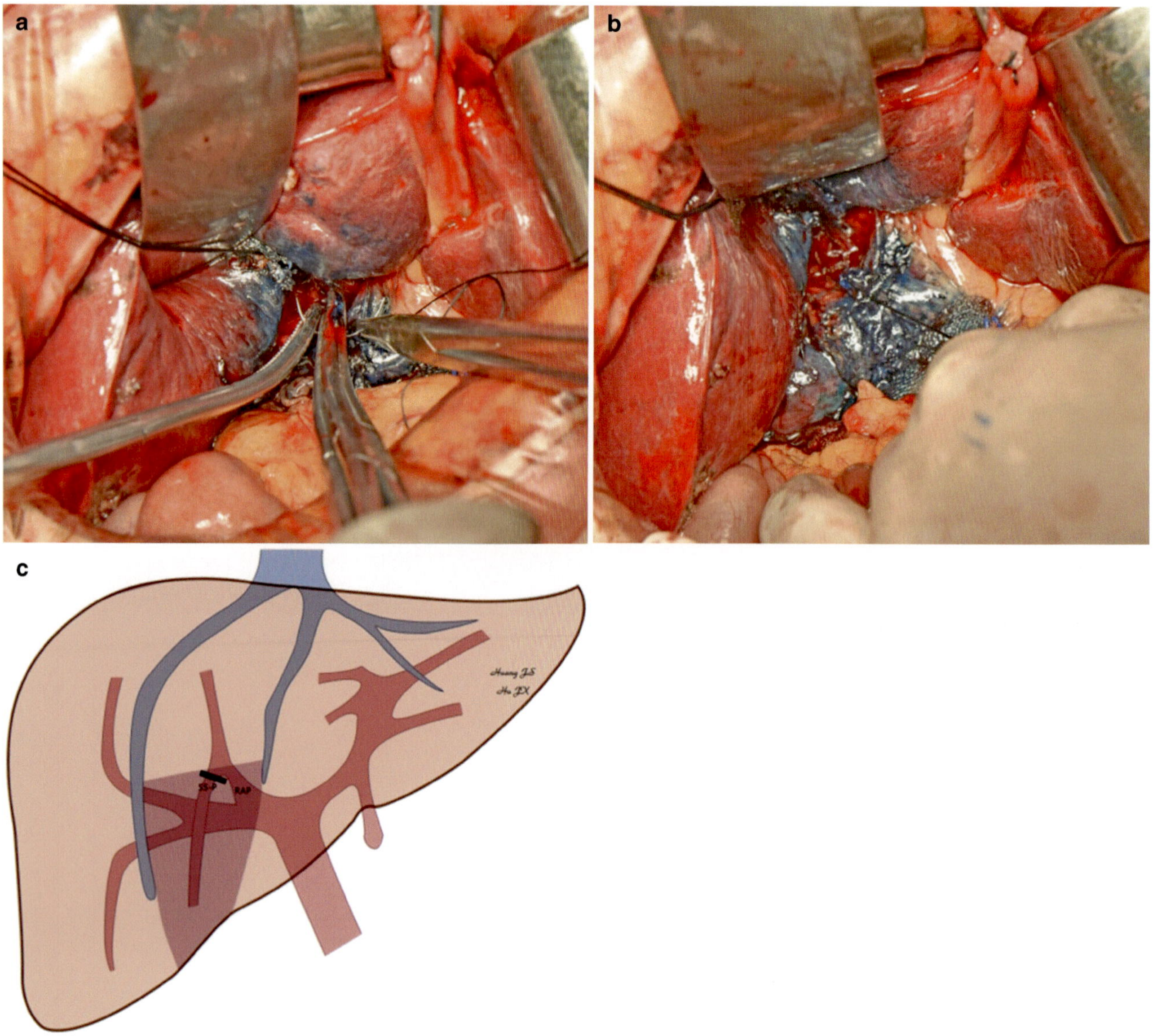

Fig. 303 (**a**, **b**) The pedicle of segment V was clamped, divided, and suture-ligated. (**c**) Schematic illustration of this procedure

Hepatic Parenchymal Transection
(Figs. 304, 305, 306, 307, 308, and 309)

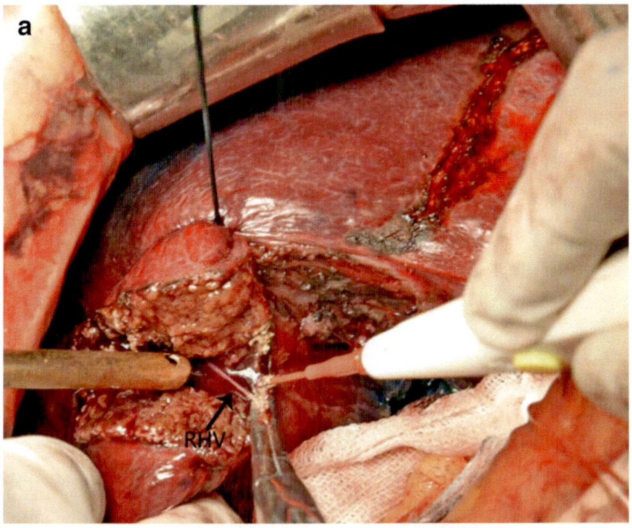

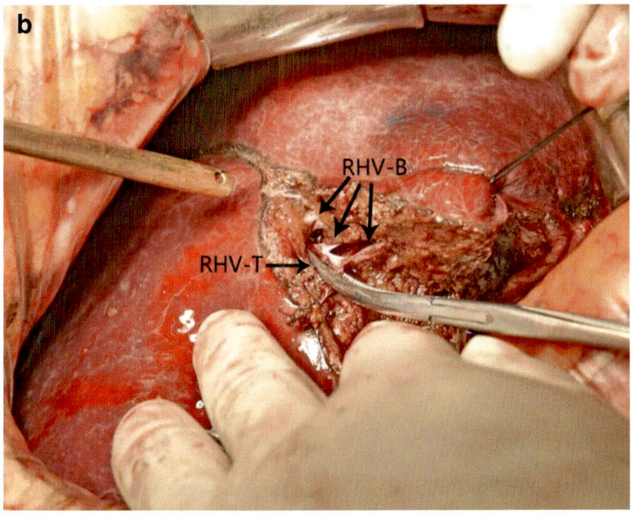

Fig. 304 (**a**, **b**) Having clamped the hepatic pedicle (Pringle maneuver), transection of the right-sided liver parenchyma was performed caudo-cranially along the demarcation line, using the clamp-crushing technique. Large branches of the right hepatic vein (RHV) were dissected and ligated. *B* branch, *T* trunk

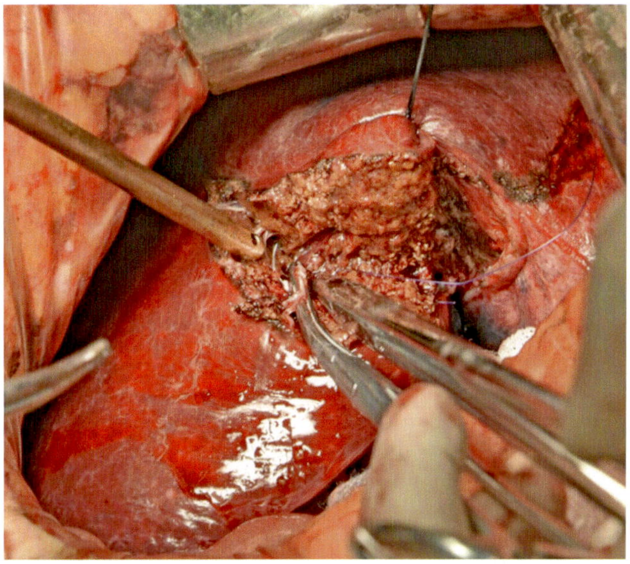

Fig. 305 Proximal stump of large branch of the RHV was suture-ligated. *RHV* right hepatic vein

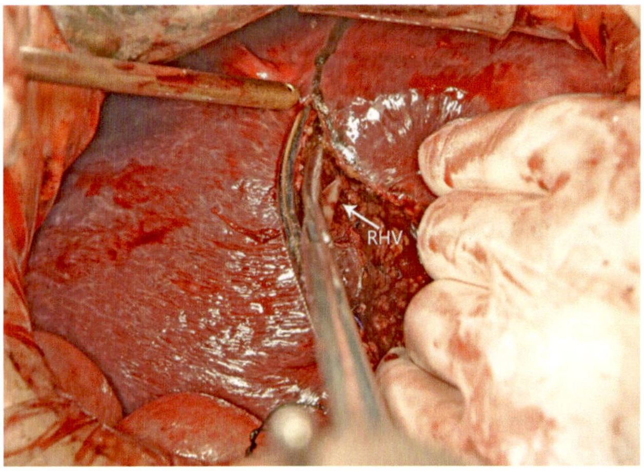

Fig. 306 Transection of the hepatic parenchyma was continued caudo-cranially. Attention should be paid to prevent injuries to the right hepatic vein (RHV)

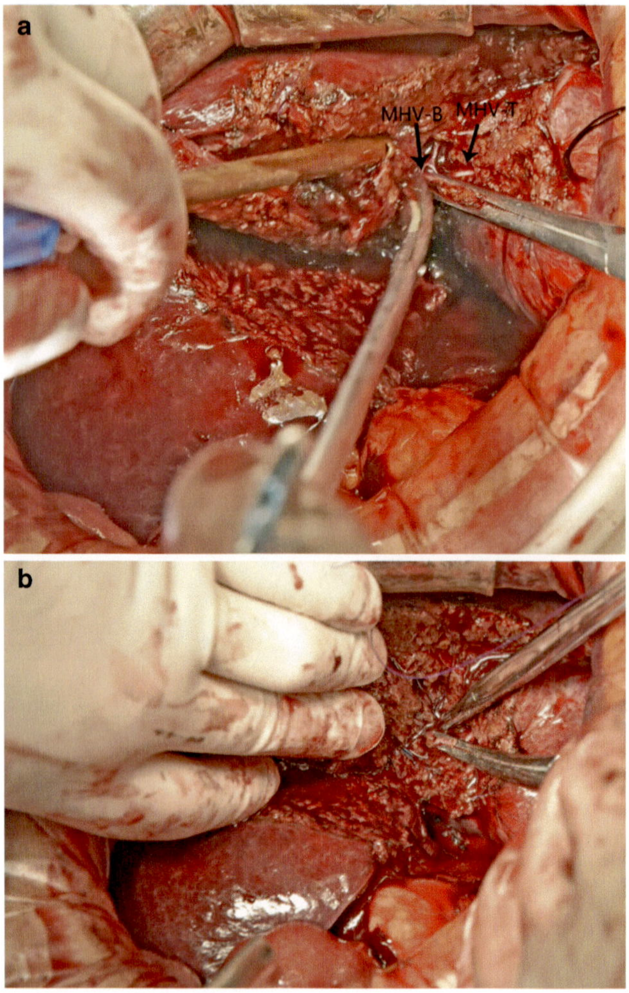

Fig. 307 (**a**, **b**) Left-sided hepatic parenchymal transection was undertaken caudo-cranially. Branch of the middle hepatic vein (MHV) was isolated, clamped, divided, and suture-ligated. *B* branch, *T* trunk

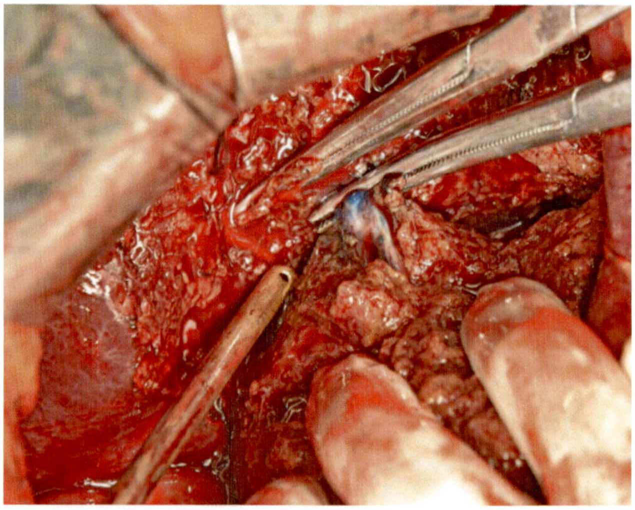

Fig. 308 Hepatic tissues around the distal stump of the pedicle of segment V was dissected

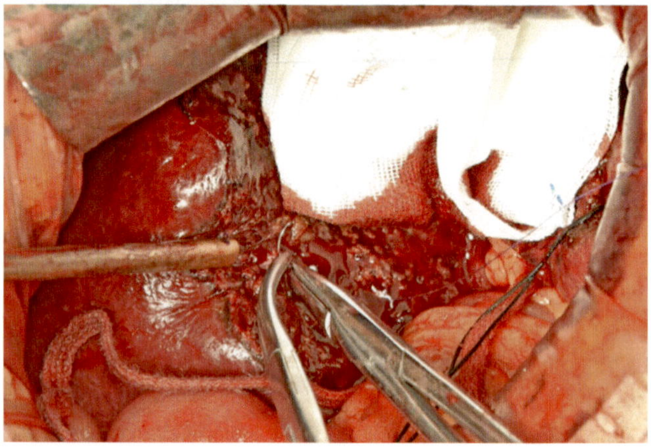

Fig. 309 Having removed the specimen and releasing the vascular tape that previously encircled the hepatic pedicle, the vascular and biliary ramifications on the cut surface of the liver remnant were sutured with 3-0 and 4-0 polypropylene, and the tiny holes on the RHV and MHV also were sutured with 5-0 polypropylene. *RHV* right hepatic vein, *MHV* middle hepatic vein

Hemostasis and Prevention of Bile Leak at the Raw Area (Figs. 310 and 311)

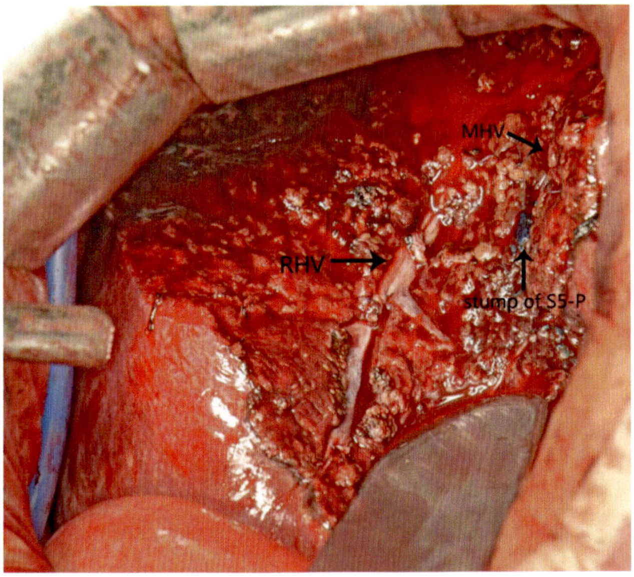

Fig. 310 The distal trunk of the right hepatic vein (RHV) was completely exposed on the right-sided cut surface of the liver remnant. *MHV* middle hepatic vein, *RHV* right hepatic vein, *S5-P* pedicle of segment V

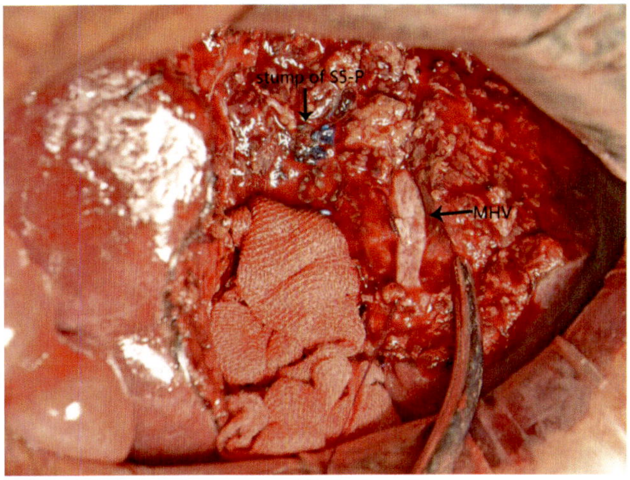

Fig. 311 The left-sided raw area of the liver remnant. The distal trunk of the middle hepatic vein was completely exposed. *MHV* middle hepatic vein, *S5-P* pedicle of segment V

Cut Surface and the Specimen
(Figs. 312, 313, and 314)

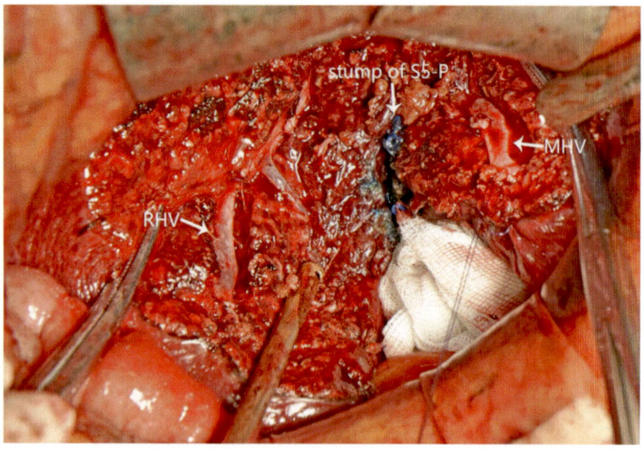

Fig. 312 Bird view of the cut surface of the liver remnant. The distal trunks of the middle hepatic vein and the right hepatic vein were completely exposed. The dye-stained proximal stump of S5-P was also clearly shown. *MHV* middle hepatic vein, *RHV* right hepatic vein, *S5-P* pedicle of segment V

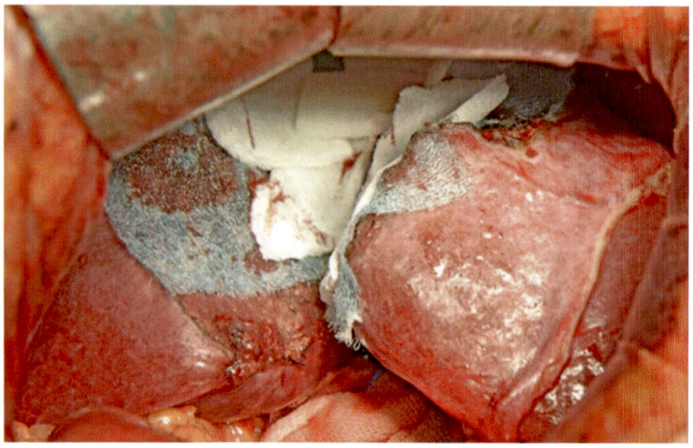

Fig. 313 The cut surface of the liver remnant was covered with fibrin glue (Neoveil®) and absorbable gelatin sponge. A drain tube close to the cut surface was placed into the Winslow hole

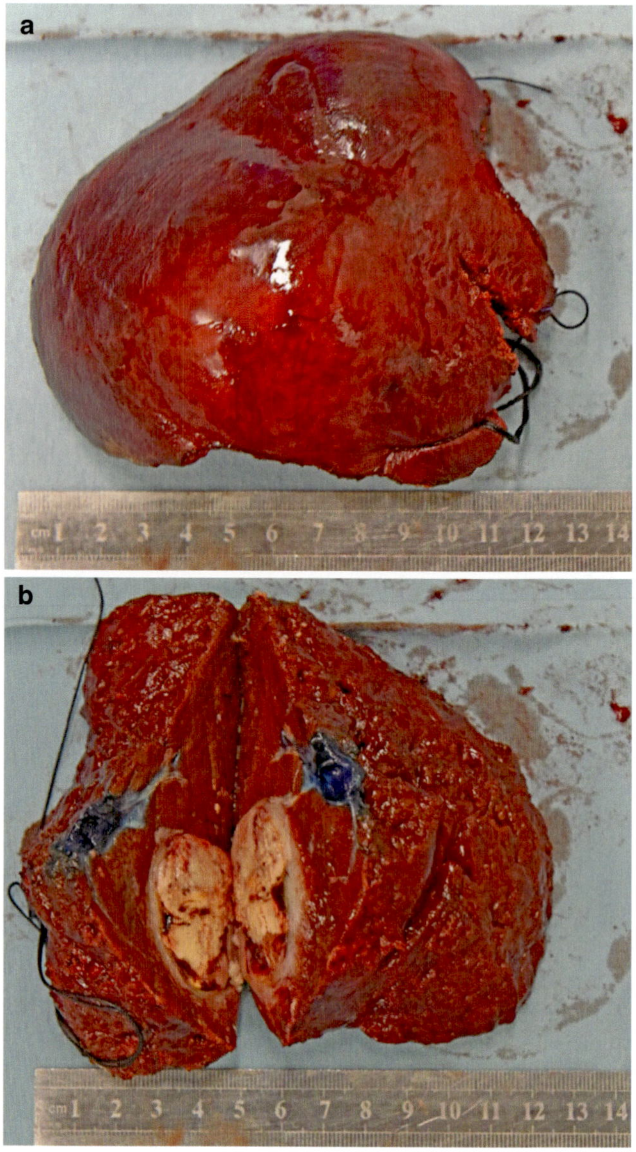

Fig. 314 (**a**, **b**) The specimen. (**a**) Anterior surface. (**b**) Surgical margin was macroscopically negative

Segmentectomy V with Resection of the Distal Trunk of the Middle Hepatic Vein (MHV)

Operative Procedures	Technical Details
Laparotomy	◀ A right subcostal incision was performed.
↓	
Preparation for total vascular exclusion	◀ The right hemiliver was dissected away from its surrounding structures. The hepatic pedicle, the supra- and infra-hepatic inferior vena cava was pre-placed with a tourniquet, respectively, because of the middle hepatic vein infiltrated by the tumor.
↓	
Marking the watershed of segment V	◀ The pedicle of the right anterior section was isolated and the clamped. The left-side ischemic demarcation line between the right anterior section and segment 5 and the line between the right anterior and posterior section was marked on the liver surface with electrocautery. The superior transverse transection line corresponds to the transverse plane thorough the hepatic hilum.
↓	
Hepatic parenchymal transection	◀ Having clamped the hepatic pedicle(Pringle maneavere), parenchymal transection was carried out using the clamp-crushing method. The several inflow pedicles of segment 5 was clamped, divided and suture-ligated, respectively.

Intraoperative Key Points

1. When the tumor confined within segment V is adequately large and/or too close to the hepatic hilum, it is technically difficult to dissect the right anterior Glissonean pedicle to access the inflow pedicle of segment V. Based on our own clinical experiences, it is advisable to isolate, divide, and suture-ligate the inflow pedicle of segment V directly originating from the right anterior Glissonean pedicle at the end of the hepatic parenchymal transection. As the inflow pedicles of segment V were not isolated occluded, its superior watershed separating segment VIII cannot be ascertained by color change on the liver surface; anatomically, this superior border between S5 and S8 corresponds to the transverse plane through the hepatic hilum.
2. Preoperative hepatic vein reconstruction image clearly shows that the distal trunk of the middle hepatic vein is infiltrated by the tumor and the hepatic vein draining segment IV exists and drains into the left hepatic vein. Thus, the distal trunk of the middle hepatic vein can be resected since the S4 vein can drain segment IV.
3. Preoperative CT portal virtual reconstruction (VR) image clearly demonstrated that a part of segment VIII was also supplied by the portal branch from the portal vein feeding the left medial section (sector). This fact was intraoperatively ascertained when the right anterior Glissonean pedicle was temporarily clamped; the left-sided and superior portion of segment VIII was not devascularized on the liver surface.
4. Just as we have previously mentioned (see section "Brief Description of the Anatomic Variations of Segment V") that segment V typically does not have a main inflow pedicle and has several inflow pedicles [4, 27], this resection of segment V shows that this segment V has three inflow Glissonean pedicles. One originates directly from the right anterior pedicle and supplies the inferior portion of segment V; another two pedicles branch off the extrasegmental trunk of the inflow pedicle of segment VIII and feed the superior ventral and dorsal portion of segment V, respectively. The anatomical resection of single Couinaud's segment is one of the key techniques in hepatobiliary surgery. Basic steps in single anatomical segmentectomy consists of (1) understanding the anatomy of the corresponding branches of the portal veins and (2) identifying segmental watersheds on the liver surface and exact intersegmental plane during hepatic parenchymal transection [126, 127]. At present, the intersegmental plane provided by preoperative image processing software cannot be referred to during hepatic parenchymal transection [27]. Glissonean pedicle clamping visualizes segmental watersheds only on the liver surface, not in the deep hepatic parenchyma, since the interface between the devascularized and the well-vascularized parenchyma will disappear when the whole or hemiliver inflow occlusion was applied during liver transection. Conventional methylene blue staining sometimes can help to identify the exact intersegmental plane during parenchymal transection if the staining can sustain for an enough long time by occluding the inflow and outflow vascular system. Unfortunately, the conventional dyeing failed in many instances because the dye was quickly washed out or the regurgitation of the dye leaded to the unwanted staining of the non-tumor-bearing segment and/or section. Consequently, anatomic resection of single segment following the exact intersegmental planes is still technically challenging. A navigation system aiming to projecting preoperative 3D images onto the real-time surgical field may facilitate to perform an anatomically precise segmentectomy [27] (Fig. 315).

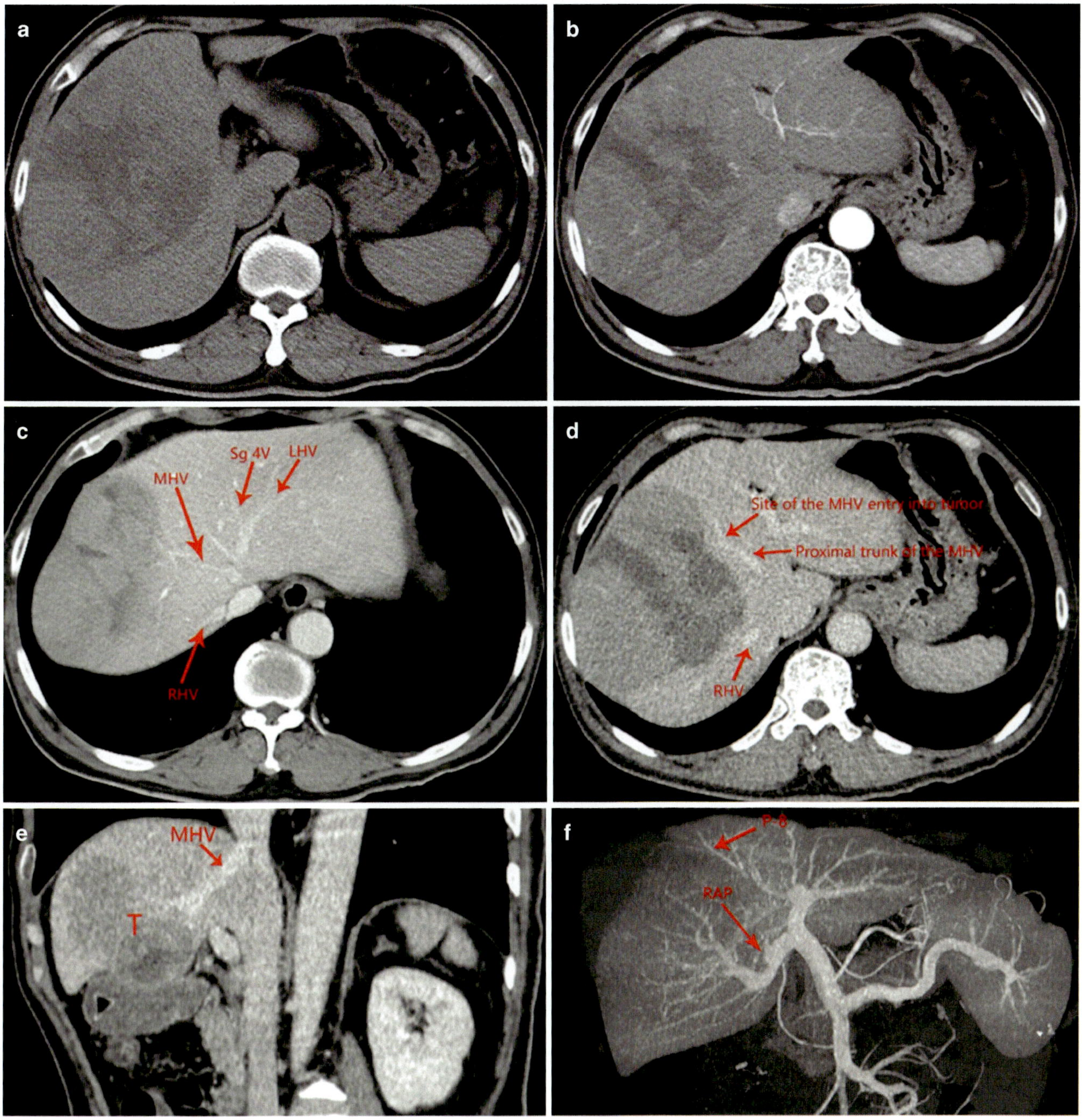

Fig. 315 (**a**) Preoperative CT (precontrast). The tumor, which appears mildly hypodense, completely occupies segment V. (**b**) Preoperative CT (hepatic arterial phase). The tumor shows heterogeneous enhancement. (**c**) The hepatic veins are shown on preoperative CT (hepatic venous phase). The tumor shows enhancement fades. (**d**) Preoperative CT (hepatic venous phase) shows that the proximal trunk of the MHV was present and the distal trunk of the MHV was involved in the tumor. The tumor shows enhancement fades. (**e**) Preoperative hepatic vein reconstruction image clearly shows that the MHV entered into the tumor. (**f**) This portal VR image clearly demonstrates that a portion of segment VIII was also supplied by the portal branch from the portal vein feeding the left medial sector. The branching point of the right anterior pedicle off the hepatic pedicle was shown. *RHV* right hepatic vein, *MHV* middle hepatic vein, *Sg 4V* segment IV vein, *LHV* left hepatic vein, *T* tumor, *P-8* branch of the portal vein supplying segment VIII, *RAP* right anterior pedicle

Abdominal Incision and Mobilization of the Right Hemiliver (Figs. 316, 317, 318, 319, 320, 321, 322, 323, 324, 325, 326, and 327)

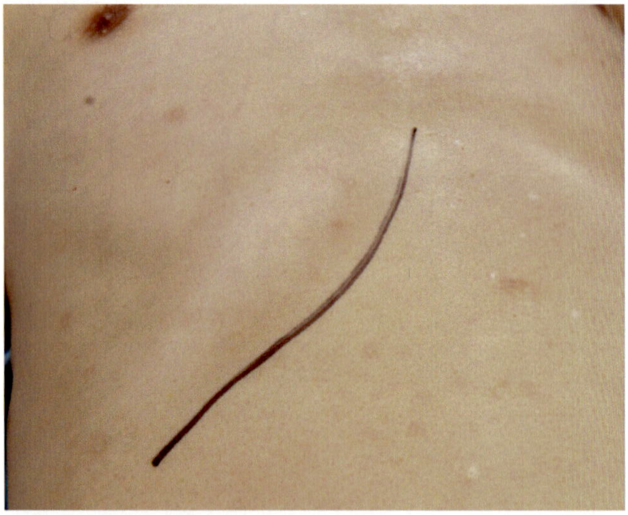

Fig. 316 A right subcostal incision was selected

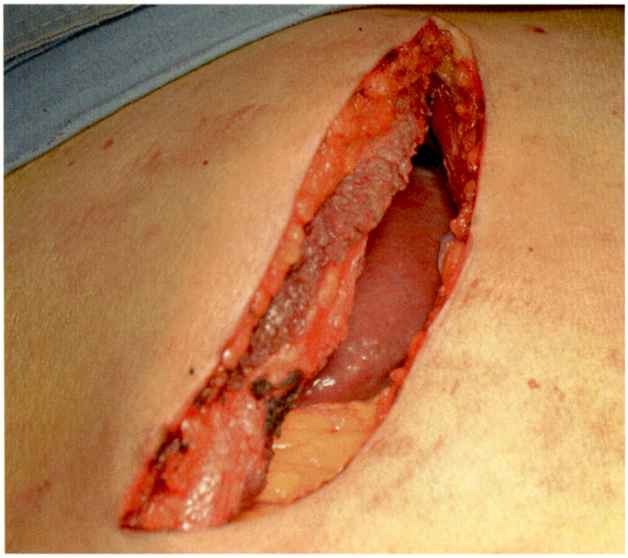

Fig. 317 A right subcostal incision was performed. Then a careful abdominal exploration was carried out

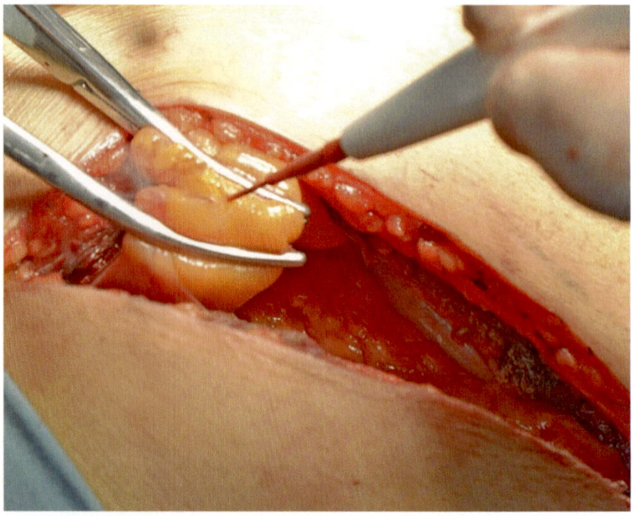

Fig. 318 Ligamentum teres was divided and ligated

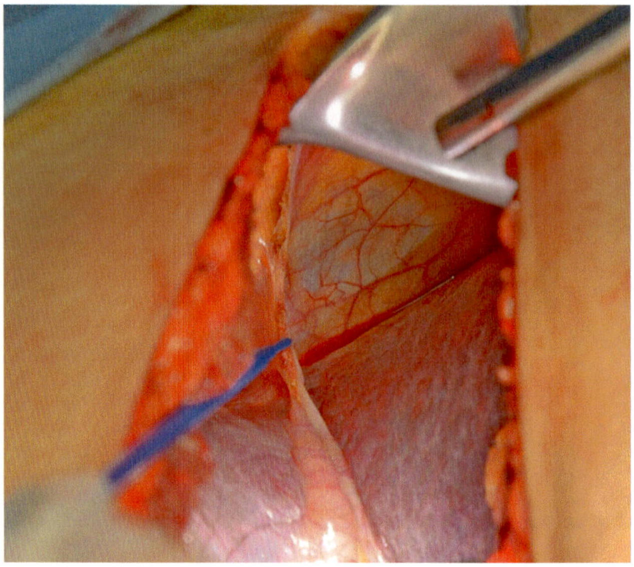

Fig. 319 Falciform ligament was divided with electrocautery

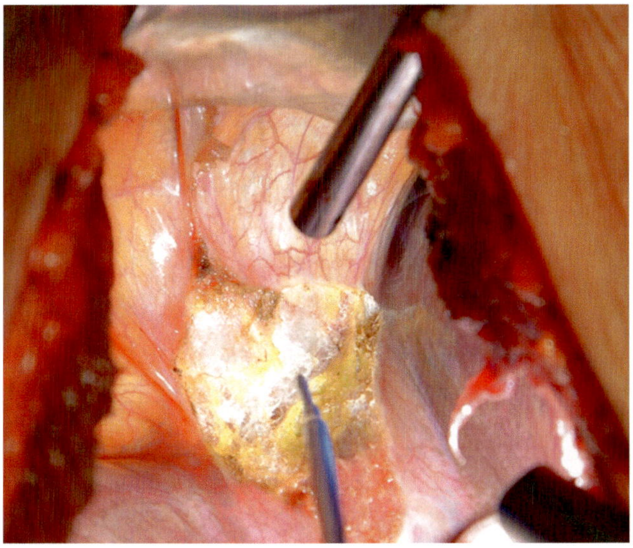

Fig. 320 Hepatocaval confluence was dissected and exposed

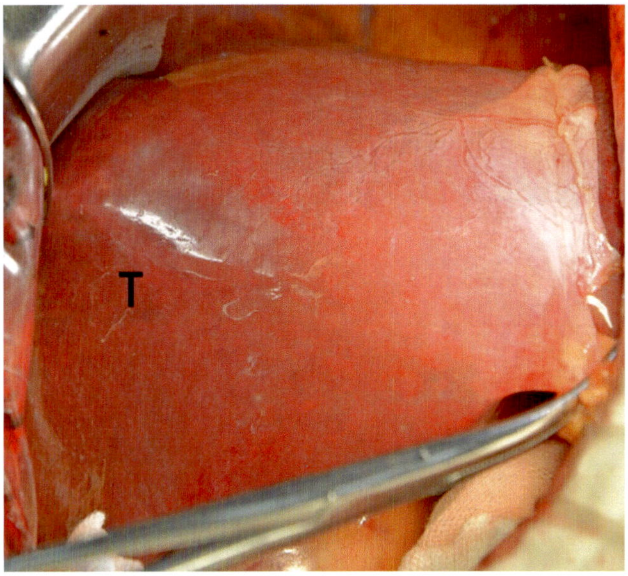

Fig. 321 Intraoperative macroscopic view. The tumor completely occupied segment V. No daughter node was found within the future liver remnant by IOUS. *IOUS* intraoperative ultrasound, *T* tumor

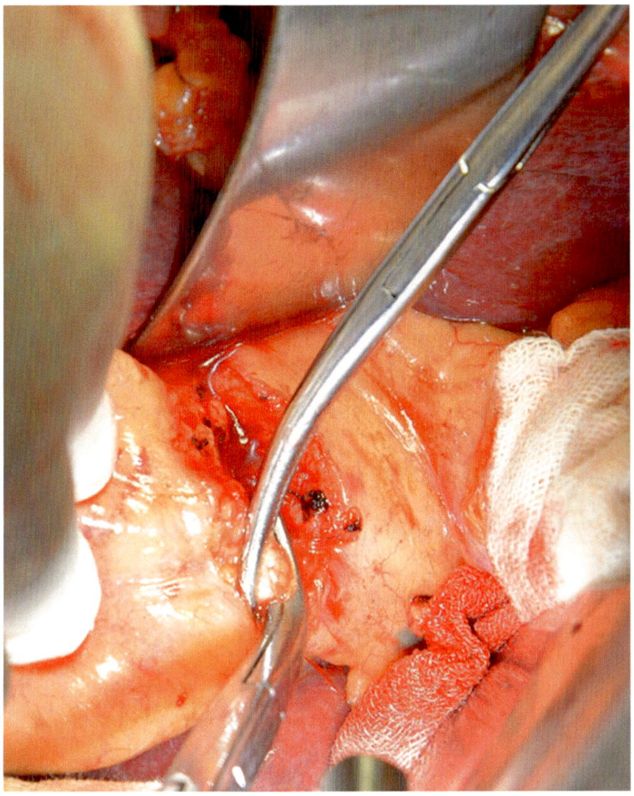

Fig. 322 Cholecystectomy was carried out

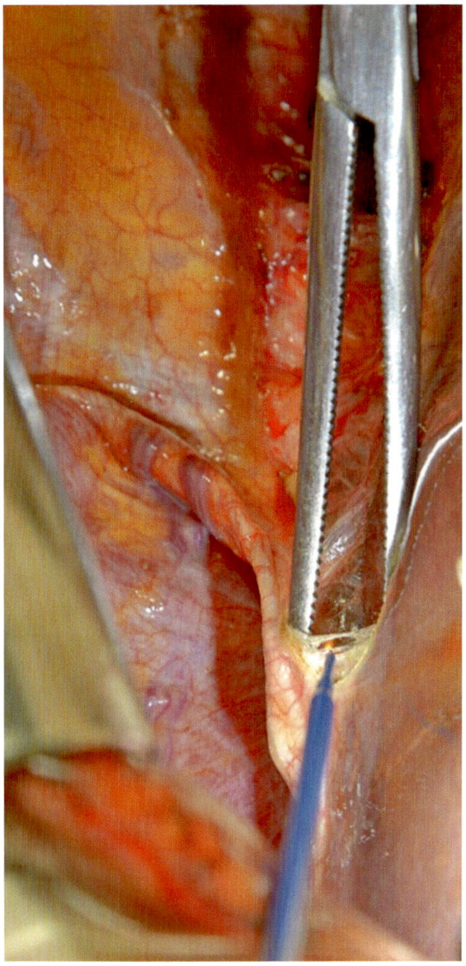

Fig. 323 The right coronary ligament was divided with electrocautery

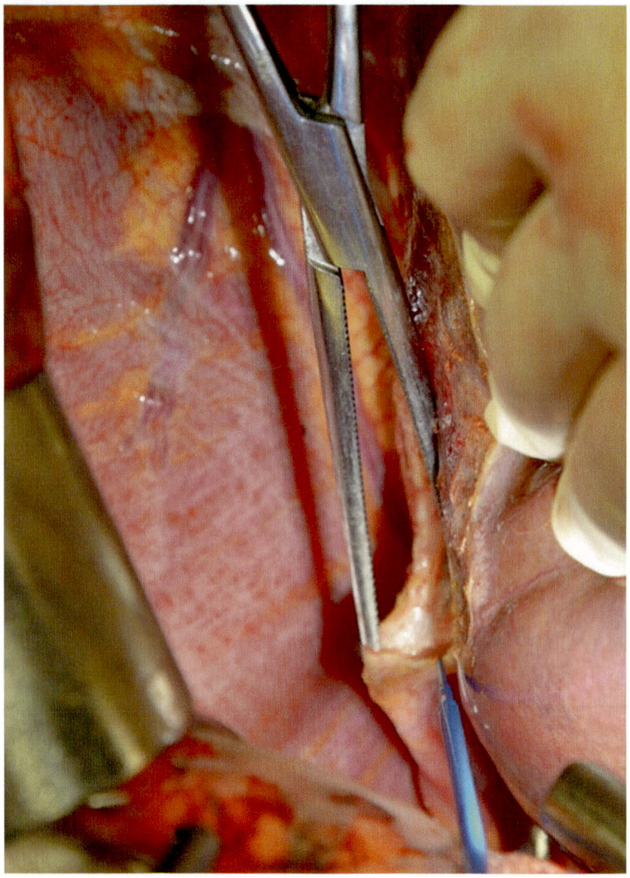

Fig. 324 The anterior layer of the right triangular ligament was divided with electrocautery

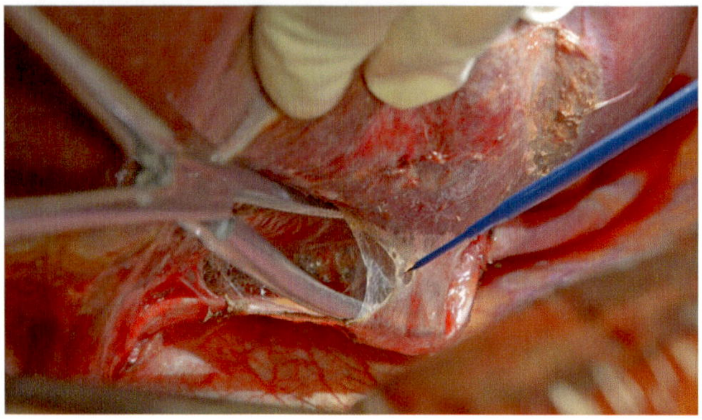

Fig. 325 The posterior layer of the right triangular ligament was divided with electrocautery

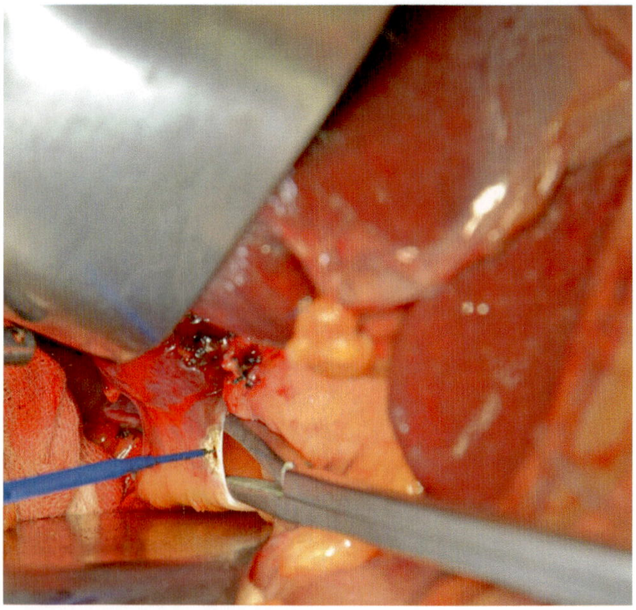

Fig. 326 The hepatocolic ligament was divided with electrocautery

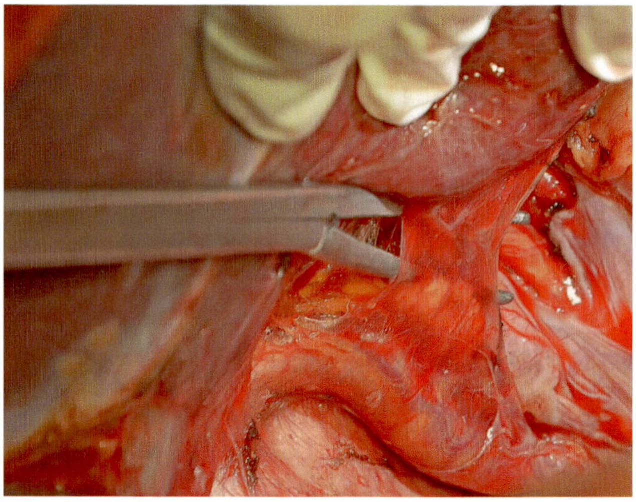

Fig. 327 The right adrenal gland was dissected away from the posterior portion of the right hemiliver with electrocautery

Preparation for Total Vascular Occlusion
(Figs. 328, 329, 330, 331, and 332)

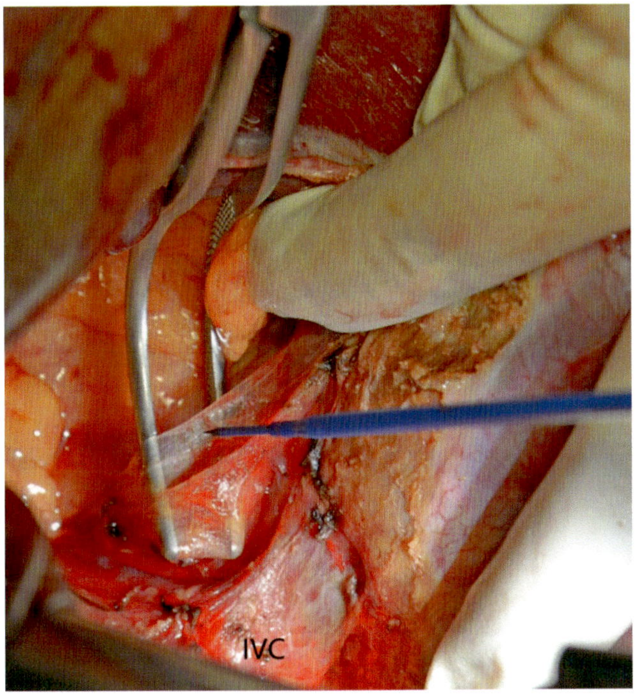

Fig. 328 The ligamentum venosum was dissected and divided. *IVC* inferior vena cava

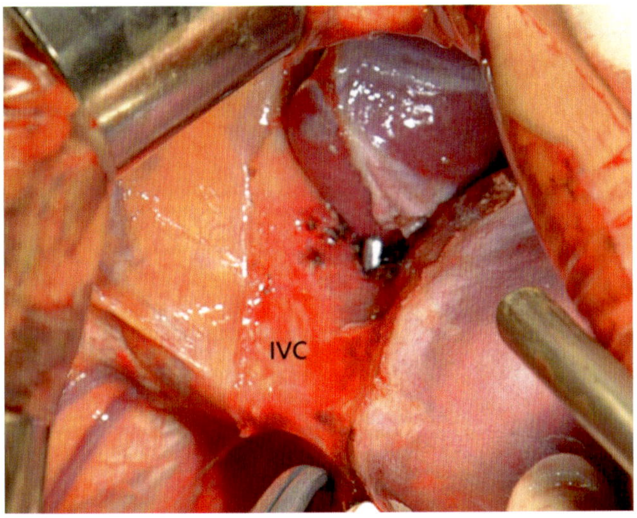

Fig. 329 The suprahepatic IVC was isolated. *IVC* inferior vena cava

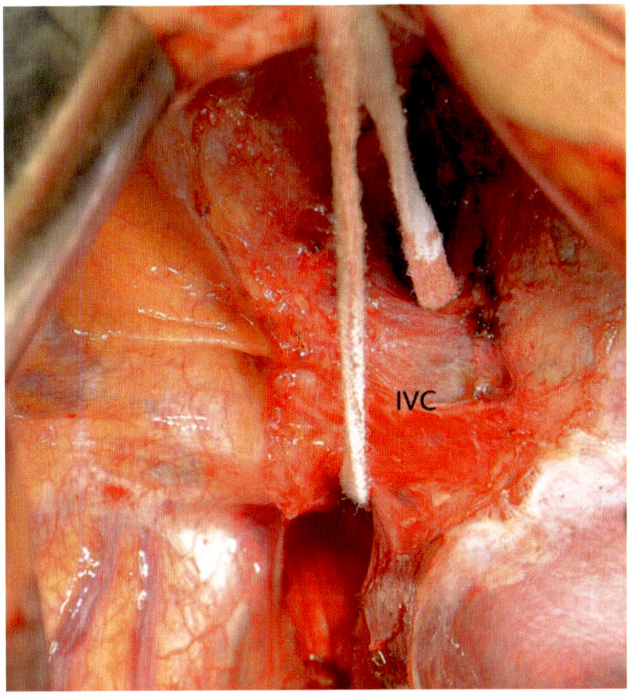

Fig. 330 The suprahepatic IVC was pre-placed with a vascular tape. *IVC* inferior vena cava

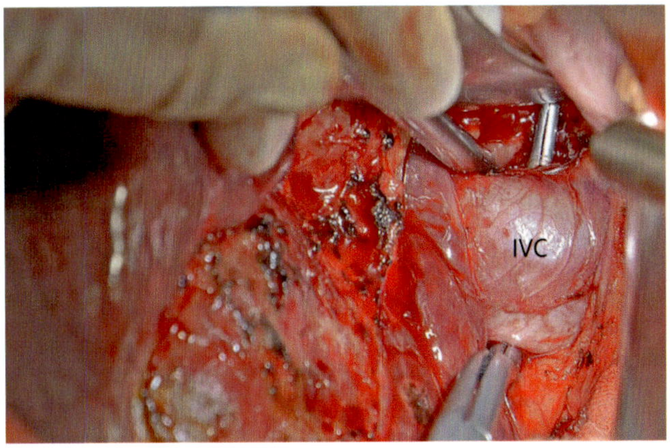

Fig. 331 The infrahepatic IVC was also isolated. *IVC* inferior vena cava

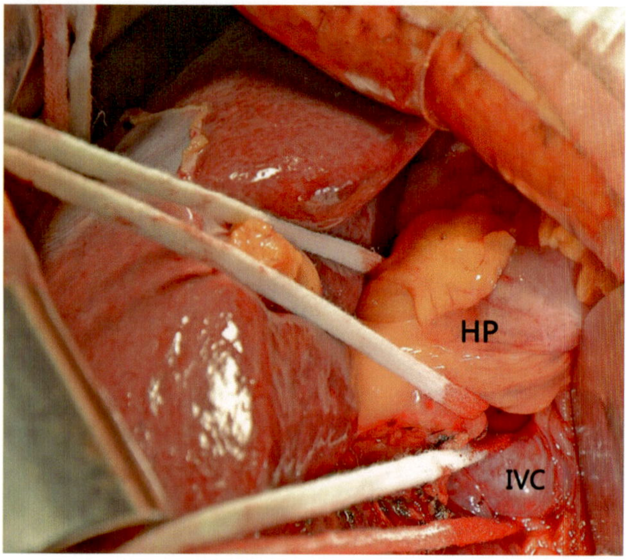

Fig. 332 The hepatic pedicle (HP) outside the liver, the supra- and subhepatic IVC was encircled with a vascular tape, respectively. *IVC* inferior vena cava

Isolation of the Right Anterior Pedicle and Marking the Cut Line
(Figs. 333, 334, 335, 336, 337, and 338)

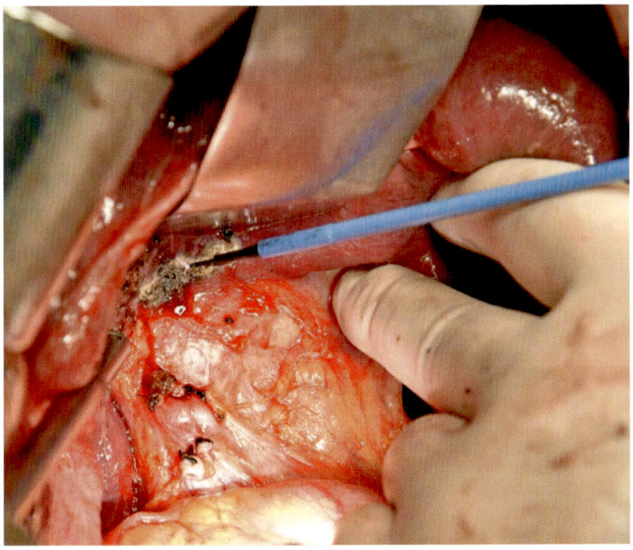

Fig. 333 One small anterior incision was made in front of the hilus, and the hepatic parenchyma around the small incision was pushed upward with blunt dissection to expose the anterior surface and bifurcation of the right hepatic Glissonean pedicle

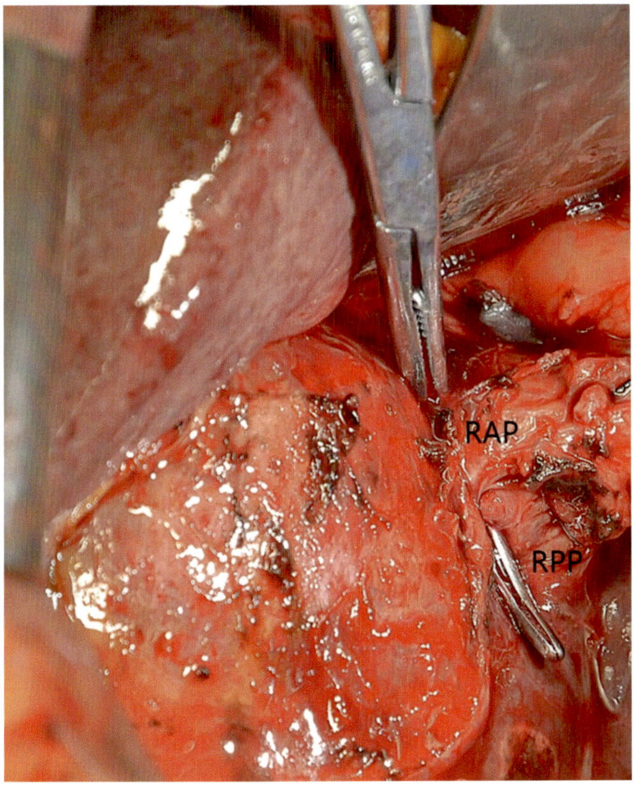

Fig. 334 Another small incision was made on the right edge of the gallbladder bed. A large curved clamp was inserted into this incision in front of the hilus and passed out of the incision on the right edge of the gallbladder bed. Thus, the right anterior pedicle (RAP) was isolated. *RPP* right posterior pedicle

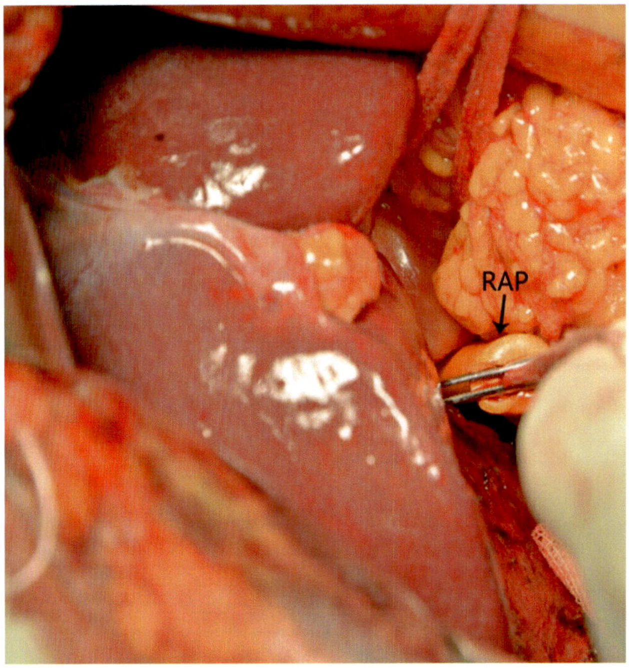

Fig. 335 The right anterior pedicle (RAP) was encircled with a vascular tape and temporarily clamped

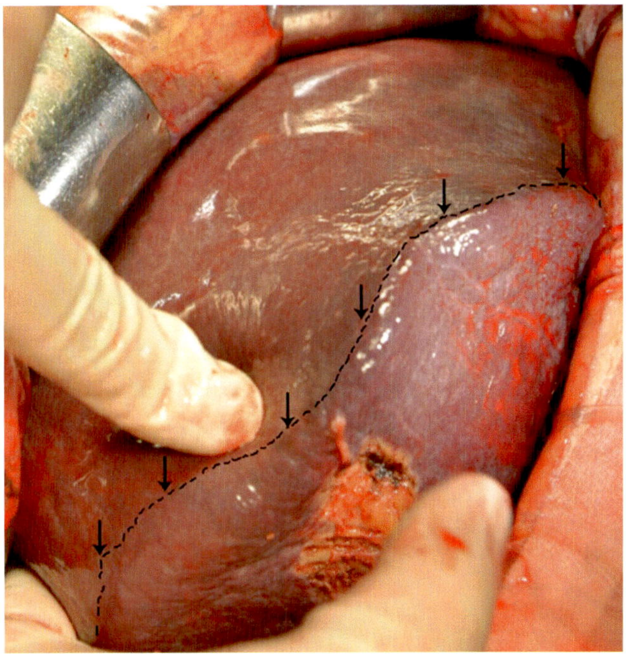

Fig. 336 Having temporarily clamped the right anterior pedicle (RAP), ischemic demarcation between the right anterior and posterior sector was obtained on the liver surface

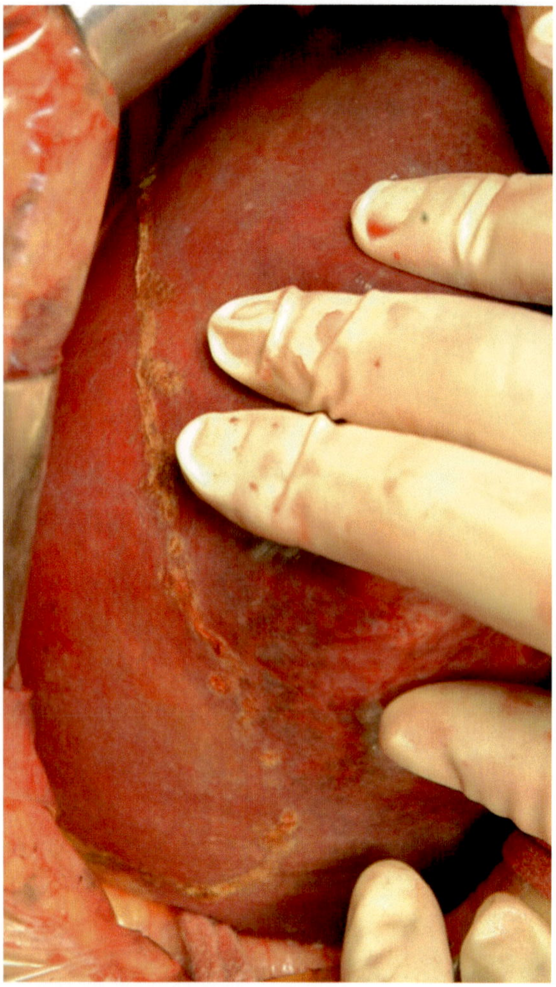

Fig. 337 The ischemic delineation between the right anterior and posterior sector was marked on the liver surface with electrocautery

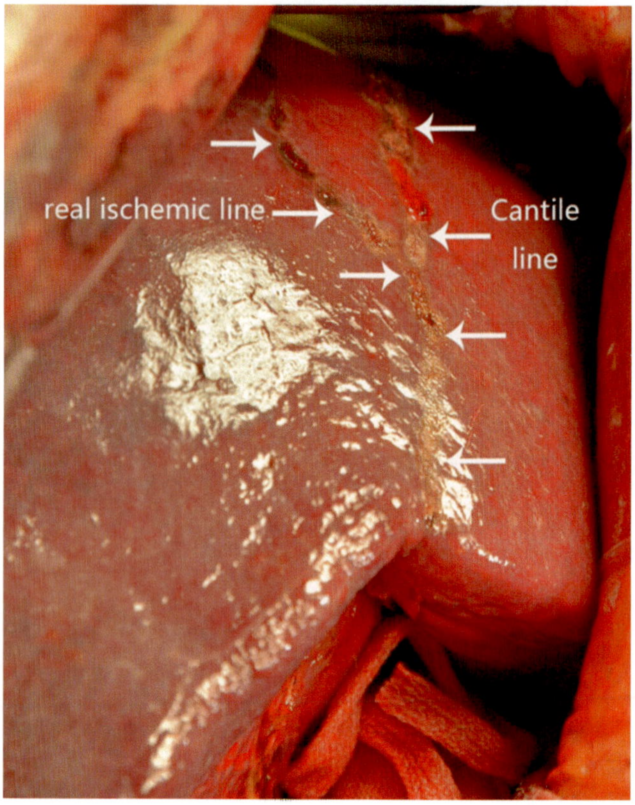

Fig. 338 The real ischemic line between the right anterior sector and segment IVA was not completely in agreement with the Cantlie line. Figure 320 showed that a part of segment VIII was also supplied by the portal branch from the left medial sector portal vein. Therefore, no color change was found on the surface of a part of segment VIII when the right anterior pedicle (RAP) was clamped

Hepatic Parenchymal Transection
(Figs. 339, 340, 341, 342, 343, 344, 345, 346, 347, 348, 349, 350, and 351)

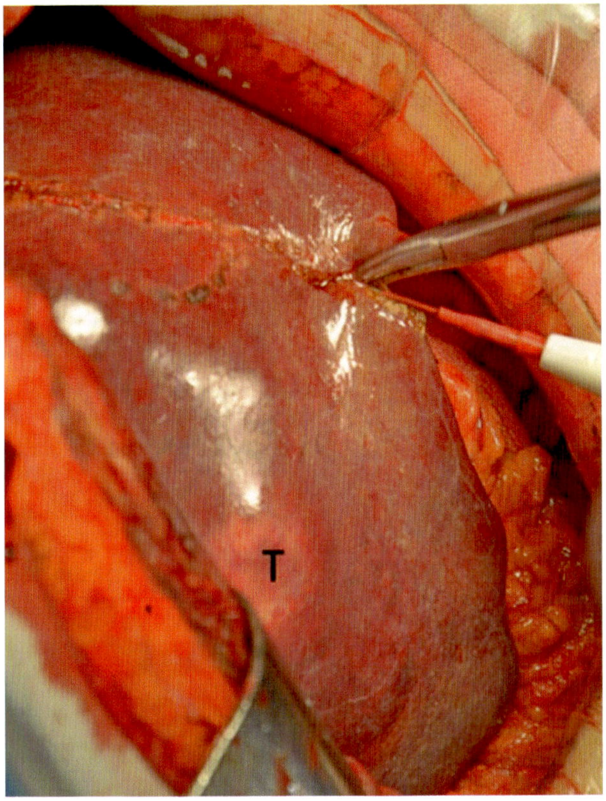

Fig. 339 The left-sided parenchymal transection was started between segment IVB and segment V caudo-cranially along the demarcation line, using a clamp-crushing technique. Small vascular structures were electrocauterized. *T* tumor

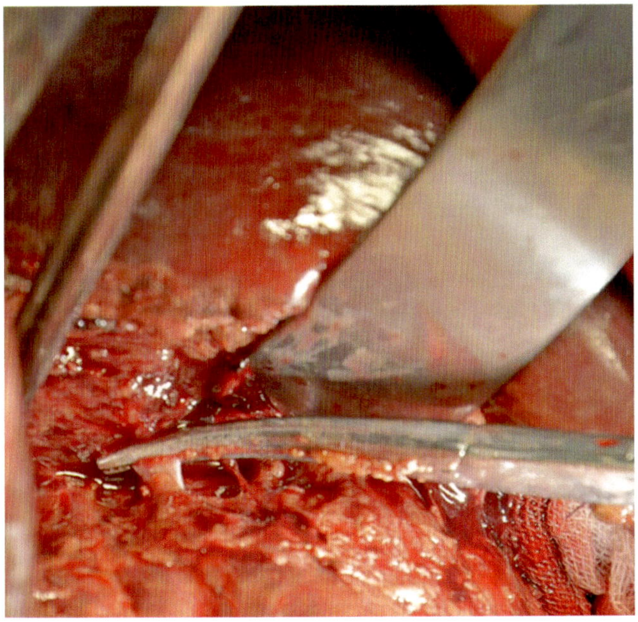

Fig. 340 A large venous branch from the middle hepatic vein (MHV) was isolated, divided, and silk-ligated

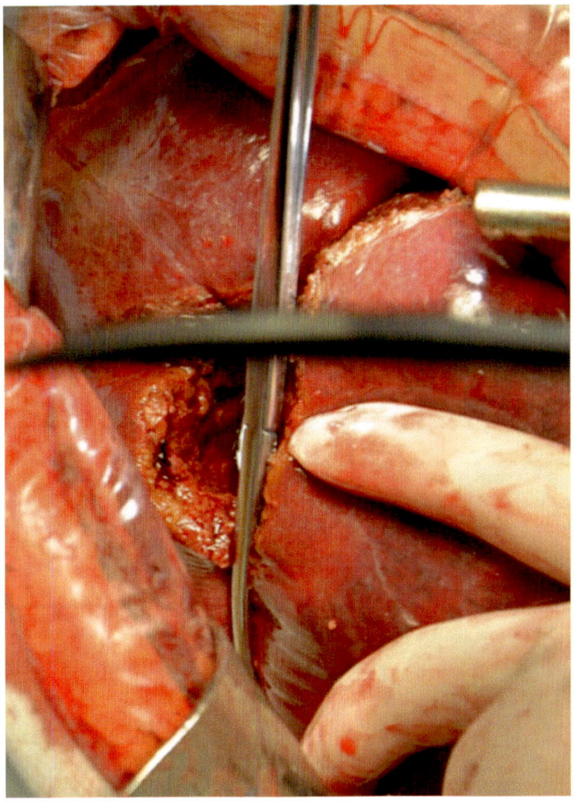

Fig. 341 Parenchymal transection was continued between segment V and segment VIII. The transectional line between segment V and segment VIII corresponded to the transverse plane through the liver hilum

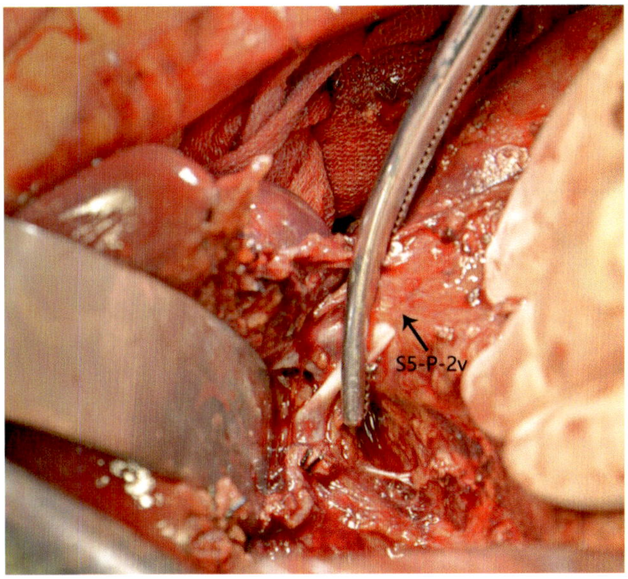

Fig. 342 A portal pedicle entering into the superior ventral portion of segment V (S5-P-2v) was identified. This pedicle was clamped, divided, and silk-sutured

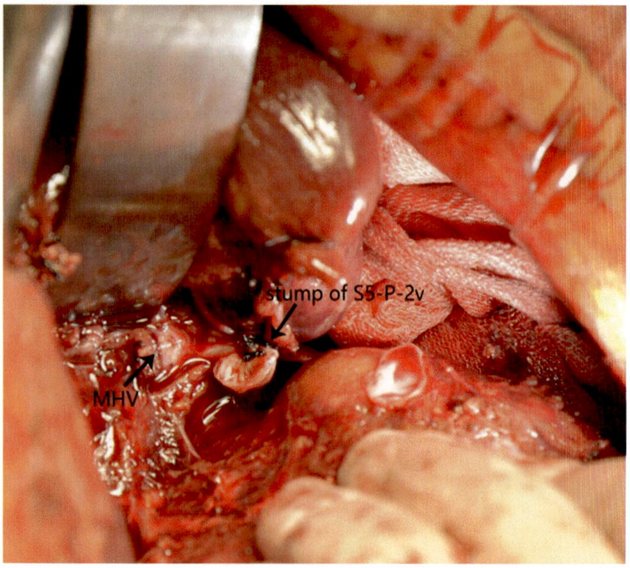

Fig. 343 The proximal stump of the superior ventral pedicle of segment V (S5-P-2v) was shown. *MHV* middle hepatic vein

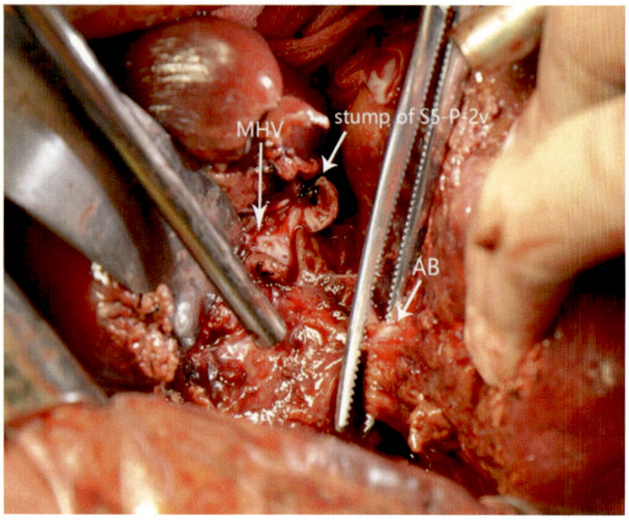

Fig. 344 The artery branch (AB) supplying superior dorsal portion of segment V was identified and clamped, divided, and ligated. *S5-P-2v* the superior ventral pedicle of segment V

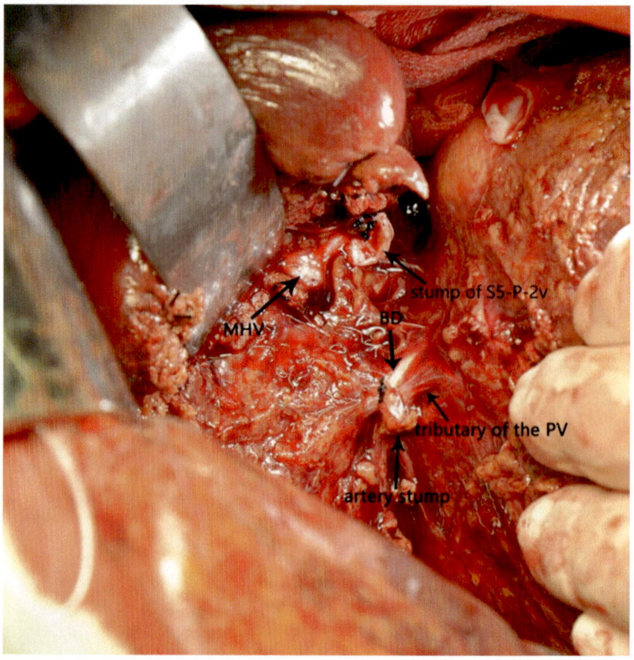

Fig. 345 The stump of the dorsal artery branch was shown. The remaining superior dorsal (S5-P-2d) pedicle [including the bile duct (BD) and a tributary of the portal vein (PV)] was clearly demonstrated. *MHV* middle hepatic vein, *S5-P-2v* the superior ventral pedicle of segment V

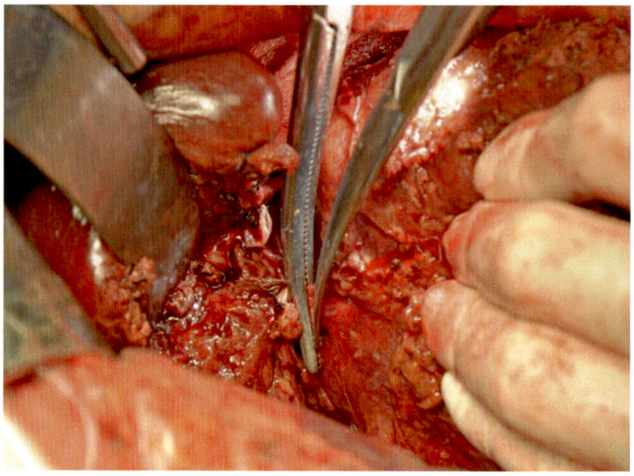

Fig. 346 The remaining superior dorsal pedicle of segment V (S5-P-2d) was clamped, divided, and silk-sutured

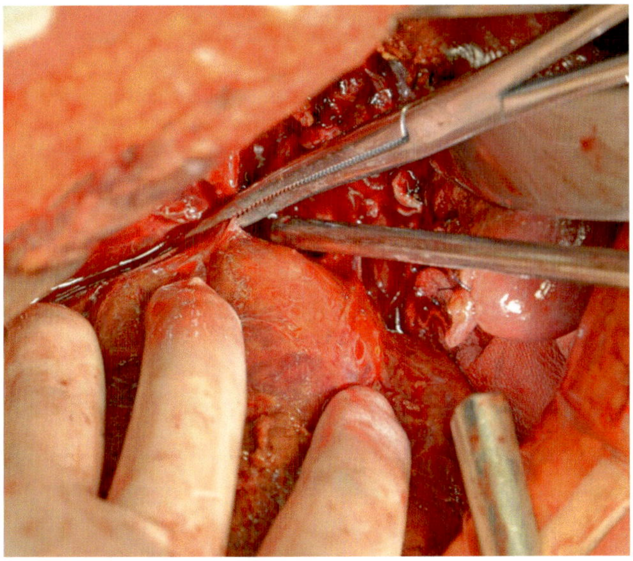

Fig. 347 The distal main trunk of the MHV was ascertained to enter into the tumor at this site parallel to the connecting area of 4A and 4B. The trunk of the MHV was clamped, divided, and silk-sutured. *MHV* middle hepatic vein

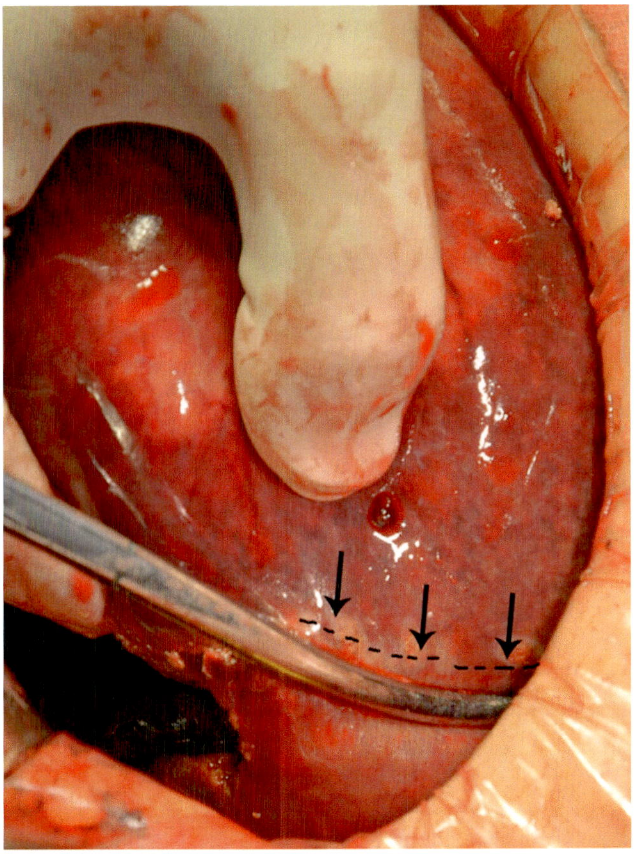

Fig. 348 Following the ischemic line, hepatic parenchymal transection was carried out between segment V and segment VI cranio-caudally

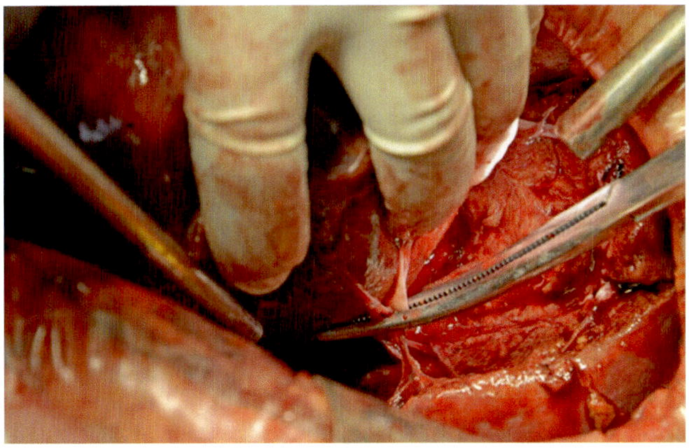

Fig. 349 Large venous branch of the RHV was clamped, divided, and ligated. *RHV* right hepatic vein

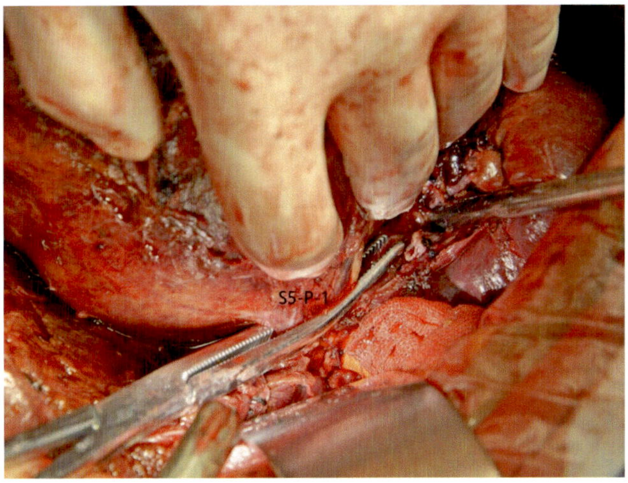

Fig. 350 At the end of hepatic parenchymal transection, the main pedicle of segment V (S5-P-1) was clamped and divided at its originating point

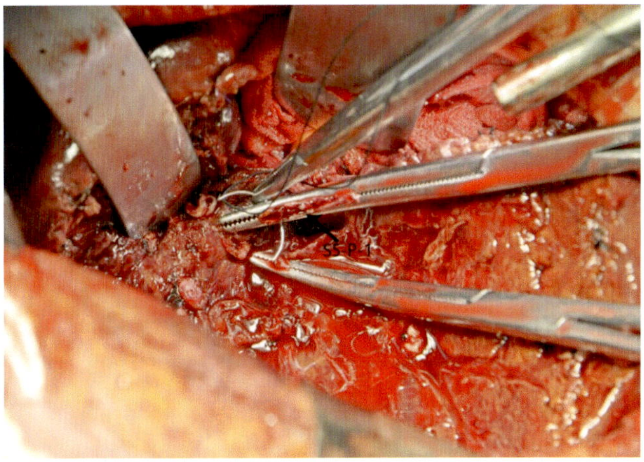

Fig. 351 Having removed the tumor, the proximal stump of the main pedicle of segment V (S5-P-1) was double silk-sutured

Hemostasis and Prevention of Bile Leak at the Cut Surface (Fig. 352)

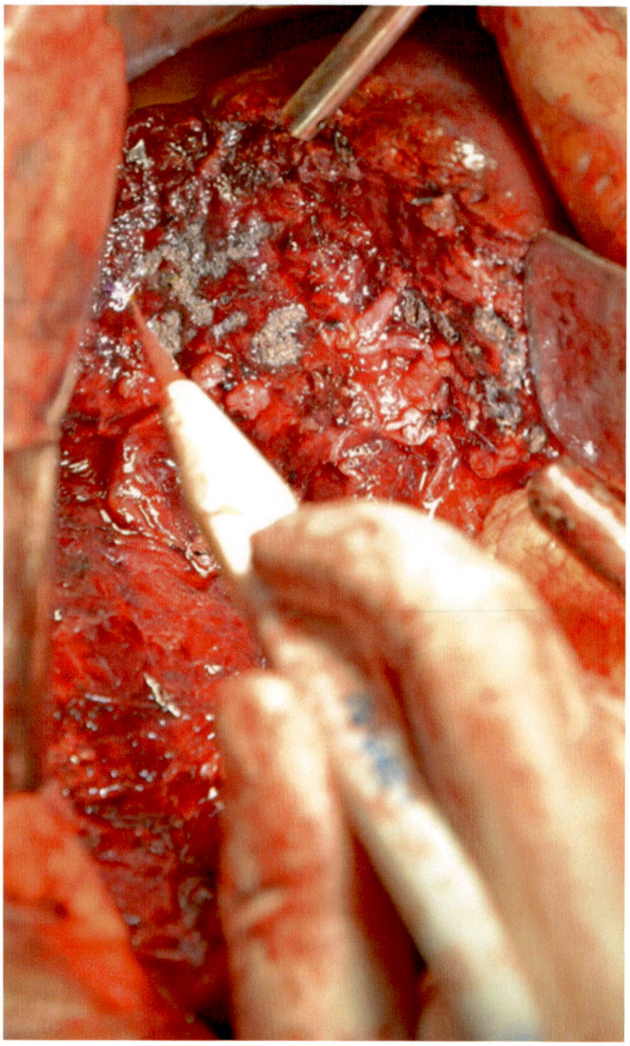

Fig. 352 The raw surface of the residual liver was electrocauterized to stop bleeding. Large stump of vascular structures were ligated or sutured. Tiny holes on the vascular structures were sutured with 4-0 and/or 5-0 polypropylene

Raw Area of the Residual Liver and the Specimen
(Figs. 353, 354, and 355)

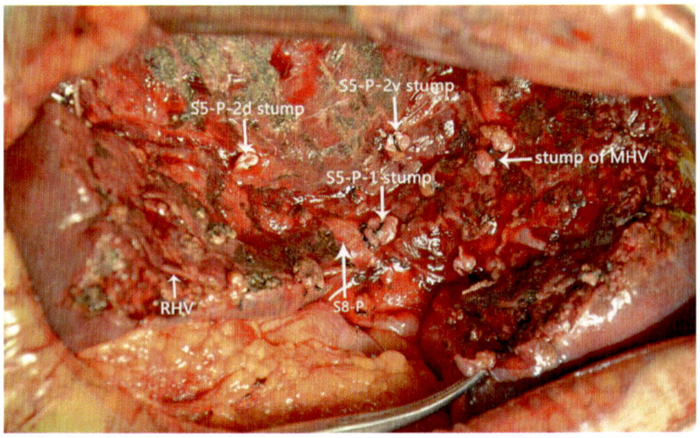

Fig. 353 Raw surface of the liver remnant. *RHV* right hepatic vein, *S5-P-2d stump* proximal stump of the superior dorsal pedicle of segment V, *S5-P-2v stump* proximal stump of the superior ventral pedicle of S5, *S5-P-1 stump* proximal stump of the main pedicle of segment V, *S8-P* pedicle of segment VIII, *MHV* middle hepatic vein

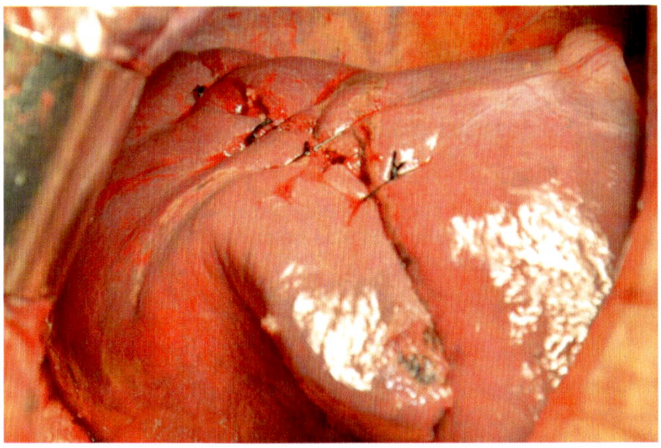

Fig. 354 Having managed the cut surface, the anterior edges of the segments VI and IV were sutured together. No abnormal color change was observed on the residual liver surface

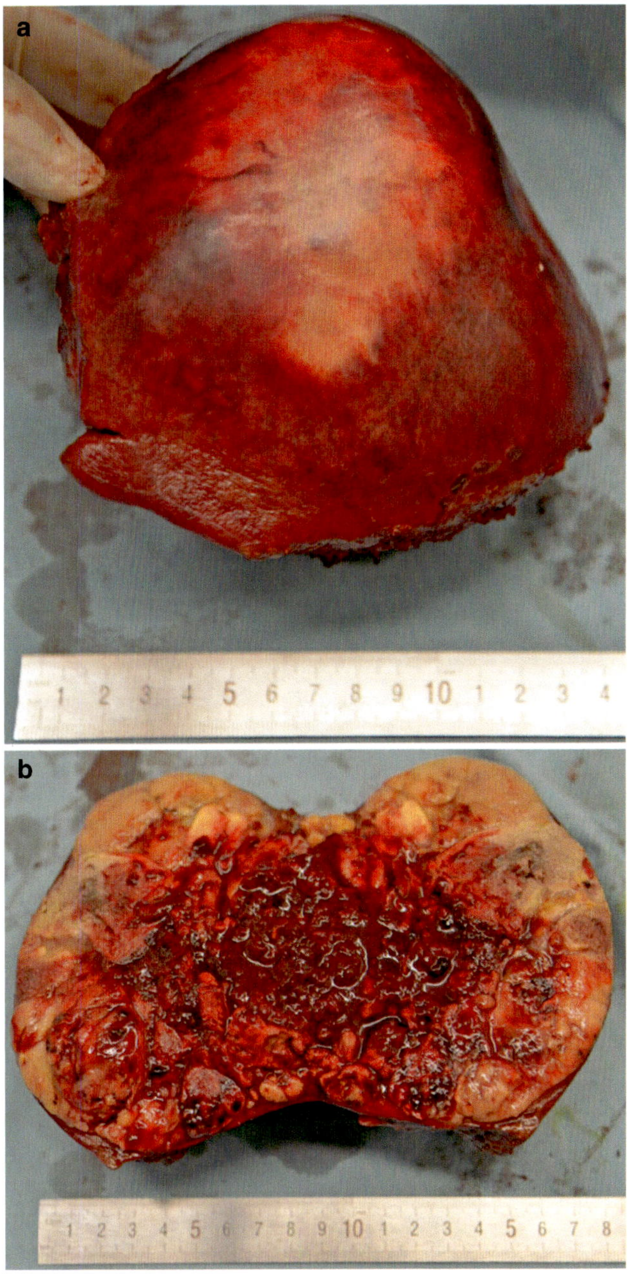

Fig. 355 (**a**) Anterior view of the specimen. (**b**) Middle cut-open plane of the specimen. The surgical margin was macroscopically negative

Segmentectomy VI

Jixiong Hu, Hongliang Yao, and Tenglong Tang

Couinaud's segments vary greatly in volume, and the watershed of each segment does not go after straight lines and varies broadly among persons [4, 60]. Single anatomical Couinaud's segment resection demands careful isolation of the inflow pedicle(s), and knowledge of common variations of the target segment is a critical prerequisite for safe segmentectomy with maximal parenchymal preservation, minimal blood loss, and oncological radicality [104, 112, 113, 115, 116, 126, 128]. The volume of segment VI accounted for 7.9% (range, 1.2–20.2%) of total liver volume (TLV) [4]. Branching types of the portal vein (P6) supplying segment VI include [4, 77] (1) bifurcation, P6 simply diverged from the trunk of the right posterior pedicle(56.1%); (2) direct bifurcation from the right portal vein, P6 diverged directly from the right portal vein (15.9%); and (3) bow-shaped, several P6 spread out into branches radially as "bow-shaped" (28.0%). Although great advancements in preoperative imaging technology have been made, single anatomical segmentectomy VI is still technically challenging in terms of anatomic variations.

Surgical Indications

The routine preoperative imaging workup included ultrasound and high-resolution helical computed tomography (CT) and MRI. For patients with HCCs confined to segment VI, systematic segmentectomy VI was preferred over non-anatomic resection (wedge resection or enucleation). Right posterior sectionectomy (RPS) or right hepatectomy was selected when the HCCs infiltrated the right posterior pedicle and the right hepatic main Glissonean pedicle [129], respectively. With respect to the evaluation to the liver function, the classification of Child-Pugh and the indocyanine green retention at 15 min (ICGR15) was used. Anatomical segmentectomy VI can be considered when the ICGR15 must be less than 30% and Child-Pugh classification is grade A.

Operative Procedures	Technical Details
Laparotomy ↓	◀ A right subcostal incision was made and an automobile retractor was used.
Isolation and looping of the pedicle of S6 ↓	◀ The right hepatic Glissonean pedicle, the right posterior sectional Glissonean pedicle and the pedicle of S6 and S7 was isolated and encircled with a vascular tape,successively.
Colorization of S6 ↓	◀ Methylene blue was injected into the pedicle of S6. Then, the pedicle of S6 was divided and suture-ligated. Color change appeared on the liver surface. According to the color change and ischemic demarcation line, the cut line was marked on the liver surface with electrocautery.
Hepatic parenchymal transection ↓	◀ Having clamped the right hepatic pedicle, parenchymal transection was undertaken using the clamp-crushing and/or finger fracture method. Having removed the specimen, the distal main trunk of the right hepatic vein (RHV) was exposed on the raw surface of the residual liver.
Drainage and closure of the abdominal cavity	◀ A drain close to the liver cut surface was used.

Intraoperative Key Points

1. The right posterior Glissonean pedicle is the most deeply placed of the right pedicles [130]. While dissecting the right posterior pedicle, attention should be paid to prevent injury to the portal pedicle(s) starting from the right main hepatic pedicle and entering into the caudate process. Further dissection is required to access to the bifurcation of the right posterior pedicle (RPP). The RPP was dissected on its anterior, superior, and inferior surface for about 1–3 cm, where it was possible to ascertain the starting point of the pedicle of segment VI and segment VII. Having isolated and looped the pedicle of segment VI, test clamping this pedicle should be attempted to ascertain this pedicle supplying the target segment and, by observing the color change on this segment surface, to determine if there is(are) another(other) pedicle(s) of segment VI, which is(are) deeply located within hepatic parenchyma, just as shown in this chapter. In addition, in order to determine if there is additional pedicle(s) of the target segment, this segment can be stained by injecting methylene blue into the already looped pedicle. Theoretically, the whole surface of segment VI should be stained blue if there is only one pedicle. When just a part of this segment surface is stained blue, it is certain that there is additional pedicle. To perform anatomical segmentectomy, this additional pedicle should also be isolated and divided from its starting point during hepatic parenchyma transectional proceedings.
2. In this segmentectomy VI, we found an anatomical anomaly, which is a pedicle originating from S7-P and supplying the superior portion of segment VI. In this operation, when the pedicle of segment VII was temporarily clamped, the superior-posterior portion of segment VI was devascularized (Fig. 381), and meanwhile, after methylene blue was injected into the pedicle of segment VI, only the superior-posterior portion was unstained (Fig. 384). Moreover, a pedicle (containing branches of artery, bile duct, and portal vein) (Fig. 392) was encountered, divided, and suture-ligated during transecting parenchyma between segment VI and segment VII. The abovementioned three facts prove that this anatomical variation truly exists. To the present author's knowledge, no report has described this variation. In this chapter, we have described three portal pedicles supplying segment VI, Mise et al. demonstrated that no portal pedicle diverged from the trunk of the pedicle of segment VII and supplied segment VI [4]. This anatomical variation once more proves that the intersegmental borders provided by preoperative imaging can only be partially referred to during hepatic parenchymal transection and that liver anatomy can be quite variable and each anatomical hepatic resection may have pitfalls about which any hepatobiliary surgeon should be kept in mind [27].
3. Having divided the pedicle of segment VI and clamped the right hepatic pedicle, parenchymal transection was carried out caudo-cranially. At the beginning of hepatic parenchymal transection, it is very important to trace the distal trunk of the right hepatic vein (RHV). After having identified the right hepatic vein, using it as a guide, the parenchymal transection was continued caudo-cranially and ventrodorsally (Fig. 356).

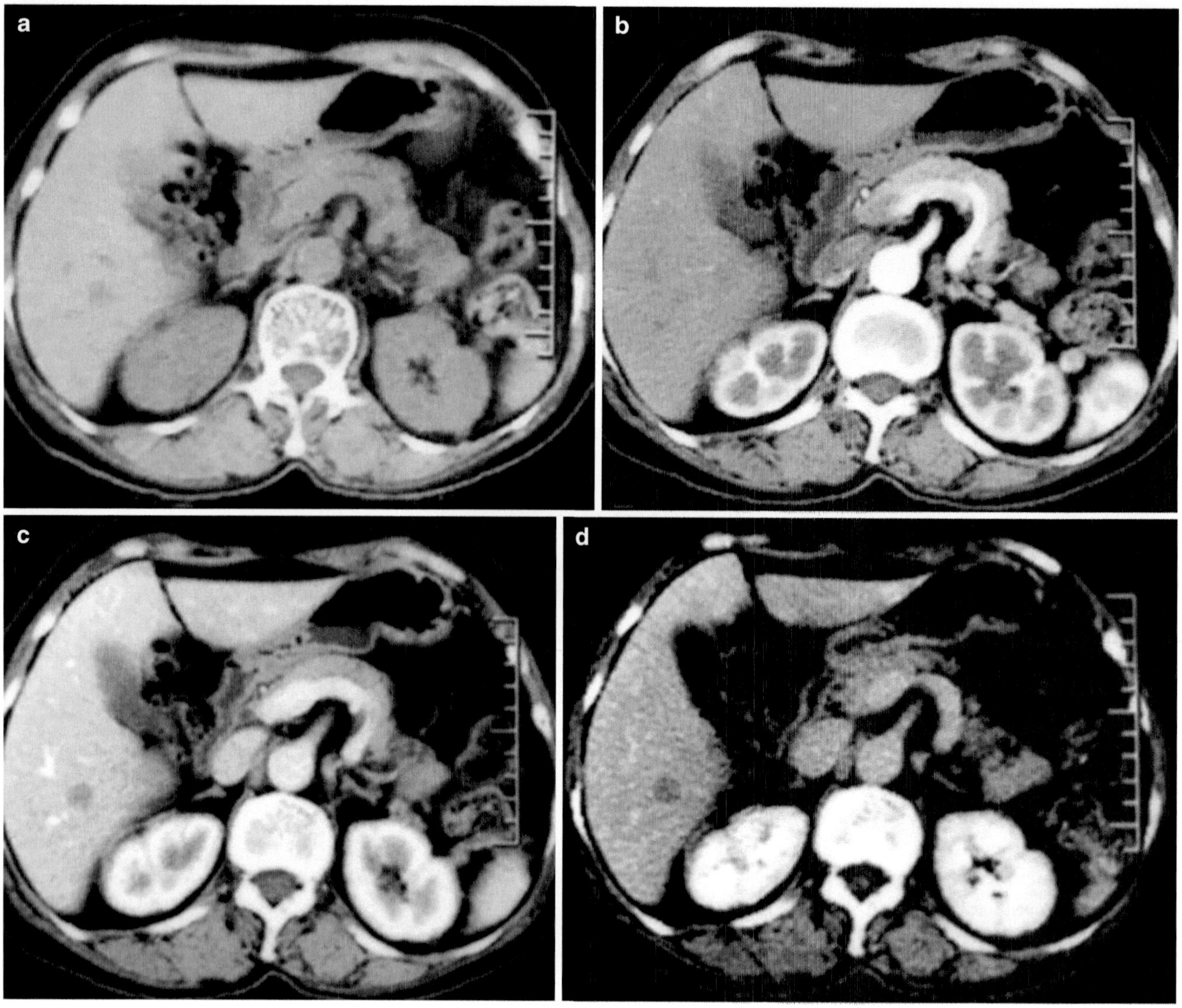

Fig. 356 (**a**) Preoperative CT (precontrast). The tumor, which appears mildly hypodense, is located in segment VI. (**b**) Preoperative CT (hepatic arterial phase). The tumor shows mild enhancement. (**c**) Preoperative CT (hepatic venous phase). The tumor shows enhancement fades. (**d**) Preoperative CT (interstitial phase). The tumor shows washout

Abdominal Incision and Mobilization of the Right Hemiliver (Figs. 357, 358, 359, 360, 361, 362, 363, and 364)

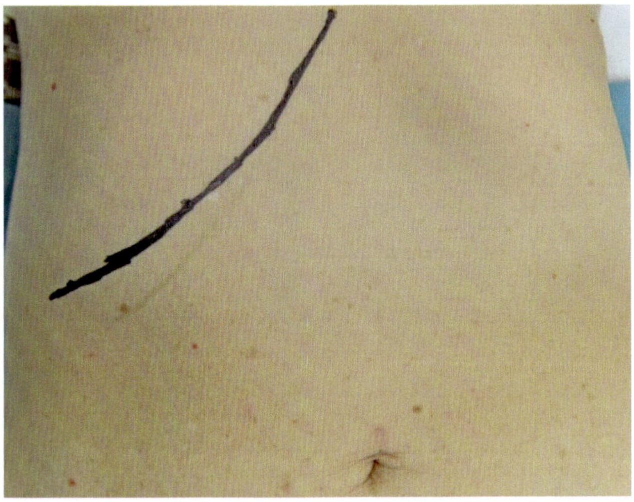

Fig. 357 A right subcostal incision was selected

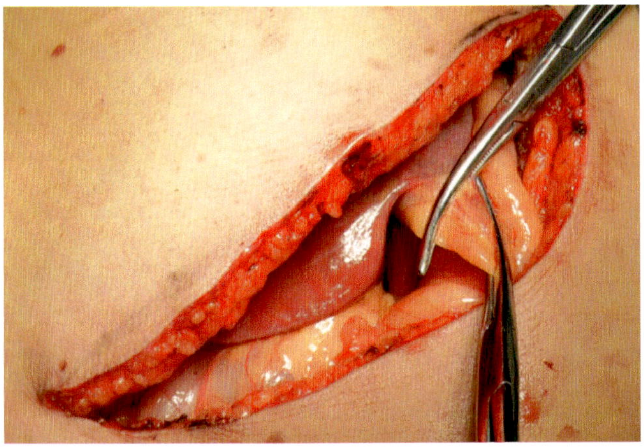

Fig. 358 Having entered into the abdominal cavity, the round ligament was divided and ligated

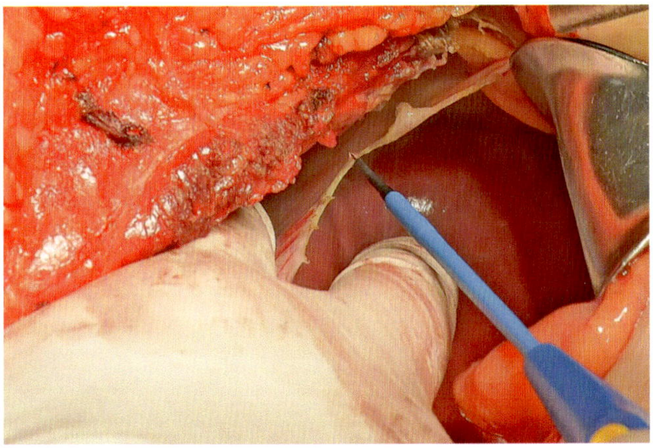

Fig. 359 The falciform ligament was electrocauterized

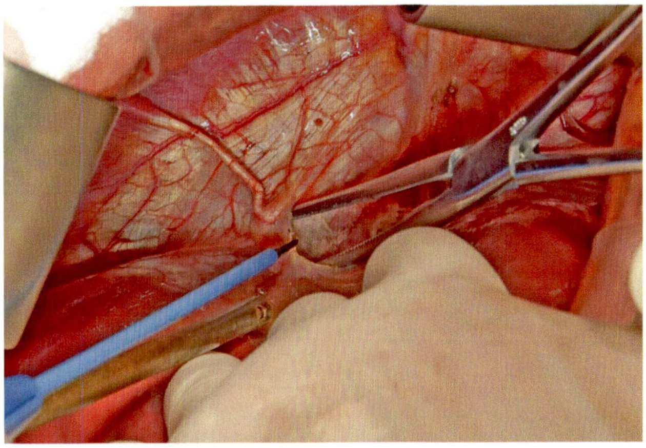

Fig. 360 The right coronary ligament was divided with electrocautery

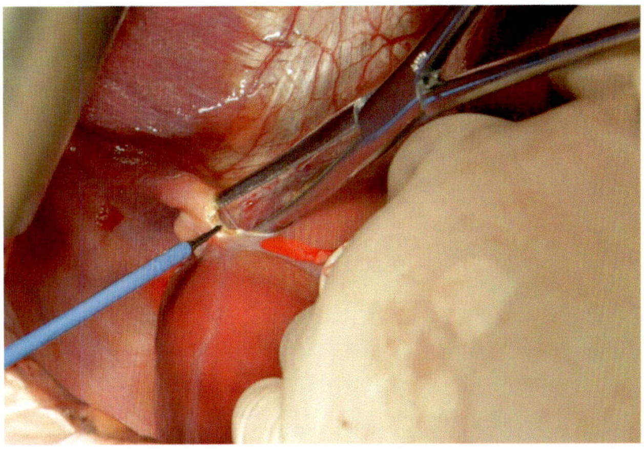

Fig. 361 The right triangular ligament was dissected

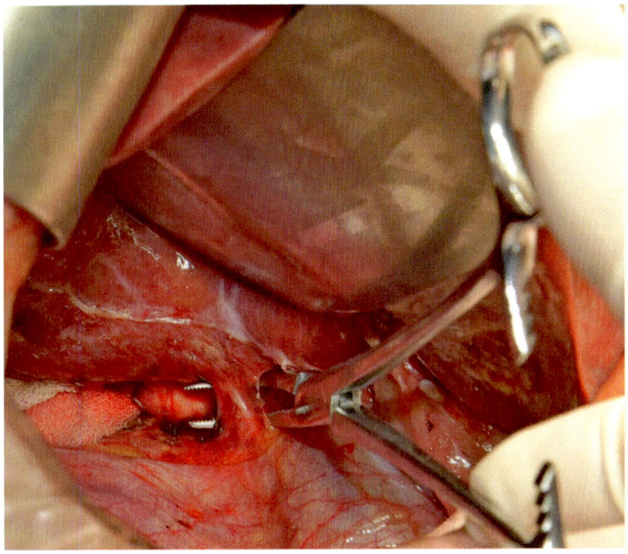

Fig. 362 The inferior right hepatic vein (IRHV) was isolated, divided, and ligated

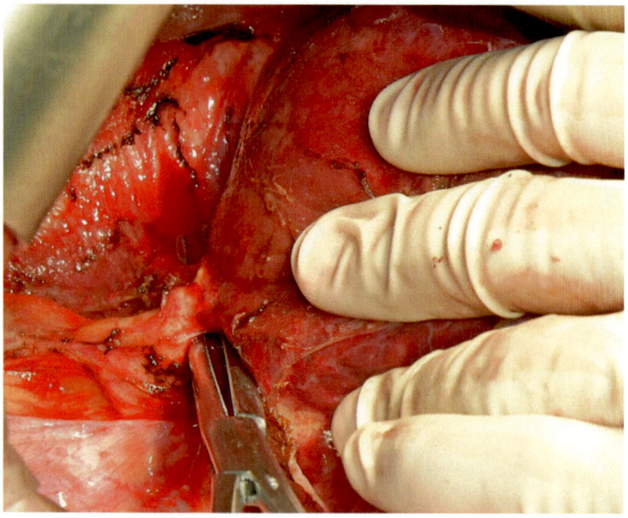

Fig. 363 The right adrenal gland was dissected away from the liver

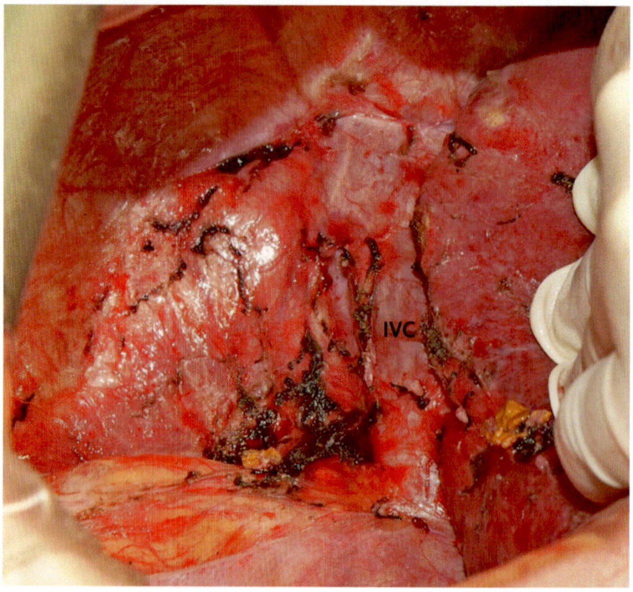

Fig. 364 The right hemiliver has been fully mobilized from its surrounding structures, and the retrohepatic inferior vena cava (IVC) was exposed

Isolation of the Right Hepatic Pedicle (RHP)
(Figs. 365, 366, 367, 368, and 369)

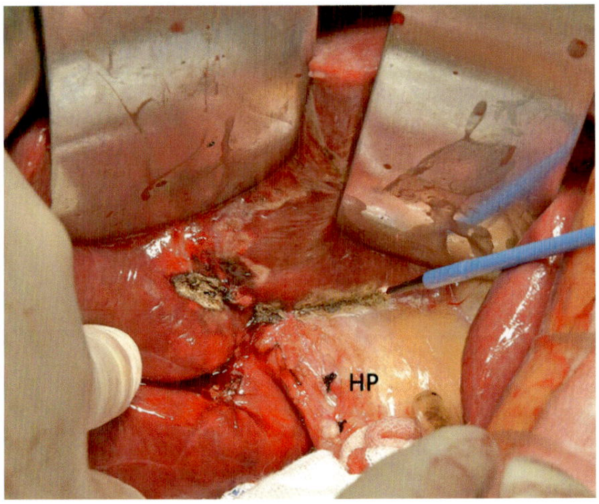

Fig. 365 Having performed cholecystectomy, one small traverse incision was made in front of the hilus. *HP* hepatic pedicle

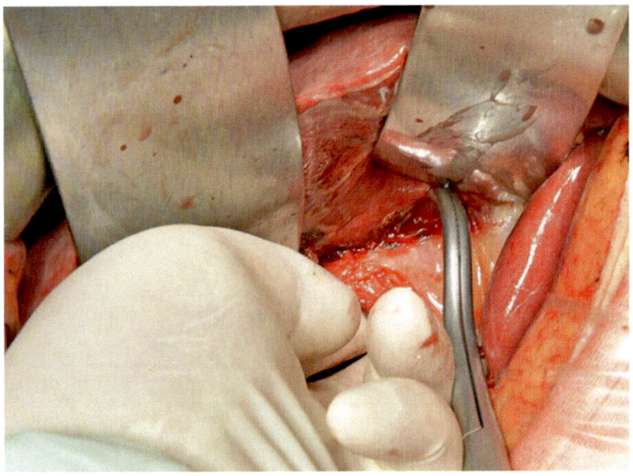

Fig. 367 The operator's left index finger was placed between the undersurface of the hilar plate and the anterior wall of the retrohepatic inferior vena cava (IVC), and then, a large curved clamp was inserted vertically into this incision and directly reached down to the tip of the index finger

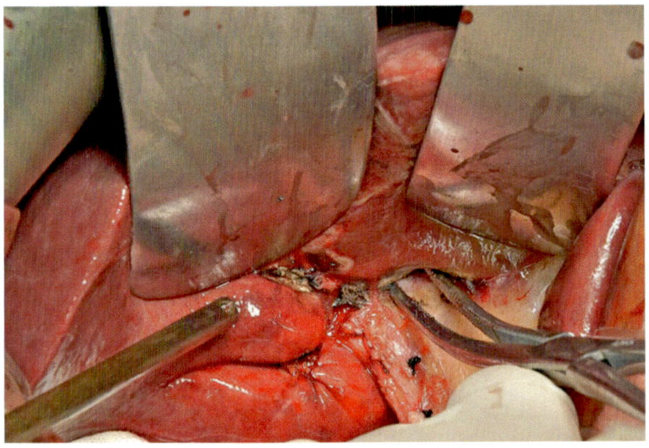

Fig. 366 Using a large curved clamp, hepatic parenchyma above this incision was pushed upward, and the hilar plate was pulled down to expose the anterior and superior surface of the right hepatic pedicle (RHP)

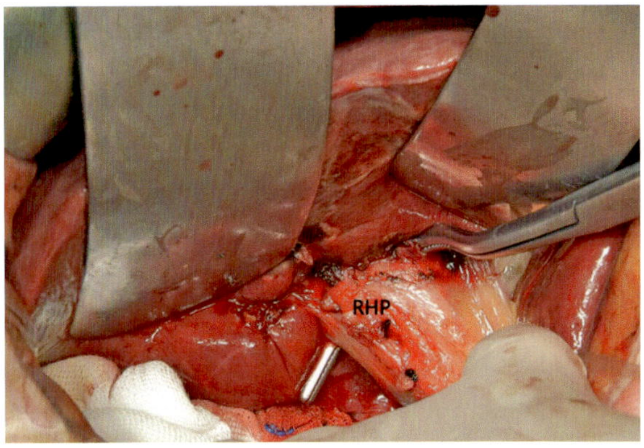

Fig. 368 Using the index finger as a guide, the large curved clamp was inserted furtherly to puncture the undersurface membrane of the hilar plate and passed out of the posterior and inferior edge of the right hepatic pedicle (RHP)

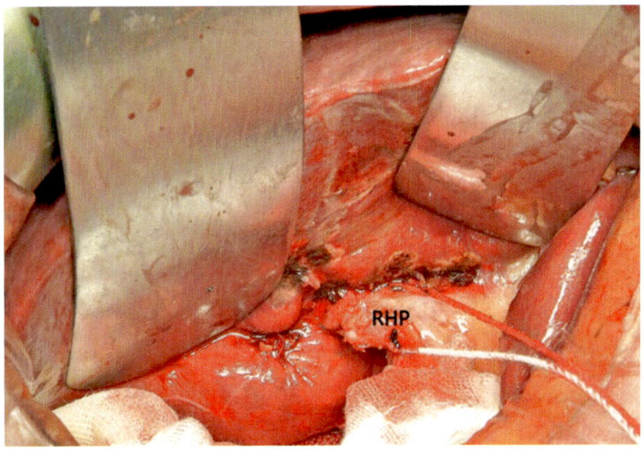

Fig. 369 Then, the right hepatic pedicle (RHP) was isolated, and a loop was encircled with it

Isolation of the Right Posterior Pedicle (RPP)
(Figs. 370, 371, 372, 373, and 374)

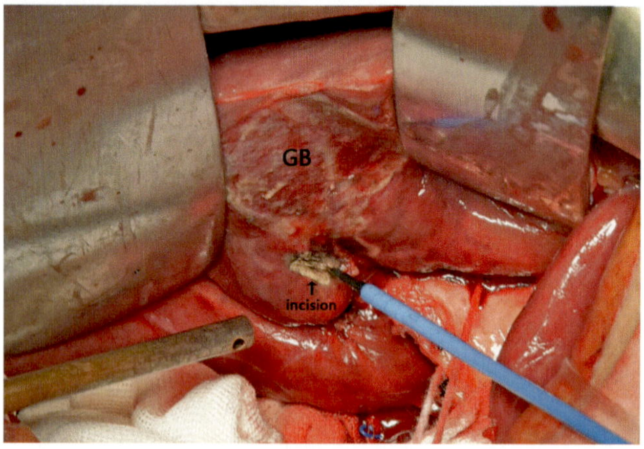

Fig. 370 Another small incision was made on the right edge of the base area of the gallbladder bed (GB), and this incision was extended using a large curved clamp

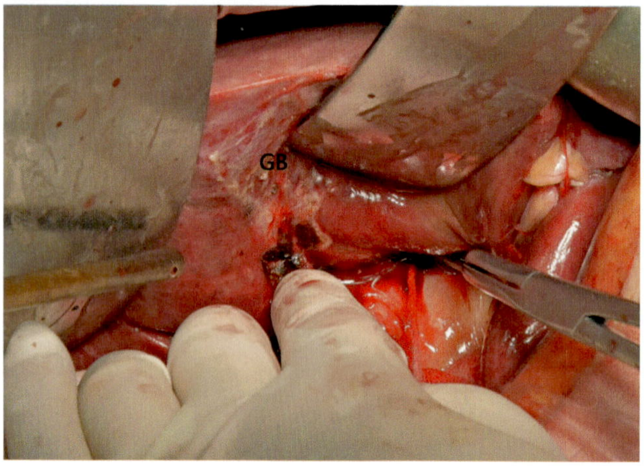

Fig. 371 A large curved clamp was inserted into this incision in front of the hilus, and the operator's index finger was covered over the second incision beside the right edge of the gallbladder bed (GB)

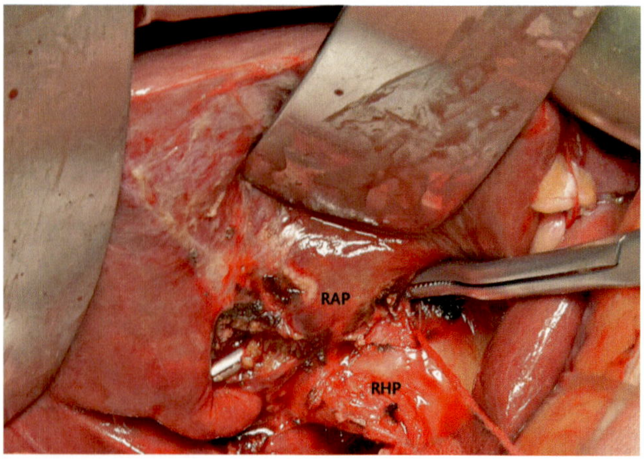

Fig. 372 Using the index finger as a guide, the clamp was passed behind the right anterior pedicle (RAP) and punched out of the second incision. Thus, the RAP was isolated. *RHP* right hepatic pedicle

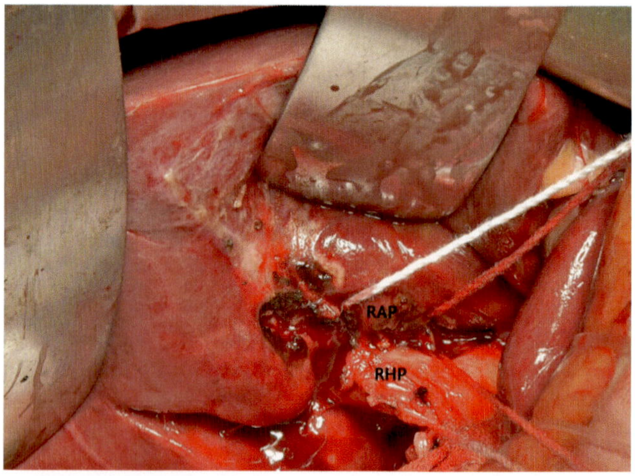

Fig. 373 The right anterior pedicle (RAP) was looped with a tourniquet. *RHP* right hepatic pedicle

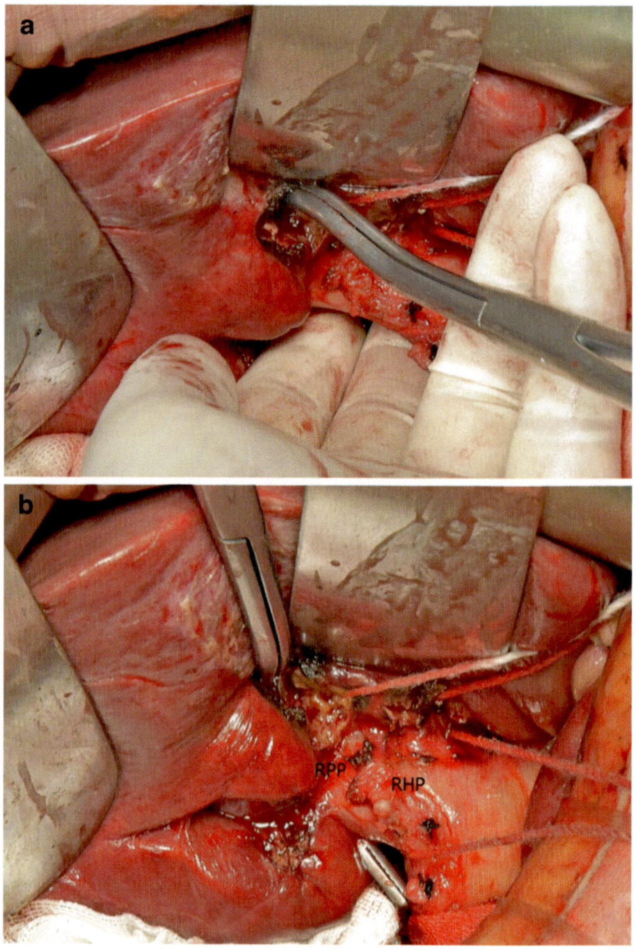

Fig. 374 (**a**, **b**) A large curved clamp was inserted into the incision at the right edge of the gallbladder, and meanwhile, the operator's left index finger was placed below the undersurface of the right hepatic pedicle; using the finger as a guide, the clamp was inserted downward and directly reached down to the fingertip and passed out of the right edge of the right hepatic pedicle. Thus, the right posterior pedicle (RPP) was isolated and encircled with a tourniquet

Isolation of the Pedicle of Segment VI and Segment VII (Figs. 375, 376, 377, 378, 379, 380, 381, and 382)

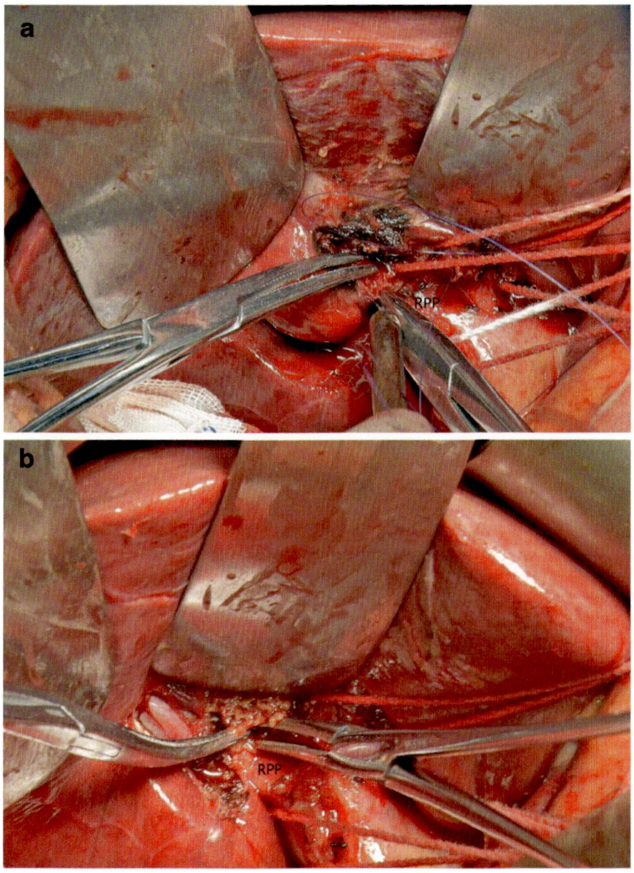

Fig. 375 (**a**, **b**) Dissection was carried out along the superior, anterior, and inferior surface of the right posterior pedicle (RPP)

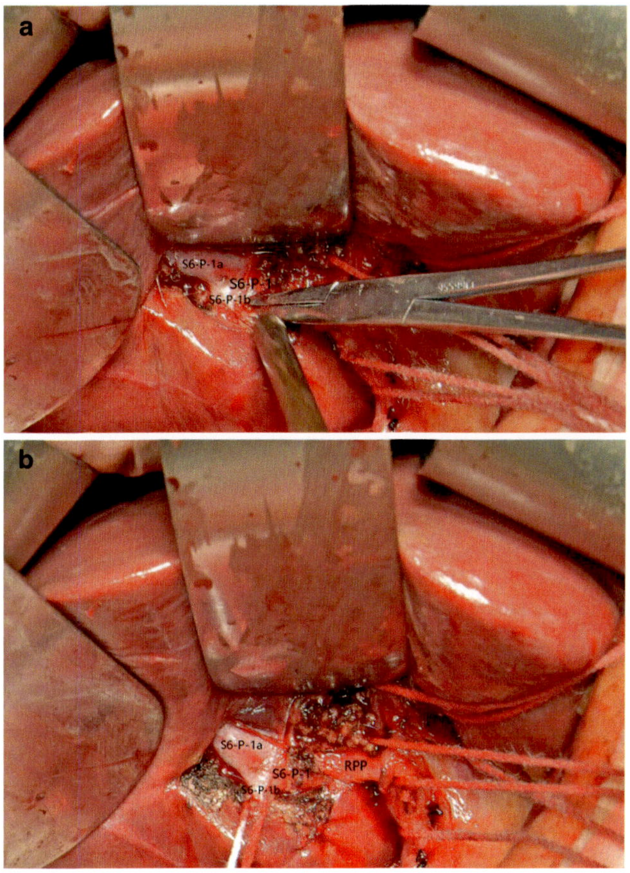

Fig. 376 (**a**, **b**) The pedicle of segment VI (S6-P-1) bifurcated into two pedicles (S6-P-1a and S6-P-1b)

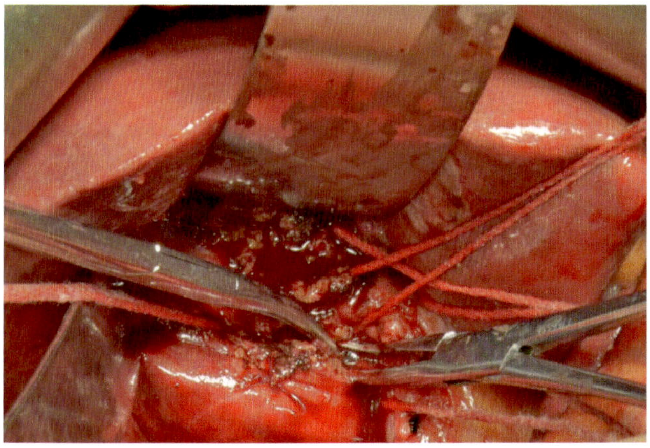

Fig. 377 Hepatic parenchyma around the start portion of the pedicle of segment VII was dissected in order to clearly expose the pedicle of segment VII

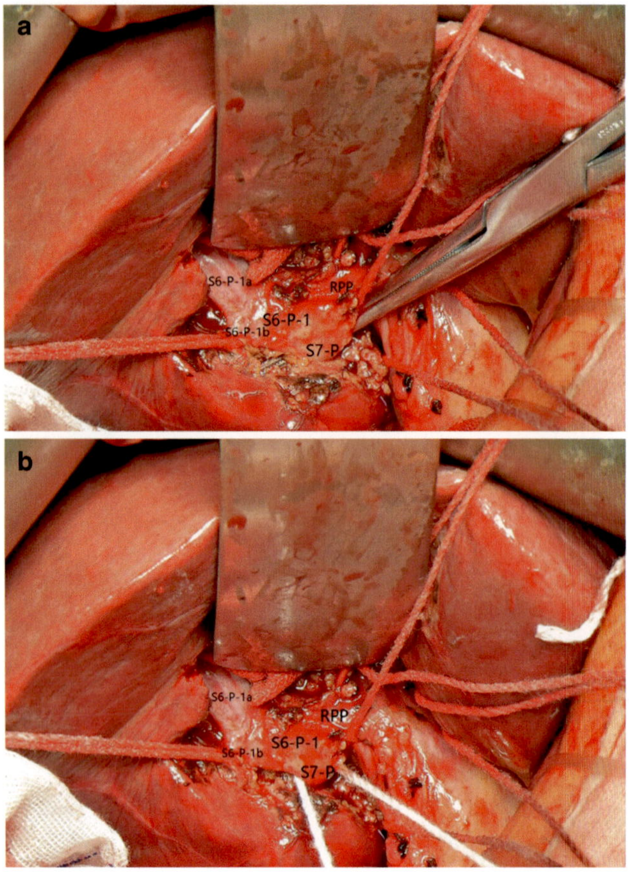

Fig. 378 (**a**, **b**) The pedicle of segment VII (S7-P) was isolated and looped with a vascular tape. *RPP* right posterior pedicle, *S6-P-1* the pedicle of segment VI, *S6-P-1a and S6-P-1b* two branches of S6-P-1

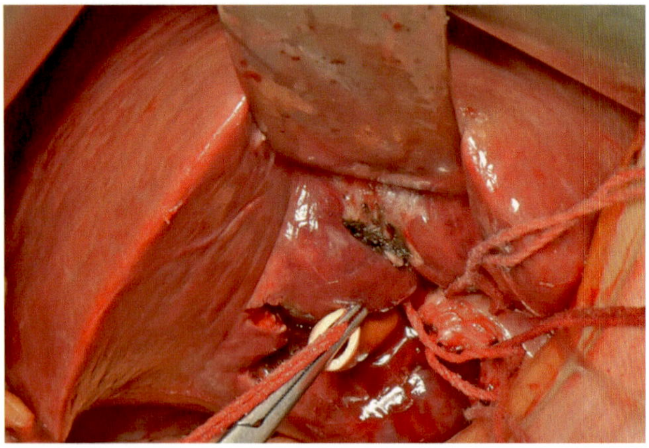

Fig. 379 The pedicle of segment VII was temporarily clamped

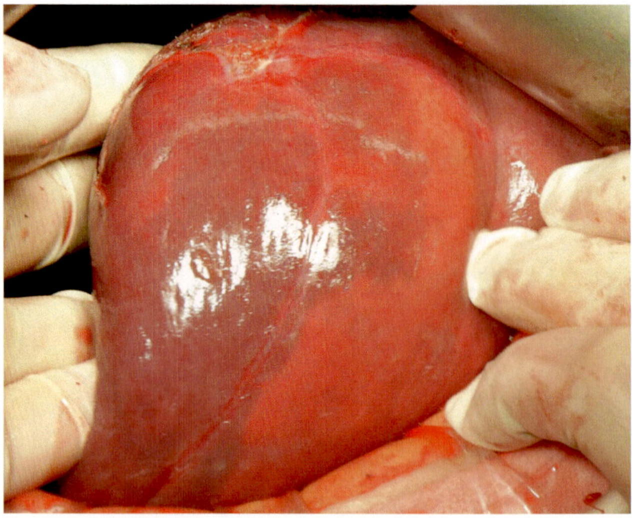

Fig. 380 The surface of segment VII showed ischemic change on the liver surface

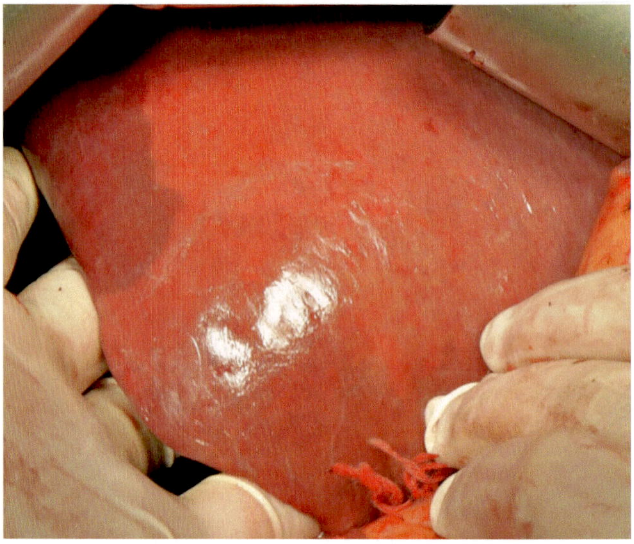

Fig. 381 The superior and posterior portion of segment VI was also under ischemic condition. This phenomenon suggested that the superior and posterior portion of segment VI was supplied by branches from segment VII pedicle

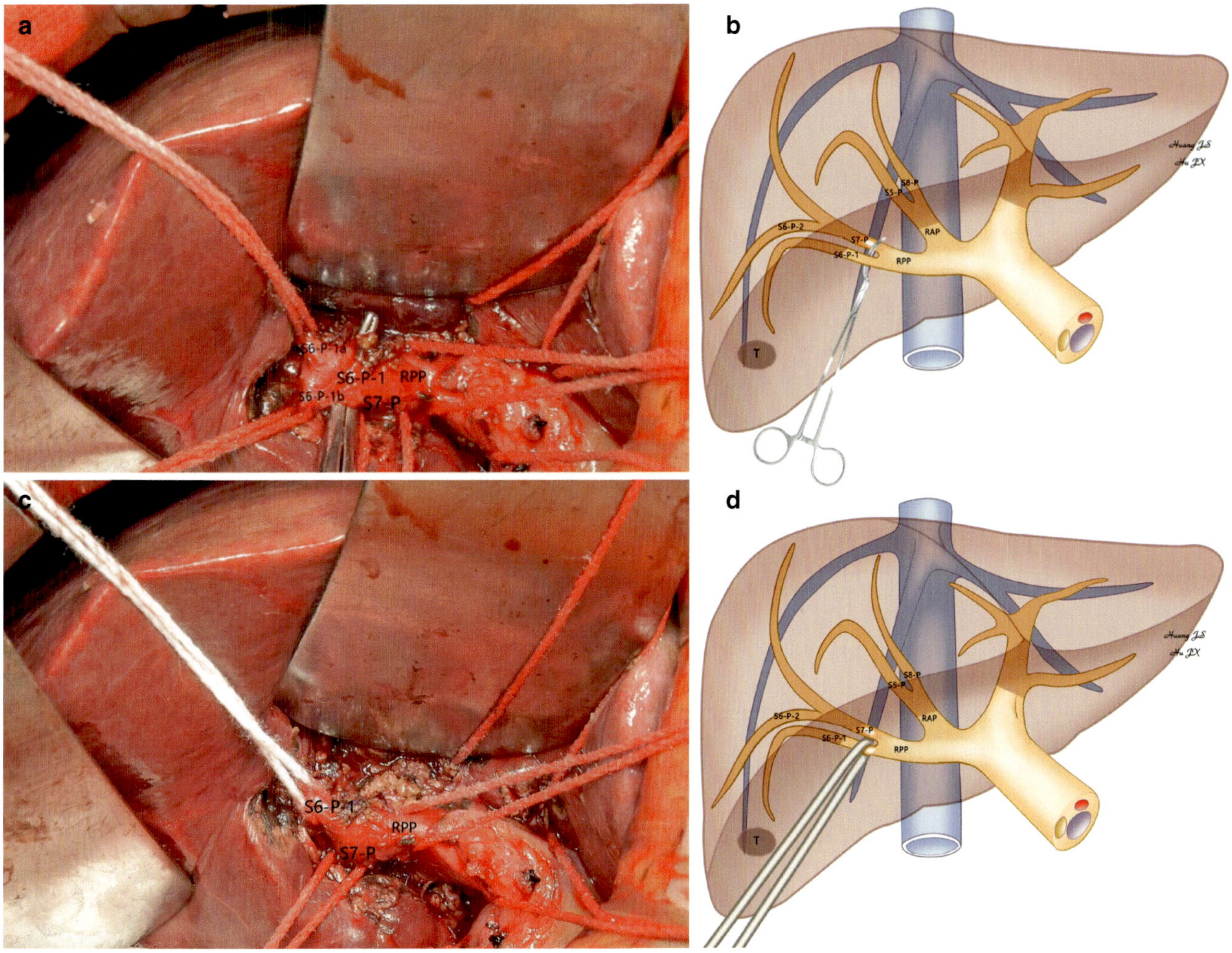

Fig. 382 (**a**, **c**) The S6-P-1 was isolated (**a**) and looped with a tourniquet (**c**). (**b**, **d**) Schematic illustration of this procedure. *RAP* right anterior pedicle, *RPP* right posterior pedicle, *S6-P-1* the pedicle of segment VI, *S6-P-1a and S6-P-1b* two branches of S6-P-1, *S7-P* pedicle of segment VII, *S5-P* pedicle of segment V, *S8-P* pedicle of segment VIII

Staining the Segments VI and Marking the Cut Line (Figs. 383, 384, 385, 386, and 387)

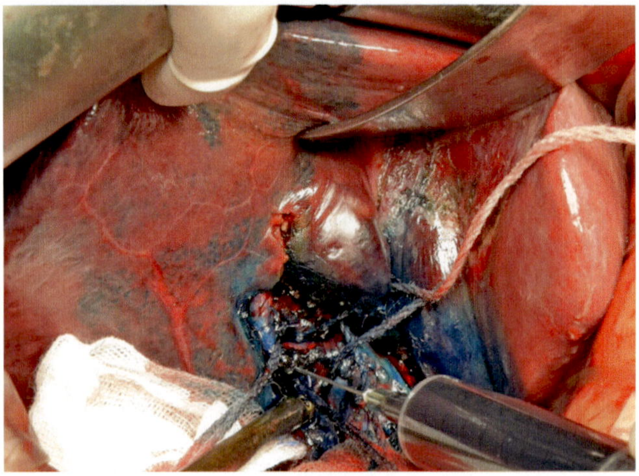

Fig. 383 Methylene blue was injected into S6-P-1. *S6-P-1* the pedicle of segment VI

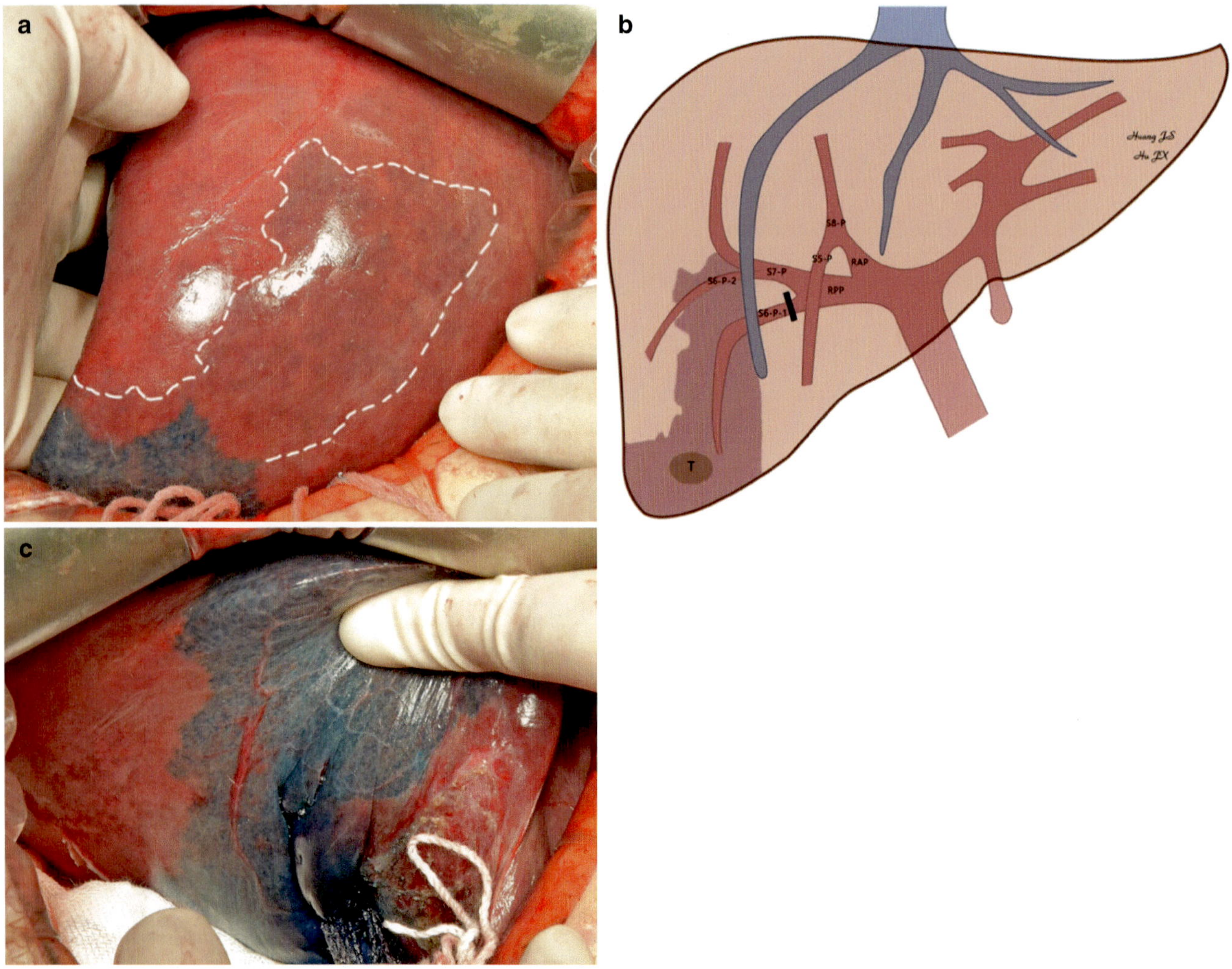

Fig. 384 (**a–c**) The superior and posterior portion of segment VI was unstained. This phenomenon was in accordance with Fig. 381

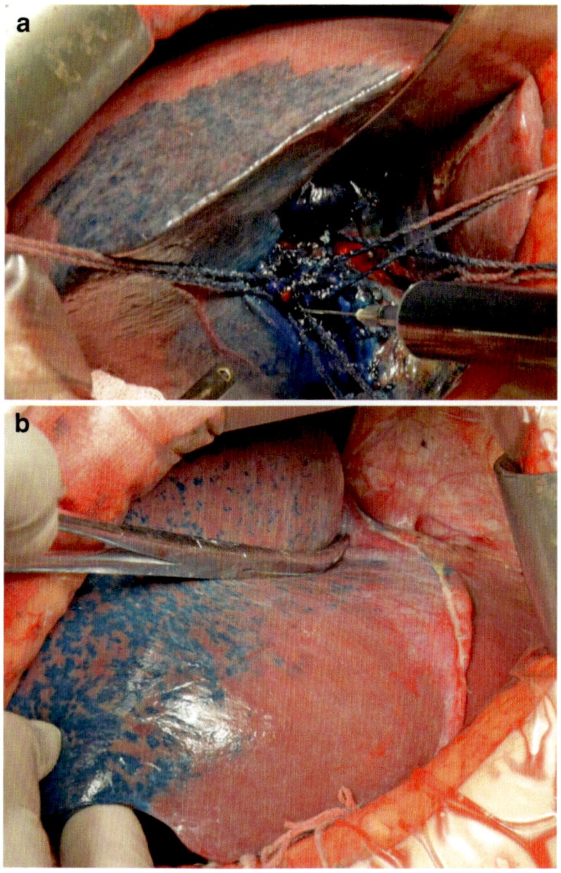

Fig. 385 (**a**, **b**) To counterstain segment VII, methylene blue was injected into the S7-P. Unfortunately, methylene blue back flowed to the right portal vein, and the right hemiliver was wholly stained. *S7-P* pedicle of segment VII

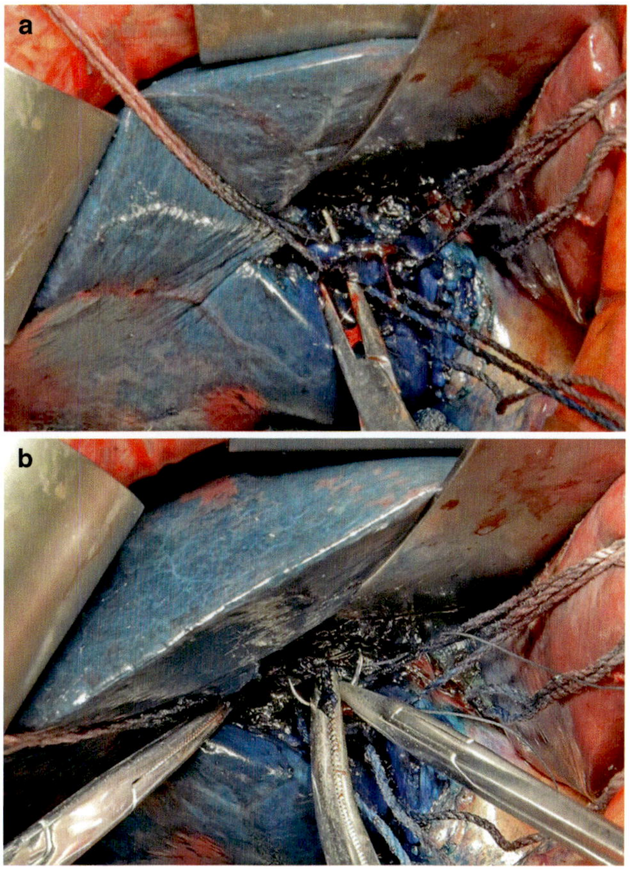

Fig. 386 (**a**, **b**) The pedicle of segment VI (S6-P-1) was divided and suture-ligated prior to hepatic parenchyma transection

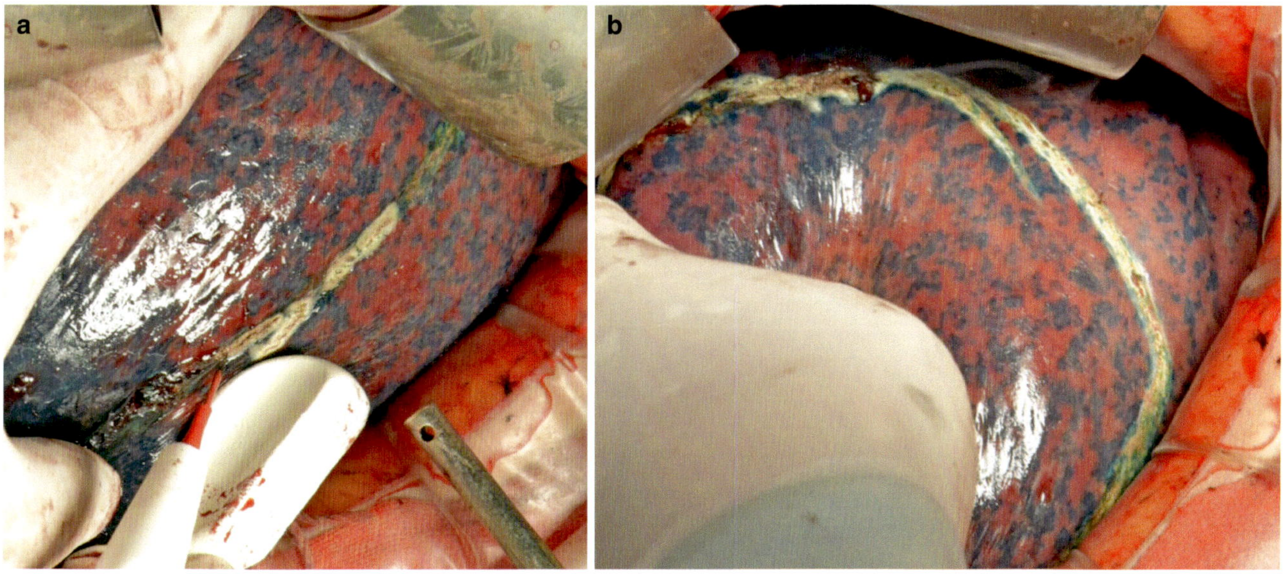

Fig. 387 (**a**, **b**) Because of unfortunate staining of the whole right hemiliver, the boundary of segment VI (caused by ischemia and staining) disappeared on the liver surface. IOUS was used to ascertain the course of the lower portion of the right hepatic vein (RHV), and the parenchymal transectional line between S5 and S6 was marked with electrocautery according to the RHV course. The superior transectional line between S6 and S7 corresponded to transverse plane through the liver hilum

Hepatic Parenchymal Transection
(Figs. 388, 389, 390, 391, and 392)

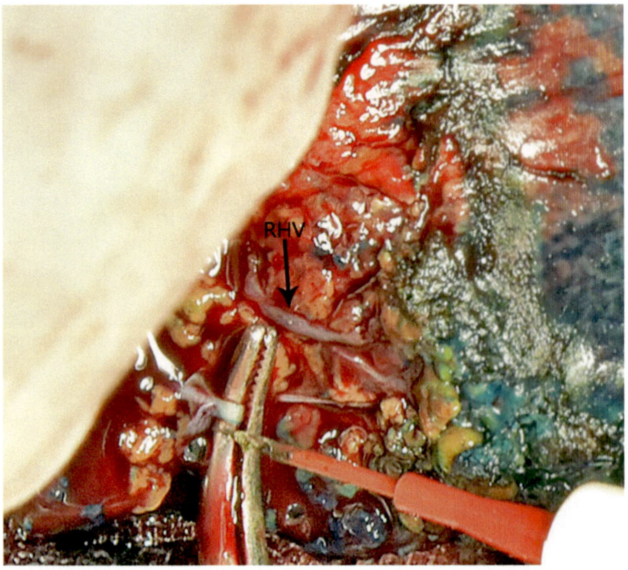

Fig. 388 Having clamped the right hepatic pedicle, hepatic parenchymal transection was initially performed between S5 and S6 caudo-cranially, using a clamp-crushing method. Attention should be paid to preserve the terminal portion of the right hepatic vein (RHV)

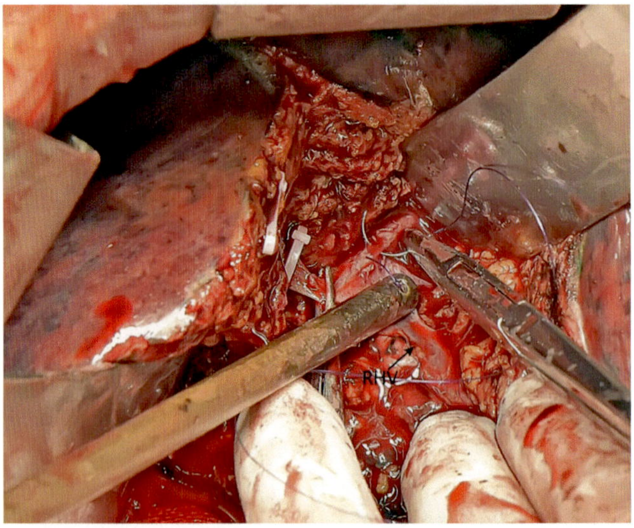

Fig. 390 A hole on the wall of the right hepatic vein (RHV) was repaired with 5-0 polypropylene

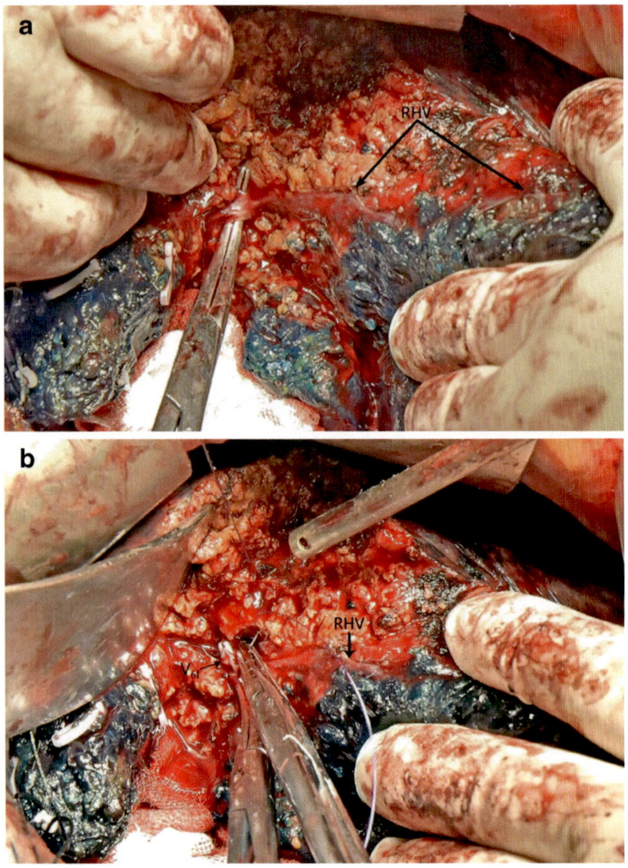

Fig. 389 (**a**, **b**) A large branch of the right hepatic vein (RHV) draining inferior portion of segment VI (V_{6I}) was isolated, divided, and ligated

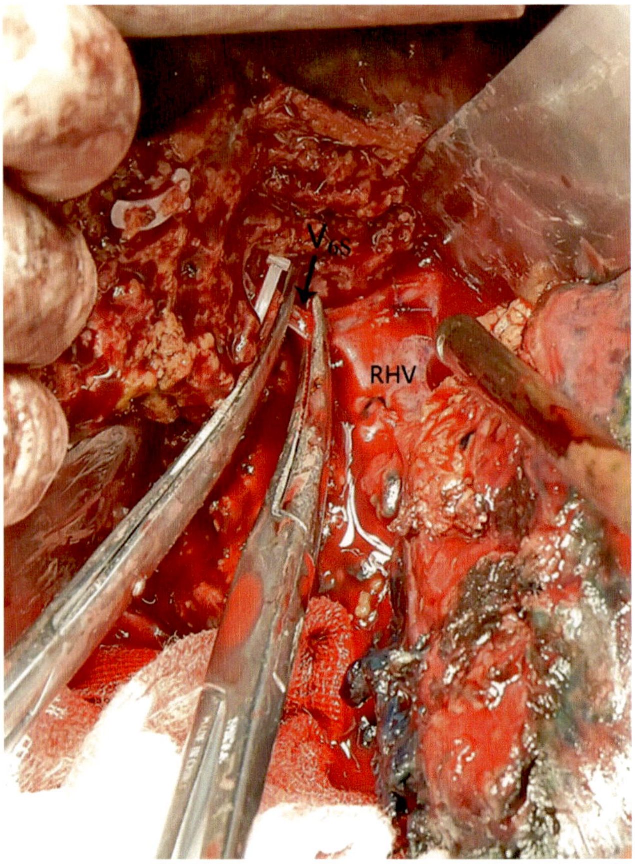

Fig. 391 Another large branch of the RHV draining superior portion of segment VI (V_{6S}) was also isolated, divided, and ligated. *RHV* right hepatic vein

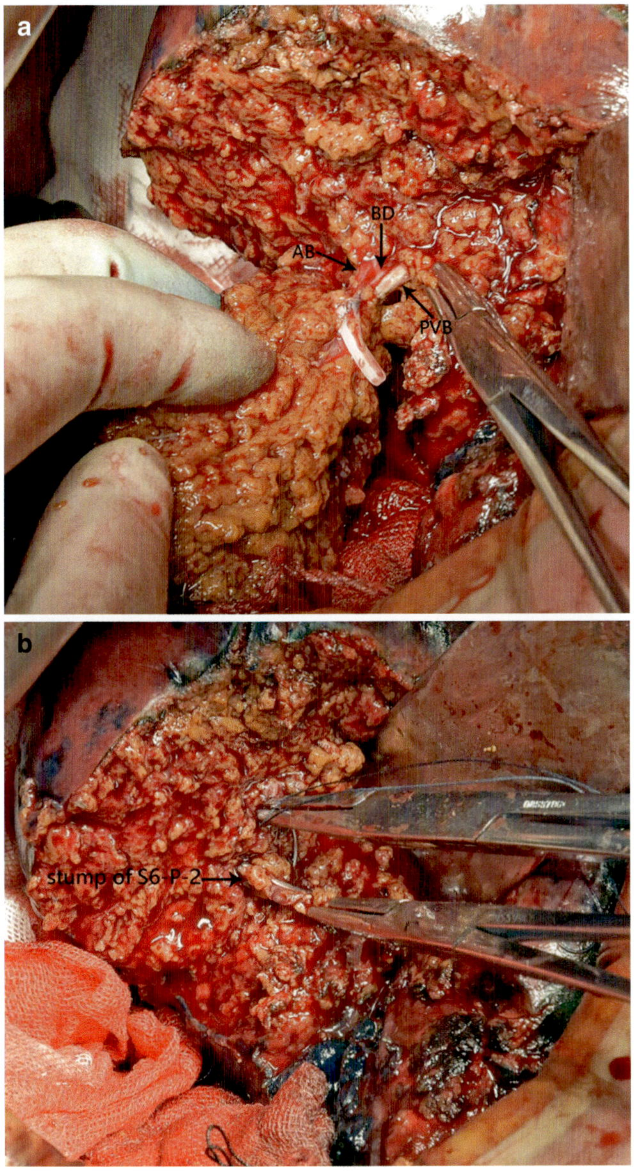

Fig. 392 (**a**, **b**) The second portal pedicle (S6-P-2) originating from the pedicle of S7 before S7-P entering into S7 parenchyma and supplying the superior and posterior portion of S6 was clamped, divided, and suture-ligated. This was in agreement with Figs. 381 and 384 in this chapter. *AB* artery branch, *BD* bile duct, *PVB* portal vein branch

Raw Area of the Residue Liver and the Specimen
(Figs. 393, 394, and 395)

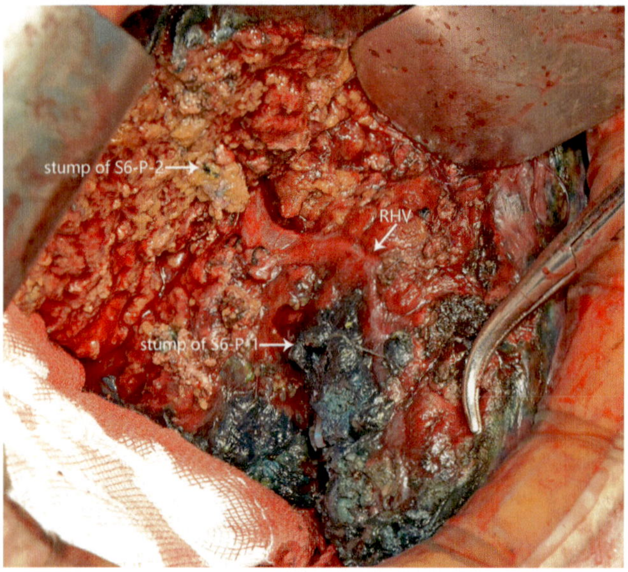

Fig. 393 Having removed the specimen and unclamped the right hepatic pedicle, the lower part of the right hepatic vein (RHV) was shown on the cut surface. The vascular and biliary ramifications on the cut surface of the residual liver were sutured with silk thread and/or polypropylene 1-0 and/or 2-0, and the tiny holes on the RHV were repaired with 4-0 and 5-0 polypropylene. *S6-P-2* the second portal pedicle originating from the start portion of the pedicle of S7 and supplying the superior and posterior portion of S6, *S6-P-1* pedicle of segment VI

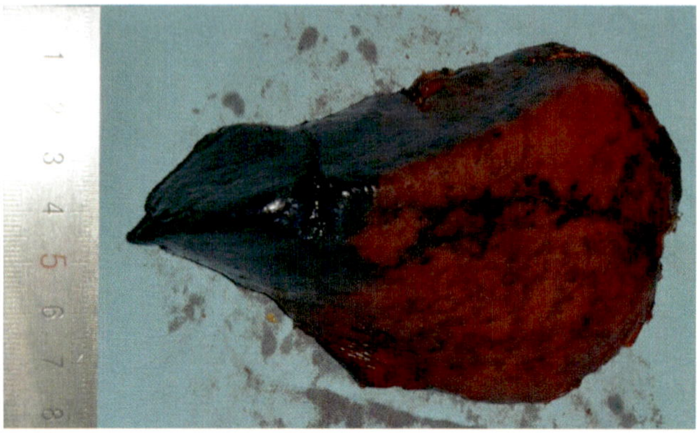

Fig. 394 Anterior surface of the specimen

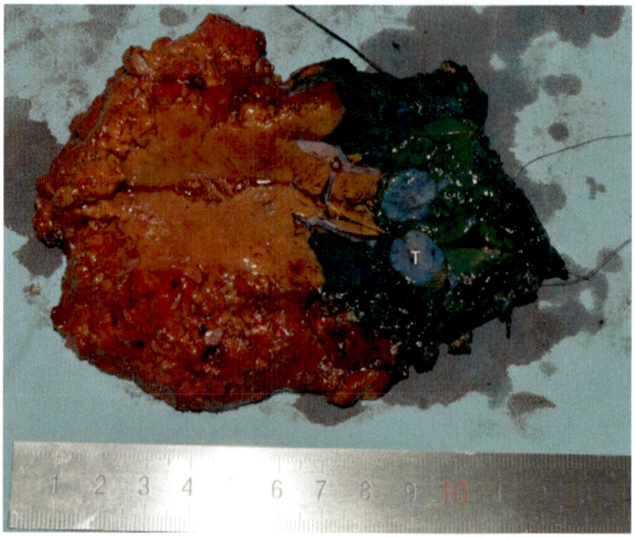

Fig. 395 Split surface of the specimen. *T* tumor

Bisegmentectomy V–VI

Jixiong Hu, Zhongkun Zuo, and Tenglong Tang

Liver resection for the treatment of hepatocellular carcinoma has progressed greatly over the last 20 years. Because of the policy of preserving maximal functioning hepatic parenchyma being widely adopted, both perioperative morbidity and mortality associated with hepatic resections have significantly decreased [131–135]. Recently, Kingham et al. reported a significant decrease in perioperative morbidity from 53.2% to 19.9% in 4152 resections for malignancy over the past 20 years. Moreover, the 90-day mortality rate in this series decreased from 5.2% to 1.6%. They believed that much of the decrease in mortality was likely associated with the decreasing number of major resections [136]. Granted the consistently high postoperative morbidity and mortality associated with major hepatectomies [137], a parenchyma-sparing policy is vital to decrease postoperative morbidity and mortality and, when possible, should be applied. This policy is furthermore supported by Kingham's data [136], which show that parenchyma-preserving resections do not compromise complete tumor clearance.

For tumors located within the right inferior segments (Couinaud's segments V and VI), right hepatectomy is usually recommended only because they are in the vicinity of the right hepatic Glissonean pedicle [88]. Anatomic right inferior bisegmentectomy (segments V and VI) could represent a valuable alternative to right hepatectomy, which may not be tolerated by hepatocellular carcinoma patients with cirrhosis. The routine preoperative imaging studies included ultrasound, high-resolution helical computed tomography (CT), MR, and CT angiography, and, if necessary, PET-CT was also selected. Right hepatectomy was adopted when the tumor confined to right inferior bisegments (segments V and VI) infiltrated the right anterior Glissonean pedicle or the right hepatic Glissonean, given this right hepatectomy tolerated by patients. In terms of the preoperative evaluation of the liver function, the so-called Makuuchi criteria [5] are used to determine the extent of safe hepatic resection. Anatomic bisegmentectomy V–VI can be considered when serum total bilirubin level was less than 1.0 mg/dl and the ICGR is less than 25%.

Operative Procedures	Technical Details
Laparotomy and mobilization of the right hemiliver	◀ A right subcostal incision was made and an automobile retractor was used. The right hemiliver was dissected off if its surrounding structures.
↓	
Isolation and looping of the pedicle of segment 5 and segment 6	◀ The right hepatic Glissonean pedicle, the right anterior and posterior Glissonean pedicle, and the pedicle of S5 and S6 was isolated and looped with a tourniquet, respectively,successively.
↓	
Division of S5-P and S6-P and marking the cut line	◀ The pedicle of segment 5 and segment 6 was clamped, divided and suture-ligated, respectively. The watershed of ischemic territory was marked on the liver surface with electrocautery.
↓	
Hepatic parenchymal transection	◀ Having occluded the right hepatic pedicle, hepatic parenchymal transection was carried out using the clamp-crushing method. The large branch of the middle hepatic vein was clamped, divided and suture-ligated. The pedicle originating from the pedicle of segment 8 and supplying the superior portion of segment 5, and the pedicle diverging from the pedicle of segment 7 and feeding the superior portion of segment 6, was identified, clamped, divided and suture-ligated, respectively.
↓	
Embedding and securing of drug delivery system(DDS), drainage and closure of the abdominal cavity	◀ DDS was embedded and secured. A drain tube was placed near to the cut surface of the liver remnant.

Intraoperative Key Points

1. Anatomic bisegmentectomy V–VI is a valuable alternative to right hepatectomy. However, it is technically more demanding to perfectly perform this resection just using simple surgical device. The individual isolation and looping of the pedicle of segment V and segment VI require minor liver transection around it; this step is a little time-consuming and demands careful and meticulous dissection. Conventionally, this step is carried out by an experienced surgeon.
2. We have previously described the anatomical variations of the Glissonean pedicle of segment V (see section "Brief Description of the Anatomic Variations of Segment V"). In this bisegmentectomy V–VI, we also encountered same branching patterns of the Glissonean pedicles of segment V as that found in segmentectomy V (see section "Segmentectomy V with Resection of the Distal Trunk of the Middle Hepatic Vein (MHV)"). These same branching patterns are as follows: a pedicle originates directly from the right anterior hepatic pedicle and supplies the inferior portion of segment V, and another two pedicles diverge from the extrasegmental pedicle of segment VIII and feed the superior ventral and dorsal portion of segment V, respectively. In this resection, our findings give a real-time and living evidence of the branching patterns of the Glissonean pedicle of segment V, which was proposed by Mise et al. using 3D image processing software [4]. Therefore, attention should be paid to prevent injury to the extrasegmental pedicle of segment VIII while transecting another two pedicles of segment V.
3. We have also previously described that a Glissonean pedicle originates directly from the extrasegmental pedicle of segment VII and supplies the superior portion of segment VI (see section "Segmentectomy VI"). In this bisegmentectomy V–VI, we also clearly show that this anatomic variation is truly existing (Fig. 432), and to the present author's knowledge, no report focusing on this variation has been found. Thus, care should be taken to identify and properly manage any possible vessels originating directly the extrasegmental pedicle of segment VII while transecting the deep parenchyma between segment VI and segment VII.
4. The right hepatic vein runs in the right portal scissura. In this resection, the distal trunk of this vein must be cross transected during dividing the hepatic parenchyma between the right superior and inferior segments. The proximal stump of the right hepatic vein must be transfix-ligated to prevent torrential backflow bleeding from this venous stump because of the slippage of the silk suture.
5. In this resection, at the beginning of parenchymal transection caudo-cranially while encountering with venous vessels, it is very important to distinguish the terminal branch of the middle hepatic vein from its trunk. Having isolating and ligating these branches, and identifying and preserving the trunk, then, parenchymal dissection is carried out along the trunk of the middle hepatic vein (Fig. 396).

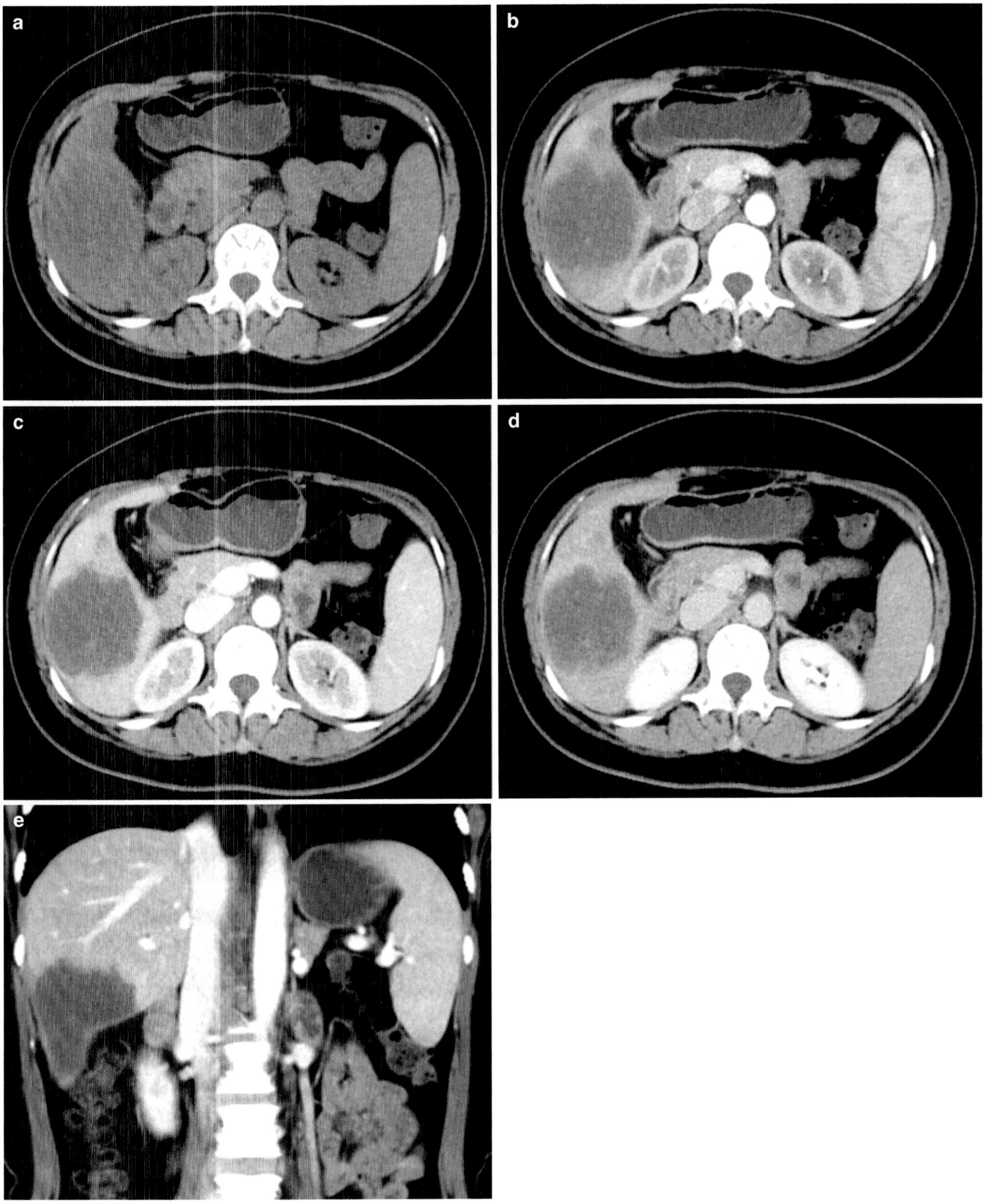

Fig. 396 (**a**) Preoperative CT (precontrast). The tumor, which appears mildly hypodense, is located in segments V and VI. (**b**) Preoperative CT (hepatic arterial phase). The tumor appears markedly hypodense due to less enhancement. (**c**) Preoperative CT (hepatic venous phase). (**d**) Preoperative CT (interstitial phase). (**e**) Preoperative CT (coronary section). The tumor was confined to segments V–VI

Abdominal Incision and Mobilization of the Right Hemiliver (Figs. 397 and 398)

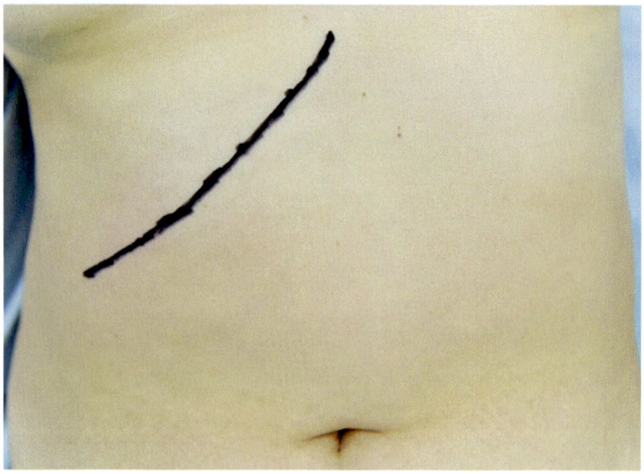

Fig. 397 A right subcostal incision was selected. No extended incision was required

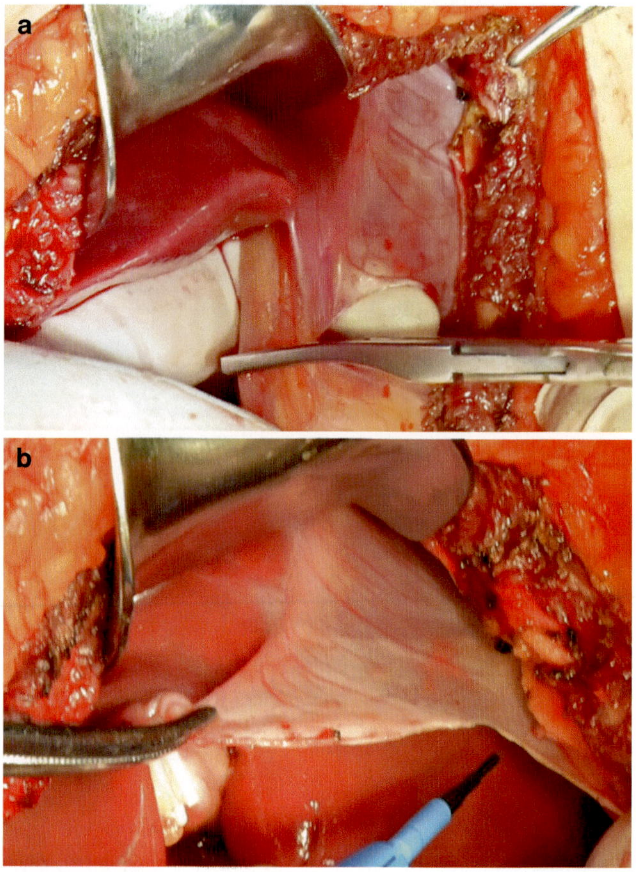

Fig. 398 (**a**, **b**) Having entered into the abdominal cavity, the round ligament was firstly divided and ligated. Then, the falciform ligament was electrocauterized. Thereafter, an incision defender was used to cover the incision. A careful peritoneal cavity exploration was performed to exclude intraabdominal tumor dissemination. Then, the right hemiliver was fully mobilized from its surrounding structures. At this time, intraoperative US (IOUS) was used to ascertain the location of the tumor and its relationship with the main vasculature and biliary tract

Isolation of the Right Anterior Pedicle (RAP) and the Right Posterior Pedicle (RPP) (Figs. 399, 400, 401, 402, 403, 404, 405, 406, 407, 408, and 409)

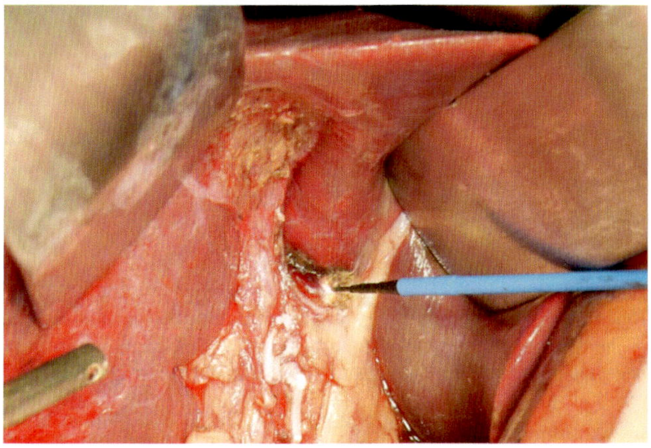

Fig. 399 Having performed cholecystectomy, a small (about 2 cm) traverse incision was made in front of the hilus

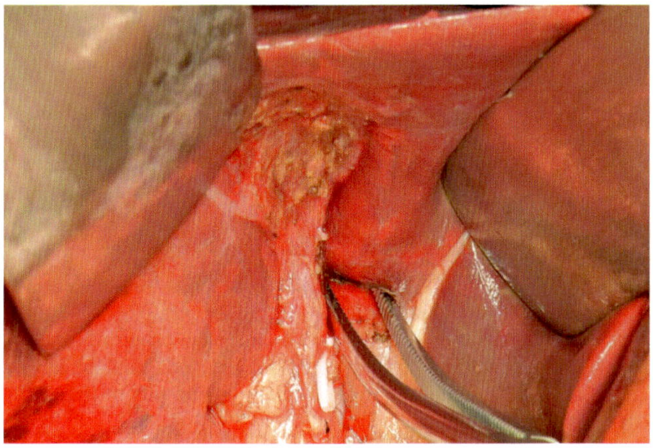

Fig. 400 Using a large curved clamp, hepatic parenchyma above this incision was pushed upward, and the hilar plate was pulled down to expose the anterior and superior surface of the right hepatic pedicle (RHV)

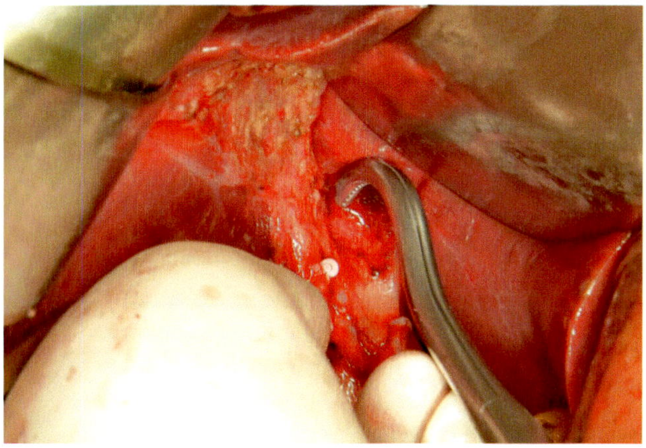

Fig. 401 The operator's left index finger was placed between the undersurface of the hilar plate and the anterior wall of the retrohepatic inferior vena cava (IVC), and then, a large curved clamp was inserted vertically into this incision and directly reached down to the tip of the index finger

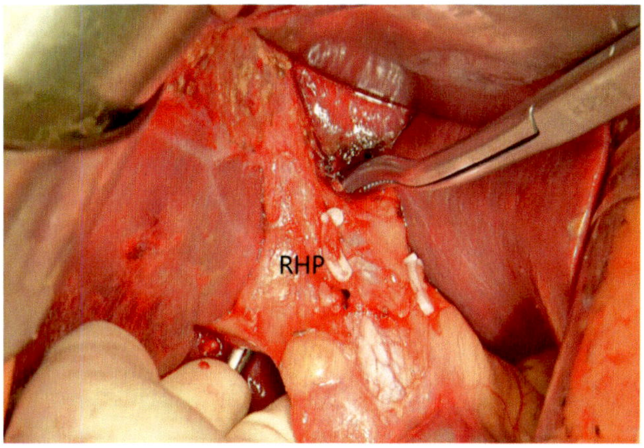

Fig. 402 Using the index finger as a guide, the large curved clamp was inserted furtherly to puncture the undersurface membrane of the hilar plate and passed out of the posterior and inferior edge of the right hepatic pedicle (RHP)

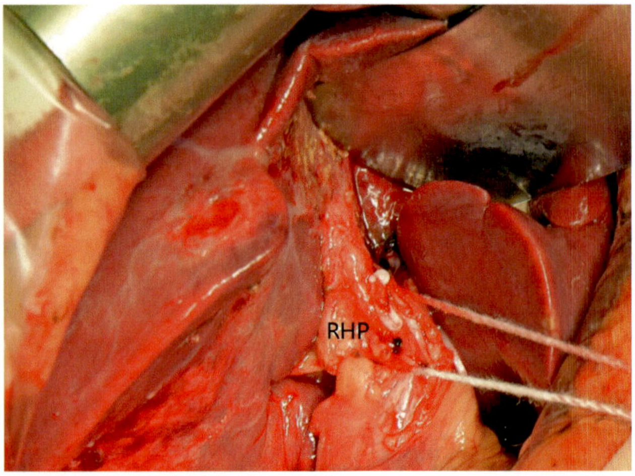

Fig. 403 As a result, the right hepatic pedicle (RHP) was isolated, and a tourniquet was looped with it

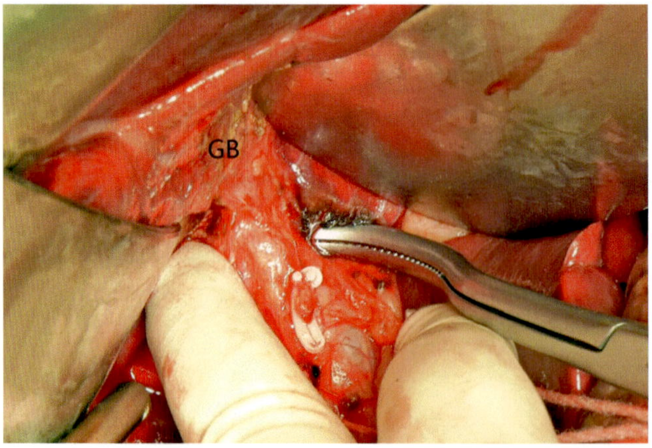

Fig. 405 A large curved clamp was inserted into this incision in front of the hilus, and the operator's middle finger was covered over the second incision beside the right edge of the gallbladder bed (GB)

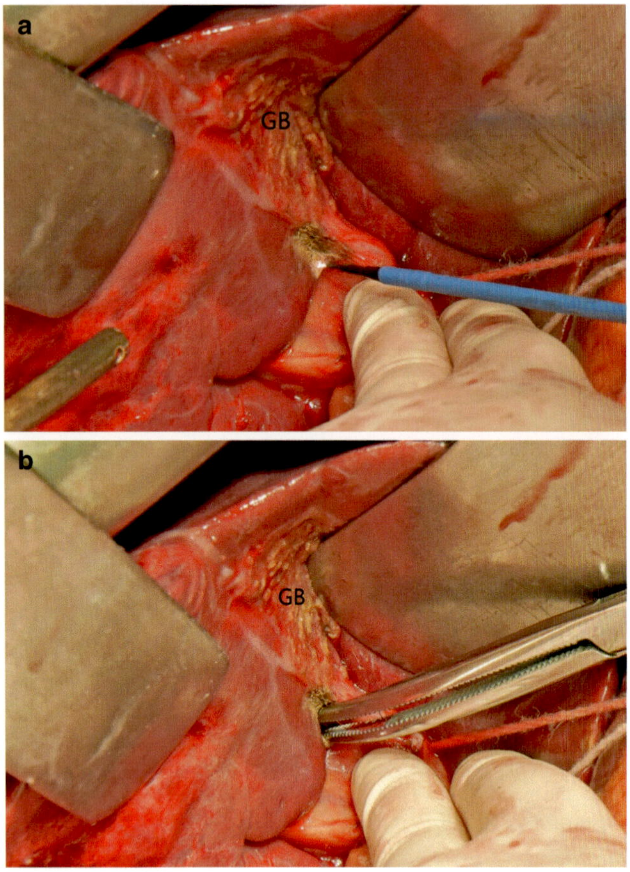

Fig. 404 (**a**, **b**) Another small incision was made on the right edge of the base area of the gallbladder bed (GB), and this incision was extended using a large curved clamp

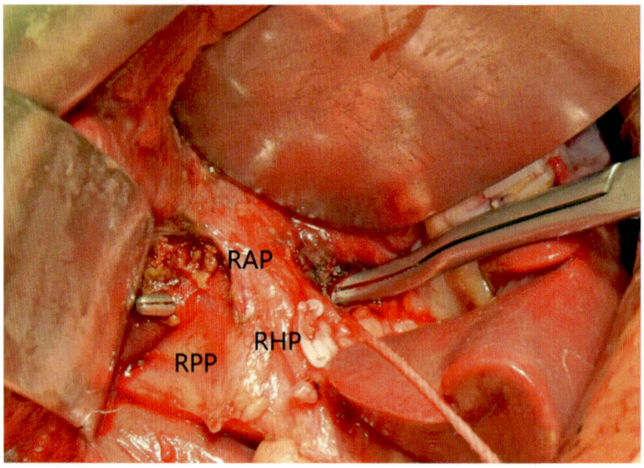

Fig. 406 Using the middle finger as a guide, the clamp was passed behind the right anterior pedicle (RAP) and punched out of the second incision. Thus, the RAP was isolated. *RHP* right hepatic pedicle, *RPP* right posterior pedicle

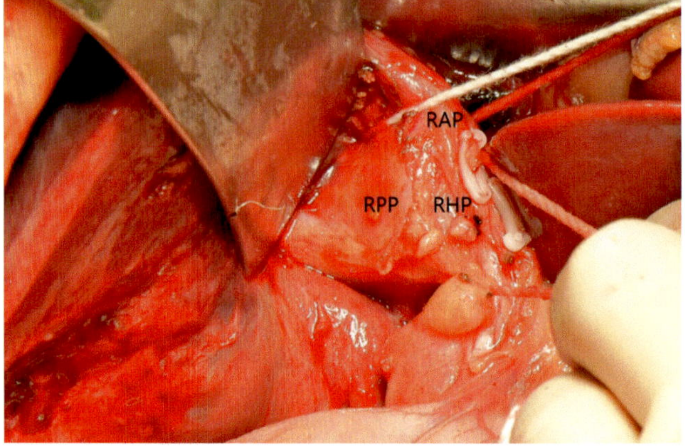

Fig. 407 The right anterior pedicle (RAP) was also encircled with a vascular tape. *RHP* right hepatic pedicle, *RPP* right posterior pedicle

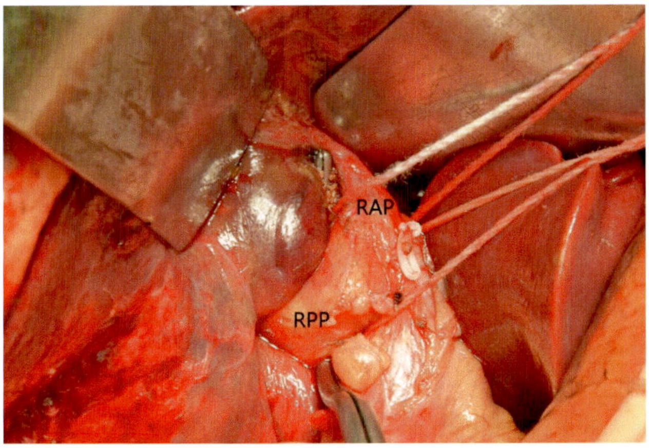

Fig. 408 A large curved clamp was inserted from the inferior and posterior edge of the right posterior pedicle (RPP), pushed upward behind the RPP, and punched out of the second incision. Thus, the RPP was isolated. *RAP* right anterior pedicle

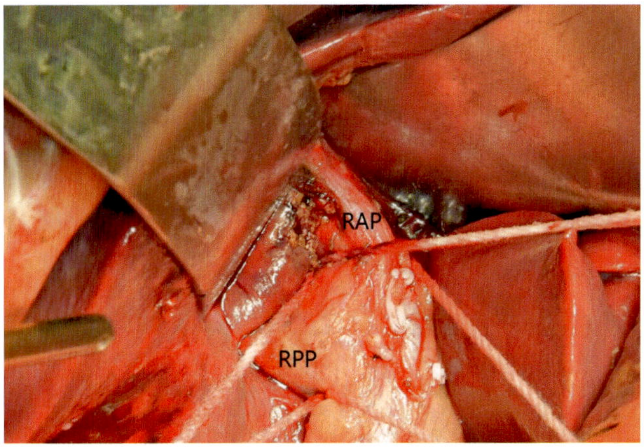

Fig. 409 The right posterior pedicle (RPP) was also looped with a tourniquet. *RAP* right anterior pedicle

Isolation of the Pedicle of Segment V (S_5-P)

(Figs. 410, 411, 412, 413, 414, and 415)

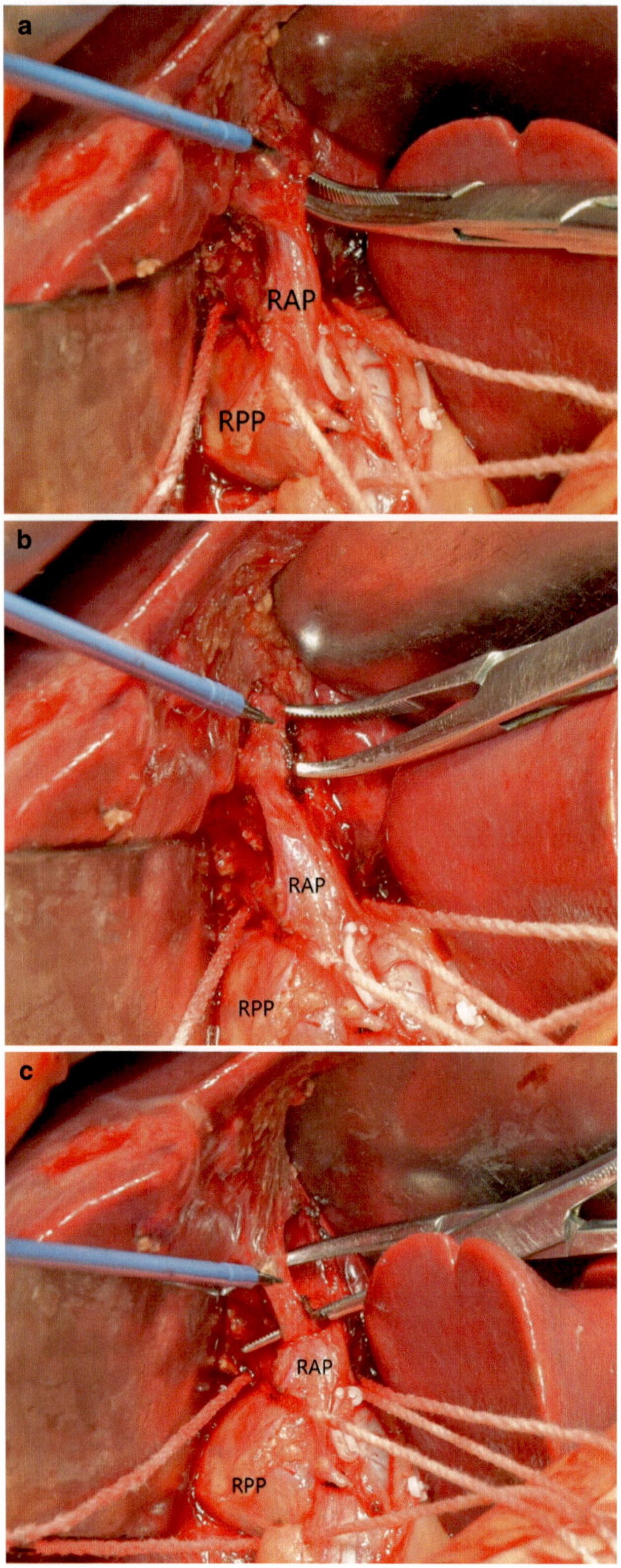

Fig. 410 (**a**–**c**) Dissection of the right anterior pedicle (RAP) was first begun. The superior (**a**), anterior (**b**), and inferior (**c**) surface was dissected. During these surgical proceedings, relatively large vessels were ligated. *RPP* right posterior pedicle

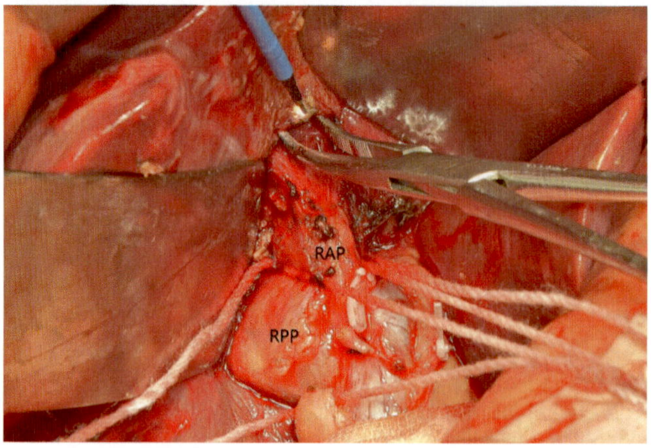

Fig. 411 To identify the bifurcation of segment V and segment VIII, further dissection was required. The hepatic parenchyma covering the anterior surface of the right anterior pedicle (RAP) was cut open with electrocautery

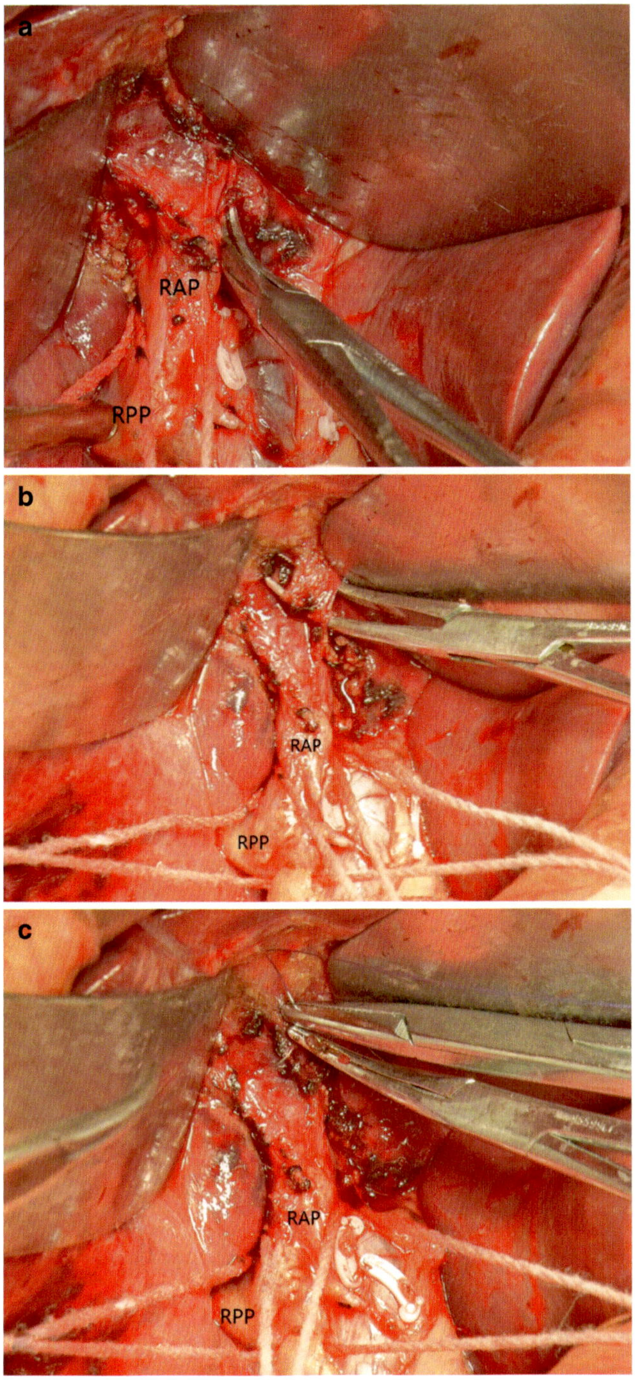

Fig. 412 (**a**–**c**) The superior surface of the right anterior pedicle (RAP) was furtherly dissected. *RPP* right posterior pedicle

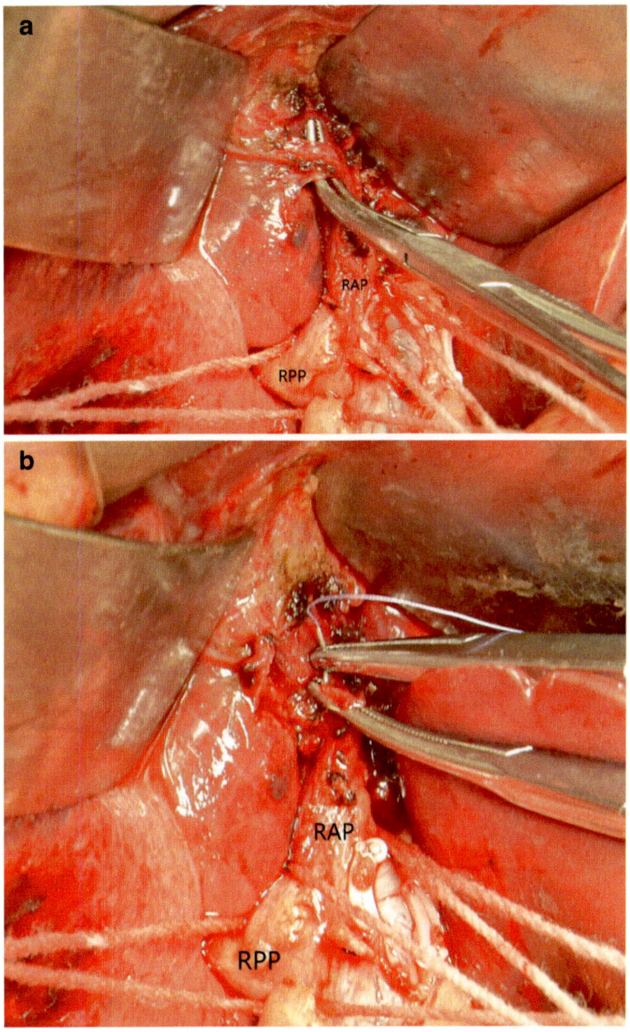

Fig. 413 (**a**, **b**) Also, the inferior surface of the right anterior pedicle (RAP) was furtherly dissected. *RPP* right posterior pedicle

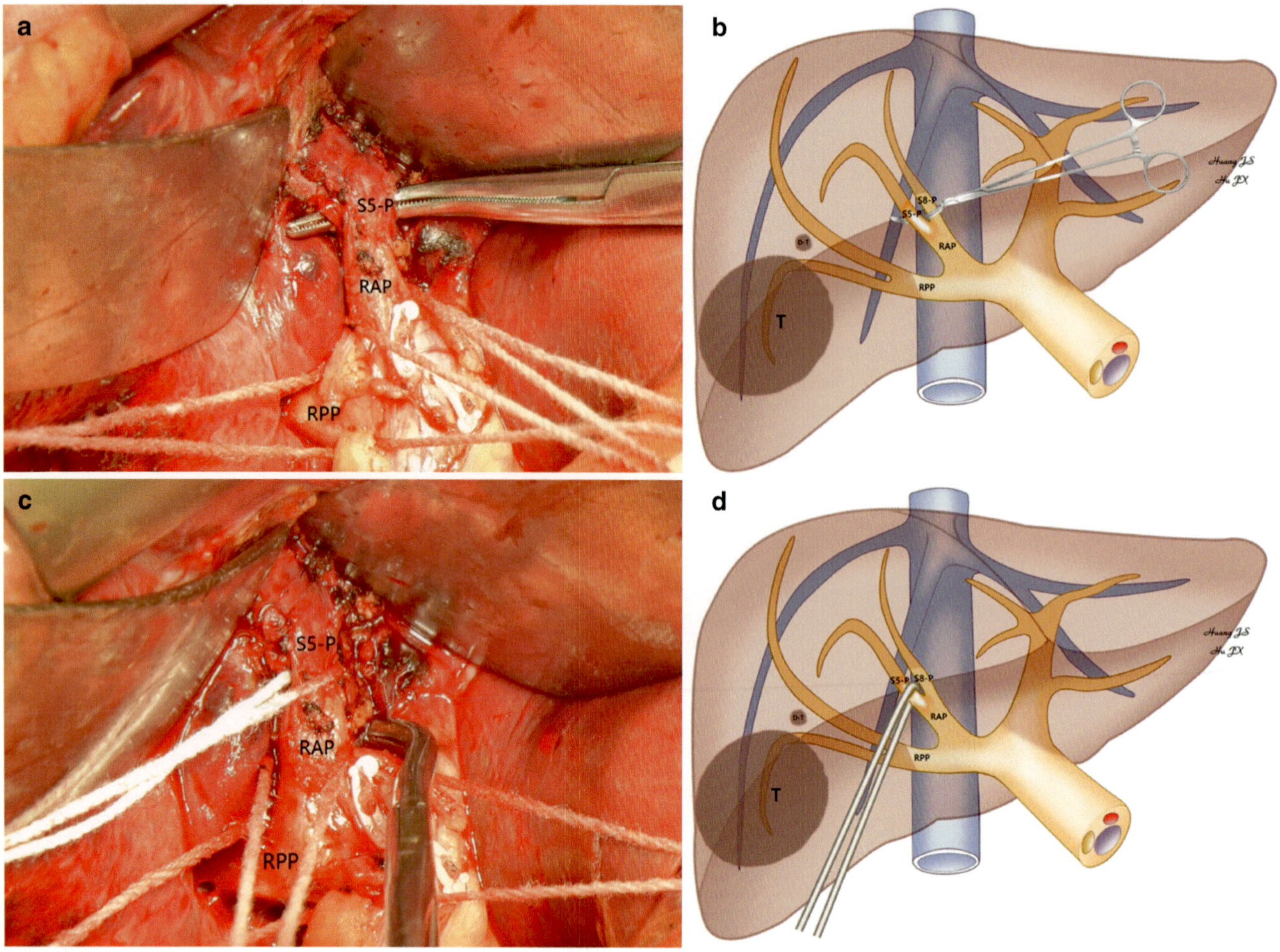

Fig. 414 Up to now, the bifurcation of segment V and segment VIII was clearly exposed. (**a** and **c**) The pedicle of segment V was isolated and encircled with a loop. (**b** and **d**) Schematic illustration of this procedure. *S5-P* pedicle of segment V, *S8-P* pedicle of segment VIII, *RPP* right posterior pedicle, *RAP* right anterior pedicle

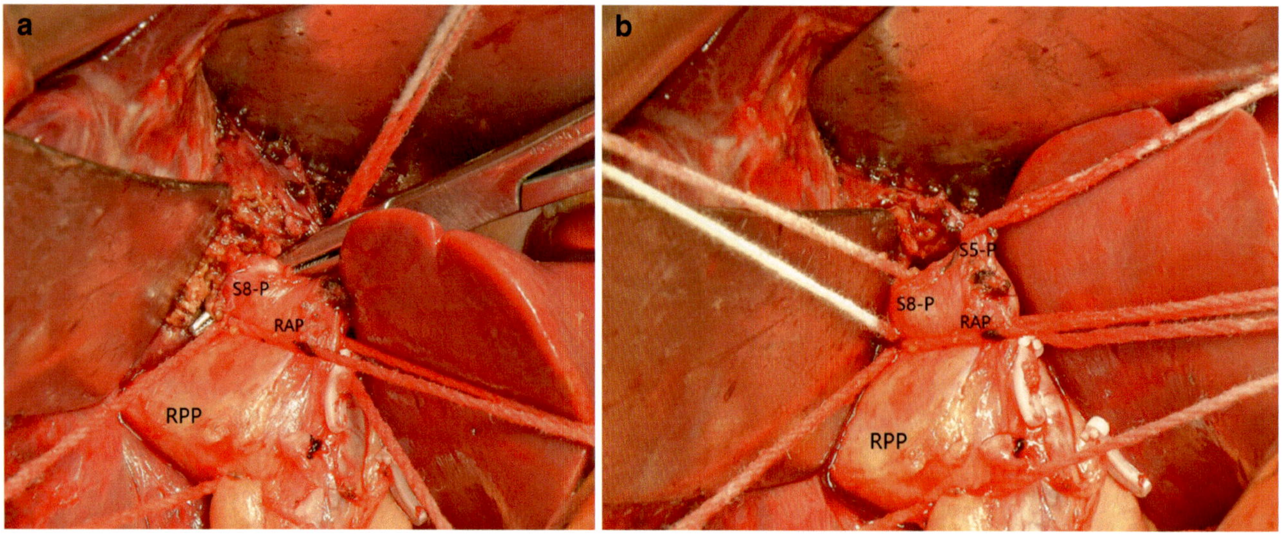

Fig. 415 (**a**, **b**) Then, to avoid inadvertent injury to the pedicle of segment VIII (S8-P), it was also isolated and looped with a tape. *RPP* right posterior pedicle, *RAP* right anterior pedicle, *S5-P* pedicle of segment V, *S8-P* pedicle of segment VIII

Isolation of the Pedicle of Segment VI (S_6-P)
(Figs. 416, 417, and 418)

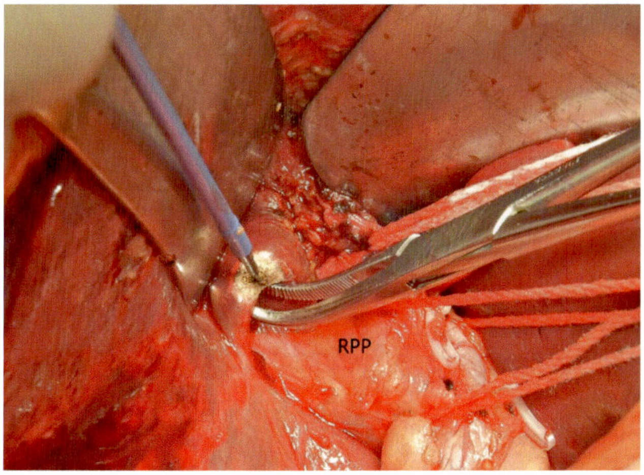

Fig. 416 Hepatic parenchyma surrounding the anterior surface of the right posterior pedicle (RPP) was incised with electrocautery to expose its anterior surface

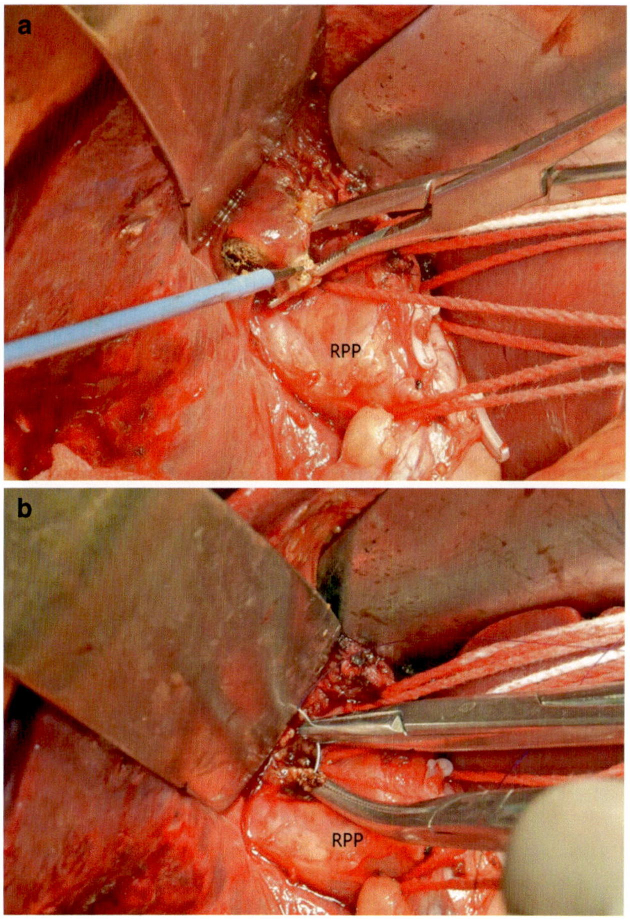

Fig. 417 (**a**, **b**) Hepatic parenchyma surrounding the superior surface of the right posterior pedicle (RPP) was dissected to expose the anterior and superior surface of the RPP

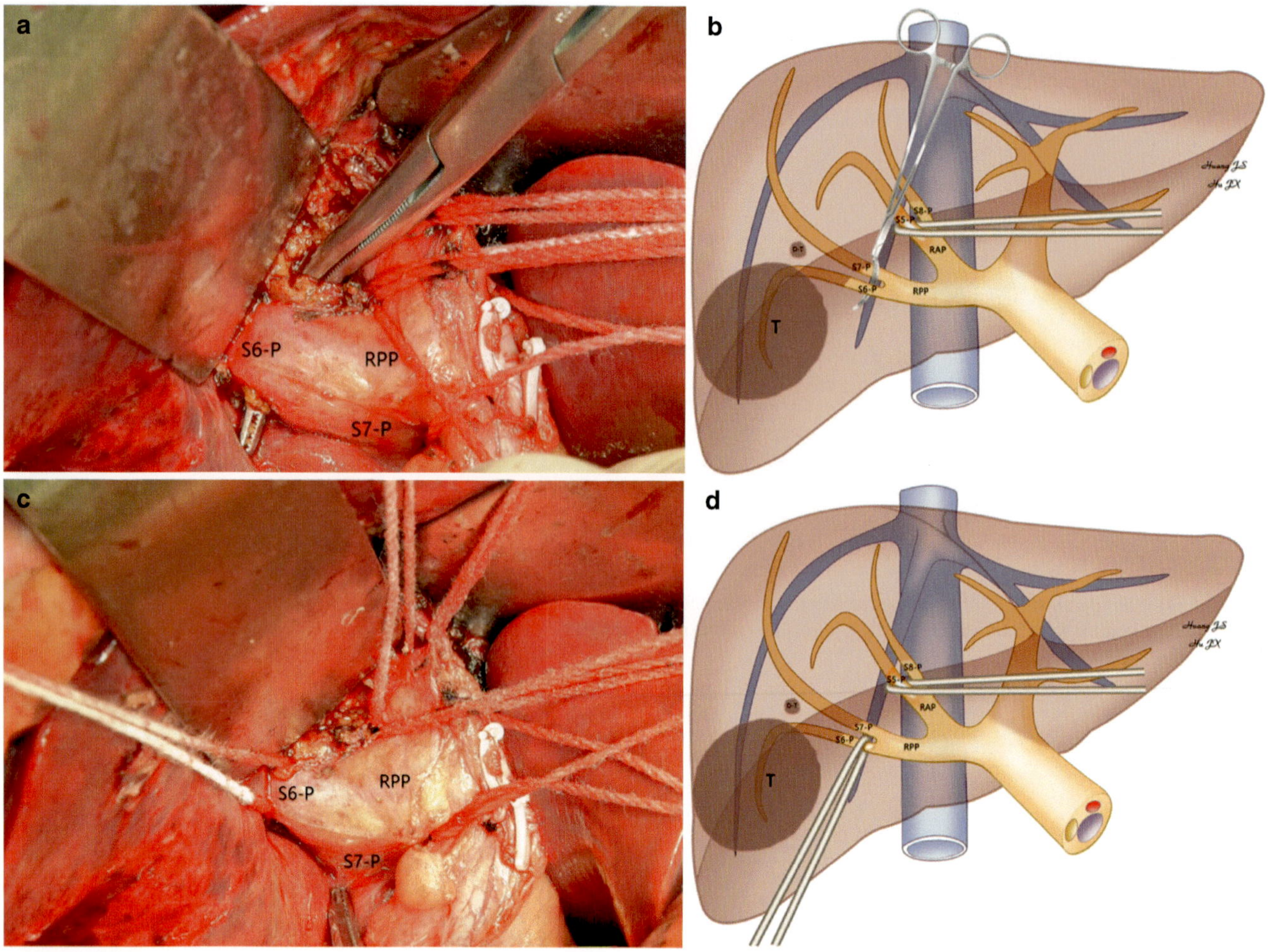

Fig. 418 (**a**, **c**) Having dissected the right posterior pedicle (RPP), the bifurcation of segment VI and segment VII can be clearly identified, and the pedicle of segment VI (S6-P) was isolated using a large curved clamp (**a**) and encircled with a loop (**c**). (**b** and **d**) Schematic illustration of this procedure. *S5-P* pedicle of segment V, *S7-P* pedicle of segment VII, *S8-P* pedicle of segment VIII

Staining Segment V (Fig. 419)

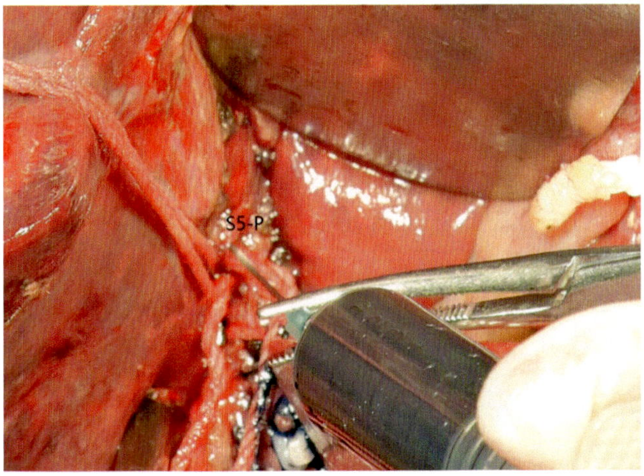

Fig. 419 In order to stain segment V, methylene blue was injected into the portal branch supplying segment V. However, the target segment was poorly stained. S5-P, pedicle of segment V

Division the Pedicle of Segment V (S_5-P) and Segment VI (S_6-P) and Marking the Cut Line

(Figs. 420, 421, and 422)

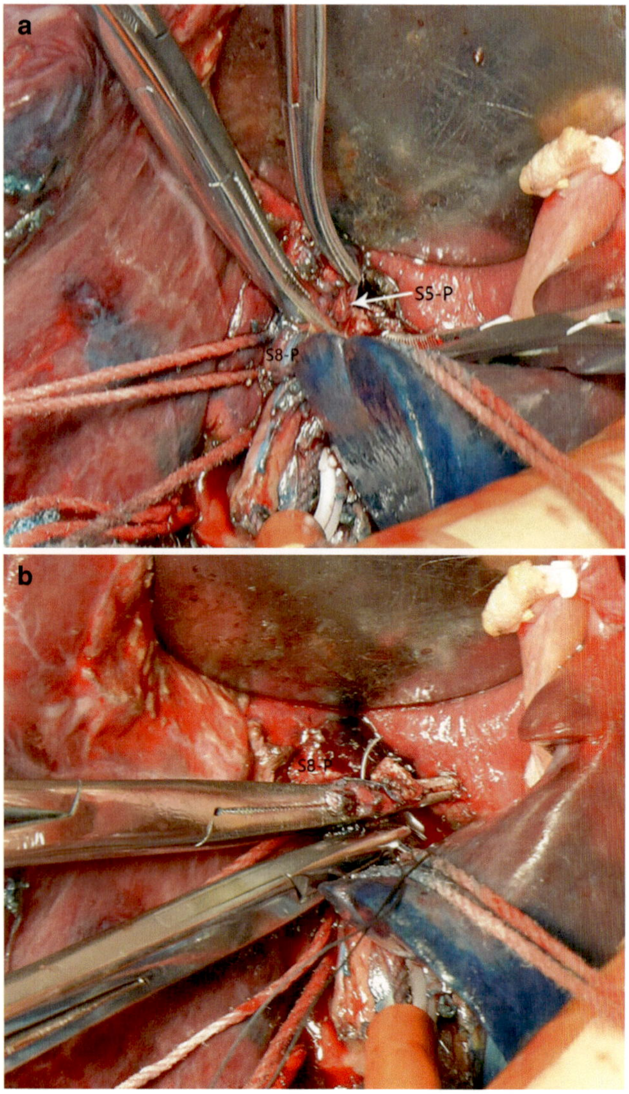

Fig. 420 (**a**, **b**) The pedicle of segment V (S5-P) was clamped and divided, and its proximal stump was suture-ligated. *S8-P* pedicle of segment VIII

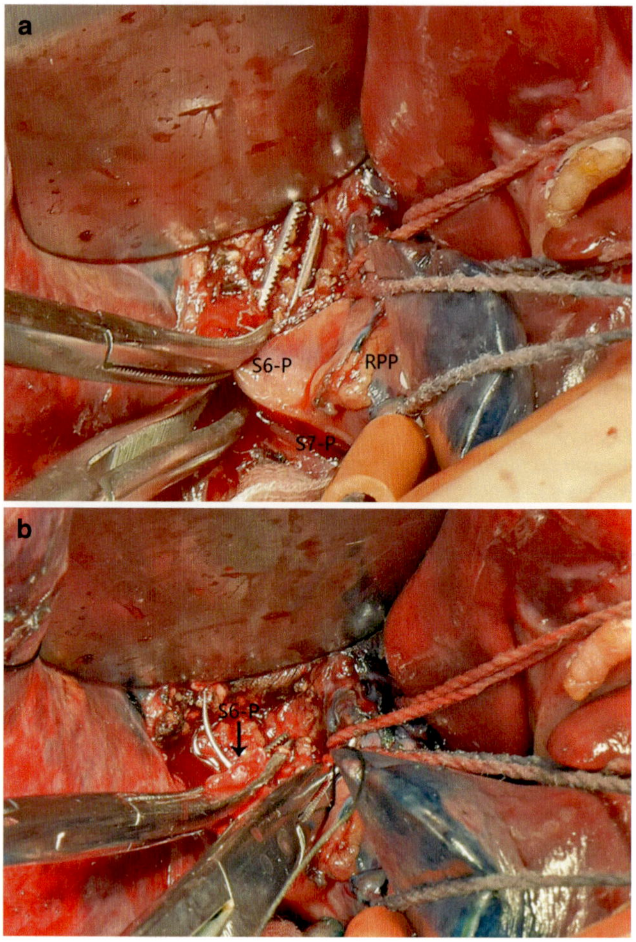

Fig. 421 (**a**, **b**) The pedicle of segment VI was also clamped and divided, and its proximal stump was suture-ligated. *S6-P* pedicle of segment VI, *S7-P* pedicle of segment VII, *RPP* right posterior pedicle

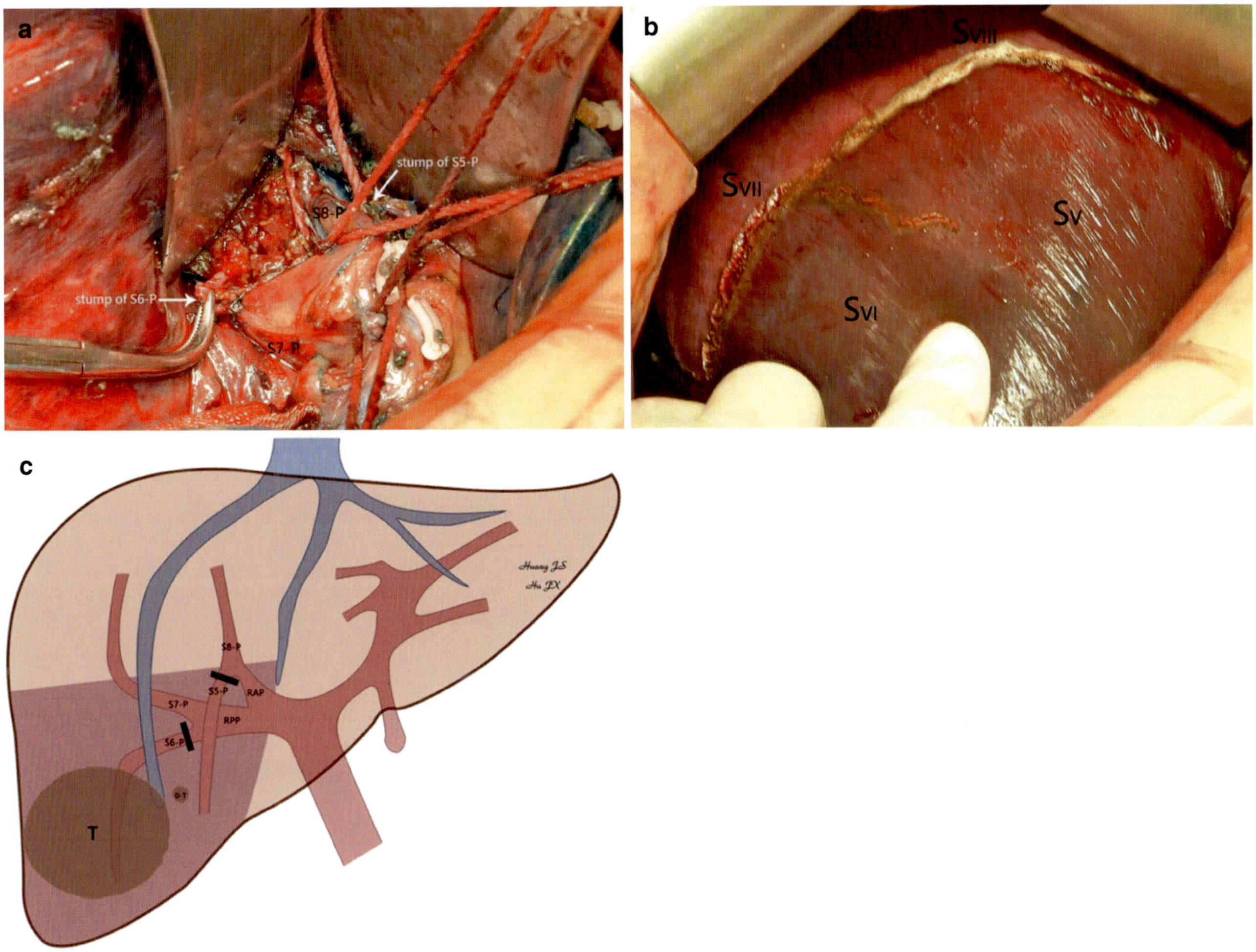

Fig. 422 (**a**, **b**) Having individually transected the pedicle of segment V and segment VI (**a**), obvious ischemic boundary appeared on the liver surface and was marked on the liver surface with electrocautery (**b**). (**c**) Schematic illustration of this procedure. *S5-P* pedicle of segment V, *S8-P* pedicle of segment VIII, *S6-P* pedicle of segment VI, *S7-P* pedicle of segment VII

Hepatic Parenchyma Transection (Figs. 423, 424, 425, 426, 427, 428, 429, 430, 431, and 432)

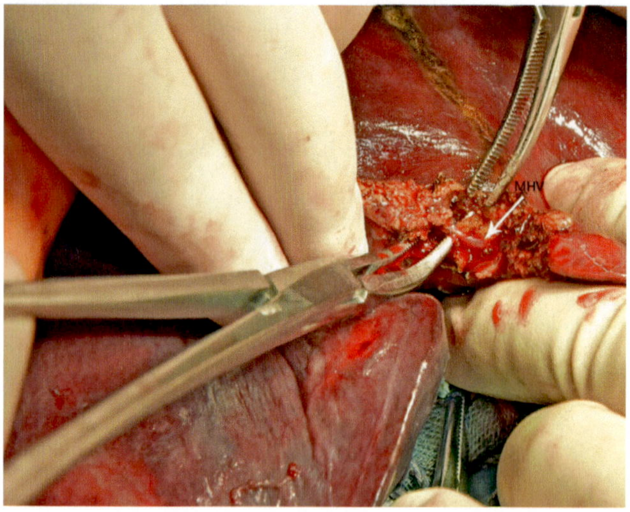

Fig. 423 Having clamped the right hepatic pedicle (RHP), hepatic parenchymal transection was initially performed along the left-sided cut line from caudal to cranial side. *MHV* middle hepatic vein

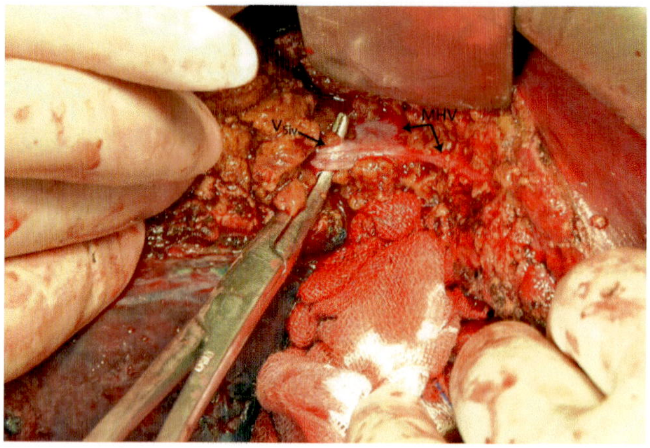

Fig. 426 A large branch (V_{5iv}) of the middle hepatic vein (MHV) draining the inferior and ventral portion of segment V was isolated, divided, and ligated

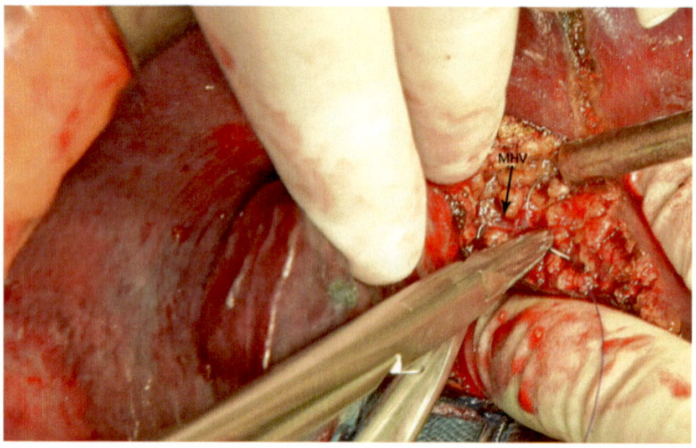

Fig. 424 A tiny hole on the middle hepatic vein (MHV) was repaired with 4-0 polypropylene

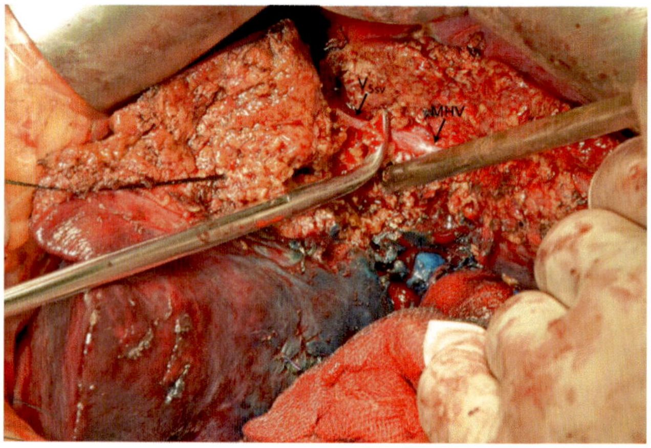

Fig. 427 Another large branch (V_{5sv}) of the middle hepatic vein (MHV) draining the superior and ventral portion of segment V was also isolated, divided, and ligated

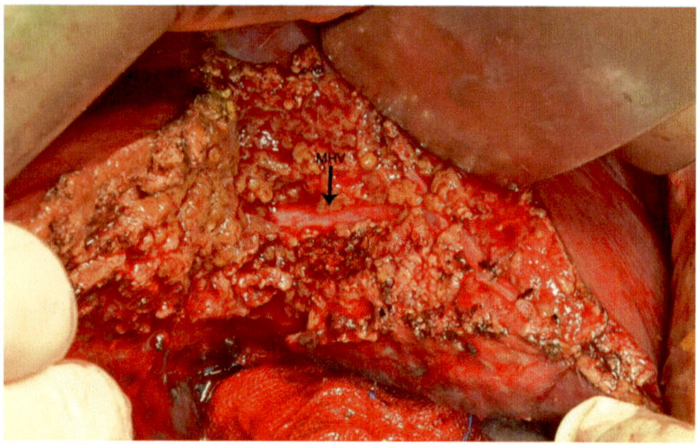

Fig. 425 The main trunk of the lower part of the middle hepatic vein (MHV) was clearly exposed on the cut surface

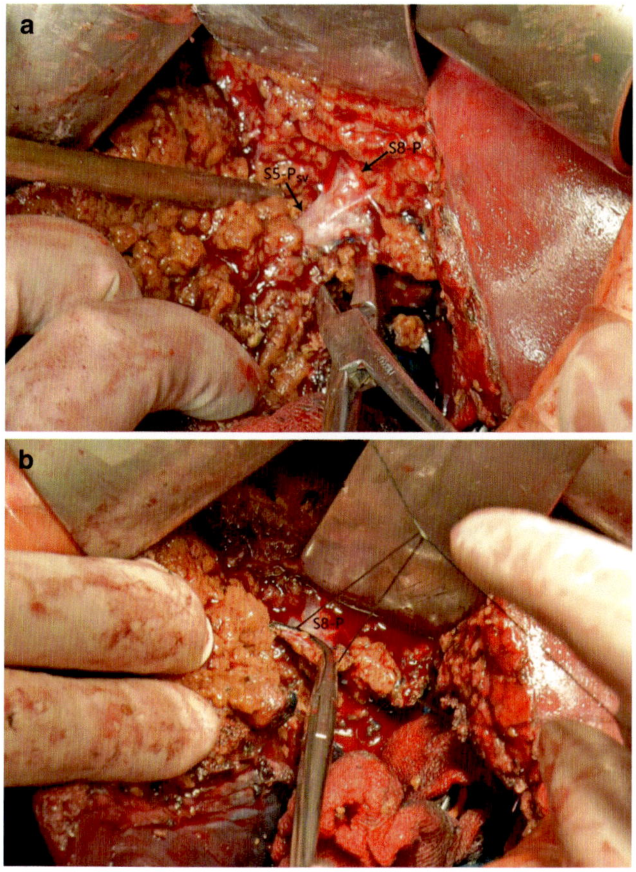

Fig. 428 (**a**, **b**) A second pedicle originating from P-8 before S8-P entering into segment VIII parenchyma and supplying the superior and ventral portion of segment V (S5-P_{sv}) was isolated, clamped, divided, and ligated. *S8-P* pedicle of segment VIII

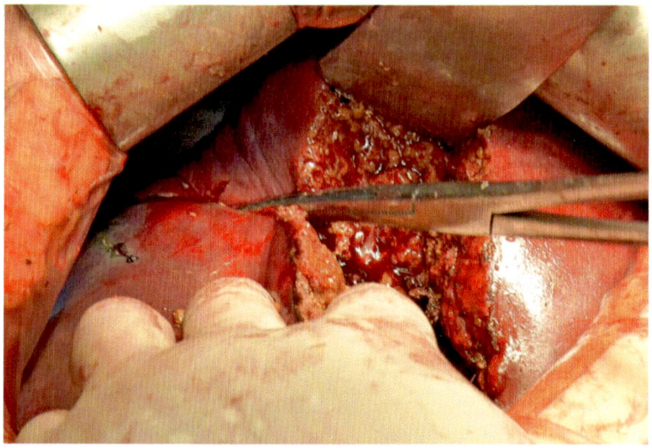

Fig. 429 Hepatic parenchymal transection was continued between segment VI and segment VII

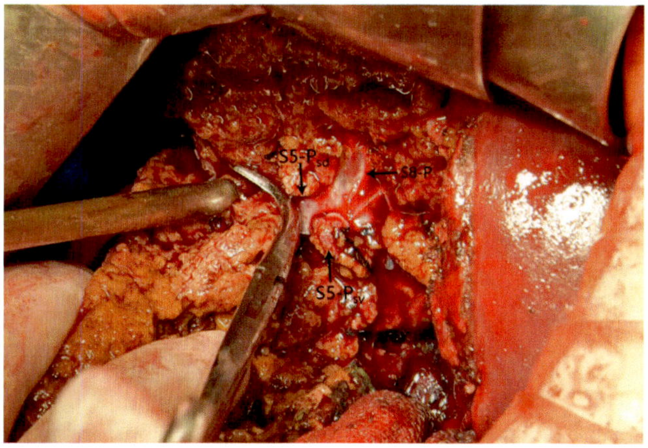

Fig.430 A third pedicle originating from S8-P before S8-P entering into segment VIII parenchyma and supplying the superior and dorsal portion of segment V (S5-P_{sd}) was isolated, clamped, divided, and ligated. *S8-P* pedicle of segment VIII

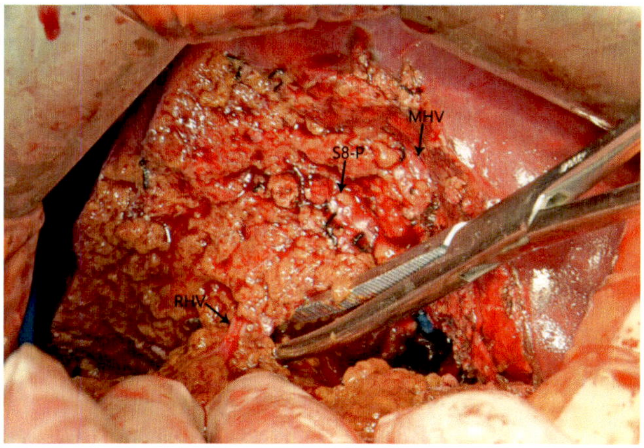

Fig. 431 The main trunk of the right hepatic vein (RHV) was transected at the. *S8-P* pedicle of segment VI segment VII segment VIII, *MHV* middle hepatic vein at the interface between segment VI and segment VII

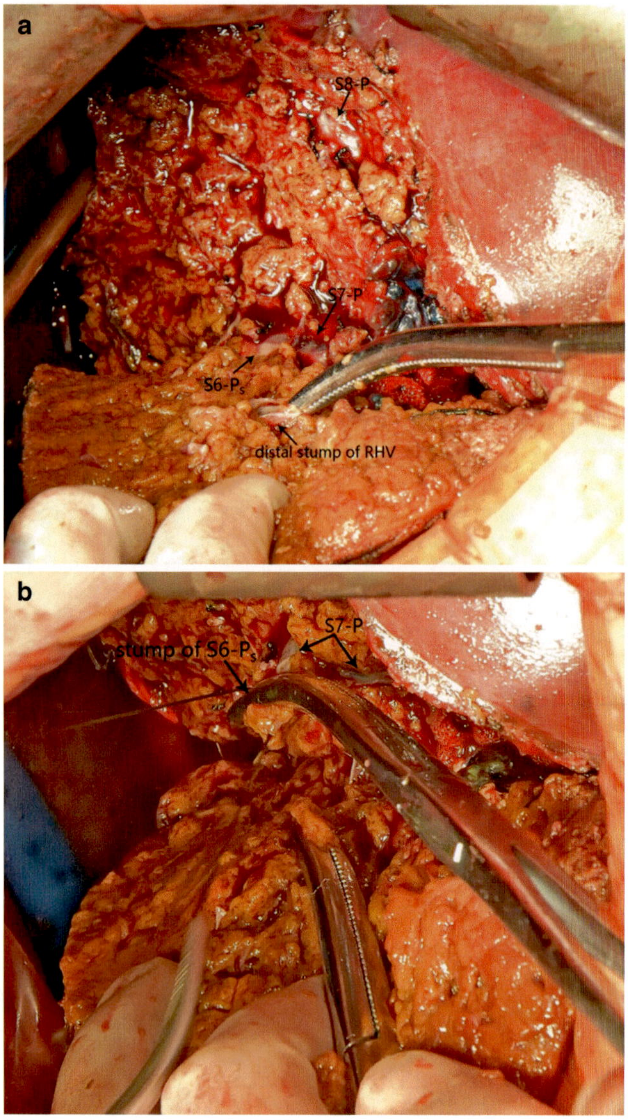

Fig. 432 (**a**, **b**) A pedicle originating from S7-P before S7-P entering into segment VII parenchyma and supplying the superior portion of segment VI (S6-P$_s$) was identified, clamped, divided, and ligated. *S7-P* pedicle of segment VII, *RHV* right hepatic vein, *S8-P* pedicle of segment VIII

Raw Area of the Remnant Liver and the Specimen
(Figs. 433, 434, and 435)

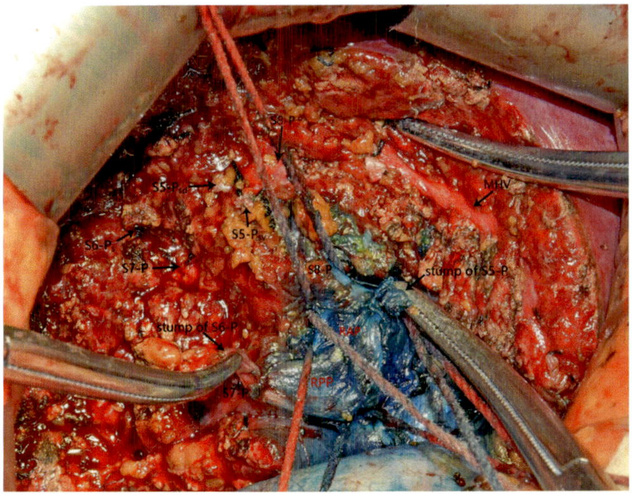

Fig. 433 Having removed the specimen and unclamped the right hepatic pedicle, the distal main trunk of the middle hepatic vein (MHV) was obviously shown on the cut surface. The vascular and biliary ramifications on the resectional surface of the residual liver were sutured with silk thread and/or polypropylene 1-0 and/or 2-0, and the tiny holes on the middle hepatic vein were repaired with 4-0 and 5-0 polypropylene. *S5-P* pedicle of segment V, *S5-P$_{sv}$* pedicle originating from S8-P and supplying the superior and ventral portion of segment V, *S5-P$_{sd}$* pedicle originating from S8-P and supplying the superior and dorsal portion of segment V, *S6-P* pedicle of segment VI, *S6-P$_{s}$* pedicle originating from S7-P and supplying the superior portion of segment VI, *S7-P* pedicle of segment VII, *S8-P* pedicle of segment VIII, *RAP* right anterior pedicle, *RPP* right posterior pedicle

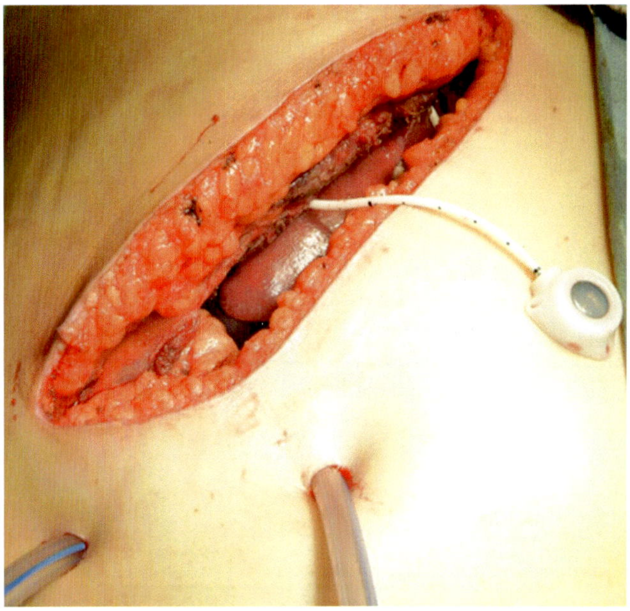

Fig. 434 A drug delivery system (DDS) was inserted into the hepatic artery and secured. A tube was placed into the right subphrenic space, and another tube was placed into the Winslow hole

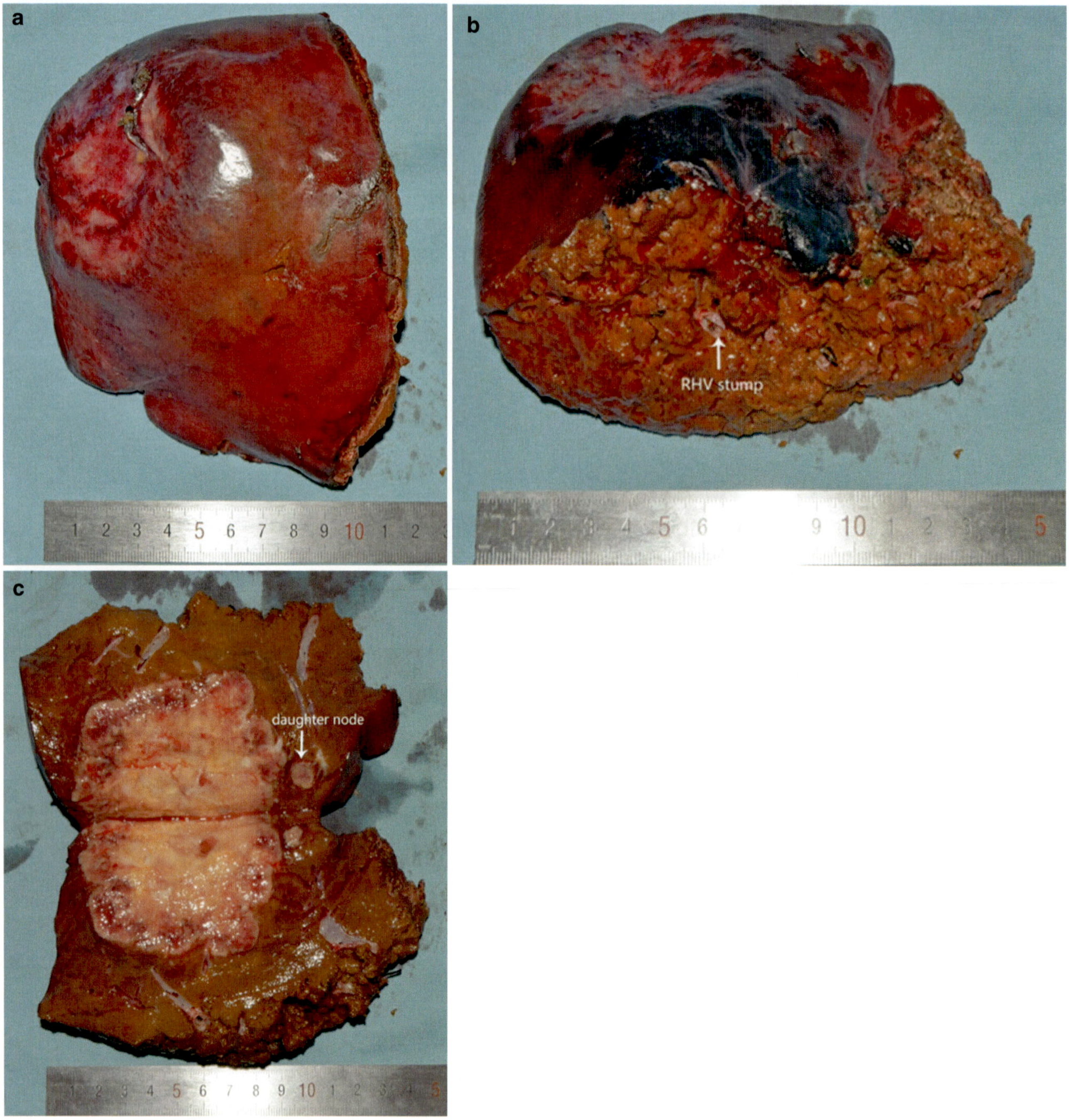

Fig. 435 The specimen. (**a**) anterior surface; (**b**) cut surface. Surgical margin was macroscopically negative; (**c**) split surface. An intrahepatic daughter node was found near the main tumor. Anatomic bisegmentectomy V–VI can simultaneously resected intrahepatic daughter node(s) located within the target segment(s). *RHV* right hepatic vein

References

1. Celinski SA, Gamblin TC. Hepatic resection nomenclature and techniques. Surg Clin North Am. 2010;90(4):737–48.
2. Terminology Committee of the IHPBA. The Brisbane terminology of the liver anatomy and resection. HPB. 2000;2:333–9.
3. Makuuchi M. Chapter 1. Right hepatectomy. In: Makuuchi M, editor. Makuuchi Kanzou Gekagaku (in Japanese)/(translated to Chinese by Yong Zeng). Beijing: People's Medical Publishing House; 2016. p. 98.
4. Mise Y, Satou S, Shindoh J, Conrad C, Aoki T, Hasegawa K, Sugawara Y, Kokudo N. Three-dimensional volumetry in 107 normal livers reveals clinically relevant inter-segment variation in size. HPB. 2013;16(5):439.
5. Makuuchi M, Kosuge T, Takayama T, Yamazaki S, Kakazu T, Miyagawa S, Kawasaki S. Surgery for small liver cancers. Semin Surg Oncol. 1993;9(4):298–304.
6. Couinaud C. Surgical anatomy of the liver revisited. Paris: C. Couinaud; 1989.
7. Honjo I, Araki C. Total resection of the right lobe of the liver. J Int Coll Surg. 1955;23(1):23–8.
8. Lortat-Jacob JL, Robert HG. Hepatectomie droite reglee. Presse Med. 1952;60:549–51.
9. Lin TY, Chem KM, Liu TK. Total right hepatic lobectomy for primary hepatoma. Surgery. 1960;48(6):1048–60.
10. Tung TT, Quang ND. Segmentary hepatectomy by transparenchymatous vascular ligation. Presse Med. 1965;73(52):3015–7.
11. Takasaki K, Kobayashi S, Tanaka S, Saito A, Yamamoto M, Hanyu F. Highly anatomically systematized hepatic resection with Glissonean sheath code transection at the hepatic hilus. Int Surg. 1990;75(2):73–7.
12. Takasaki K. Glissonean pedicle transection method for hepatic resection: a new concept of liver segmentation. J Hepato-Biliary-Pancreat Surg. 1998;5(3):286–91.
13. Launois B, Sutherland FR, Harissis HA. A new technique of Hepp–Couinaud hepaticojejunostomy using the posterior approach to the hepatic hilum. J Am Coll Surg. 1999;188(1):59–62.
14. Machado MA, Herman P, Machado MC. A standardized technique for right segmental liver resections. Arch Surg. 2003;138(8):918–20.
15. Yamamoto M, Katagiri S, Ariizumi S, Kotera Y, Takahashi Y. Glissonean pedicle transection method for liver surgery (with video). J Hepatobiliary Pancreat Sci. 2012;19(1):3–8.
16. Yamamoto M, Katagiri S, Ariizumi S, Kotera Y, Takahashi Y, Egawa H. Tips for anatomical hepatectomy for hepatocellular carcinoma by the Glissonean pedicle approach (with videos). J Hepatobiliary Pancreat Sci. 2014;21(8):E53–6.
17. Figueras J, Llado L, Ruiz D, Ramos E, Busquets J, Rafecas A, Torras J, Fabregat J. Complete versus selective portal triad clamping for minor liver resections: a prospective randomized trial. Ann Surg. 2005;241(4):582–90.
18. Figueras J, Lopez-Ben S, Llado L, Rafecas A, Torras J, Ramos E, Fabregat J, Jaurrieta E. Hilar dissection versus the 'Glissonean' approach and stapling of the pedicle for major hepatectomies: a prospective, randomized trial. Ann Surg. 2003;238(1):111–9.
19. Giordano M, Lopez-Ben S, Codina-Barreras A, Pardina B, Falgueras L, Torres-Bahi S, Albiol M, Castro E, Figueras J. Extra-Glissonian approach in liver resection. Hepatol Pancreatol Biliary Surg. 2010;12(2):94–100.
20. Machado MA, Herman P, Figueira ER, Bacchella T, Machado MC. Intrahepatic Glissonian access for segmental liver resection in cirrhotic patients. Am J Surg. 2006;192(3):388–92.
21. Regimbeau JM, Mauvais F. Liver resection; the approach via Glisson's capsule. J Chir (Paris). 2008;145(4):355–62.
22. Katagiri S, Ariizumi SI, Kotera Y, Takahashi Y, Yamamoto M. Right hepatectomy using Glissonean pedicle transection method with anterior approach (with video). J Hepatobiliary Pancreat Sci. 2012;19(1):25–9.
23. Mouly C, Fuks D, Browet F, Mauvais F, Potier A, Yzet T, Quentin Q, Regimbeau JM. Feasibility of the Glissonian approach during right hepatectomy. HPB. 2013;15(8):638–45.
24. Madoff D, Hicks M, Vauthey JN, Charnsangavej C, Morello JF, Ahrar K, Wallace MJ, Gupta S. Transhepatic portal vein embolization: anatomy, indications, and technical considerations. Radiographics. 2002;22(5):1063–76.
25. Nakai T, Koh K, Funai S, Kawabe T, Okuno K, Yasutomi M. Comparison of controlled and Glisson's pedicle transections of hepatic hilum occlusion for hepatic resection. J Am Coll Surg. 1999;189(3):300–4.
26. Takasaki K. Procedures for hepatic resection. Anterior approach technique. In: Glissonean pedicle transection method for hepatic resection. Tokyo: Springer; 2007. p. 76–82.
27. Lowe MC, D'Angelica MI. Anatomy of hepatic resectional surgery. Surg Clin N Am. 2016;96(2):183–95.
28. Lau WY, et al. Chapter 10. Other techniques in controlling haemorrhage during liver resection. In: Lau WY, editor. Applied anatomy in liver resection and liver transplantation. Beijing: People's Medical Publishing House; 2010. p. 92.
29. Takayama C. Chapter 2. Left Sectionectomy (S1~S4). In: Makuuchi M, editor. Makuuchi Kanzou Gekagaku (in Japanese)/(translated to Chinese by Yong Zeng). Beijing: People's Medical Publishing House; 2016. p. 110–21.
30. Kamiyama T, Kakisaka T, Orimo T, Wakayama K. Hepatectomy for hepatocellular carcinoma with portal vein tumor thrombus. World J Hepatol. 2017;9(36):1296–304.
31. Lau WY, et al. Chapter 6. Introhepatic Glissonian triad: anatomy relevant to liver resection and liver transplantation. In: Lau WY, editor. Applied anatomy in liver resection and liver transplantation. Beijing: People's Medical Publishing House; 2011. p. 49.
32. Kim SH, Kim YK. Hanging manoeuver for a left hepatectomy using Glisson's approach with a focus on tape position in liver hilum. HPB. 2013;15(9):681–6.
33. Fredet M, Bernier E. Hepatectomie segmentaire droite reglee pour volumineux hemangiome caverneus defoie. Mem Acad Chir. 1956;82:1060–2.
34. Kim KH, Kim HS, Lee YJ, Park KM, Hwang S, Ahn CS, Moon DB, Ha TY, Kim YD, Kim KK, Song KW, Choi ST, Kim DS, Jung DH, Lee SG. Clinical analysis of right anterior segmentectomy for hepatic malignancy. Hepato-Gastroenterology. 2006;53(72):836.
35. Figueroa R, Laurenzi A, Laurent A, Cherqui D. Perihilar Glissonian approach for anatomical parenchymal sparing liver resections: technical aspects: the taping game. Ann Surg. 2018;267(3):537–43.
36. Kirchner VA, Kim KH, Kim SH, Lee SK. Pure laparoscopic right anterior sectionectomy for hepatocellular carcinoma with great vascular exposure. Surg Endosc. 2017;31(8):3349–50.
37. Makuuchi M, Hashikura Y, Kawasaki S, Tan D, Kosuge T, Takayama T. Personal experience of right anterior segmentectomy (segments V and VIII) for hepatic malignancies. Surgery. 1993;114(1):52–8.
38. Nakayama H, Tadatoshi T. Management before hepatectomy for hepatocellular carcinoma with cirrhosis. World J Hepatol. 2015;7(20):2292–302.
39. Malassagne B, Cherqui D, Alon R, Brunetti F, Humeres R, Fagniez PL. Safety of selective vascular clamping for major hepatectomies. J Am Coll Surg. 1998;187(5):482.
40. Miao XY, Hu JX, Dai WD, Zhong DW, Huang SF, Wen Y, Xiong SZ. Anatomic mesohepatectomy with extrahepatic control of hepatic veins. Hepato-Gastroenterology. 2009;56(96):1730–4.

41. Hashimoto T. Chapter 4. Right anterior sectionectomy. In: Makuuchi M, editor. Makuuchi Kanzou Gekagaku (in Japanese)/(translated to Chinese by Yong Zeng). Beijing: People's Medical Publishing House; 2016. p. 122–33.
42. Yamashita YI, Imai K, Tsujita E, Kaida T, Yamao T, Umezaki N, Nakagawa S, Hashimoto D, Chikamoto A, Baba H. Selective venous occlusions for reducing blood loss during right anterior sectionectomy of the liver for hepatocellular carcinoma. J Am Coll Surg. 2017;224(2):e5–9.
43. Cheng YF, Huang TL, Lee TY, Chen TY, Chen CL. Variation of the intrahepatic portal vein; angiographic demonstration and application in living-related hepatic transplantation. Transplant Proc. 1996;28(3):1667–8.
44. Couinaud C. Liver anatomy: portal (and suprahepatic) or biliary segmentation digestive. Surgery. 1999;16(6):459.
45. Covey AM, Brody LA, Getrajdman GI, Sofocleous CT, Brown KT. Incidence, patterns, and clinical relevance of variant portal vein anatomy. AJR Am J Roentgenol. 2004;183(4):1055–64.
46. Koç Z, Oğuzkurt L, Ulusan S. Portal vein variations: clinical implications and frequencies in routine abdominal multidetector CT. Diagn Interv Radiol. 2007;13(2):75.
47. Germain T, Favelier S, Cercueil JP, Denys A, Krausé D, Guiu B. Liver segmentation: practical tips. Diagn Interv Imaging. 2014;95(11):1003–16.
48. Iqbal S, Iqbal R, Iqbal F. Surgical implications of portal vein variations and liver segmentations: a recent update. J Clin Diagn Res. 2017;11(2):AE01.
49. Atasoy C, Ozyürek E. Prevalence and types of main and right portal vein branching variations on MDCT. AJR Am J Roentgenol. 2006;187(3):676–81.
50. Fujimoto J, Hai S, Hirano T, Iimuro Y, Yamanaka J. Anatomic liver resection of right paramedian sector: ventral and dorsal resection. J Hepatobiliary Pancreat Sci. 2015;22(7):538–45.
51. Shimizu H, Sawada S, Kimura F, Yoshidome H, Ohtsuka M, Kato A, Miyazaki M. Clinical significance of biliary vascular anatomy of the right liver for hilar cholangiocarcinoma applied to left hemihepatectomy. Ann Surg. 2009;249(3):435–9.
52. Jia CK, Weng J, Chen YK, Fu Y. Anatomic resection of liver segments 6-8 for hepatocellular carcinoma. World J Gastroenterol. 2014;20(15):4433–9.
53. Chun YS, Ribero D, Abdalla EK, Madoff DC, Mortenson MM, Wei SH, Vauthey JN. Comparison of two methods of future liver remnant volume measurement. J Gastrointest Surg. 2008;12(1):123–8.
54. Yip VSK, Poon RTP, Chok KSH, Chan AC, Dai WC, Tsang SH, Chan SC, Lo CM, Cheung TT. Comparison of survival outcomes between right posterior sectionectomy and right hepatectomy for hepatocellular carcinoma in cirrhotic liver: a single-centre experience. World J Surg. 2015;39:2764–70.
55. Lim C, Ishizawa T, Miyata A, Mise Y, Sakamoto Y, Hasegawa K, Sugawara Y, Kokudo N. Surgical indications and procedures for resection of hepatic malignancies confined to segment VII. Ann Surg. 2016;263:529–37.
56. Pugh RN, Murray-Lyon IM, Dawson JL, Pietroni MC, Williams R. Transection of the oesophagus for bleeding oesophageal varices. Br J Surg. 1973;60(8):646–9.
57. Cai SW, Yang SZ, Lv WP, Yamazaki S, Kakazu T, Miyagawa S, Kawasaki S. Sustained methylene blue staining toguide anatomic hepatectomy forhepatocellular carcinoma: initial experience and technical details. Surgery. 2015;158(1):121–7.
58. Ahn KS, Kang KJ, Park TJ, Kim YH, Lim TJ, Kwon JH. Benefit of systematic segmentectomy of the hepatocellular carcinoma: revisiting the dye injection method for various portal vein branches. Ann Surg. 2013;258(6):1014–21.
59. Fischer L, Cardenas C, Thorn M, Benner A, Grenacher L, Vetter M, Lehnert T, Klar E, Meinzer HP, Lamadé W. Limits of Couinaud's liver segment classification: a quantitative computer-based three-dimensional analysis. J Comput Assist Tomogr. 2002;26:962–7.
60. Shindoh J, Mise Y, Satou S, Sugawara Y, Kokudo N. The intersegmental plane of the liver is not always flat-tricks for anatomical liver resection. Ann Surg. 2010;251:917–22.
61. Torzilli G, Donadon M, Marconi M, Botea F, Palmisano A, Del Fabbro D, Procopio F, Montorsi M. Systematic extended right posterior sectionectomy: a safe and effective alternative to right hepatectomy. Ann Surg. 2008;247(4):603.
62. Torzilli G, Procopio F, Donadon M, Palmisano A, Del Fabbro D, Montorsi M. Anatomical right posterior sectionectomy: a further expansion of the ultrasound-guided compression technique. Updat Surg. 2011;63(2):91–5.
63. Fisher SB, Kneuertz PJ, Dodson RM, Patel SH, Maithel SK, Sarmiento JM, Russell MC, Cardona K, Choti MA, Staley CA 3rd, Pawlik TM, Kooby DA. A comparison of right posterior sectorectomy with formal right hepatectomy: a dual-institution study. HPB. 2013;15(10):753–62.
64. Lau WY. Chapter 2. Liver Segments. In: Lau WY, editor. Applied anatomy in liver resection and liver transplantation. Beijing: People's Medical Publishing House; 2010. p. 21.
65. Nakayama H. Chapter 5. Left lateral sectionectomy. In: Makuuchi M, editor. Makuuchi Kanzou Gekagaku (in Japanese)/(translated to Chinese by Yong Zeng). Beijing: People's Medical Publishing House; 2016. p. 146–55.
66. Ikai I, Arii S, Okazaki M, Okita K, Omata M, Kojiro M, Takayasu K, Nakanuma Y, Makuuchi M, Matsuyama Y, Monden M, Kudo M. Report of the 17th nationwide follow-up survey of primary liver cancer in Japan. Hepatol Res. 2007;37(9):676–91.
67. Arii S, Tanaka J, Yamazoe Y, Minematsu S, Morino T, Fujita K, Maetani S, Tobe T. Predictive factors for intrahepatic recurrence of hepatocellular carcinoma after partial hepatectomy. Cancer. 1992;69(4):913–9.
68. Ikai I, Arii S, Kojiro M, Ichida T, Makuuchi M, Matsuyama Y, Nakanuma Y, Okita K, Omata M, Takayasu K, Yamaoka Y. Reevaluation of prognostic factors for survival after liver resection in patients with hepatocellular carcinoma in a Japanese nationwide survey. Cancer. 2004;101(4):796–802.
69. Llovet JM, Ricci S, Mazzaferro V, Hilgard P, Gane E, Blanc JF, de Oliveira AC, Santoro A, Raoul JL, Forner A, Schwartz M, Porta C, Zeuzem S, Bolondi L, Greten TF, Galle PR, Seitz JF, Borbath I, Häussinger D, Giannaris T, Shan M, Moscovici M, Voliotis D, Bruix J, SHARP Investigators Study Group. Sorafenib in advanced hepatocellular carcinoma. N Engl J Med. 2008;359(23):378–90.
70. Kudo M, Izumi N, Kokudo N, Matsui O, Sakamoto M, Nakashima O, Kojiro M, Makuuchi M, HCC Expert Panel of Japan Society of Hepatology. Management of hepatocellular carcinoma in Japan: consensus-based clinical practice guidelines proposed by the Japan Society of Hepatology (JSH) 2010 updated version. Dig Dis. 2011;29(3):339–64.
71. Minagawa M, Makuuchi M, Takayama T, Ohtomo K. Selection criteria for hepatectomy in patients with hepatocellular carcinoma and portal vein tumor thrombus. Ann Surg. 2001;233(3):379–84.
72. Nagano H, Sakon M, Eguchi H, Kondo M, Yamamoto T, Ota H, Nakamura M, Wada H, Damdinsuren B, Marubashi S, Miyamoto A, Takeda Y, Dono K, Umeshit K, Nakamori S, Monden M. Hepatic resection followed by IFN-alpha and 5-FU for advanced hepatocellular carcinoma with tumor thrombus in the major portal branch. Hepato-Gastroenterology. 2007;54(73):172–9.
73. Cho JY, Han HS, Yoon YS, Shin SH. Feasibility of laparoscopic liver resection for tumors located in the posterosuperior segments of the liver, with a special reference to overcoming current limitations on tumor location. Surgery. 2008;144(1):32.
74. Cherqui D, Husson E, Hammoud R, Malassagne B, Stéphan F, Bensaid S, Rotman N, Fagniez PL. Laparoscopic liver resections: a feasibility study in 30 patients. Ann Surg. 2000;232(6):753.

75. Han HS, Cho JY, Yoon YS. Techniques for performing laparoscopic liver resection in various hepatic locations. J Hepato-Biliary-Pancreat Surg. 2009;16(4):427–32.
76. Iguchi K, Hatano E, Yamanaka K, Tanaka S, Taura K, Uemoto S. Validation of the conventional resection criteria in patients with hepatocellular carcinoma in terms of the incidence of posthepatectomy liver failure and long-term prognosis. Dig Surg. 2015;32(5):344–51.
77. Lau WY, et al. Chapter 6. Intrahepatic Glissonian triad: anatomy relevant to liver resection and liver transplantation. In: Lau WY, editor. Applied anatomy in liver resection and liver transplantation. Beijing: People's Medical Publishing House; 2010. p. 45–9.
78. Dina C, Bordei P, Beşleagă A, Bordei L. Aspects de la vascularisation segmentaire veineuse du foie. Morphologie. 2005;89(287):176.
79. Couinaud C. Le foie: Etudes anatomiques et chirurgicales. Paris: Masson; 1957.
80. Blumgart LH, Baer HU, Czerniak A, Zimmermann A, Dennison AR. Extended left hepatectomy: technical aspects of an evolving procedure. Br J Surg. 1993;80(7):903–6.
81. Vauthey JN, Pawlik TM, Abdalla EK, Arens JF, Nemr RA, Wei SH, Kennamer DL, Ellis LM, Curley SA. Is extended hepatectomy for hepatobiliary malignancy justified? Ann Surg. 2004;239(5): 722–32.
82. Wu CC, Ho WL, Chen JT, Tang CS, Yeh DC, Liu TJ, P'eng FK. Mesohepatectomy for centrally located hepatocellular carcinoma: an appraisal of a rare procedure. J Am Coll Surg. 1999;188(5):508–15.
83. Lee JG, Choi SB, Kim KS, Choi JS, Lee WJ, Kim BR. Central bisectionectomy for centrally located hepatocellular carcinoma. Br J Surg. 2008;95(8):990–5.
84. Dai WD, Hu JX, Miao XY, Zhong DW, Wen Y, Xiong SZ. Intrahepatic Glissonian access for mesohepatectomy in cirrhotic patients. Hepato-Gastroenterology. 2008;55(85):1153–7.
85. Miao XY, Hu JX, Dai WD, Zhong DW, Xiong SZ. Null-margin mesohepatectomy for centrally located hepatocellular carcinoma in cirrhotic patients. Hepato-Gastroenterology. 2011;58(106):575–82.
86. Scudamore CH, Buczkowski AK, Shayan H, Ho SG, Legiehn GM, Chung SW, Owen DA. Mesohepatectomy. Am J Surg. 2000;179(5):356–60.
87. McBride CM, Wallace S. Cancer of the right lobe of the liver: a variety of operative procedures. Arch Surg. 1972;105(2):289–96.
88. Chouillard E, Cherqui D, Tayar C, Brunetti F, Fagniez PL. Anatomical bi- and trisegmentectomies as alternatives to extensive liver resections. Ann Surg. 2003;238(1):29–34.
89. Jacobs M, McDonough J, ReMine SG. Resection of central hepatic malignant lesions. Am Surg. 2003;69(3):186–9.
90. Ogura Y, Matsuda S, Sakurai H, Kawarada Y, Mizumoto R. Central bisegmentectomy of the liver plus caudate lobectomy for carcinoma of the gallbladder. Dig Surg. 1988;15(3):218–23.
91. Hu RH, Lee PH, Chang YC, Ho MC, Yu SC. Treatment of centrally located hepatocellular carcinoma with central hepatectomy. Surgery. 2003;133(3):251–6.
92. Yu WB, Rao A, Vu V, Xu L, Rao JY, Wu JX. Management of centrally located hepatocellular carcinoma: update 2016. World J Hepatol. 2017;9(13):627–34.
93. Wu CC. Progress of liver resection for hepatocellular carcinoma in Taiwan. Jpn J Clin Oncol. 2017;47(5):375–80.
94. Qiu J, Chen S, Wu H, Du C. The prognostic value of a classification system for centrally located liver tumors in the setting of hepatocellular carcinoma after mesohepatectomy. Surg Oncol. 2016; 25(4):441–7.
95. Yang LY, Chang RM, Lau WY, Ou DP, Wu W, Zeng ZJ. Mesohepatectomy for centrally located large hepatocellular carcinoma: indications, techniques, and outcomes. Surgery. 2014; 156(5):1177–87.
96. Li J, Wang C, Song J, Chen N, Jiang L, Yang J, Yan L. Mesohepatectomy versus extended hemihepatectomies for centrally located liver tumors: a meta-analysis. Sci Rep. 2017;7(1):9329.
97. Li W, Li L, Minigalin D, Wu H. Anatomic mesohepatectomy versus extended hepatectomy for patients with centrally located hepatocellular carcinoma. HPB. 2018. pii: S1365-182X(17):31166-8.
98. Billingsley KG, Jarnagin WR, Fong Y, Blumgart LH. Segment-oriented hepatic resection in the management of malignant neoplasms of the liver. J Am Coll Surg. 1998;187(5):471–81.
99. Mazziotti A, Maeda A, Ercolani G, Cescon M, Grazi GL, Pierangeli F. Isolated resection of segment 8 for liver tumors: a new approach for anatomical segmentectomy. Arch Surg. 2000;135(10):1224–9.
100. Hu JX, Dai WD, Miao XY, Zhong DW, Huang SF, Wen Y, Xiong SZ. Anatomic resection of segment VIII of liver for hepatocellular carcinoma in cirrhotic patients based on an intrahepatic Glissonian approach. Surgery. 2009;146(5):854–60.
101. Kishi Y, Hasegawa K, Kaneko J, Aoki T, Beck Y, Sugawara Y, Makuuchi M, Kokudo N. Resection of segment VIII for hepatocellular carcinoma. Br J Surg. 2012;99(8):1105–12.
102. Launois B, Tay KH. Intrahepatic Glissonian approach in hepatocellular carcinoma. Singapore: World Scientific Publishing; 2008. p. 429–46.
103. Yoshida H, Katayose Y, Rikiyama T, Motoi F, Onogawa T, Egawa S, Unno M. Segmentectomy of the liver. J Hepatobiliary Pancreat Sci. 2012;19(1):67–71.
104. Hasegawa K, Kokudo N, Imamura H, Matsuyama Y, Aoki T, Minagawa M, Sano K, Sugawara Y, Takayama T, Makuuchi M. Prognostic impact of anatomic resection for hepatocellular carcinoma. Ann Surg. 2005;242(2):252–9.
105. Nakayama H. Chapter 9. S7 resection. In: Makuuchi M, editor. Makuuchi Kanzou Gekagaku (in Japanese)/(translated to Chinese by Yong Zeng). Beijing: People's Medical Publishing House; 2016. p. 188–95.
106. Tanaka K, Shimada H, Matsumoto C, Matsuo K, Nagano Y, Endo I, Togo S. Anatomic versus limited nonanatomic resection for solitary hepatocellular carcinoma. Surgery. 2008;143(5):607–15.
107. Kang KJ, Ahn KS. Anatomical resection of hepatocellular carcinoma: a critical review of the procedure and its benefits on survival. World J Gastroenterol. 2017;23(7):1139–46.
108. Lui WY, Chau GY, Loong CC, Tsay SH, Wu JC, King KL, Chiu JH, Lai CR, P'eng FK. Hepatic segmentectomy for curative resection of primary hepatocellular carcinoma. Arch Surg. 1995;130(10):1090–7.
109. Makuuchi M, Imamura H, Sugawara Y, Takayama T. Progress in surgical treatment of hepatocellular carcinoma. Oncology. 2002;62(1):74–81.
110. Liau KH, Blumgart LH, Dematteo RP. Segment-oriented approach to liver resection. Surg Clin North Am. 2004;84(2):543.
111. Shou-Wang C, Shi-Zhong Y, Wen-Ping L, Geng C, Wan-qing G, Wei-dong D, Wei-yi W, Zhi-qiang H, Jia-hong D. Sustained methylene blue staining to guide anatomic hepatectomy for hepatocellular carcinoma: initial experience and technical details. Surgery. 2015;158(1):121–7.
112. Eguchi S, Kanematsu T, Arii S, Okazaki M, Okita K, Omata M, Ikai I, Kudo M, Kojiro M, Makuuchi M. Comparison of the outcomes between an anatomical subsegmentectomy and a non-anatomical minor hepatectomy for single hepatocellular carcinomas based on a Japanese nationwide survey. Surgery. 2008;143(4):469–75.
113. Regimbeau JM, Kianmanesh R, Farges O, Dondero F, Sauvanet A, Belghiti J. Extent of liver resection influences the outcome in patients with cirrhosis and small hepatocellular carcinoma. Surgery. 2002;131(3):311–7.
114. Torzilli G, Procopio F, Cimino M, Del Fabbro D, Palmisano A, Donadon M, Montorsi M. Anatomical segmental and subsegmental resection of the liver for hepatocellular carcinoma: a new

approach by means of ultrasound-guided vessel compression. Ann Surg. 2009;251(2):229–35.
115. Wakai T, Shirai Y, Sakata J, Kaneko K, Cruz PV, Akazawa K, Hatakeyama K. Anatomic resection independently improves long-term survival in patients with T1-T2 hepatocellular carcinoma. Ann Surg Oncol. 2007;14(4):1356–65.
116. Imamura DH, Matsuyama Y, Miyagawa Y, Ishida K, Shimada R, Miyagawa S, Makuuchi M, Kawasaki S. Prognostic significance of anatomical resection and des-γ-carboxy prothrombin in patients with hepatocellular carcinoma. Br J Surg. 1999;86(8):1032–8.
117. Castaing D, Garden OJ, Bismuth H. Segmental liver resection using ultrasound-guided selective portal venous occlusion. Ann Surg. 1989;210(1):20–3.
118. Cho A, Okazumi S, Takayama W, Takeda A, Iwasaki K, Sasagawa S, Natsume T, Kono T, Kondo S, Ochiai T. Anatomy of the right anterosuperior area (segment 8) of the liver: evaluation with helical CT during arterial portography. Radiology. 2000;214(2):491–5.
119. Ohashi I, Ina H, Okada Y, Yoshida T, Gomi N, Himeno Y, Hanafusa K, Shibuya H. Segmental anatomy of the liver under the right diaphragmatic dome: evaluation with axial CT. Radiology. 1996;200(3):779–83.
120. van Leeuwen MS, Noordzij J, Fernandez MA, Hennipman A, Feldberg MA, Dillon EH. Portal venous and segmental anatomy of the right hemiliver: observations based on three-dimensional spiral CT renderigs. AJR Am J Roentgenol. 1994;163(6):1395–404.
121. Makuuchi M. Intrahepatic architecture of the portal vein in right anterior sector of the liver by ultrasound imaging approach. Kanzo. 1986;27:391. [In Japanese].
122. Couinaud C. Surgical anatomy of the liver revised. Paris: Acheve D'imprimer Sur Les Presses; 1989.
123. Miyagawa S. Surgical strategy for HCC using ICG test. Liver Cancer. 2013;2:108–9.
124. Nakayama H. Chapter 10. S5 resection. In: Makuuchi M, editor. Makuuchi Kanzou Gekagaku (in Japanese)/(translated to Chinese by Yong Zeng). Beijing: People's Medical Publishing House; 2016. p. 196–205.
125. Huang JS, Dai WD, Miao XY, Zhong DW, Xiong SZ, Hu JX. Null-margin bisegmentectomy VII-VIII for hepatocellular carcinoma in cirrhotic patients. Hepato-Gastroenterology. 2012;59(118):1706–9.
126. Makuuchi M, Hasegawa H, Yamazaki S. Ultrasonically guided subsegmentectomy. Surg Gynecol Obstet. 1985;161(4):346–50.
127. Takayama T, Makuuchi M, Watanabe K, Kosuge T, Takayasu K, Yamazaki S, Hasegawa H. A new method for mapping hepatic subsegment: counterstaining identification technique. Surgery. 1991;109(2):226–9.
128. Cucchetti A, Cescon M, Ercolani G, Bigonzi E, Torzilli G, Pinna AD. A comprehensive meta-regression analysis on outcome of anatomic resection versus non-anatomic resection for hepatocellular carcinoma. Ann Surg Oncol. 2012;19(12):3697–705.
129. Lim C, Ishizawa T, Miyata A, Sakamoto Y, Hasegawa K, Sugawara Y, Kokudo N. Surgical indications and procedures for resection of hepatic malignancies confined to segment VII. Ann Surg. 2015;263(3):529–37.
130. Launois B, Tay KH. Introhepatic Glissonian approach. In: Lau WY, editor. Hepatocellular carcinoma. Singapore: World Scientific Publishing; 2008. p. 429–46.
131. Zimmitti G, Roses RE, Andreou A, Shindoh J, Curley SA, Aloia TA, Vauthey JN. Greater complexity of liver surgery is not associated with an increased incidence of liver-related complications except for bile leak: an experience with 2,628 consecutive resections. J Gastrointest Surg. 2013;17(1):57–64.
132. Sadamori H, Yagi T, Shinoura S, Umeda Y, Yoshida R, Satoh D, Nobuoka D, Utsumi M, Fujiwara T. Risk factors for major morbidity after liver resection for hepatocellular carcinoma. Br J Surg. 2013;100(1):122–9.
133. Dokmak S, Fteriche FS, Borscheid R, Cauchy F, Farges O, Belghiti J. Liver resections in the 21st century: we are far from zero mortality. HPB (Oxford). 2013;15(11):908–15.
134. Poon RT, Fan ST, Lo CM, Liu CL, Lam CM, Yuen WK, Yeung C, Wong J. Improving perioperative outcome expands the role of hepatectomy in management of benign and malignant hepatobiliary diseases: analysis of 1222 consecutive patients from a prospective database. Ann Surg. 2004;240(4):698–708.
135. Mullen JT, Ribero D, Reddy SK, Donadon M, Zorzi D, Gautam S, Abdalla EK, Curley SA, Capussotti L, Clary BM, Vauthey JN. Hepatic insufficiency and mortality in 1,059 noncirrhotic patients undergoing major hepatectomy. J Am Coll Surg. 2007;204(5):854–62.
136. Kingham TP, Correa-Gallego C, D'Angelica MI, Gönen M, DeMatteo RP, Fong Y, Allen PJ, Blumgart LH, Jarnagin WR. Hepatic parenchymal preservation surgery: decreasing morbidity and mortality rates in 4,152 resections for malignancy. J Am Coll Surg. 2015;220(4):471–9.
137. Shindoh J, Vauthey JN, Zimmitti G, Curley SA, Huang SY, Mahvash A, Gupta S, Wallace MJ, Aloia TA. Analysis of the efficacy of portal vein embolization for patients with extensive liver malignancy and very low future liver remnant volume, including a comparison with the associating liver partition with portal vein ligation for staged hepatectomy approach. J Am Coll Surg. 2013;217(1):126–33.

Other Types of Hepatic Resection for HCC

Jixiong Hu, Weidong Dai, Chun Liu, and Tenglong Tang

Resection of the Caudate Lobe for Hepatocellular Carcinoma

Jixiong Hu, Yu Wen, Zhongkun Zuo, and Tenglong Tang

Anatomy of the Caudate Lobe and Surgical Approach for Resection of the Caudate Lobe

The caudate lobe lies between major vascular structures: the inferior vena cava posteriorly and the portal triad inferiorly and the right and the middle and left hepatic veins at the upper part [1]. Couinaud's definition of the caudate lobe is based on morphological segmentation but not on portal perfusion. Thus, Kumon's definition of the caudate lobe was widely accepted and applied, in which the caudate lobe was divided into three parts: the Spiegel lobe, paracaval portion, and caudate process based on portal perfusion [2, 3]. The branches of the paracaval portion were defined as the branches originating from the first-order branches of the portal vein and passing toward the cranial side, along with the retrohepatic inferior vena cava. Many other small vessels from the portal vein go into the caudate lobe, but usually there is one large trunk. The large vein is about 1 mm in diameter and 5 mm in length. Isolation and division of this branch is an important step in the dissection of the caudate blood supply at the base of the umbilical fissure [4].

Commonly the posterior edge of the caudate lobe on the left has a fibrous attachment which extends posterior behind the vena cava to join segment VII. It is noteworthy to realize that in up to 50% of individuals, this fibrous component is replaced, partly or completely, by hepatic parenchyma [5]. And the caudate lobe may thus completely embrace the retrohepatic inferior vena cava and join segment VII on the right side. Such a circumstance may pose additional technical difficulty in the resection of the entire caudate lobe by the anterior approach. The caudate venous drainage is unique in that it is the only hepatic segment which drains directly into the retrohepatic inferior vena cava.

Because of its deep location behind the liver parenchyma and its proximity to its surrounding major vascular vessels, elective complete isolated caudate lobectomy is probably the most demanding resection from a technical point of view [6], and limited literature addresses this subject [6–19]. Meanwhile, nonsurgical treatment modalities, including percutaneous ethanol ablation and radiofrequency ablation, are difficult because of probable inaccessibility and difficulties encountered in accurately imaging the tumors in the caudate lobe, and the results are less certain than with surgery [4]. Experience with transarterial chemotherapy embolization (TACE) in treating tumors in the caudate lobe is also discouraging as a result of the

The corresponding author of section "Resection of the Caudate Lobe for Hepatocellular Carcinoma" is Zhongkun Zuo, Email: arthasreal@csu.edu.cn.
The corresponding author of section "Bisegmentectomy VII–VIII" is Weidong Dai, Email: 494489457@qq.com.
The corresponding author of section "Non-anatomic Mesohepatectomy for HCC" is Chun Liu, Email: liuchun504@163.com.
The corresponding author of section "Hepatic Resection for Hepatocellular Carcinoma with Bile Duct Tumor Thrombus" is Weidong Dai, Email: 494489457@qq.com.

J. X. Hu · W. D. Dai (✉) · C. Liu
Department of Hepatobiliary Surgery and Hunan Provincial Key Laboratory of Hepatobiliary Disease Research, The Second Xiangya Hospital, Central South University, Changsha, Hunan, PR China
e-mail: 13908459086@163.com; 494489457@qq.com; liuchun504@163.com

T. L. Tang
Department of Minimally Invasive Surgery, The Second Xiangya Hospital, Central South University, Changsha, Hunan, PR China
e-mail: tangtenglong@csu.edu.cn

J. S. Huang et al. (eds.), *Atlas of Anatomic Hepatic Resection for Hepatocellular Carcinoma*, https://doi.org/10.1007/978-981-13-0668-6_5

small size of supplying arteries [8, 20, 21]. Therefore, surgical resection is almost the only available choice for treatment of hepatocellular carcinoma in this unique location.

According to the literature [22–24], there are probably four types of surgical approach for resection of the caudate lobe. The first approach entails a left lateral sectionectomy or left hemihepatectomy or left trisectionectomy en bloc with the caudate lobectomy. This approach is often taken. The second approach requires a right hemihepatectomy or a right trisectionectomy combined with the caudate lobectomy. The third approach is a central or anterior transhepatic approach. Although this technique could provide a safe strategic alternative for isolated complete caudate lobectomy, it is technically challenging, is time-consuming, and may be associated with a significant amount of blood loss [4, 19]. The fourth approach is the anterior approach for isolated partial or complete caudate lobectomy without removal of other hepatic lobes, with which our surgical technique is in agreement.

Surgical Indications for Hepatocellular Carcinoma Confined to the Caudate Lobe

For tumors confined to the caudate lobe, the selection of the surgical approach should be based on the liver function reserve and the location, size of the tumor, and its relationship with its adjacent liver lobe. In terms of liver function evaluation, serum total bilirubin level is less than 1 mg/dl, and ICGR15 is less than 20%; either the left-side or the right-side approach can be applied, combined with partial or complete resection of the caudate lobe. In contrast, 20% < ICGR15 < 30% and 1 mg/dl < serum TBIL <2 mg/dl may allow isolated partial or complete resection of the caudate lobe. If 30% < ICGR15 < 40%, just wedge or elucleation resection is indicated. In addition, its proximity to the retrohepatic inferior vena cava and its venous drainage directly into the vena cava decides that any type of caudate lobectomy is technically more demanding, and intraoperative massive bleeding should be rapidly controlled by tightening the tourniquets, which have been encircled around the hepatic pedicle and infra- and suprahepatic inferior vena cava, respectively, to achieve total vascular exclusion.

Anterior Approach for Complete Isolated Caudate Lobectomy (Fig. 1)

Operative Procedures	Technical Details
Laparotomy and mobilization of the right hemiliver ↓	◀ A right subcostal incision can provide a good surgical view. The right hemiliver was dissected away from its surrounding structures.
Mobilization of the caudate process ↓	◀ The several portal triads arising from the right hepatic pedicle and entering into the caudate process was isolated, clamped, divided and suture-ligated.
Mobilization of the left hemiliver ↓	◀ The left hemiliver was completely freed off from its surrounding structures.
Mobilization of the spiegel lobe and the paracaval portion ↓	◀ The Spiegel Lobe and the Paracaval Portion was dissected away from the retrohepatic inferior vena cava.
The right edge of the caudate process ↓	◀ IOUS was used on the inferior surface of the right liver to ascertain the proximal trunk of the middle hepatic vein and the right hepatic vein.
Hepatic parenchymal transection ↓	◀ Using IOUS as a guide, parenchymal transection was carried out using the clamp-crushing methodas close to the root of the right hepatic vein and the middle hepatic vein as possible. Havingremoved the specimen, the root of the righthepatic veinwas exposed on the cut surface.
Closure of the abdominal cavity and drainage	◀ He mostasis and biliostasis were achieved by electrocautory, ligation or suture-ligated.Arubber tube was placed in the infrahepatic space and secured.

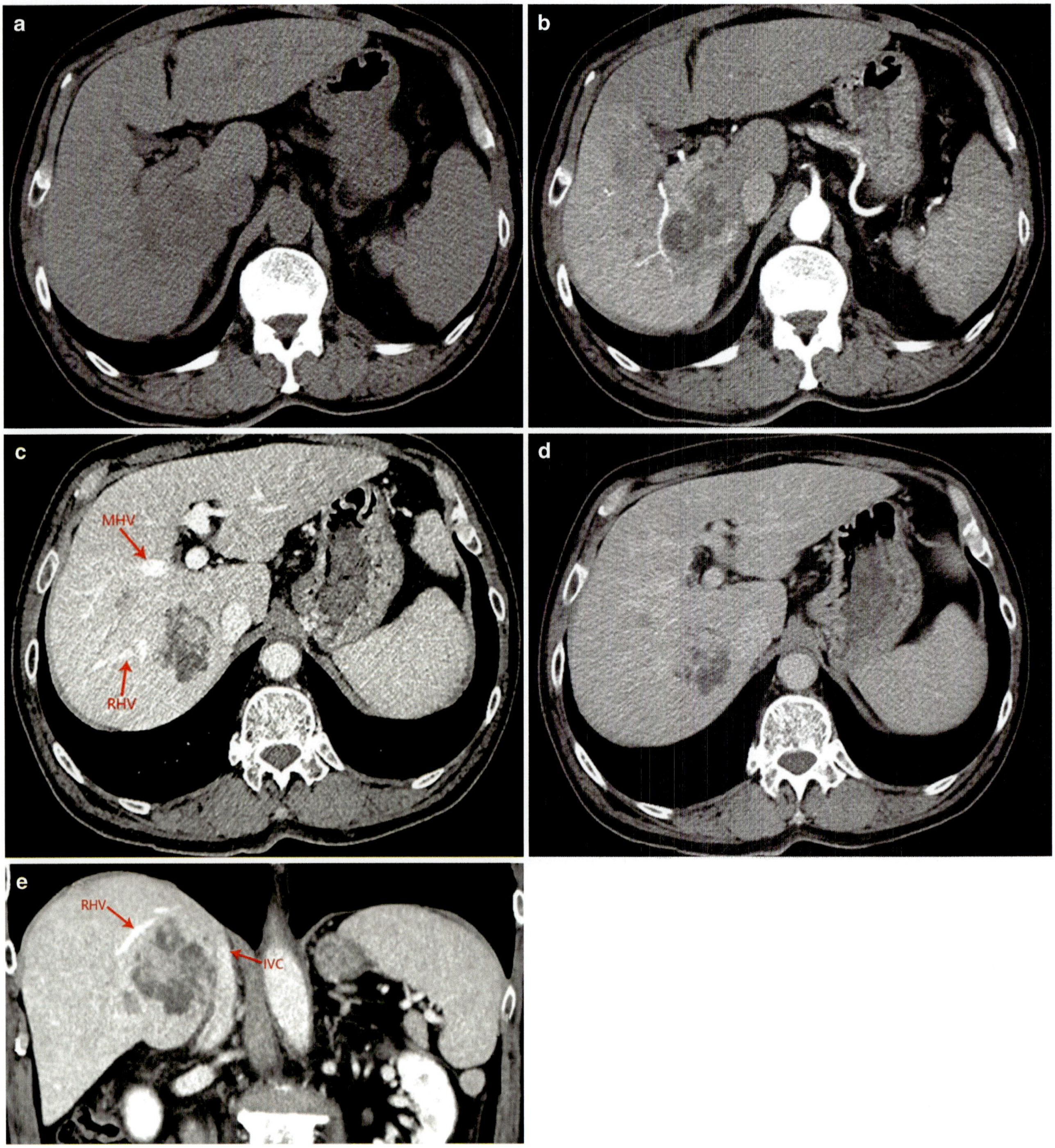

Fig. 1 (**a**) Preoperative CT (precontrast). The tumor, which appears mildly hypodense, is located in the caudate process. (**b**) Preoperative CT (hepatic arterial phase). The tumor shows heterogeneous enhancement. (**c**) Preoperative CT (hepatic venous phase). The tumor shows enhancement fades. (**d**) Preoperative CT (interstitial phase). The tumor shows subtle washout. (**e**) Preoperative CT (coronal section of the tumor). *RHV* right hepatic vein, *MHV* middle hepatic vein, *IVC* inferior vena cava

Abdominal Incision and Mobilization of the Right Hemiliver (Figs. 2, 3, 4, and 5)

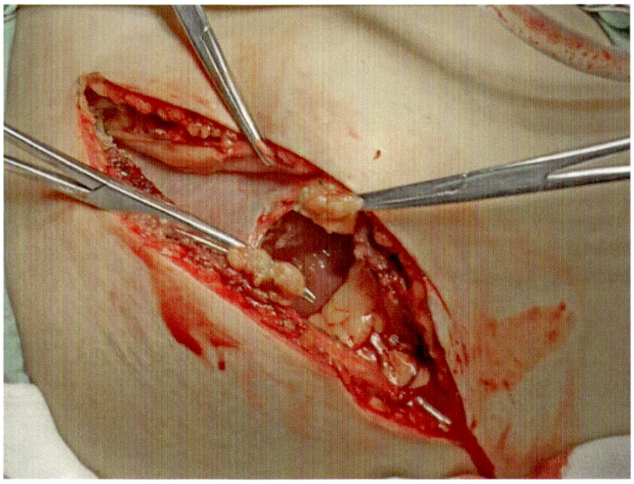

Fig. 2 The ligamentum teres was isolated, divided, and sutured near to the umbilicus

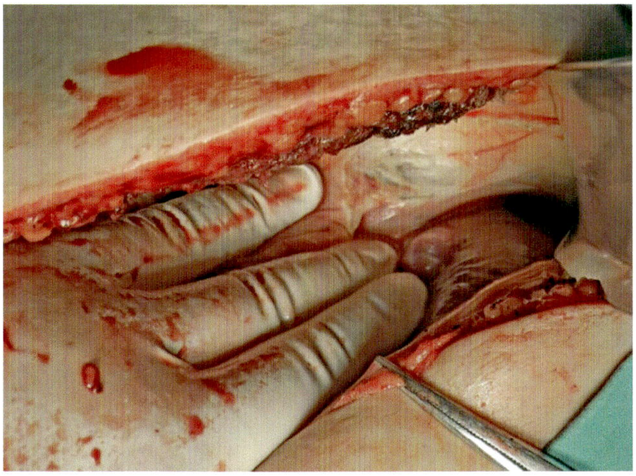

Fig. 3 The falciform ligament was divided up to the anterior surface of the suprahepatic IVC, and the roots of the RHV, MHV, and LHV or the common trunk of the MHV and LHV were dissected anteriorly and completely exposed. *IVC* inferior vena cava, *RHV* right hepatic vein, *MHV* middle hepatic vein, *LHV* left hepatic vein

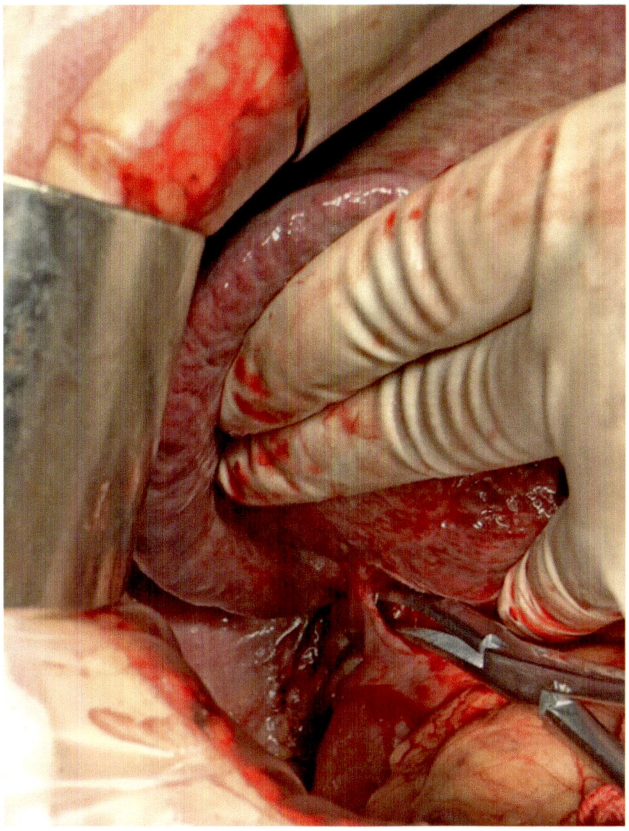

Fig. 4 The hepatocolic ligament was dissected and divided with electrocautery

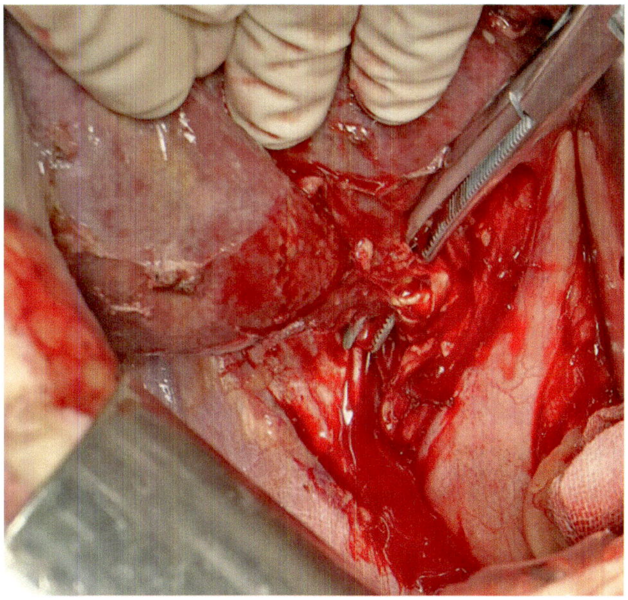

Fig. 5 The right adrenal gland was dissected away from the posterior portion of the right hemiliver

Mobilization of the Caudate Process

(Figs. 6, 7, 8, and 9)

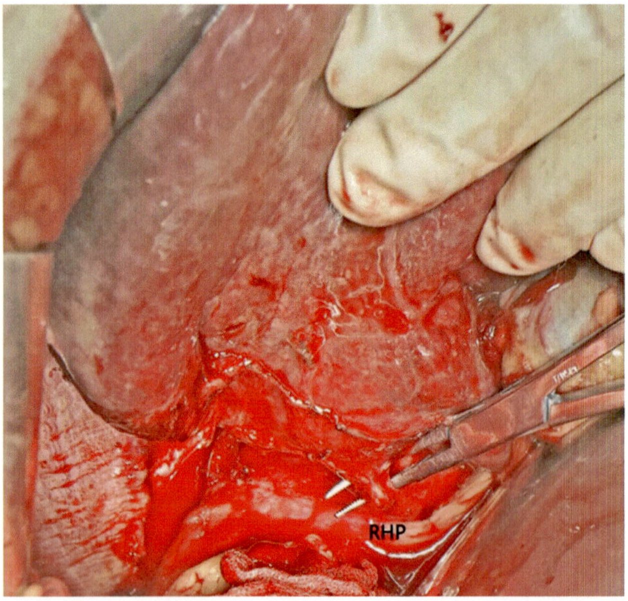

Fig. 6 Having freeing the right liver away from the surrounding structures, the right liver was lifted upward to expose the right hepatic pedicle. The portal triad arising from the right hepatic pedicle (RHP) to the caudate process was isolated

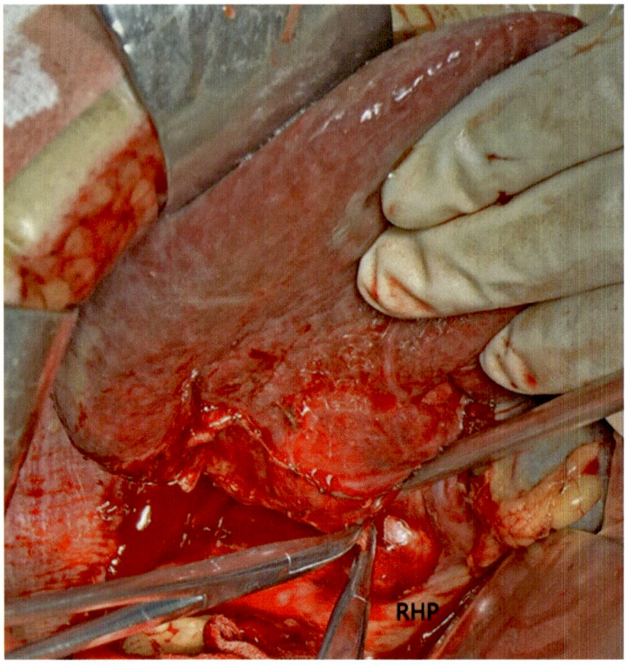

Fig. 7 The portal triad entering into the caudate process was clamped. *RHP* right hepatic pedicle

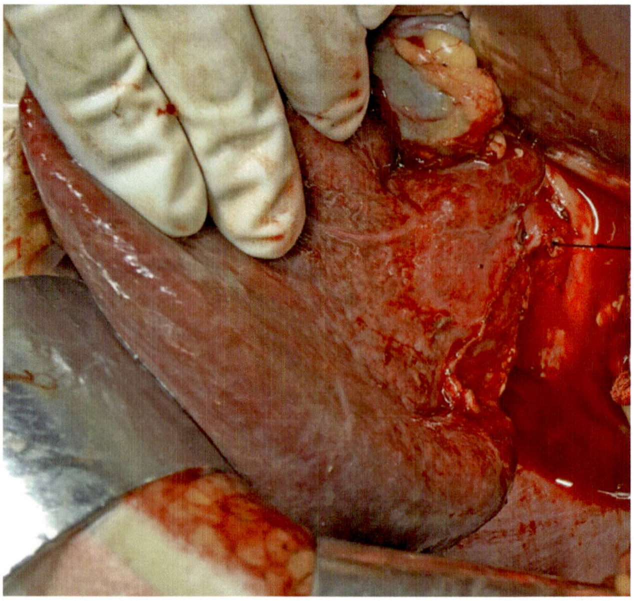

Fig. 8 The portal triad to the caudate process was divided and the distal and proximal stump was sutured separately

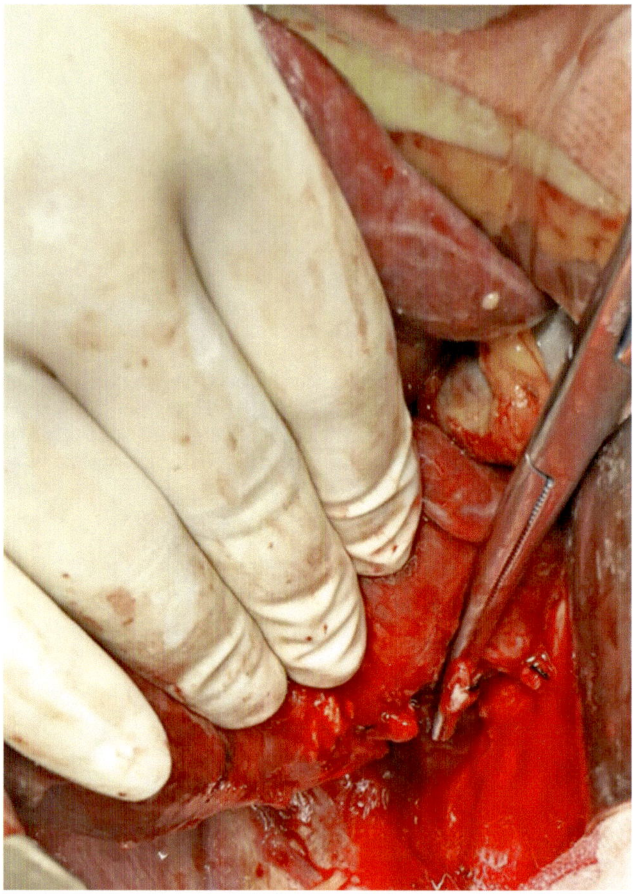

Fig. 9 The inferior right hepatic vein (IRHV) was divided and sutured

Mobilization of the Left Hemiliver
(Figs. 10, 11, 12, 13, and 14)

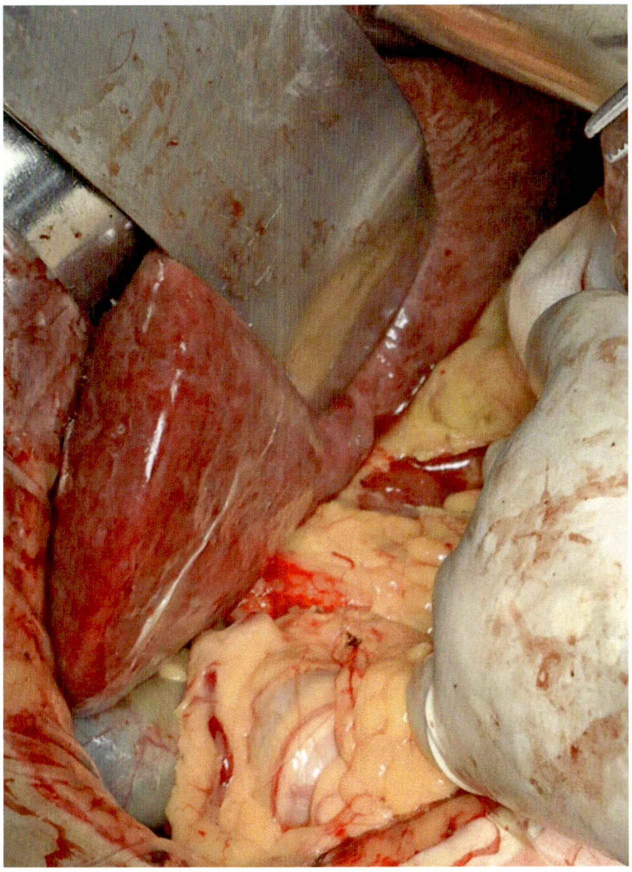

Fig. 10 Dissection was turned to the left liver. The less omentum was cut open

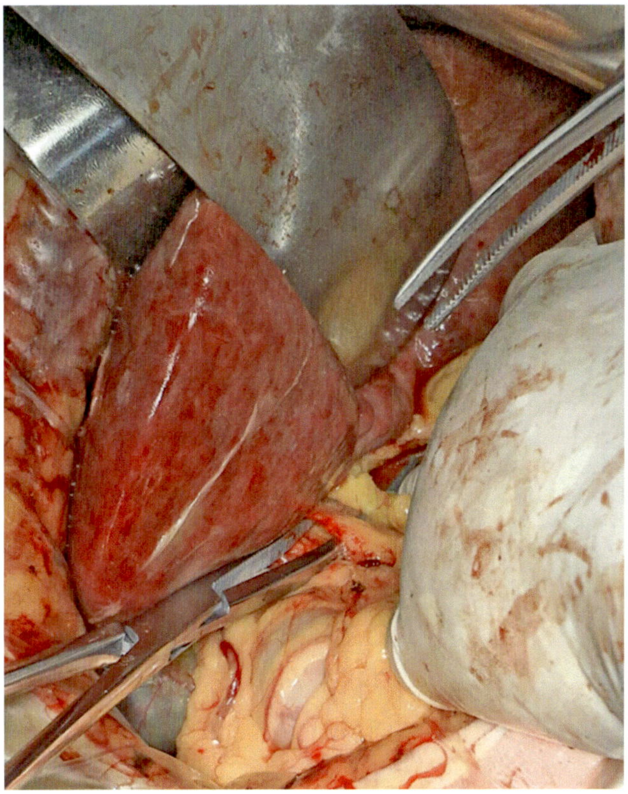

Fig. 11 The gastrohepatic ligament was divided

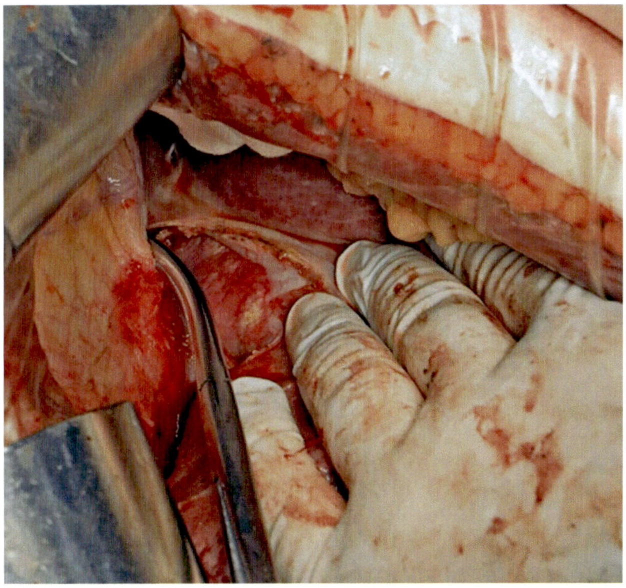

Fig. 12 The left liver was turned over upward and medially and the ligamentum venosum was incised at the level of the tip of the Spiegel lobe

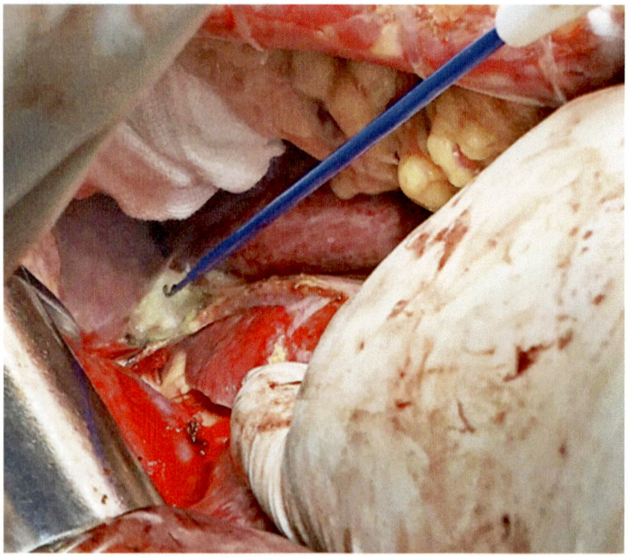

Fig. 13 The left coronary ligament was widely incised with electrocautery toward the left triangular ligament

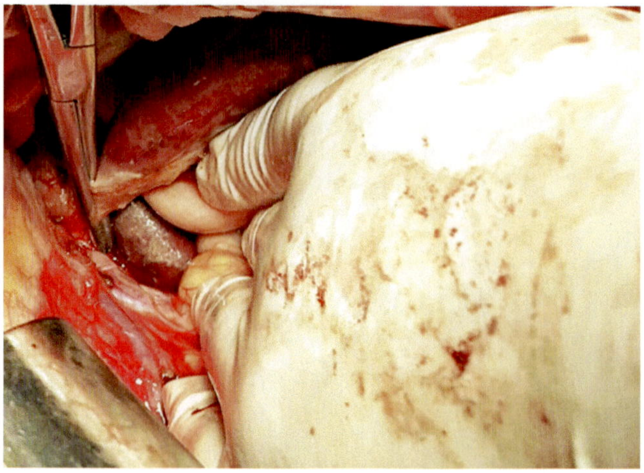

Fig. 14 The left triangular ligament was clamped and divided with electrocautery

Mobilization of the Spiegel Lobe and the Paracaval Portion (Figs. 15, 16, 17, 18, and 19)

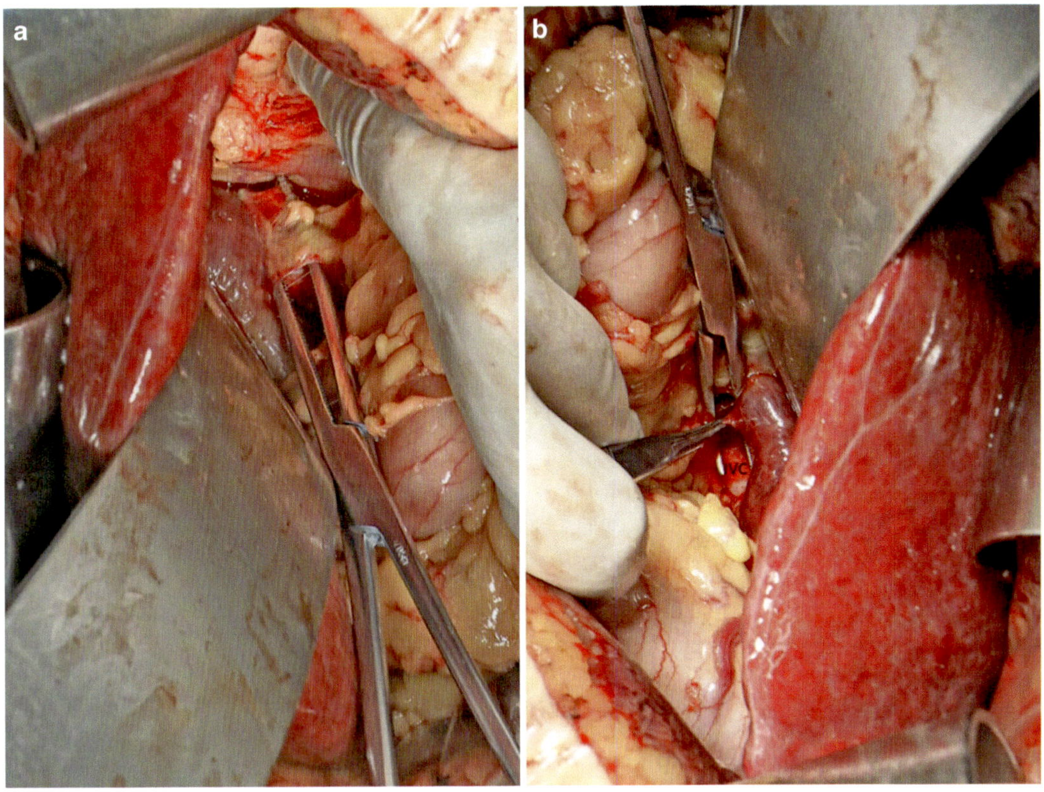

Fig. 15 (**a**, **b**) The Spiegel lobe was turned over upward and medially, the hepatocaval ligament was widely incised. *IVC* inferior vena cava

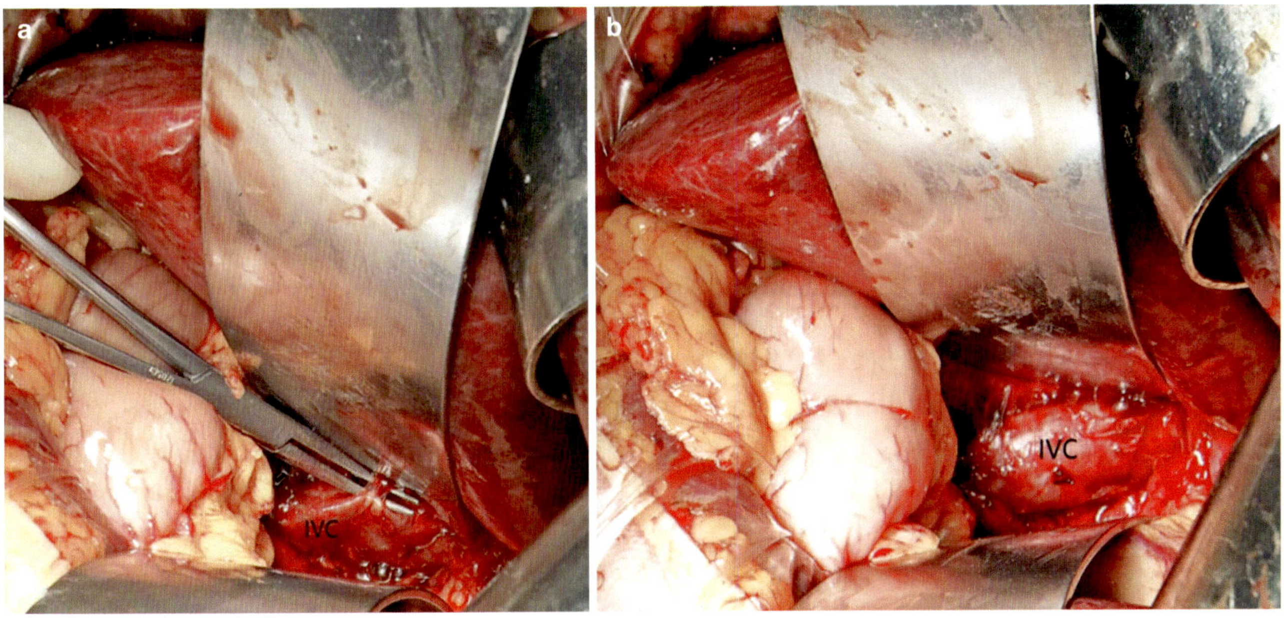

Fig. 16 (**a**, **b**) The Spiegel lobe was continuously lifted upward and medially to expose the left-sided and anterior wall of the retrohepatic IVC; the left-sided short veins were isolated, divided, and ligated one by one. *IVC* inferior vena cava

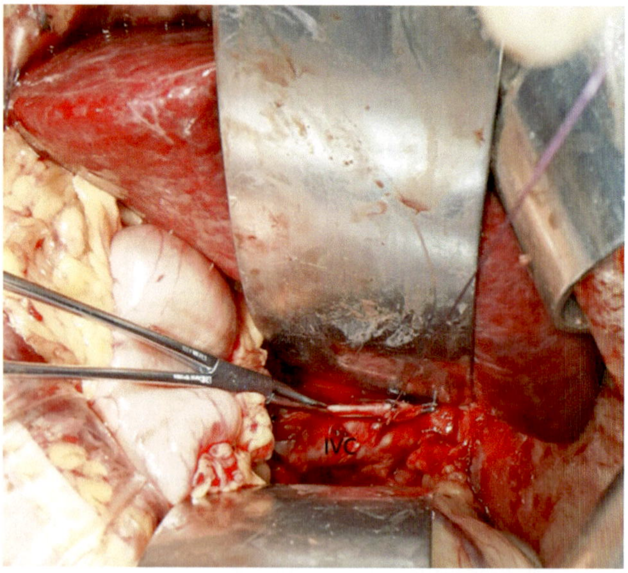

Fig. 17 The anterior wall of the retrohepatic IVC was lacerated and repaired with 4-0 polypropylene. *IVC* inferior vena cava

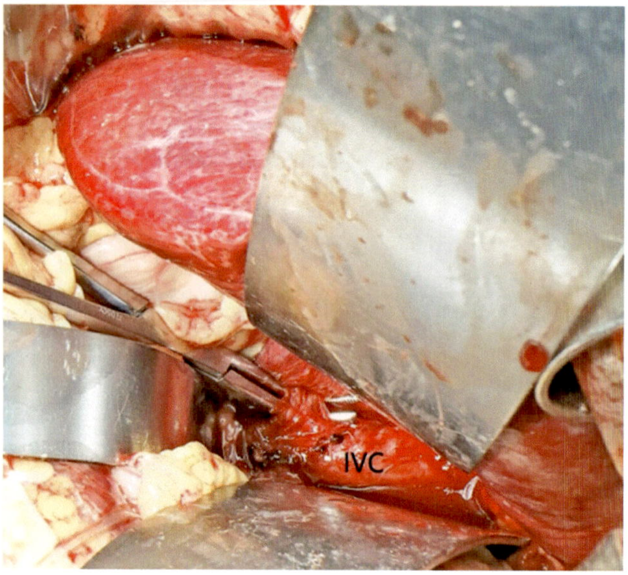

Fig. 18 The right-sided retrohepatic short veins were isolated, divided, and ligated caudal-cranially, respectively. *IVC* inferior vena cava

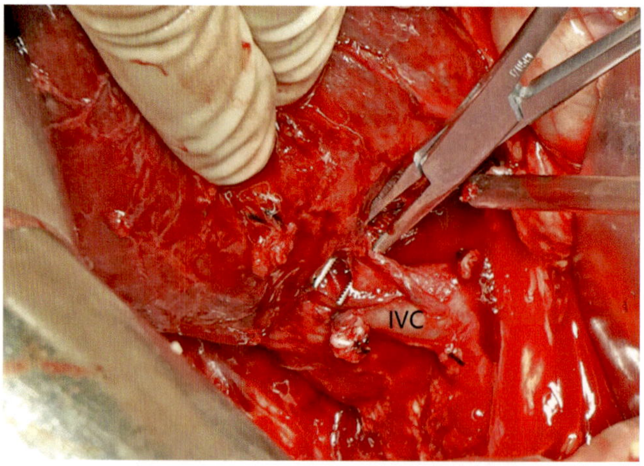

Fig. 19 To continue to free the paracaval portion from the retrohepatic IVC upward to the hepatocaval confluence, all of the retrohepatic short veins were continually isolated, divided, and ligated caudal-cranially, respectively. *IVC* inferior vena cava

Further Mobilization of the Caudate Process (Fig. 20)

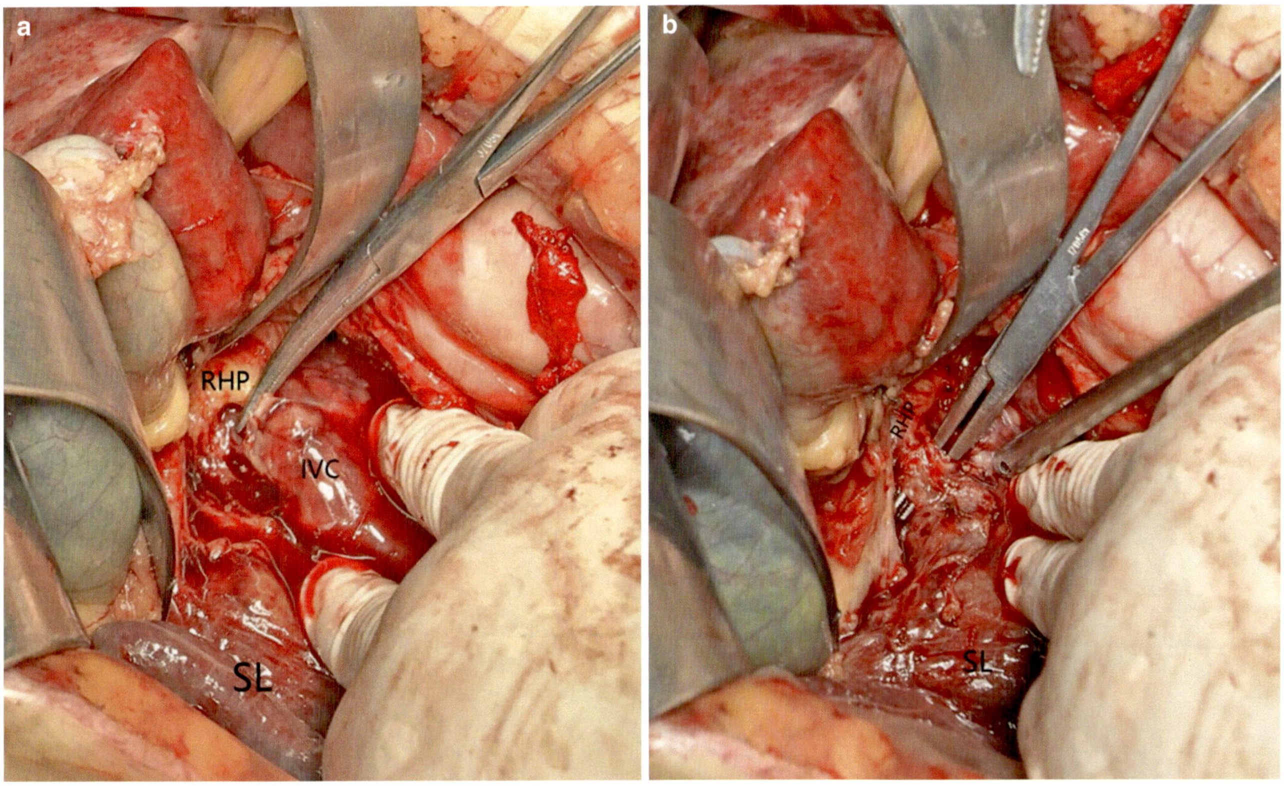

Fig. 20 (**a**, **b**) The Spiegel lobe (SL) was completely dissected off of the vena cava and was turned over the retrohepatic IVC to the right infrahepatic space; the branches from the right hepatic pedicle (RHP) into the caudate process were further isolated, divided, and ligated. *IVC* inferior vena cava

Hepatic Parenchymal Transection (Fig. 21)

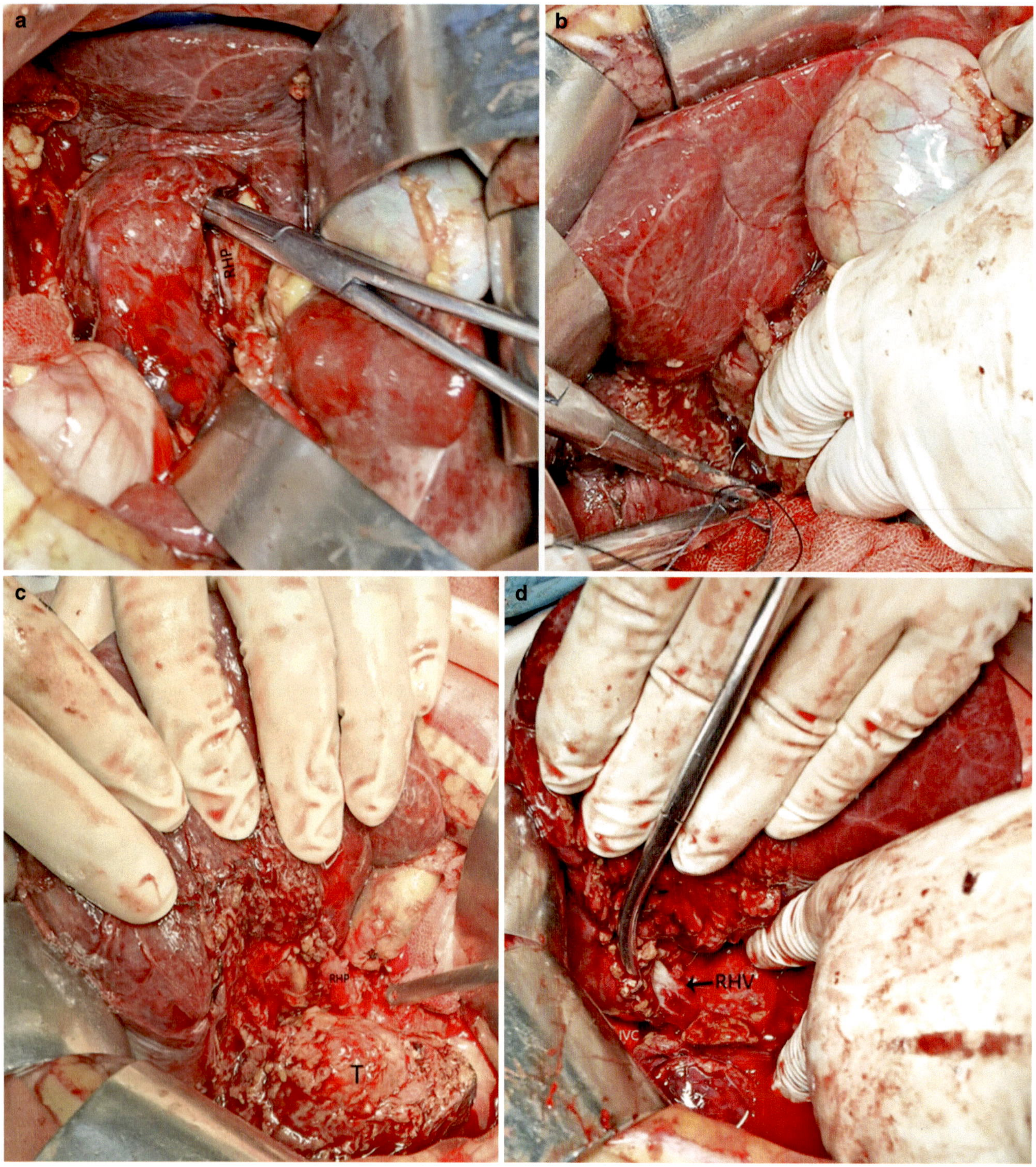

Fig. 21 (**a**–**f**) Having used intraoperative ultrasound (IOUS) to decide the transectional plane within the liver substance, the hepatic parenchymal transection was carried out between the caudate process and segments V, VI, and VII, using clamp crushing method. *RHP* right hepatic pedicle, *T* tumor, *RHV* right hepatic vein, *IVC* inferior vena cava

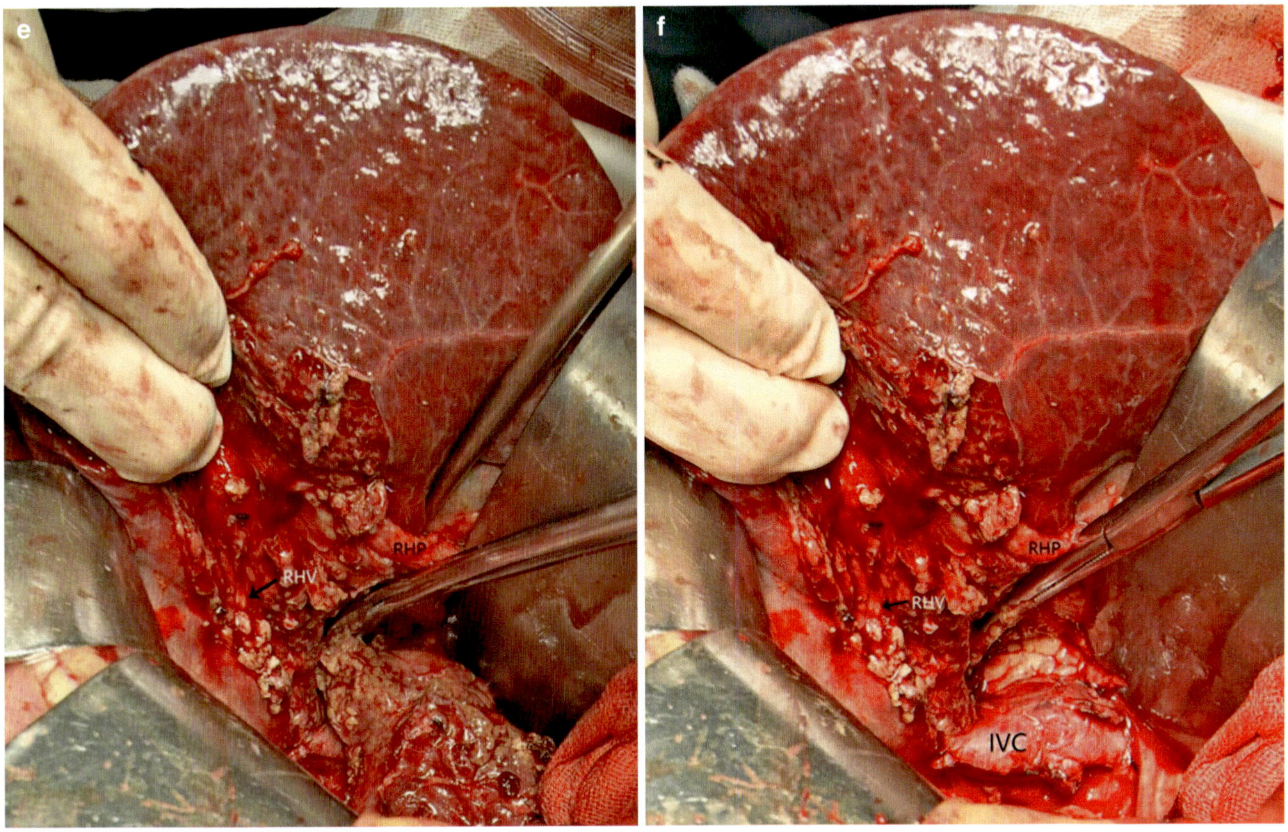

Fig. 21 (continued)

Raw Area of the Residual Liver and the Specimen (Fig. 22)

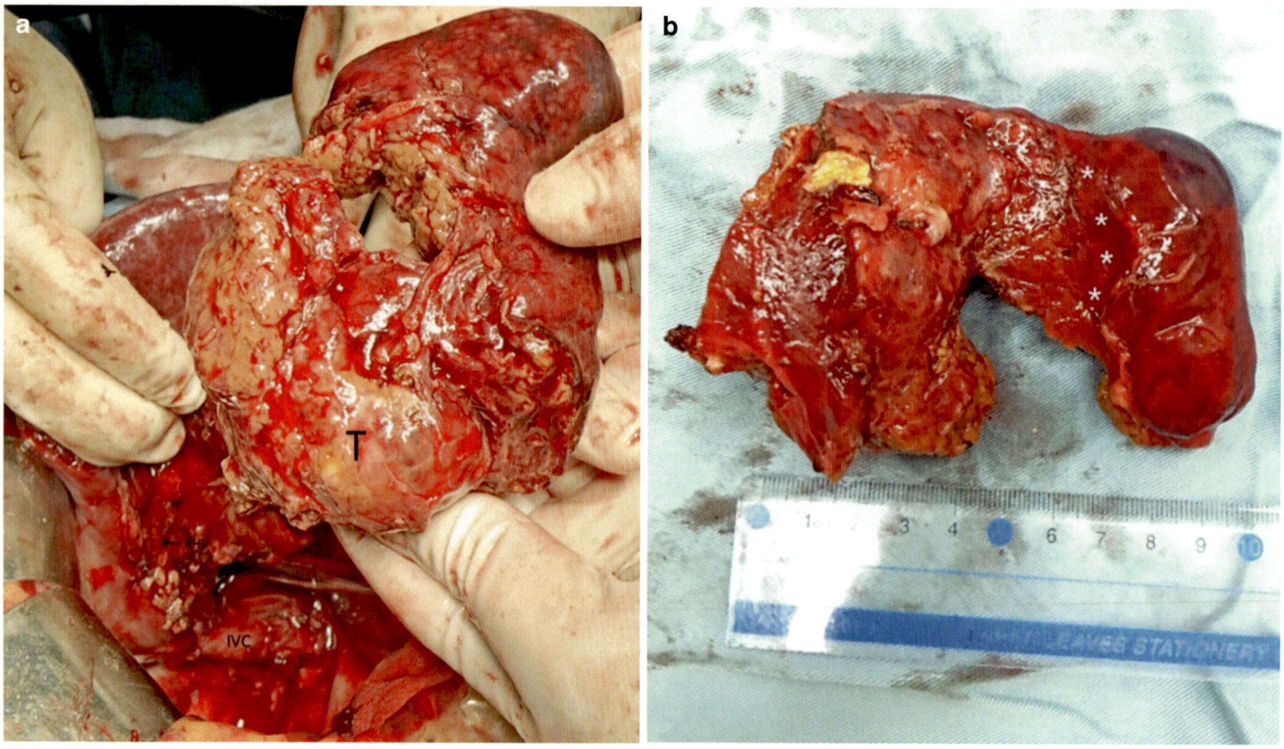

Fig. 22 To remove the specimen. (**a**) Cut surface. (**b**) Dorsal face. *RHV* right hepatic vein, *IVC* inferior vena cava, *T* tumor, * impression of the retrohepatic IVC

Anterior Transhepatic Approach for Resection of HCC Confined to the Paracaval Portion of the Caudate Lobectomy (Fig. 23)

Operative Procedures	Technical Details
Laparotomy and mobilization of the liver ↓	◀ A right subcostal incision was made.The right and left hemiliver was dissected away from its surrounding structures.
Preparation for total vascular exclusion (TVE) ↓	◀ The hepatic pedicle, the infra-and suprahepatic inferior vena cava was encircled with a tourniquet, respectively.
Marking the cut line and hepatic parenchymal transection ↓	◀ The anterior transhepatic parenchymal transection line (corresponding to the main portal fissure) was identified by IOUS and marked on the liver surface. Along the cut line, the parenchymal transection was undertaken caudal-cranially,using the clamp-crushing method.
Closure of the abdominal cavity and drainage	◀ Having removed the specimen, hemostasis and biliostasis were achieved by electrocautory, ligation or suture-ligated. A rubber tube was placed at the Winslow hole and secured.

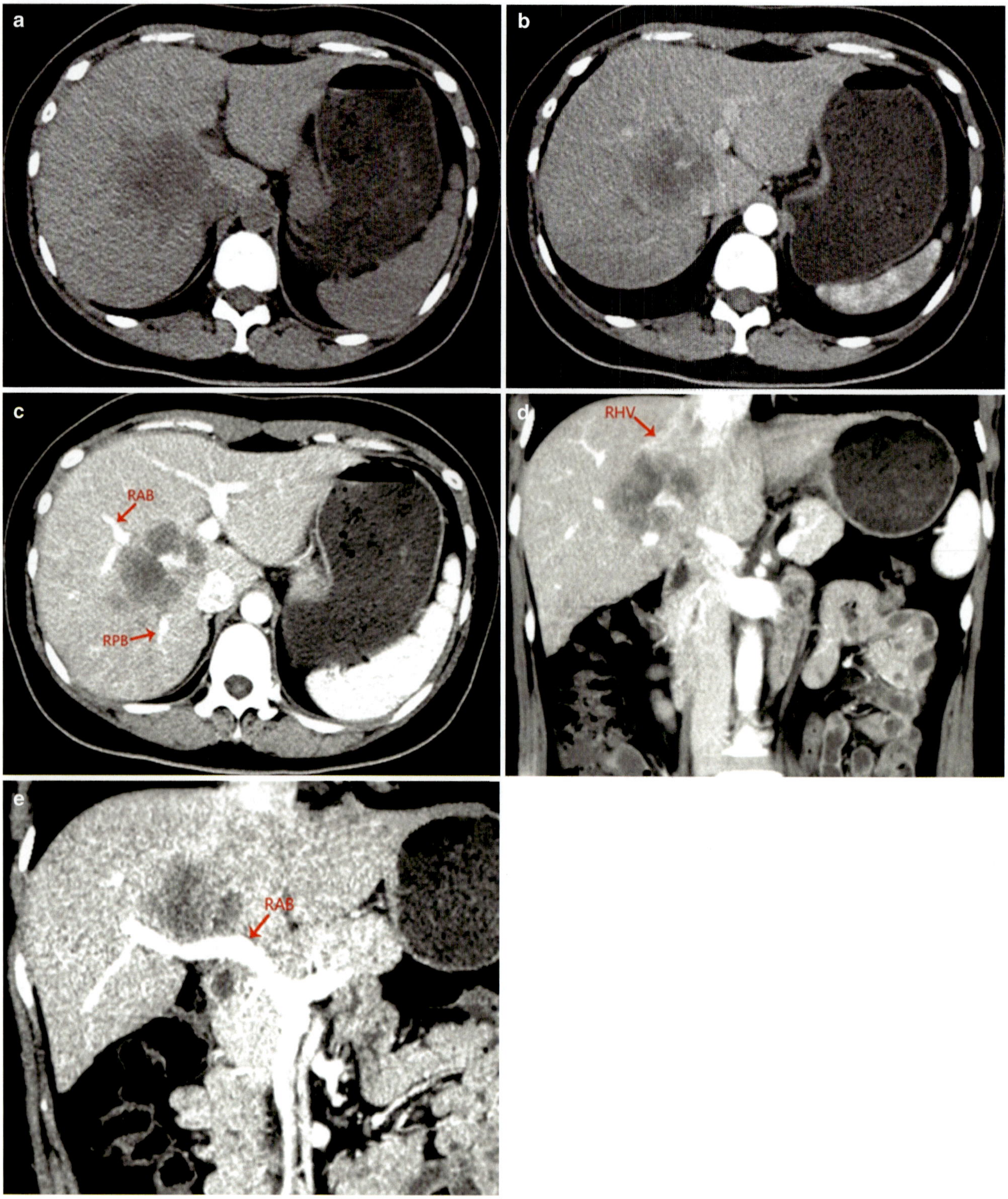

Fig. 23 (**a**) Preoperative CT (precontrast). The tumor, which appears mildly hypodense, is located in the paracaval portion. (**b**) Preoperative CT (hepatic arterial phase). The tumor shows heterogeneous enhancement. (**c**) Preoperative CT (hepatic venous phase). The tumor shows enhancement fades. (**d**) Preoperative CT (coronal section of the tumor). The relationship between the RHV and the tumor. (**e**) Preoperative CT (coronal section of the tumor). The relationship between the RAB and the tumor. *RHV* right hepatic vein, *RAB* right anterior branch of portal vein, *RPB* right posterior branch of portal vein

Abdominal Incision and Mobilization of the Liver
(Figs. 24, 25, 26, 27, 28, 29, 30, 31, and 32)

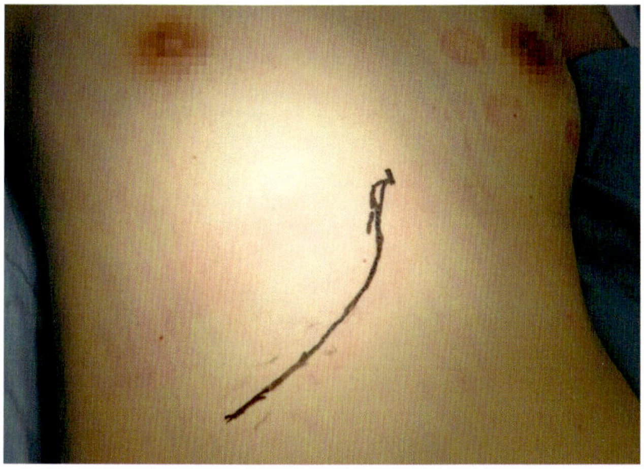

Fig. 24 Right subcostal incision was marked on the abdominal wall

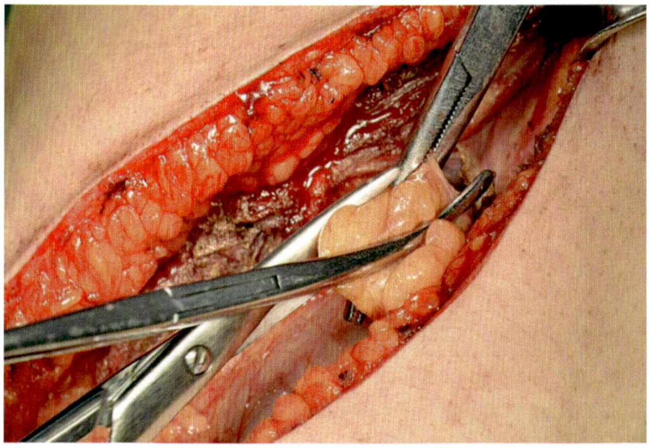

Fig. 25 Having entered the peritoneal cavity, the round ligament was divided and ligated near the umbilicus

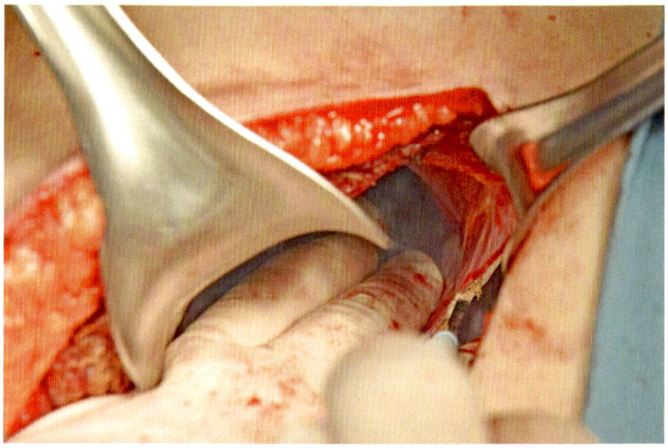

Fig. 26 The falciform ligament was divided with electrocautery

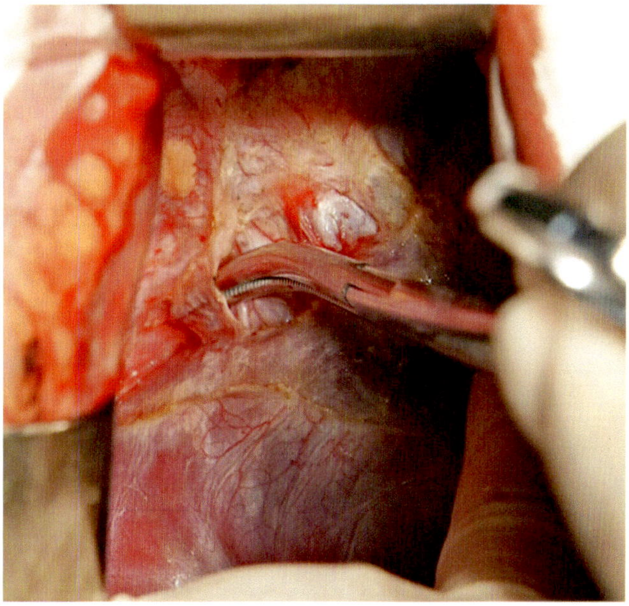

Fig. 27 The dissection was carried out upward to expose the hepatocaval confluence

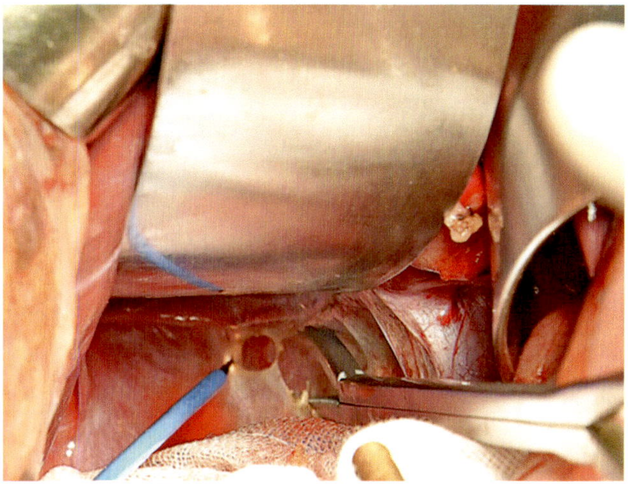

Fig. 28 The hepatocolic ligament was divided

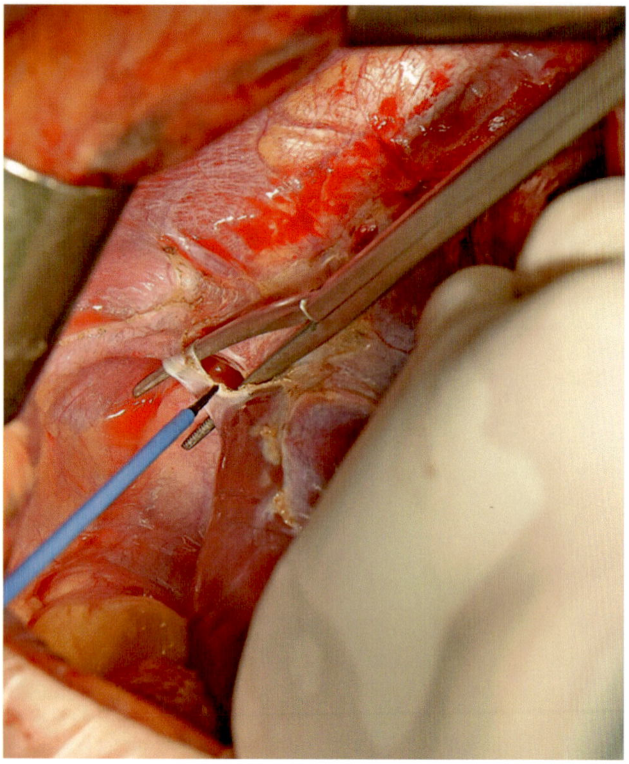

Fig. 29 The right triangular ligament was divided with electrocautery

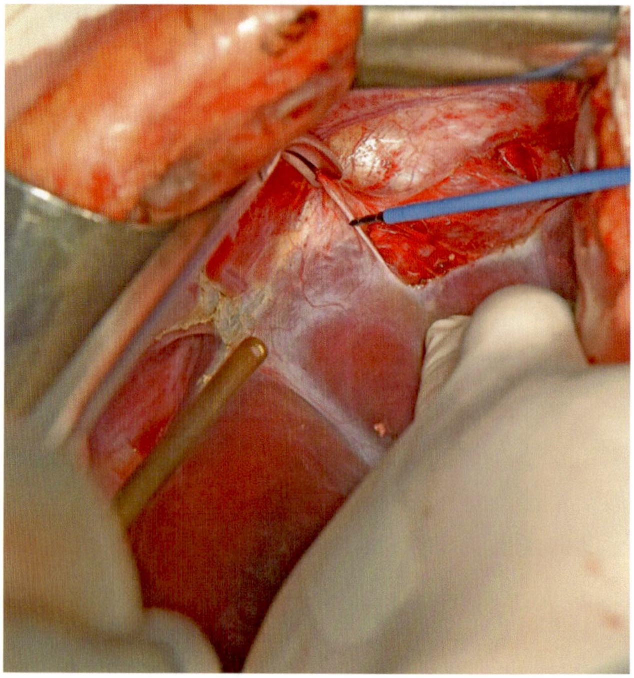

Fig. 30 The right coronary ligament was electrocauterized

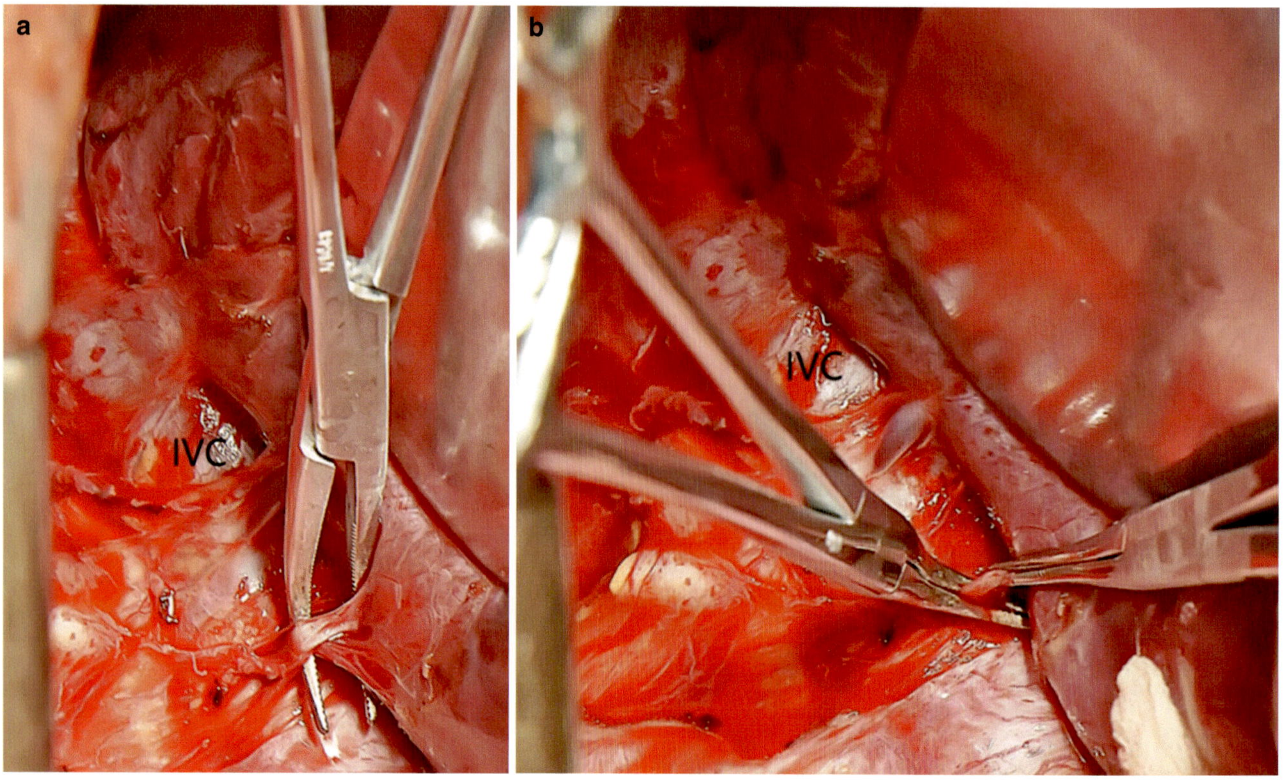

Fig. 31 (**a**–**c**) The inferior right hepatic vein (IRHV) was isolated (**a**), divided (**b**), and suture-ligated (**c**). *IVC* inferior vena cava

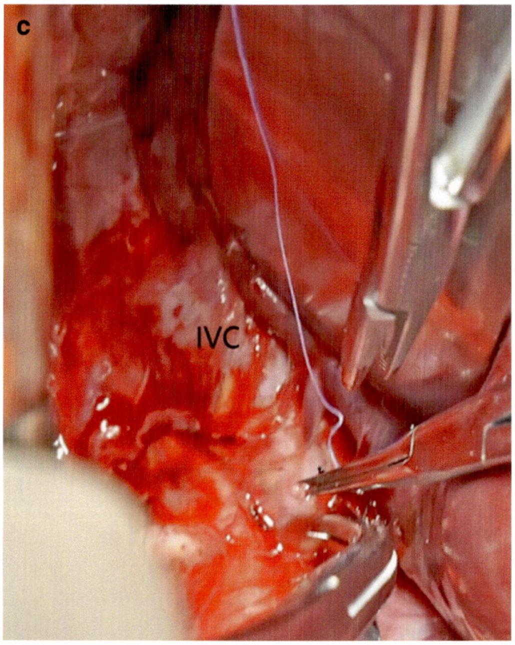

Fig. 31 (continued)

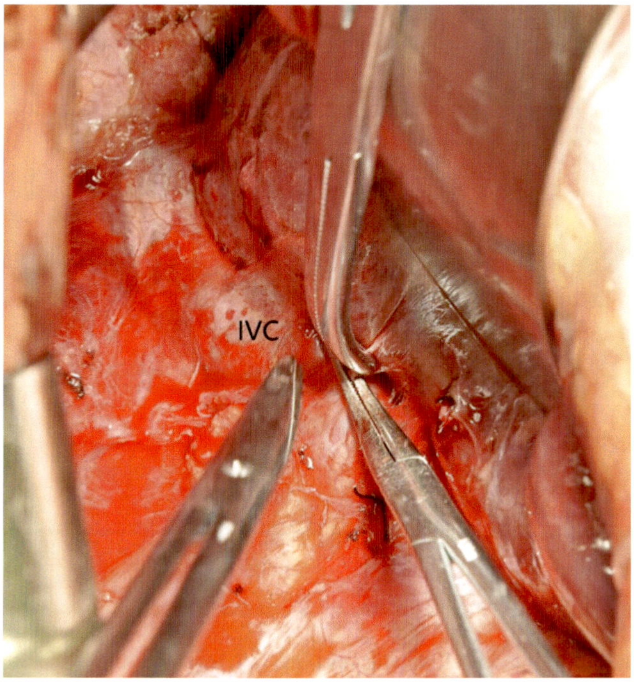

Fig. 32 The right-sided retrohepatic short veins were isolated, divided, and ligated, respectively. *IVC* inferior vena cava

Preparation for Total Vascular Occlusion
(Figs. 33 and 34)

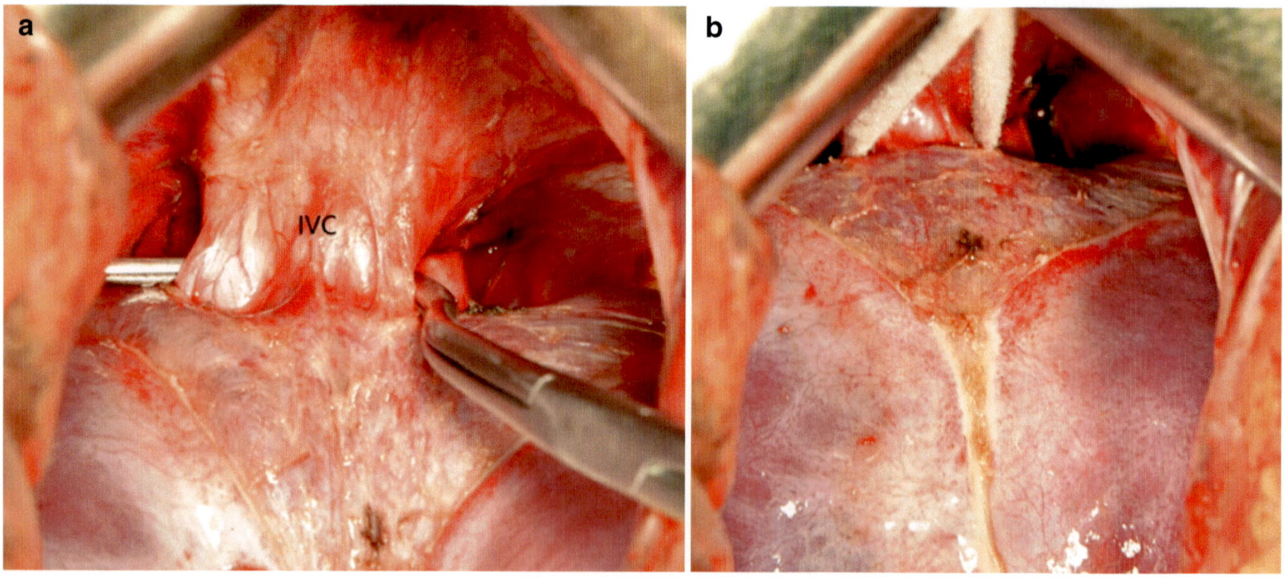

Fig. 33 (**a**, **b**) The suprahepatic IVC was isolated (**a**) and encircled (**b**) with a vascular tape. *IVC* inferior vena cava

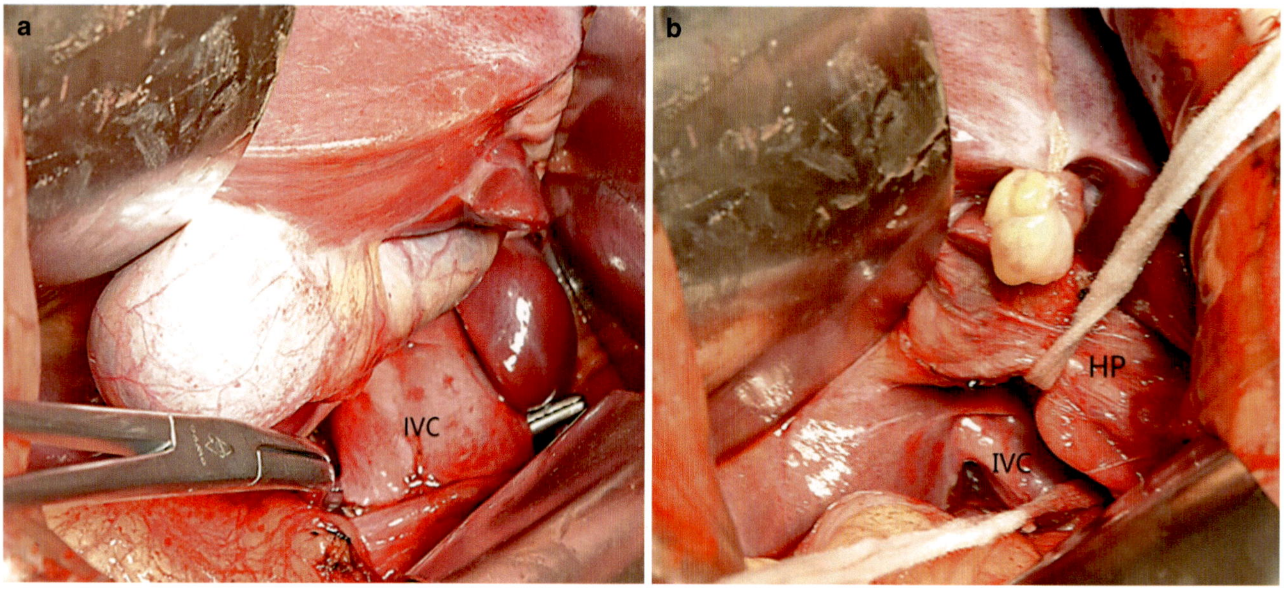

Fig. 34 (**a**, **b**) The infrahepatic IVC was isolated (**a**) and encircled (**b**) with a vascular tape. *IVC* inferior vena cava, *HP* hepatic pedicle

Marking the Cut Line and Hepatic Parenchymal Transection (Figs. 35, 36, 37, 38, 39, and 40)

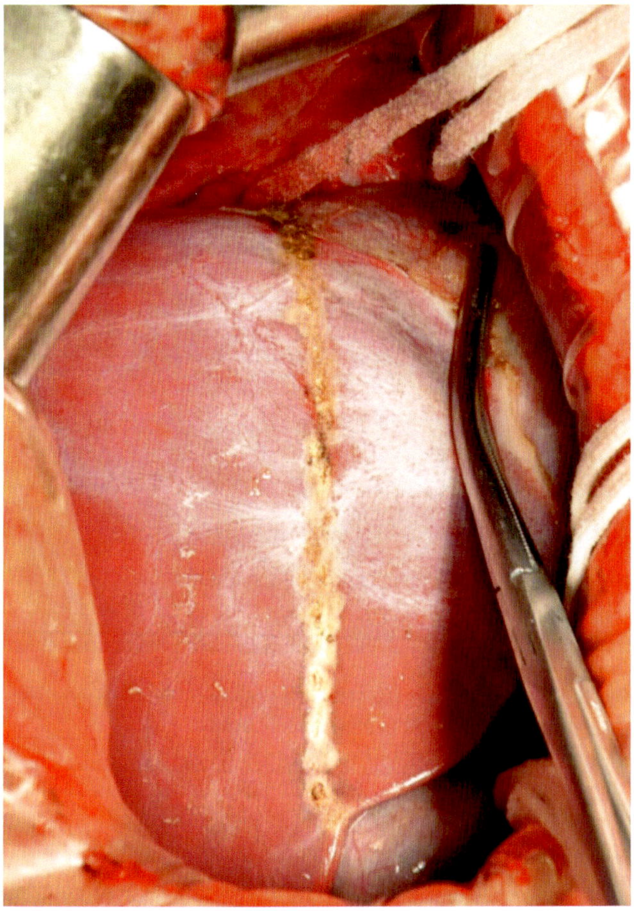

Fig. 35 The anterior transhepatic parenchymal transection line (corresponding to the main portal fissure) was ascertained by intraoperative ultrasound (IOUS) and marked on the liver surface. The line runs from the fossa between the right hepatic vein (RHV) and the middle hepatic vein (MHV) or the common trunk of the MHV and left hepatic vein (LHV) to the gallbladder fossa

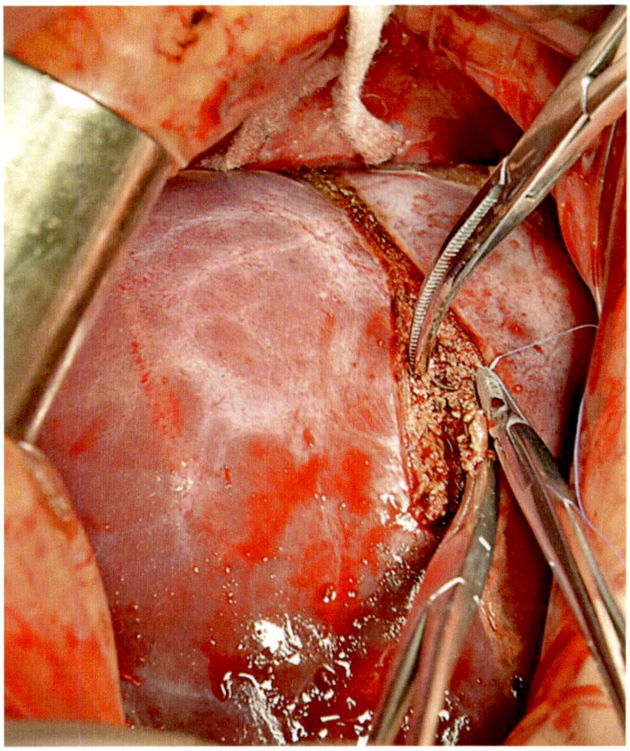

Fig. 36 Along the cut line, the hepatic parenchymal transection was carried out caudal-cranially, using clamp crushing method. Large vessels were divided and ligated

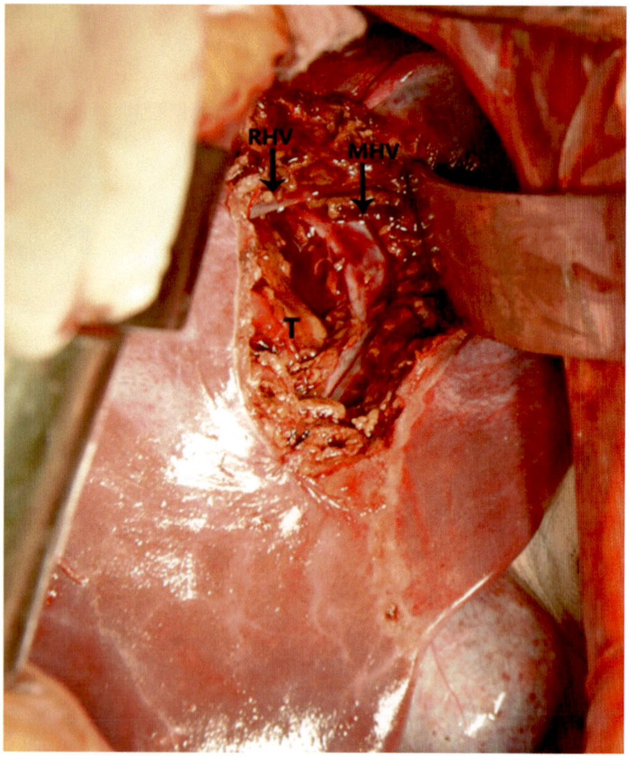

Fig. 37 The tip and left-side edge of the tumor was meticulously dissected away from the MHV and RHV. *RHV* right hepatic vein, *MHV* middle hepatic vein

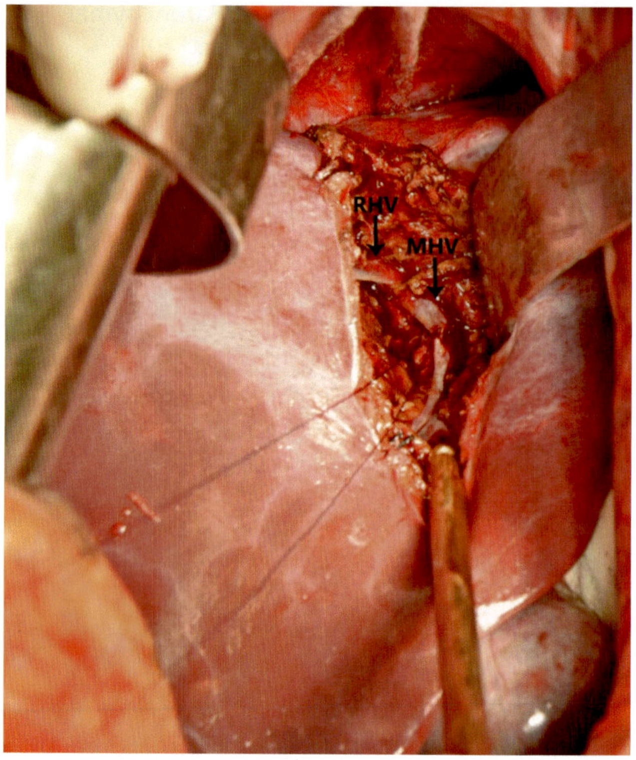

Fig. 38 The tiny holes in the MHV were repaired with 5-0 polypropylene. *RHV* right hepatic vein, *MHV* middle hepatic vein

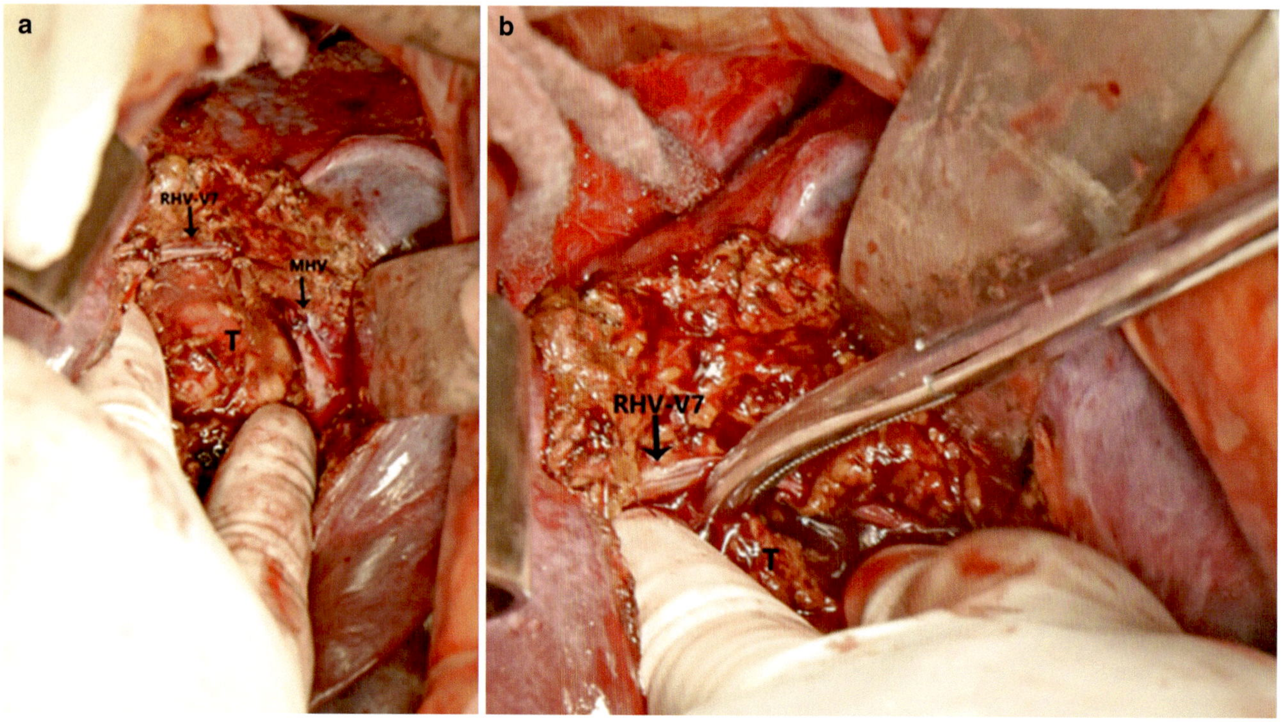

Fig. 39 (a–d) The operator's left index finger was used as a guide, the right-sided edge of the tumor was peeled off from the RHV. *RHV* right hepatic vein, *MHV* middle hepatic vein, *T* tumor, *RHV-V7* venous branch of the RHV draining segment 7

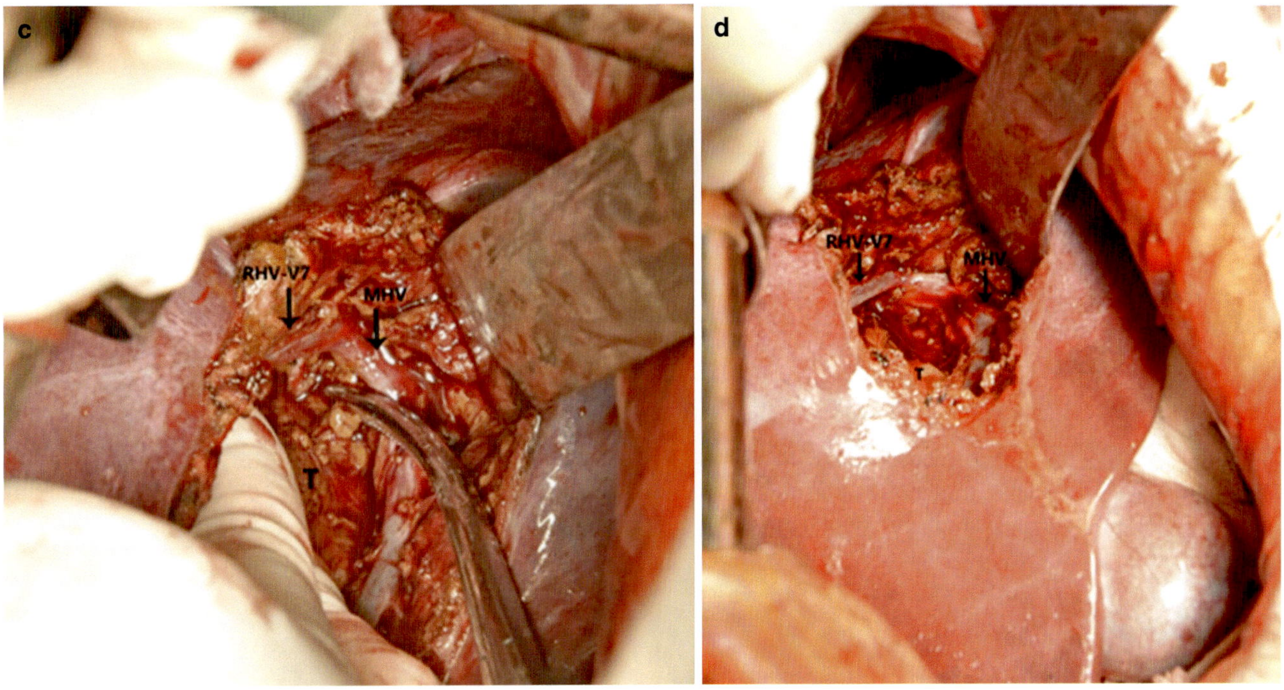

Fig. 39 (continued)

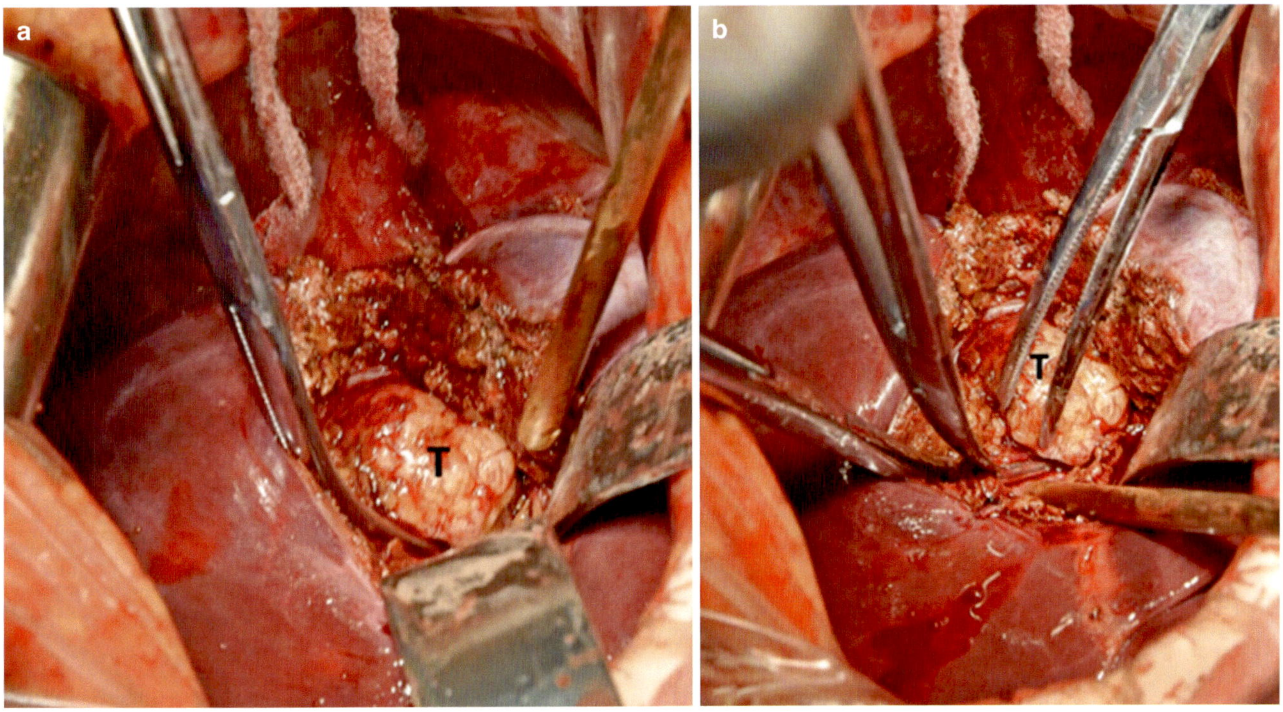

Fig. 40 (**a**–**f**) The inferior edge of the tumor was dissected. Right-sided and left-sided pedicles of the tumor from the right and left hepatic pedicle (RHV, LHV) were isolated, divided, and ligated/suture-ligated, respectively. *T* tumor

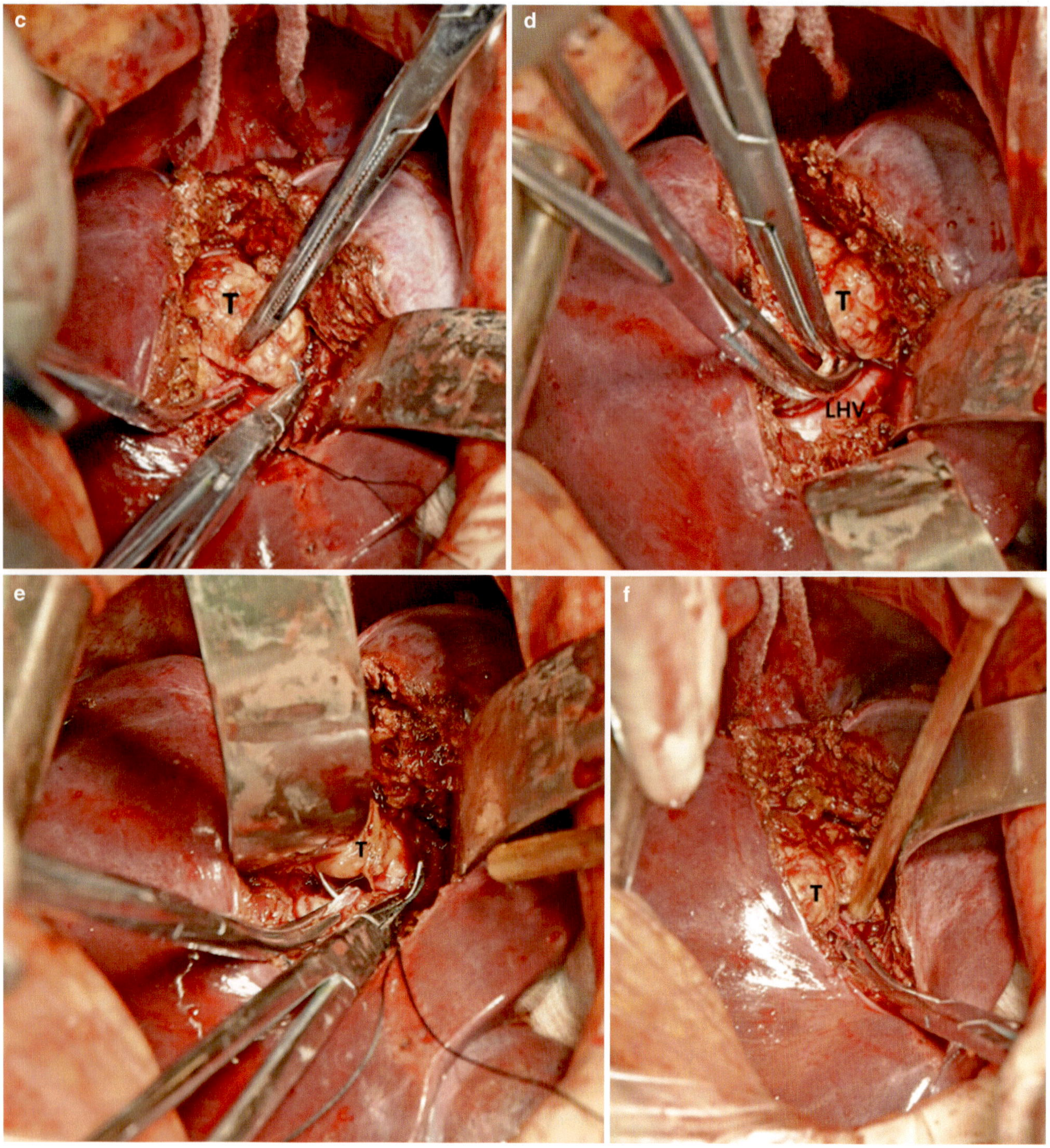

Fig. 40 (continued)

Cut Surface of the Remnant Liver and the Specimen (Figs. 41, 42, 43, and 44)

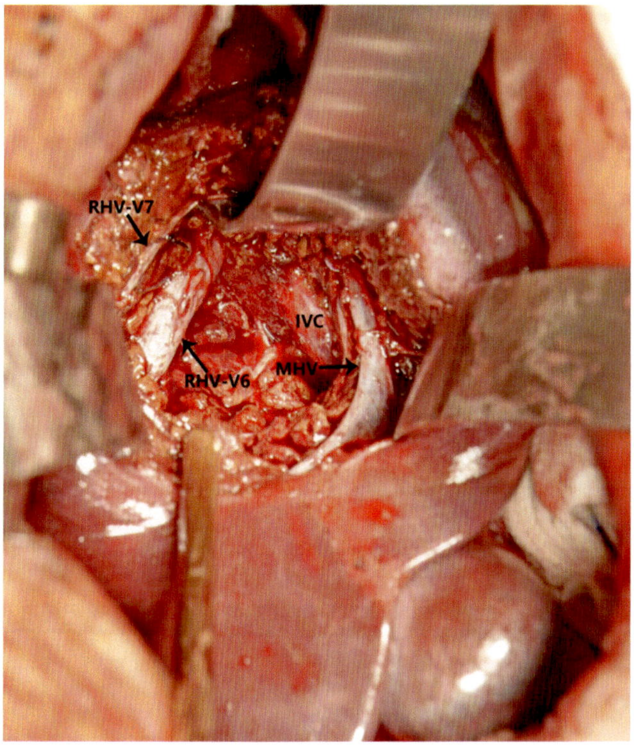

Fig. 41 Having removed the specimen, the upper portion of the raw area was shown. *RHV-V7* venous branch of the right hepatic vein draining segment 7, *RHV-V6* venous branch of the right hepatic vein draining segment 6, *IVC* inferior vena cava, *MHV* middle hepatic vein

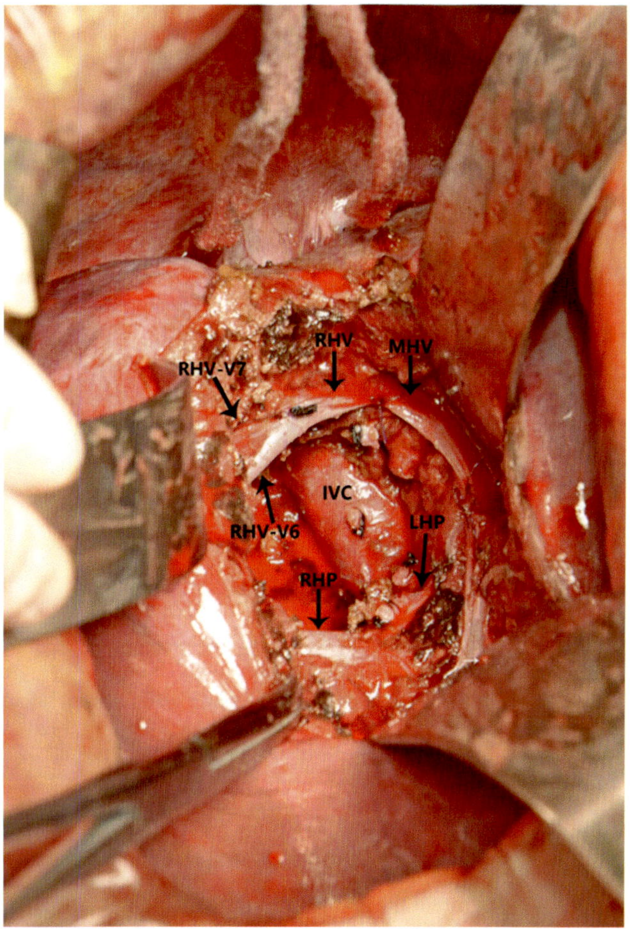

Fig. 42 Bird's-eye view of the whole raw area. *RHV-V7* venous branch of the right hepatic vein draining segment 7, *RHV-V6* venous branch of the right hepatic vein draining segment 6, *IVC* inferior vena cava, *MHV* middle hepatic vein, *RHP* right hepatic pedicle, *LHP* left hepatic pedicle

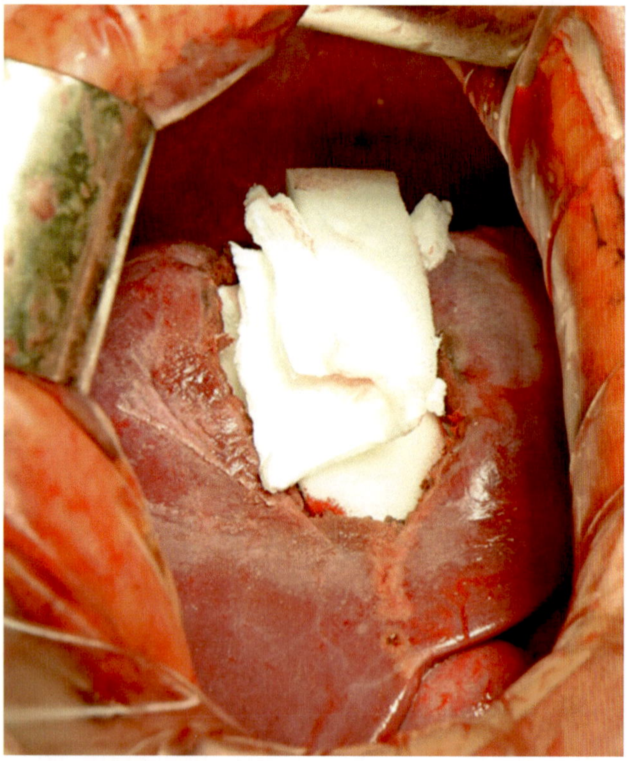

Fig. 43 The cut surface was covered with fibrin glue (Neoveil®) and absorbable gelatin sponge

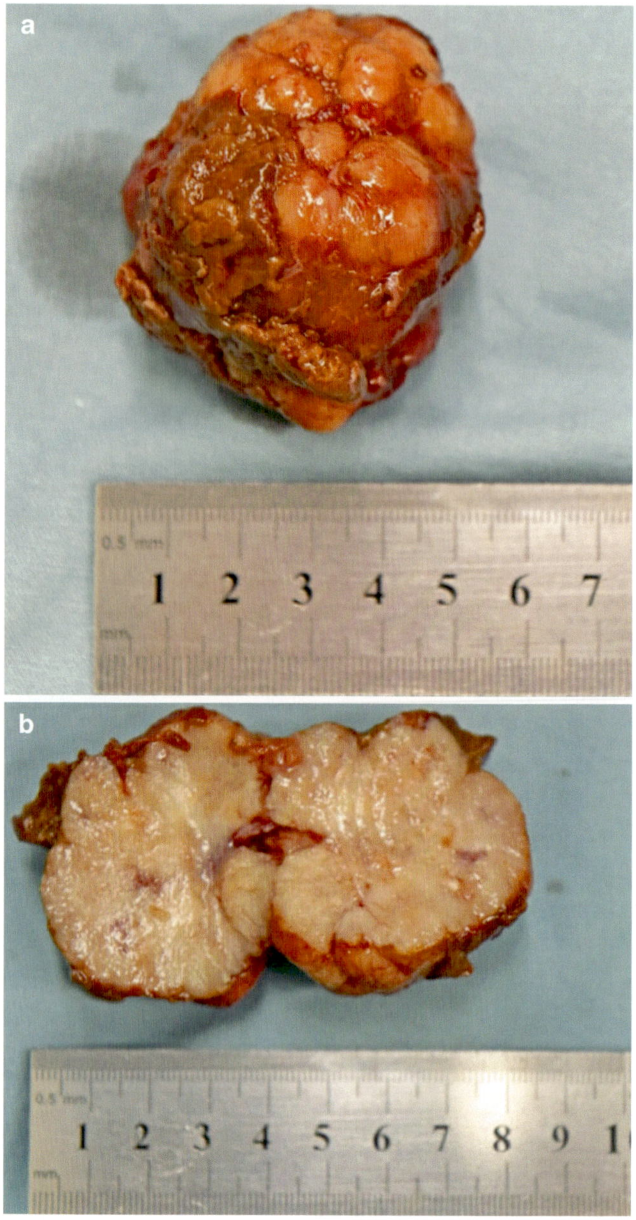

Fig. 44 (**a**, **b**) The specimen. Surgical margin was null

Anterior Approach for Resection for HCC Located Within the Paracaval Portion of the Caudate Lobectomy (Fig. 45)

Operative Procedures	Technical Details
Laparotomy and mobilization of the liver ↓	◀ A Benz incision was made and two automobile retractors were used. The right hemiliver was freed away from its surrounding tissues. The retrohepatic short veins were dissected individually and caudal-cranially, up to the hepatocaval confluence.
Preparation for total vascular exclusion (TVE) ↓	◀ The hepatic pedicle, the infra- and suprahepatic inferior vena cava was isolated and looped with a vascular tape, respectively.
Hepatic parenchymal transection ↓	◀ Having performed TVE, the hepatic parenchymal transection was carried out,using the clamp-crushing method.
Repairing the right hepatic vein and the middle hepatic vein ↓	◀ Because the tumor was closely adjacent to the roots of the right hepatic vein and the middle hepatic vein, the tumor was peeled away from the roots of the RHV and the MHV. Many holes on the roots were repaired with 4-0/5-0 polypropylene.
Closure of the abdominal cavity and drainage	◀ Having unloosened the vascular tapes, hemostasis and biliostasis were achieved by electrocautory, ligation or suturing on the cut surface. A rubber tube was placed below the right subdiaphragmatic space and secured.

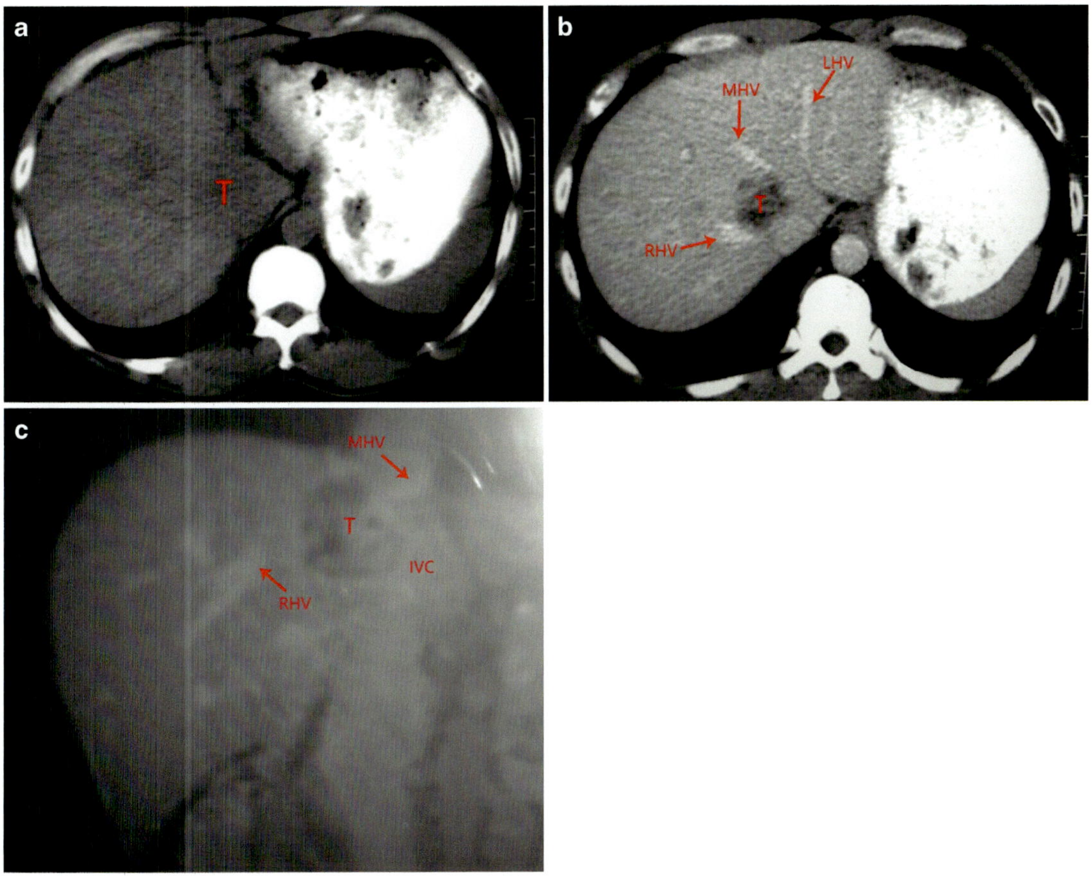

Fig. 45 (**a**) Preoperative CT (precontrast). The tumor (T) appears mildly hypodense. (**b**) Preoperative CT (hepatic venous phase). The lesion shows heterogeneously enhancement. (**c**) Preoperative CT. The tumor is closely adjacent to the RHV, MHV, and retrohepatic IVC. *RHV* right hepatic vein, *MHV* middle hepatic vein, *LHV* left hepatic vein, *IVC* inferior vena cava, *T* tumor

Abdominal Incision and Mobilization of the Right Hemiliver (Figs. 46 and 47)

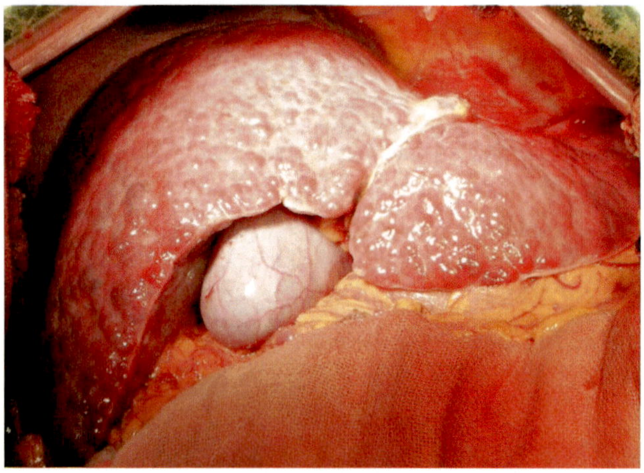

Fig. 46 A Benz incision was made, and two automobile retractors were used to adequately expose the surgical field

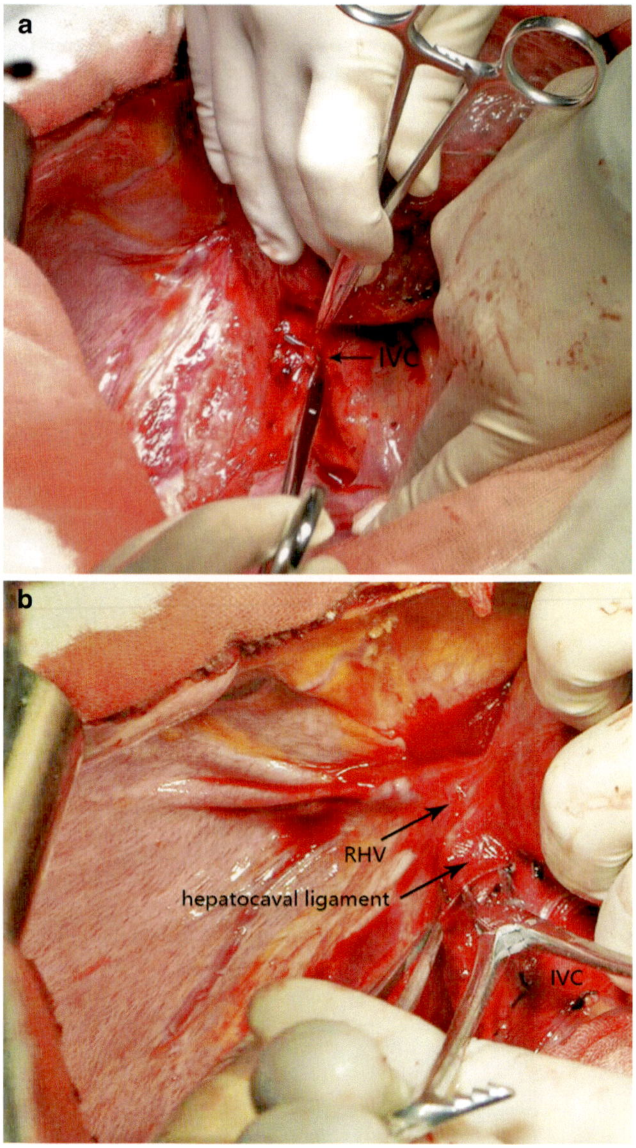

Fig. 47 (**a**, **b**) Having freed the right hemiliver away from its surrounding tissues, the right hemiliver was rotated upward and medially, the retrohepatic short veins were dissected and ligated individually and caudal-cranially. The hepatocaval ligament was also divided. *RHV* right hepatic vein, *IVC* inferior vena cava

Preparation for Total Vascular Exclusion (Fig. 48)

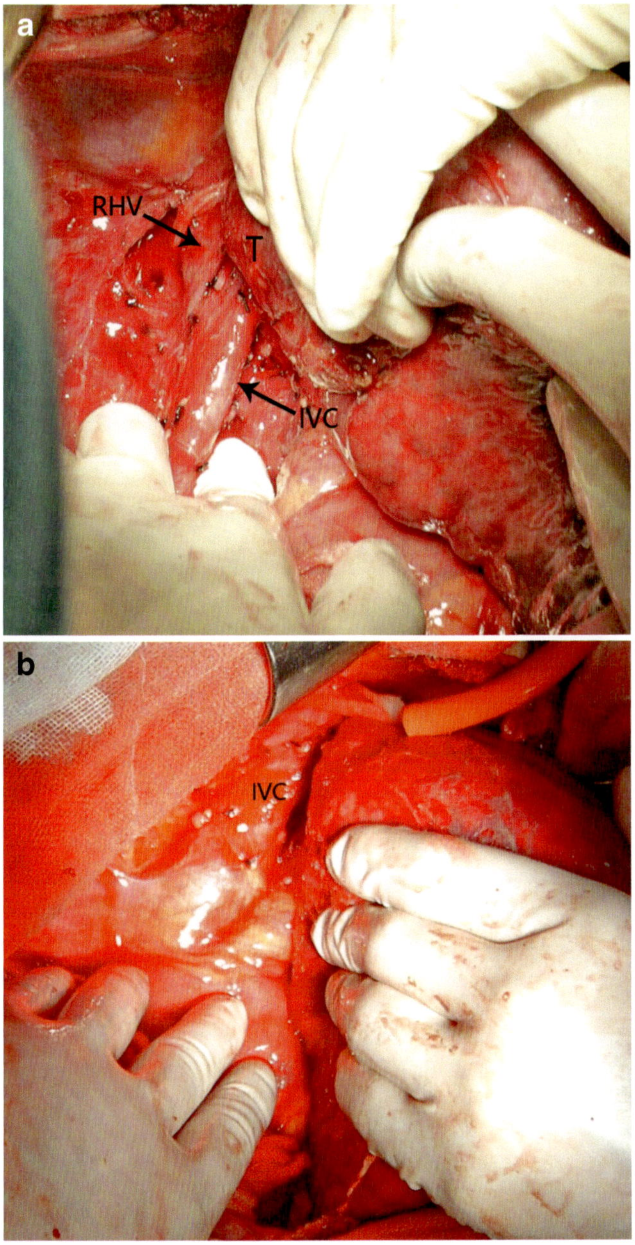

Fig. 48 (**a**, **b**) Hepatocaval confluence was dissected, and a vascular tape was encircled with the suprahepatic IVC. Then, the infrahepatic IVC and the hepatic pedicle were also encompassed by a vascular tape, respectively. *IVC* inferior vena cava

Hepatic Parenchymal Transection (Fig. 49)

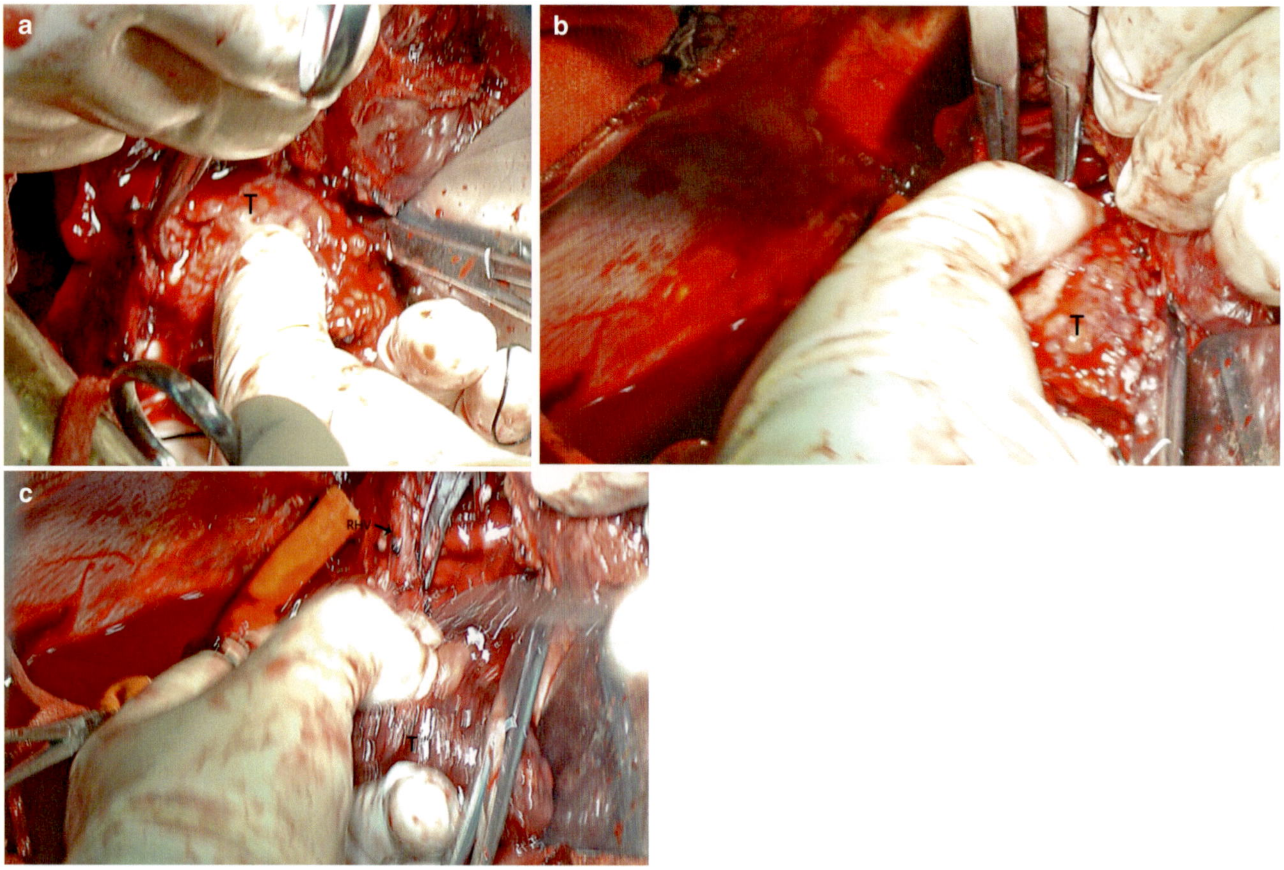

Fig. 49 (**a**–**c**) Having occluded the inflow and outflow blood of the liver, hepatic parenchyma transection was performed, using the clamp crushing method. Attention should be paid to prevent injury to the RHV and MHV. *RHV* right hepatic vein, *MHV* middle hepatic vein

Repairing the Right Hepatic Vein (RHV) and the Middle Hepatic Vein (MHV) (Figs. 50 and 51)

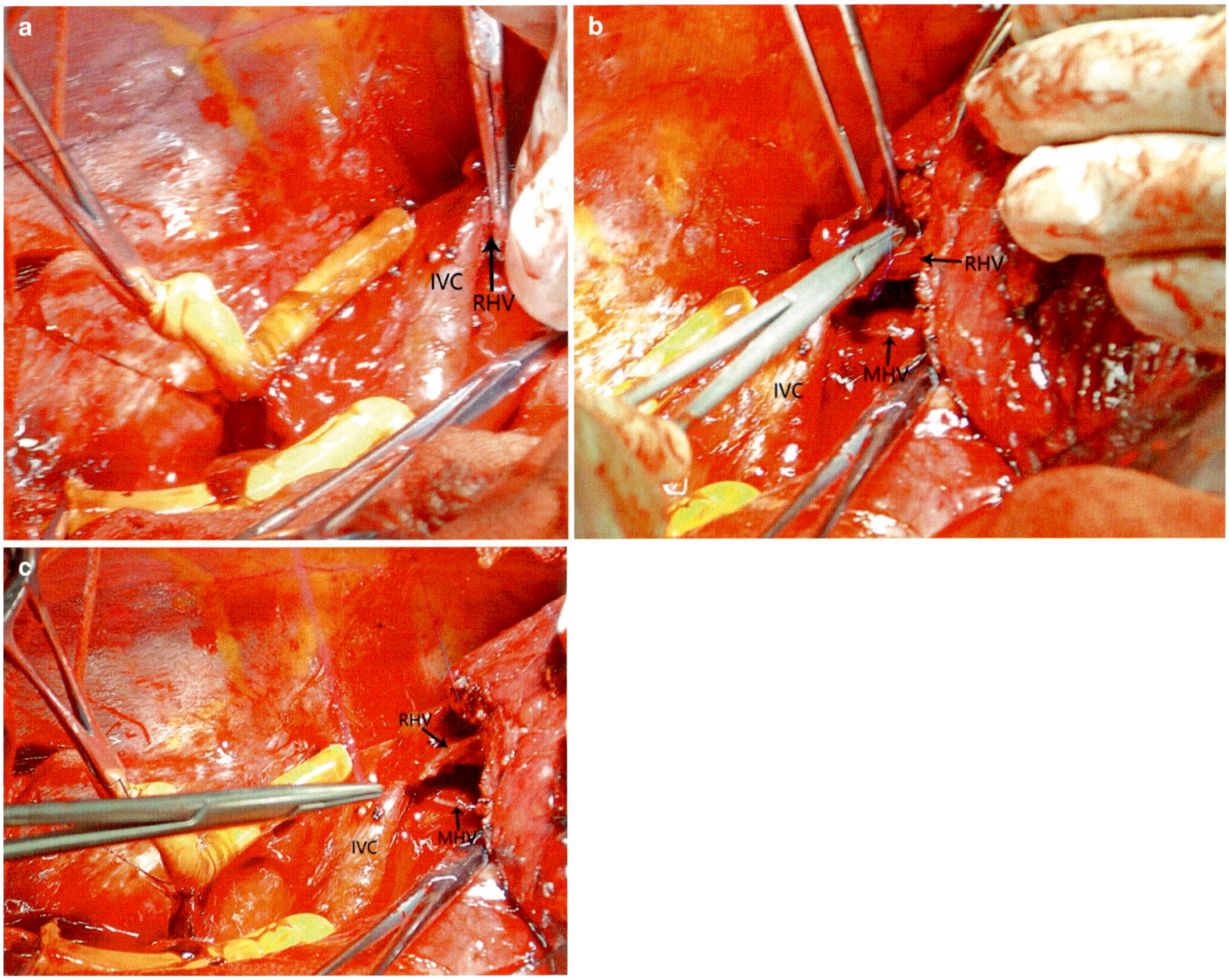

Fig. 50 (**a**–**c**) Having removed the specimen, the tiny holes on the RHV and MHV were repaired with 4-0 polypropylene. *RHV* right hepatic vein, *MHV* middle hepatic vein

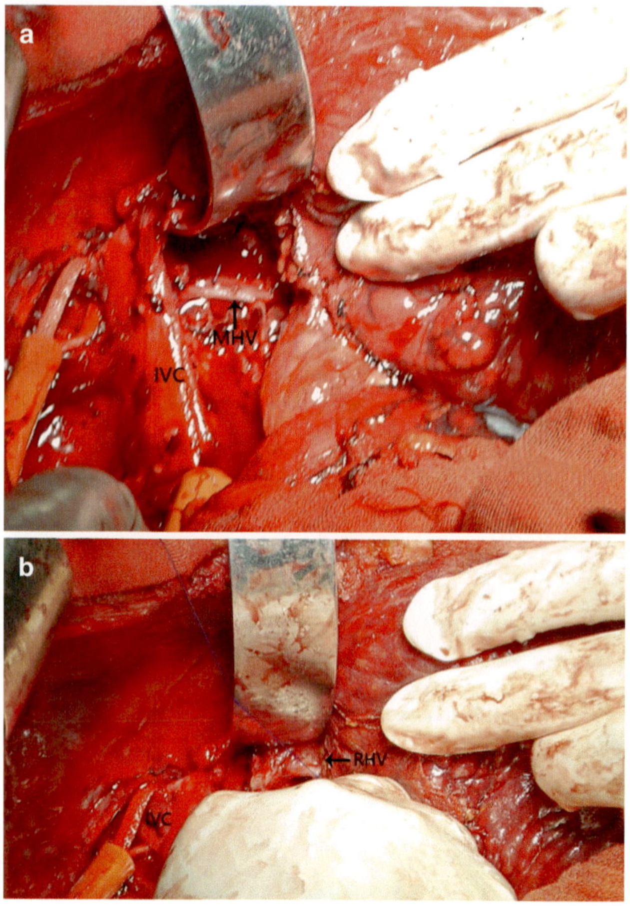

Fig. 51 (**a**, **b**) Having unloosened the vascular tapes, vascular and biliary ramifications on the cut surface were ligated or suture-ligated. *RHV* right hepatic vein, *MHV* middle hepatic vein, *IVC* inferior vena cava

Raw Area of the Remnant Liver and the Specimen
(Figs. 52 and 53)

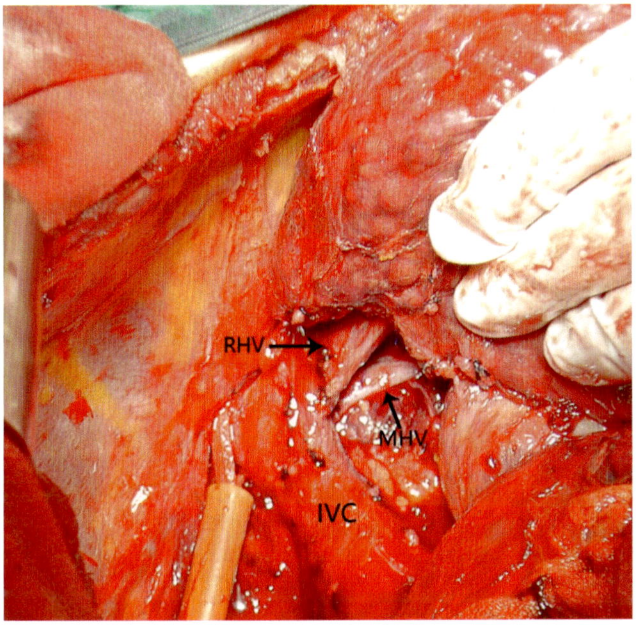

Fig. 52 Raw area of the residual liver

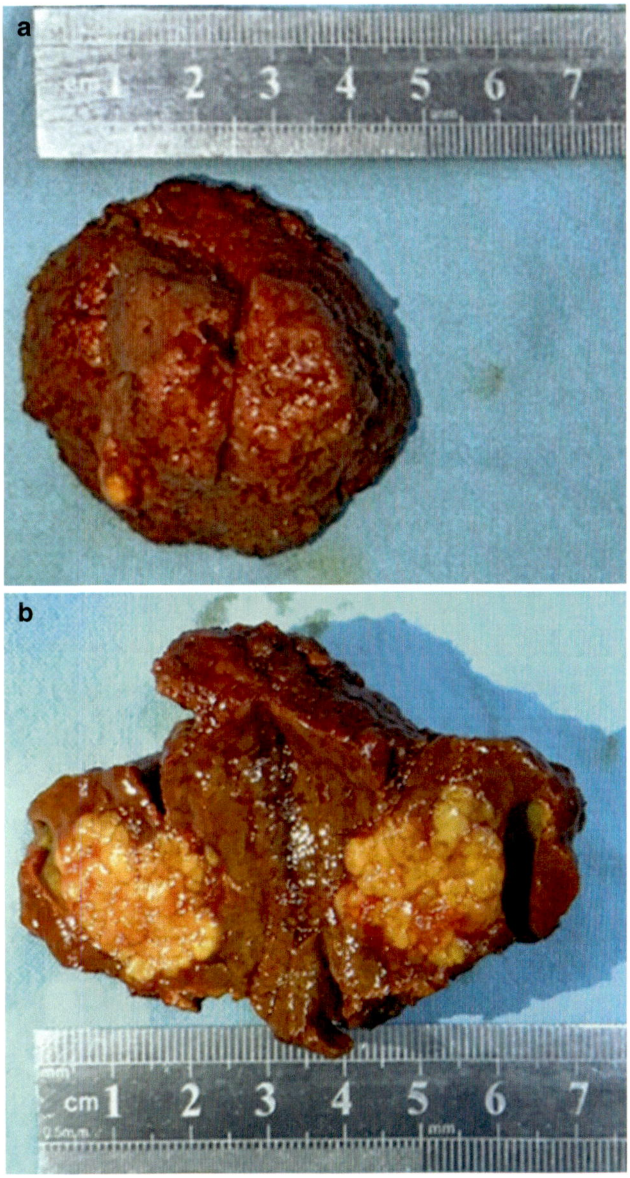

Fig. 53 (**a**, **b**) The specimen. Surgical margin was macroscopically negative

Anterior Approach for Complete Caudate Lobectomy with Reconstruction of the Trunk of the Portal Vein (Fig. 54)

Operative Procedures	Technical Details
Laparotomy	◀ A Benz incision was made. Two automobile retractors were used.
↓	
Peritoneal exploration and dissection of the tumor	◀ Peritoneal exploration was performed to exclude extrahepatic metastasis. The tumor was dissected away from its surrounding tissues. The portal triad was infiltrated by the tumor, among them, the trunk of the portal vein was completely destructed by the tumor.
↓	
Hepatic parenchymal transection	◀ Hepatic parenchymal transection of the caudate lobe was approached anteriorly, using the clamp-crushing method. The portal triad was also resected
↓	
Reconstruction of the portal vein and drainage of the common hepatic duct	◀ The resected trunk of the portal vein was reconstructed with artificial vascular graft. The proximal stump of the common hepatic duct was drained by a tube. There months later, the biliary tract was reconstructed
↓	◀ Vascular and biliary ramifications on the raw area were electrocauterized, ligated or suture-ligated. A rubber tube was placed at the Winslow hole and secured.
Closure of the abdominal cavity and drainage	

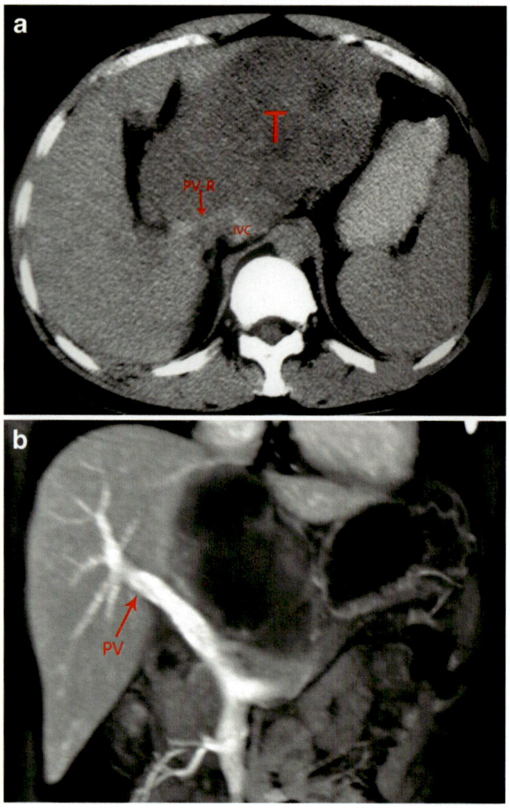

Fig. 54 (**a**) Preoperative CT (precontrast). The tumor, which appears mildly hypodense, completely occupies the whole caudate lobe. (**b**) The tumor is closely adjacent to the main trunk of the portal vein. *PV* portal vein, *IVC* inferior vena cava, *PV-R* right trunk of the portal vein, *T* tumor

Abdominal Incision and Exploration and Dissection of the Tumor (Figs. 55, 56, and 57)

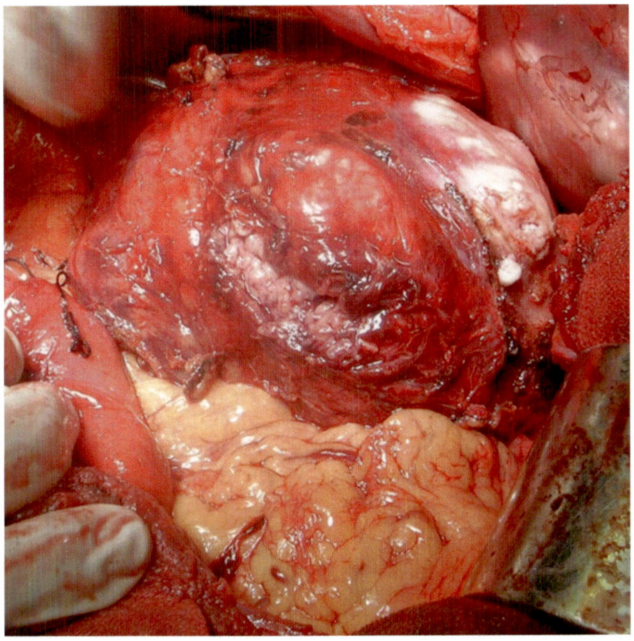

Fig. 55 Having entered into the peritoneal cavity, the tumor was shown

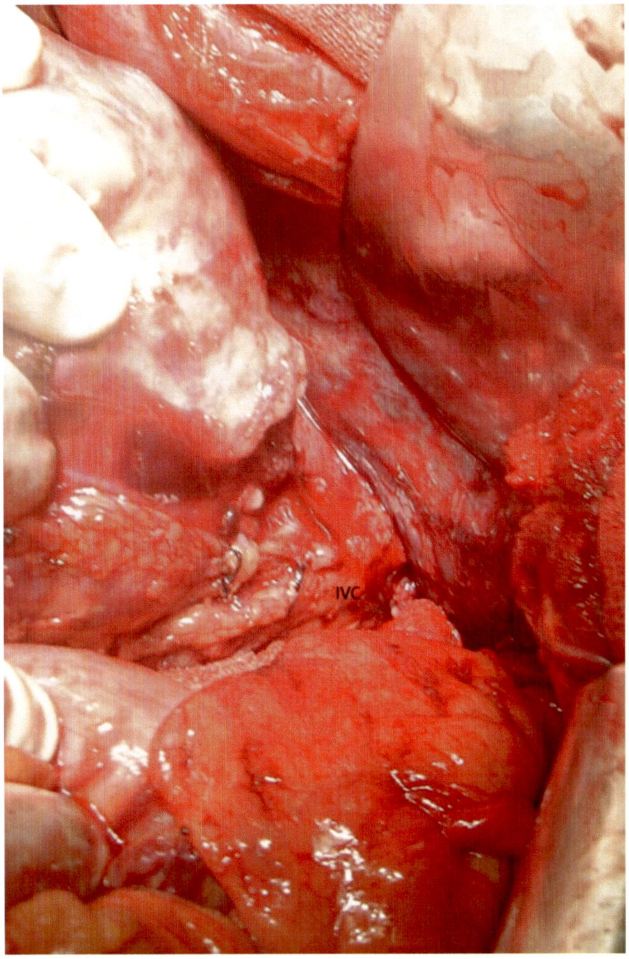

Fig. 56 Having explored the peritoneal cavity to exclude extrahepatic metastasis, dissection of the tumor from its surrounding tissues was carried out. *IVC* inferior vena cava

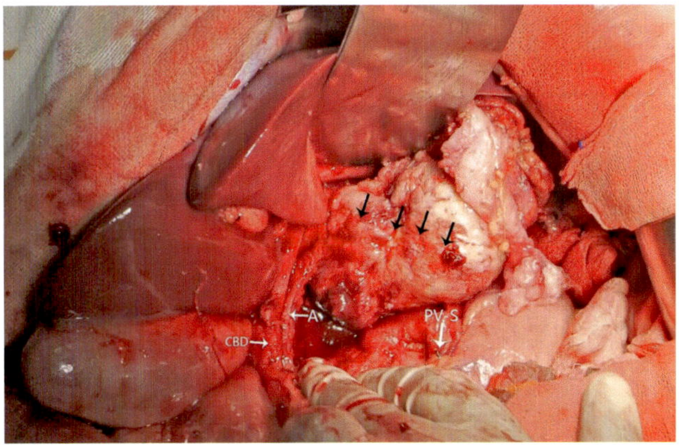

Fig. 57 The main trunk of the portal vein (PV) was infiltrated by the tumor (black arrows indicated to the main trunk of the PV). Besides, the hepatic artery (A) and the common bile duct (CBD) were also infiltrated by the tumor. The decision was made to completely resect the portal triad and to reconstruct it. *PV-S* distal stump of the portal vein

Hepatic Parenchymal Transection (Figs. 58 and 59)

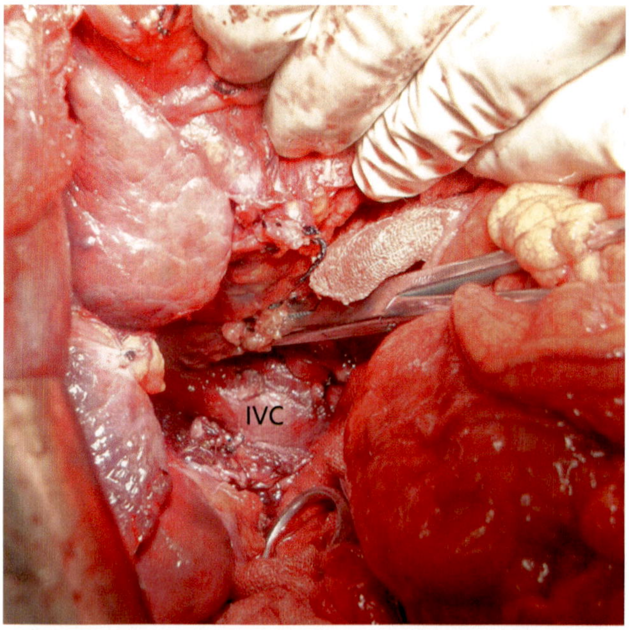

Fig. 58 Hepatic parenchymal transection of the caudate lobe was approached anteriorly, using the clamp crushing method. *IVC* inferior vena cava

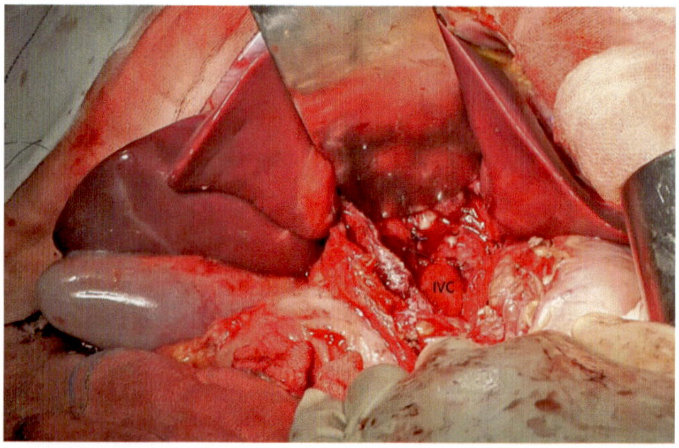

Fig. 59 The vascular and biliary vessels originating from the right and left hepatic pedicle were divided and suture-ligated. Having removed the specimen, cholecystectomy was performed, and the infiltrated common bile duct (CBD) and hepatic artery were also resected

Reconstruction of the Portal Vein and Drainage of the Common Hepatic Duct (CHD) (Fig. 60)

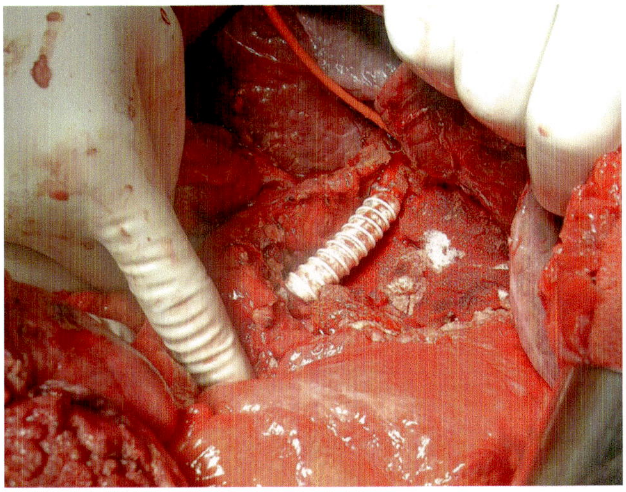

Fig. 60 The resected trunk of the portal vein (PV) was reconstructed with artificial vascular graft. The proximal stump of the common hepatic duct (CHD) was inserted into a 14# urine catheter to drain the bile. Three months later, the proximal stump of the CBD was anastomosed with the jejunal loop

The Specimen (Figs. 61 and 62)

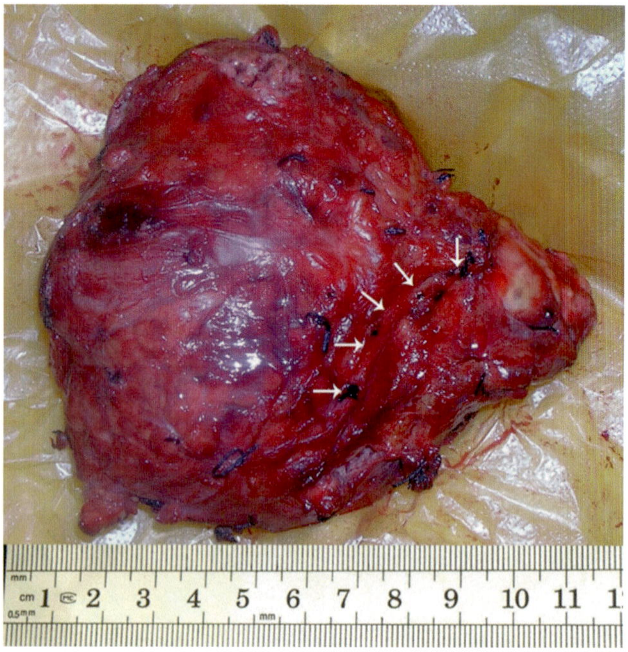

Fig. 61 White arrows indicated the resected main trunk of the portal vein (PV)

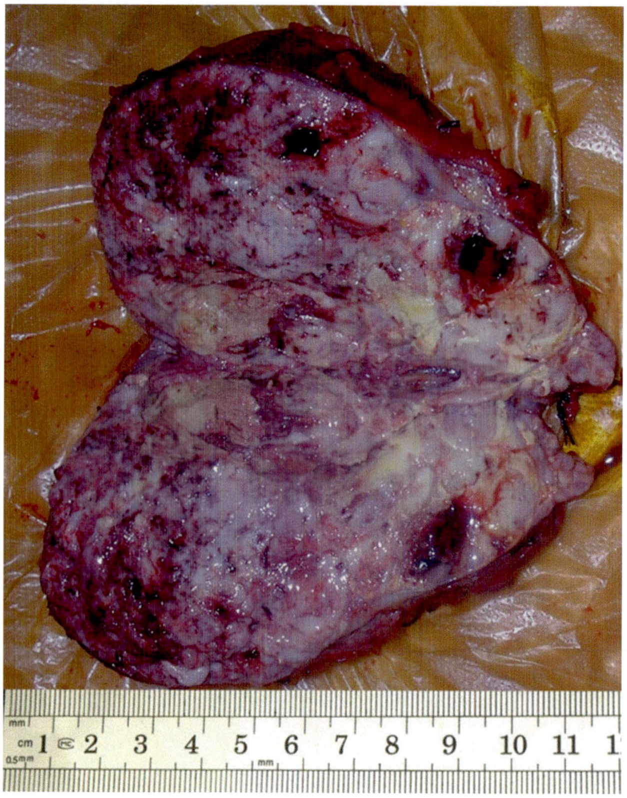

Fig. 62 The cutoff face of the specimen

Intraoperative Key Points During Partial or Complete Isolated Caudate Lobectomy

1. The appropriate surgical approach is critical to the success of caudate lobectomy. As the paracaval portion is located between the Spiegel lobe and the caudate process, and overrides the retrohepatic inferior vena cava, this portion cannot be accessed easily by the left or the right approach. In addition, the paracaval portion is surrounded by major vascular vessels, with the middle hepatic vein anteriorly, the hepatocaval confluence superiorly, the hepatic hilum inferiorly and anteriorly, and the retrohepatic inferior vena cava dorsally. This anatomical characteristic determines that tumors located within this portion are often in close proximity to main vascular vessels. Hepatic resection for tumors confined to this area tends to cause uncontrollable bleeding and even intraoperative mortality. Thus, total vascular exclusion should be prepared for such a hepatic resection, no matter which surgical approach is applied. In order to fully expose the tumor, and conserve as much functioning hepatic parenchyma as possible, anterior transhepatic or only anterior approach is recommended to resect tumors located within this paracaval portion [7, 19, 25]. In this chapter, these two kinds of hepatic resections for tumors in the paracaval portion are performed with narrow and even null resection margins. These tumors are almost peeled away from the major vascular vessels due to their unique locations; thus, it is logical that such a resection cannot obtain a surgical resection margin of more than 1 cm. Many studies have reported that patients with HCCs located within the caudate lobe had a similar prognosis to that in those patients with HCCs in other areas of the liver, regardless of surgical margin width [26–30].
2. It is our experience that the approach to resection from the anterior side is sometimes technically more demanding. We think that if the tumor in the caudate lobe is smaller and no signs show that the inferior vena cava or the main hepatic veins are involved with the tumor, hepatic inflow occlusion (Pringle maneuver) or total vascular exclusion is not necessary as advocated by others [30]. Should the tumor in the caudate lobe be large and the inferior vena cava or the main hepatic veins are invaded by the malignance, then the surgeons must be careful and cautious, and preparation for total vascular exclusion should be made. For isolated complete caudate lobectomy, the most dangerous and difficult manipulation is the parenchymal transection of its anterosuperior portion, where the roots of major hepatic veins are running near to the dissection line [5, 13, 23]. Division of the anterosuperior portion from other segments may pose the danger that may arise from massive hemorrhage from the major hepatic veins, should they be torn or lacerated posteriorly. In this instance, bleeding could often be temporarily controlled by local compression using the index finger or a sheet of wet gauze, and if not, Pringle maneuver or total vascular exclusion should be employed. After having removed the specimen, the posterior laceration of the middle hepatic vein was repaired with fine monofilament suture [7].
3. Aside from the abovementioned problems, intensive invasion of the tumor within the caudate lobe (especially the paracaval portion) into the retrohepatic inferior vena cava is another one. Since part of the retrocaudate short hepatic veins could not be previously be isolated and divided safely, we had to use total vascular exclusion and resect a part of the anterior wall of the inferior vena cava in them. Although total vascular exclusion could prevent bleeding and air embolism, such a strategy would result in hemodynamic disturbances and cause damage to the liver in up to 40% of patients [31] and, therefore, should be used as little as possible. In addition, there is also an important surgical procedure during mobilizing the Spiegel lobe. After the gastrohepatic ligament was widely incised, the left hepatic vein or the main trunk of the middle and left hepatic veins was exposed by transecting the left triangular ligament and the ligamentum venosum. The fibrous retrocaval attachment joining the Spiegel lobe and segment VII was incised. This step was very crucial in fully freeing the Spiegel lobe to expose the retrocaudate veins along the anterior surface of the retrohepatic inferior vena cava [12].
4. For the surgical treatment of huge hepatocellular carcinoma, some investigators suggest that HCC larger than 10 cm represents more aggressive tumor [32] and is associated with higher rates of vascular invasion [33] and the hepatic resection for HCC larger than 10 cm is often associated with various complications, which brings into question the value of surgery as a therapeutic option. According to the literature [34–37] and based on our own experiences [12], caudate lobectomy for huge HCC, sometimes even associated with resection and reconstruction of the portal vein, is a technically demanding but safe procedure, although this procedure is sometimes extremely difficult and time-consuming.

Bisegmentectomy VII–VIII

Jixiong Hu, Weidong Dai, and Tenglong Tang

The extent of hepatic resection is often defined by the main trunks of the major hepatic veins and their relationship to the tumor. For tumors located within the right superior segments (Couinaud's segments VII, VIII) [38] and infiltrating the main trunk of the right hepatic vein (RHV) close to its caval confluence, right hepatectomy is traditionally adopted [39]. This surgical procedure unavoidably resects the noncancerous right inferior segments (Couinaud's segments V, VI) and may lead to postoperative liver function failure and even death. Fortunately, anatomic studies have shown that a stout inferior right hepatic vein (IRHV) draining segment VI is present in about 25% of patients [40–42] and that segment VI has multiple veins presenting several anastomosis with the surrounding hepatic veins [43, 44]. Consequently, the maintenance of the IRHV and of the veins from segment 5 that ultimately drain into the middle hepatic vein (MHV) can be enough to assure venous drainage of both segments V and VI. In fact, it has been reported that bisegmentectomy VII–VIII is clinically feasible, irrespective of the presence of a large IRHV [45].

One of the intentions of hepatectomy for hepatocellular carcinoma (HCC) is to completely remove the tumor with an adequate surgical margin to prevent postoperative recurrence at the cut stump. Nevertheless, in cases of right superiorly located and RHV-involved HCCs which adhere to or compress the MHV near to its caval confluence, bisegmentectomy VII–VIII is difficult to undertake with adequate resection margins. Under such circumstances, to avoid postoperative liver failure for patients with cirrhosis by preserving segments V and VI, bisegmentectomy VII–VIII with exposure of the tumor surface at the cut stump with no resection margins has to be performed. Null-margin bisegmentectomy VII–VIII entails the tumor in its entirety being peeled from the right wall of the MHV and leaves the exposed proximal main trunk of the middle hepatic vein near its caval confluence along the cut surface intact [26].

Surgical Indications

The routine imaging studies carried out preoperatively included ultrasonography and helical contrast-enhanced computed tomography (CT), magnetic resonance (MR), and, if necessary, PET-CT. Concerning the evaluation of the liver function, the classification of Child-Pugh and the indocyanine green retention rate at 15 min (ICGR 15) were adopted. Bisegmentectomy VII–VIII for tumor located within the right superior segments and infiltrating the main trunk of the RHV close to its caval confluence was indicated only for patients with Child-Pugh Class A and with an ICGR 15 < 20%.

Operative Procedures	Technical Details
Laparotomy ↓	◀ A right subcostal incision was made.
Isolation and clamping of the right hepatic pedicle ↓	◀ The right hepatic pedicle was isolated and clamped using perihilar Glissonean approach. The right hemiliver was occluded and the ischemic demarcation line between segment VIII and segment IVA was marked on the liver surface with electrocautery.
Mobilization of the right hemiliver ↓	◀ The right hepatic ligaments were dissected with electrocautery. The retrohepatic short veins were isolated, clamped, divided and suture-ligated individually. If the inferior right hepatic vein (IRHV) is stout, it should be kept intact. The right hepatic vein (RHV) was isolated, divided and suture-ligated.
Hepatic parenchymal transection ↓	◀ The inferior boundary of segments VII and VIII corresponded to the transverse plane through the hepatic hilum and was marked on the liver surface with electrocautery. Under the right hepatic pedicle clamping and venous outflow control, the parenchymal transection was carried out along the cut line, using the clamp crushing method. During the transectional proceedings, the pedicles to segment VII, VIII were isolated, divided and suture-ligated, respectively. After delivery of the specimen, hemorrhage and bile leakage from the traumatic liver surface were treated by electrocautery, ligating and suture-ligating. Any injury to large vessels or bile duct was repaired with polypropylene sutures 4-0 or 5-0 on the cut surface. Then, the cut liver surface was covered with fibrin glue and other hemostatic agents.
Drainage and closure of the peritoneal cavity	◀ A tube was placed below the right subphrenic space and secured with silk-suture.

Intraoperative Key Points

1. Hemorrhage control remains the most important problem in high-risk hepatic resection. For a right superiorly located tumor that compresses or adheres to the middle hepatic vein (MHV), severe backflow bleeding from the MHV may occur at any time and may even lead to operative mortality during hepatic parenchymal transection. Preliminary extrahepatic isolation and looping of the MHV or the common trunk of the MHV and the left hepatic vein are recommended prior to parenchymal transection [46, 47]. During the process of transecting hepatic parenchyma, in case of injury to the MHV and sever backflow bleeding from the MHV, clamping the tourniquet circling the MHV allows total control of bleeding and repair of the injury to the MHV in a bloodless surgical field.
2. In clinical practice, we often encounter patients with impaired liver functional reserve and with right superiorly located and RHV-involved tumors adhering to or compressing the main trunk of the MHV at/near its caval confluence; we have to dissect and peel the tumor away from the right wall of the main trunk of the MHV, and this leads to exposure of the tumor surface on the liver cut surface at the site of vascular contact and also exposure of the main trunk of the MHV along the plane of parenchymal transection. In order to avoid postoperative liver failure by preserving segments V and VI, this bisegmentectomy with no resection margin has to be carried out [26] (Fig. 63).

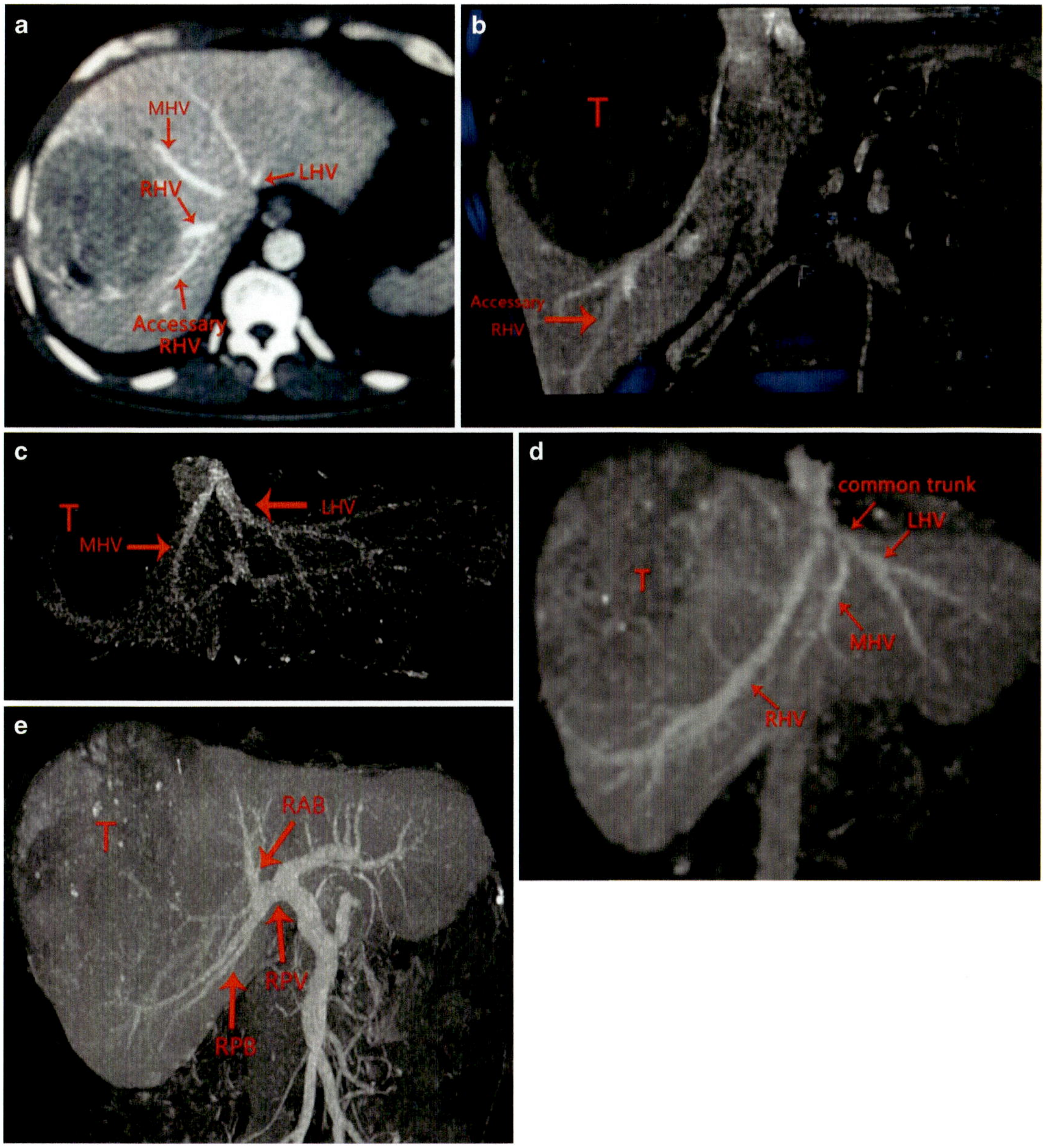

Fig. 63 Preoperative CT (hepatic venous phase and its reconstruction) shows the tumor (T) appears markedly hypodense. *RHV* right hepatic vein, *MHV* middle hepatic vein, *LHV* left hepatic vein, *RPB* right posterior branch of the portal vein, *RPV* right portal vein, *RAB* right anterior branch of the portal vein

Abdominal Incision and Mobilization of the Liver (Figs. 64, 65, and 66)

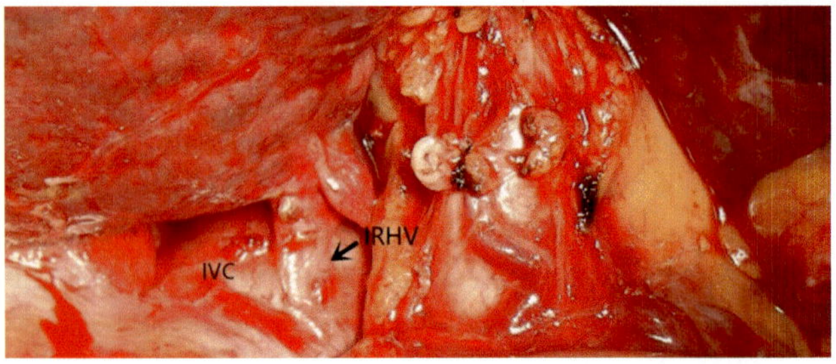

Fig. 64 A right subcostal incision was made. Having entered into the abdominal cavity, peritoneal tumor dissemination was excluded. The right hemiliver was fully mobilized. Then, IOUS was performed to evaluate the location of the tumor and its relationship with the main vasculatures. Thereafter, dissection of the retrohepatic short veins was carried out. The inferior right hepatic vein (IRHV) was not obviously enlarged, and if no accessory RHV existed, it should be kept intact. *IVC* inferior vena cava, *RHV* right hepatic vein

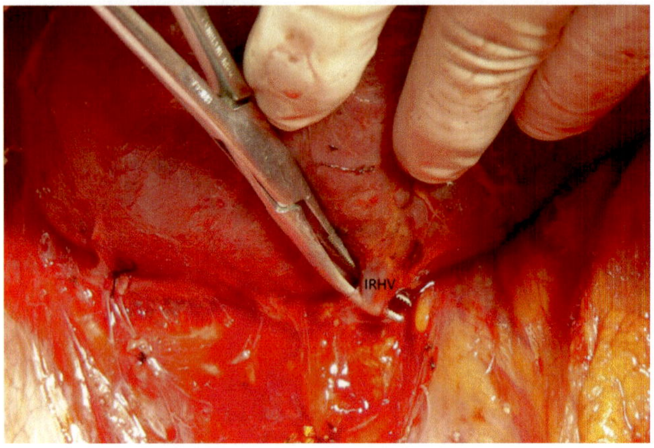

Fig. 65 The IRHV was clamped and divided, and the proximal stump was suture-ligated to prevent bleeding from the retrohepatic IVC. *IRHV* inferior right hepatic vein, *IVC* inferior vena cava

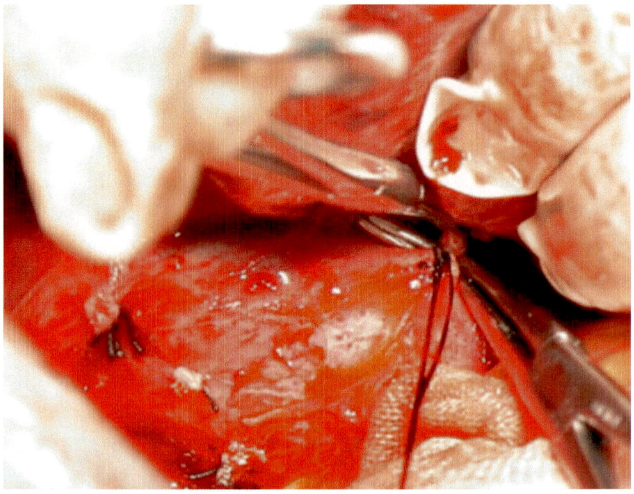

Fig. 66 Isolation and division of a left-side short hepatic vein was carried out

Extrahepatic Management of the Right Hepatic Vein (RHV) (Figs. 67, 68, and 69)

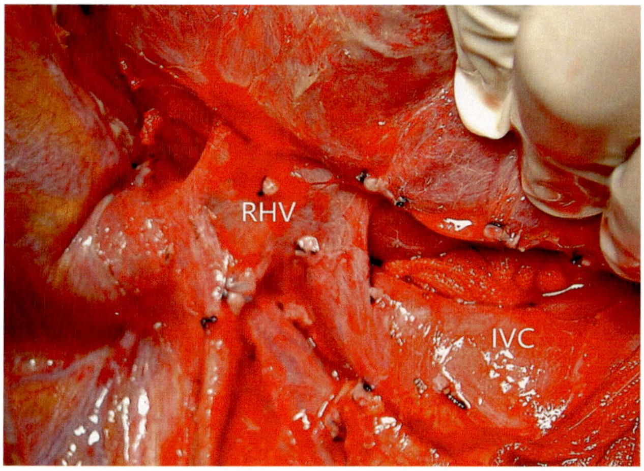

Fig. 67 The RHV was isolated. *RHV* right hepatic vein, *IVC* inferior vena cava

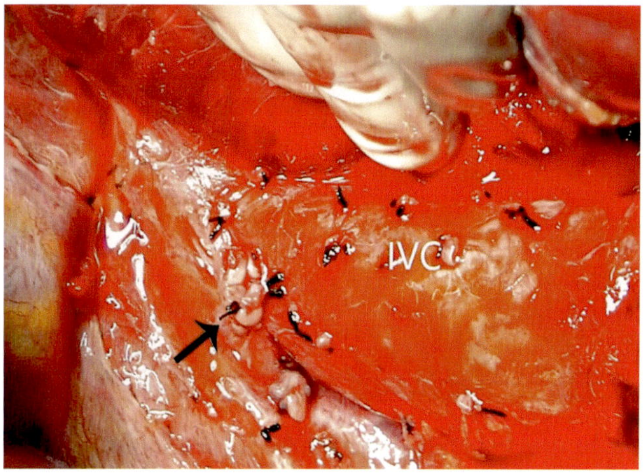

Fig. 69 Black arrow indicated to the proximal stump of the RHV. *RHV* right hepatic vein, *IVC* inferior vena cava

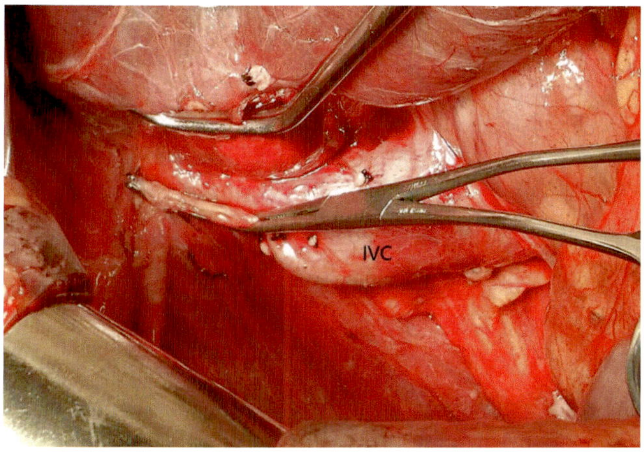

Fig. 68 The RHV was extrahepatically clamped, divided, and suture-ligated. *RHV* right hepatic vein

Marking the Cut Line (Fig. 70)

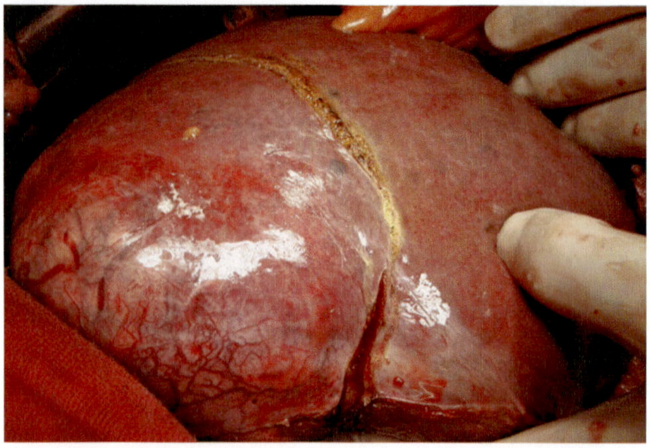

Fig. 70 The right hepatic pedicle (RHP) was temporarily clamped, and ischemic boundary between segment 8 and segment 4A appeared on the liver surface. The left-sided hepatic parenchyma transection line (based on the ischemic demarcation line) was marked on the liver surface with electrocautery, and the base parenchymal transectional line corresponded to the transverse plane through the liver hilum and was also marked on the liver surface

Hepatic Parenchymal Transection
(Figs. 71, 72, 73, and 74)

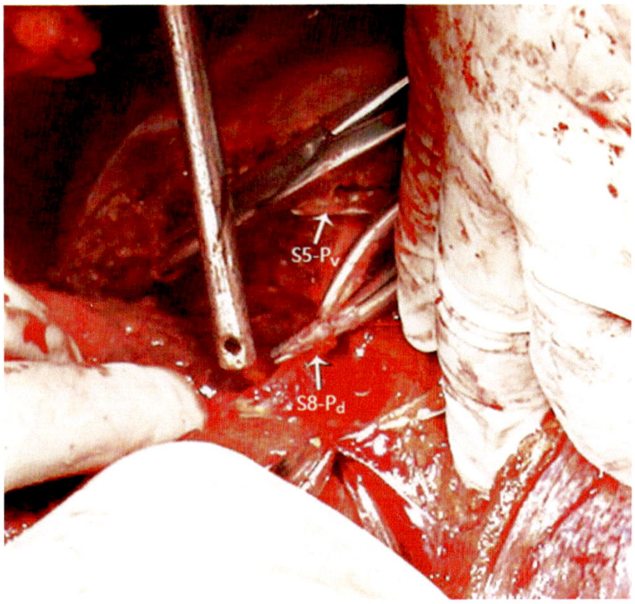

Fig. 71 Hepatic parenchymal transection between segment 8 and segment 4A was initially performed cranial-caudally, using finger fracture and clamp crushing method. Then, parenchymal transection between segment 8 and segment 5 was continued along the cut line. *S8-*P_v ventral pedicle of segment 8, *S8-*P_d dorsal pedicle of segment 8

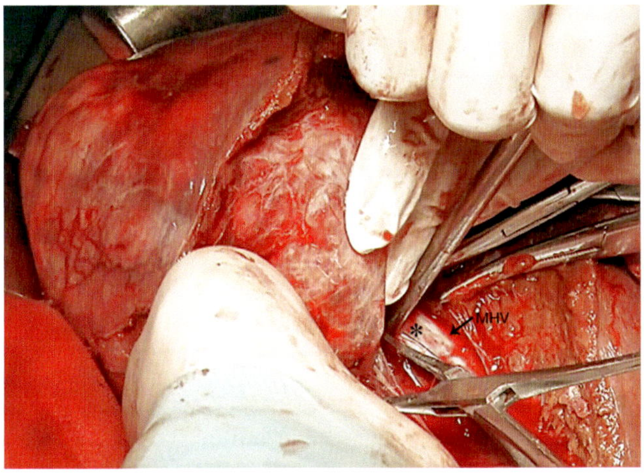

Fig. 72 Parenchymal transection was continued between segment 7 and segment 6. The tumor was peeled away from the MHV, and a longitudinal (asterisk) laceration was made on the right-side wall of the MHV. Immediately, the laceration was sutured using 5-0 polypropylene. *MHV* middle hepatic vein

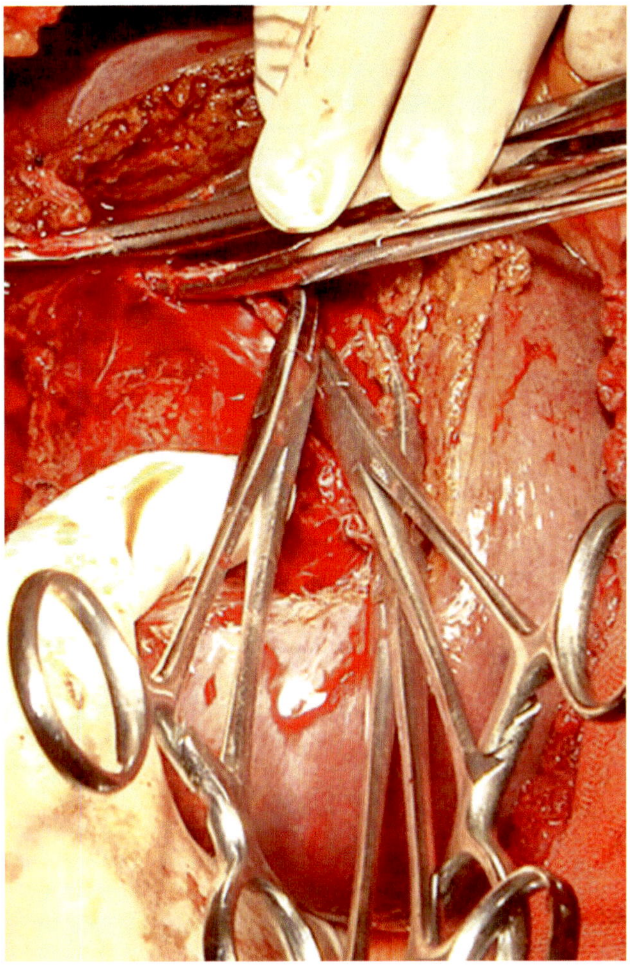

Fig. 73 The specimen was removed, and the proximal stump of the pedicle of segments 7 and 8 was silk-sutured, respectively

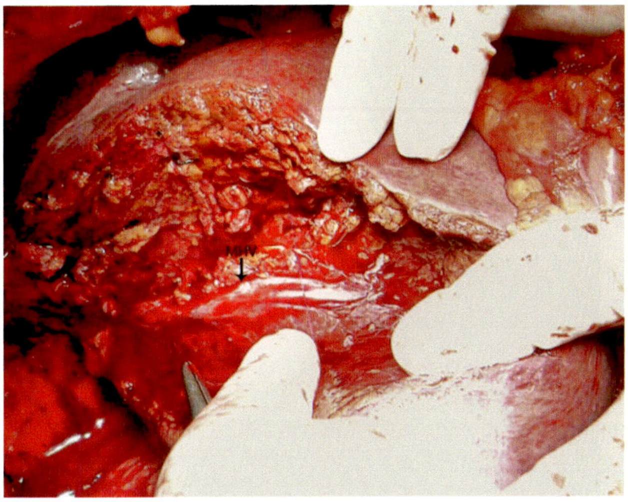

Fig. 74 The tiny holes on the MHV were sutured using 5-0 polypropylene. *MHV* middle hepatic vein

Raw Area of the Remnant Liver and the Specimen (Figs. 75 and 76)

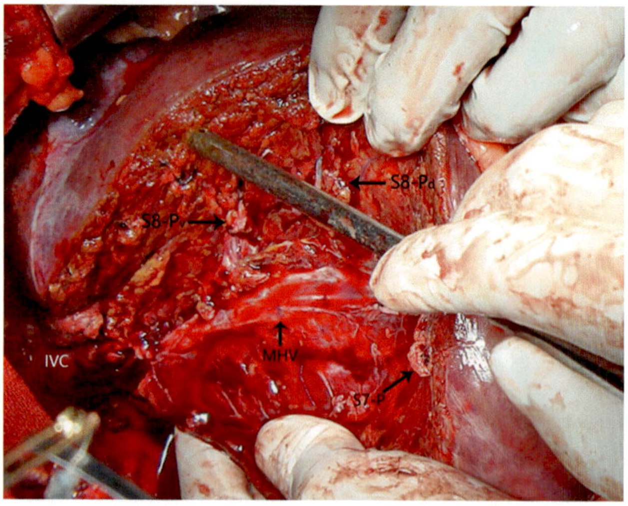

Fig. 75 Raw area after complete resection of segments VII–VIII. *S7-P* pedicle of segment 7, *S8-P*$_v$ ventral pedicle of segment 8, *S8-P*$_d$ dorsal pedicle of segment 8, *IVC* inferior vena cava, *MHV* middle hepatic vein

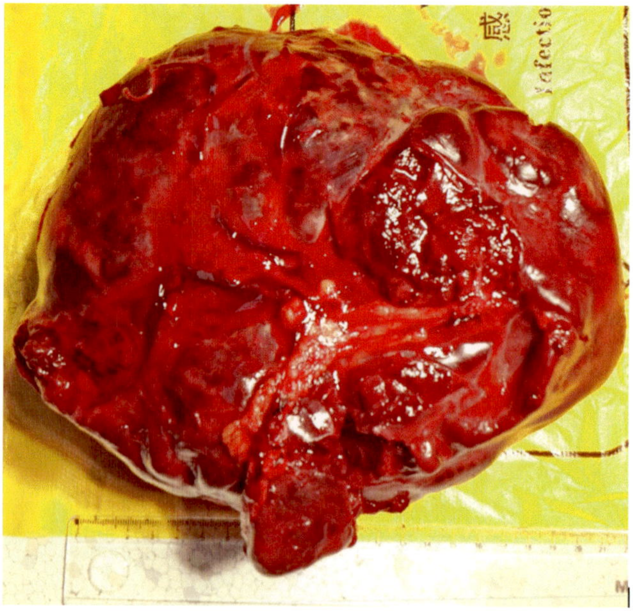

Fig. 76 The specimen was completed

Non-anatomic Mesohepatectomy for HCC

Jixiong Hu, Chun Liu, and Zhongkun Zuo

For HCCs located centrally within the liver (Couinaud's segments IV, V, and VIII), anatomical mesohepatectomy is preferred over traditional extended right or left hepatectomy [27, 48–51]. Although anatomic liver resection is preferred when resecting hepatocellular carcinoma, evidence that it is associated with more good prognosis when compared with a nonanatomic resection is lacking [52]. Anatomical hepatic resection was introduced in the 1980s. Although several studies have shown perceptible benefits of anatomic resection for HCC, these benefits are still debated [53].

Surgical Indications

For HCCs located within the central segments of the liver, anatomic mesohepatectomy was performed when the future liver remnant volume was estimated to be adequate. Preoperative imaging and evaluation of the liver reserve function were previously described [27, 50, 51] (see Section "Mesohepatectomy (S4 + S5 + S8 Resection)" in the Chapter "Types of Segment-Oriented Hepatic Resection by the Glissonean Pedicle Approach"). In case of serum total bilirubin level less than 1 mg/dl, anatomic mesohepatectomy for centrally located HCC was indicated only for patients with ICGR15 less than 10%. In this resection, the preoperative ICGR15 was 15%, and preoperative 3D simulation showed that postoperative liver remnant volume is not adequate. Moreover, preoperative image demonstrated that partial portions of segment IVA and superior portion of segment VIII were not involved with the tumor. Therefore, tumor capsule-oriented resection for this central tumor was planned to preserve the uninvolved central superior portion parenchyma.

Operative Procedures	Technical Details
Laparotomy and mobilization of the liver ↓	◀ A right subcostal incision. The whole liver was dissected away from its surrounding structures.
Preparation for total vascular exclusion (TVE) ↓	◀ The hepatic pedicle, the infra- and suprahepatic inferior vena cava was isolated and looped with a tourniquet, respectively.
Marking the cut line ↓	◀ The right-side and left-side hepatic parenchymal transection line was marked on the liver surface with electrocautery. The line runs 2cm away from the edge of the tumor
Hepatic parenchymal transection ↓	◀ Having occluded the portal triad and the infrahepatic inferior vena cava, hepatic parenchymal transection was performed along the cut line, using the clamp-crushing method.
Management of the raw area of the liver remnant ↓	◀ The residual liver was closely intermittently suture-ligated together to stop bleeding.
Closure of the abdominal cavity and drainage	◀ A rubber tube was placed at the Winslow hole and secured.

Intraoperative Key Points

1. For huge HCCs (diameter >10 cm) located centrally, due to its close proximity to the intrahepatic major vascular vessels and the retrohepatic inferior vena cava, control of the intraoperative bleeding is the key to success of this surgery. Therefore, precautionary total vascular exclusion should be prepared for; in case of torrential bleeding, rapid and effective hemostasis can be achieved (see Section "Mesohepatectomy (S4 + S5 + S8 Resection)" in the Chapter "Types of Segment-Oriented Hepatic Resection by the Glissonean Pedicle Approach").
2. In liver surgery, the liver volume to be resected and the volume of the future liver remnant must be assessed preoperatively for safe hepatic resection, especially for patients with either borderline liver function or a small-for-size future liver remnant (see Chapter 2.1.2) [54–56]. Meanwhile, using three-dimensional (3D) image processing software [57, 58], volumetric analysis facilitates selection of the optional and precise parenchymal transection plane.
3. In this resection, nonanatomic resection must be undertaken to preserve the uninvolved central superior hepatic parenchyma, in order to prevent postoperative liver failure caused by insufficient functional liver tissue. No matter anatomic versus limited nonanatomic resection for this solitary hepatocellular carcinoma is oncologically superior or not, the safety of the liver resection is the most paramount goal, which all surgeons must always keep in mind [59, 60].
4. In liver resection with large cut surface associated with stubborn errhysis, intermittent close suture ligation is an effective and safe method to achieve hemostasis (Fig. 77).

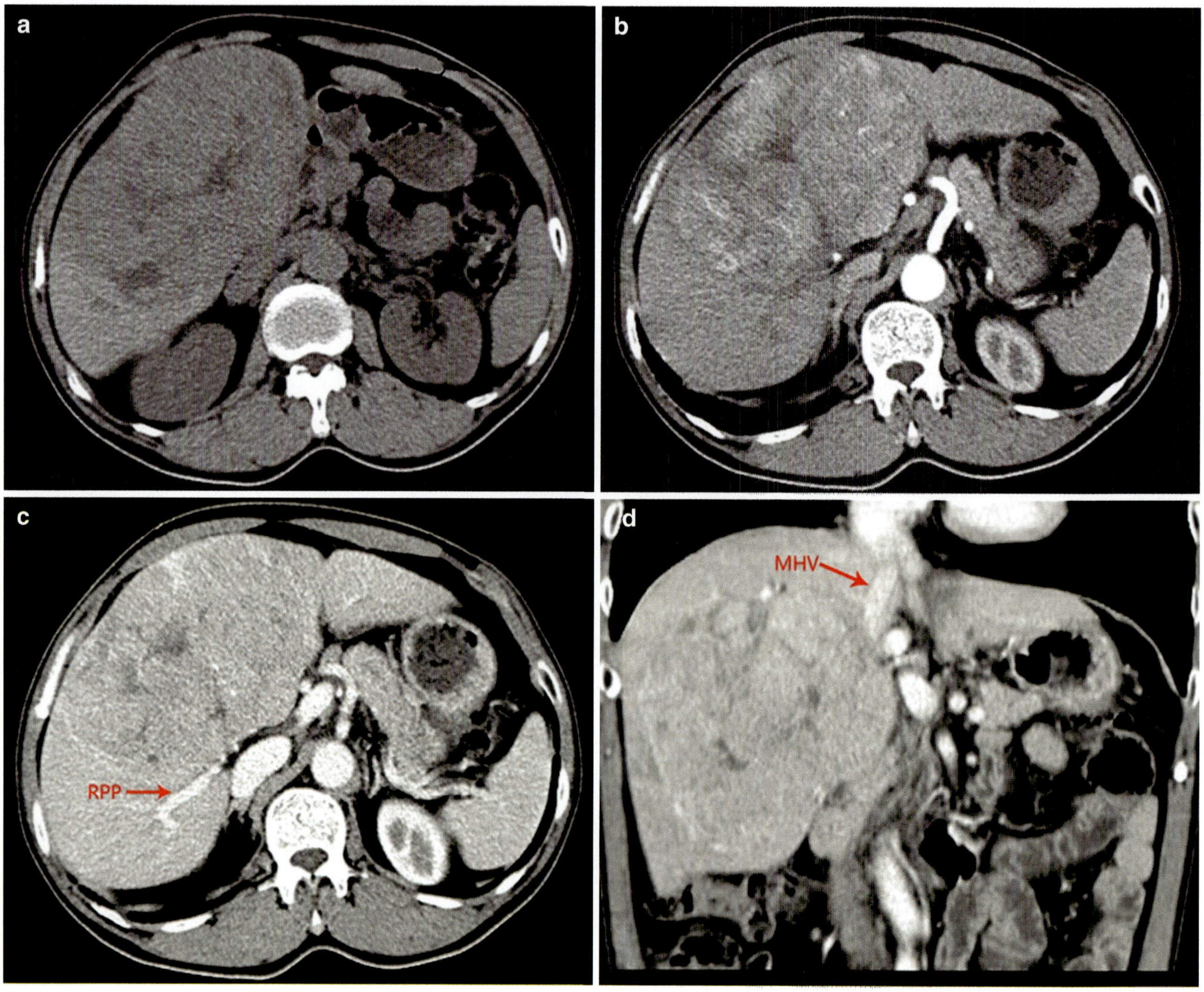

Fig. 77 (**a**) Preoperative CT (precontrast). The tumor, which appears mildly hypodense, occupies the central segments. (**b**) Preoperative CT (hepatic arterial phase). The tumor shows heterogeneous enhancement. (**c**) Preoperative CT (hepatic venous phase). The right posterior branch of the portal vein is obviously normal. The tumor shows enhancement fades. (**d**) Preoperative CT (coronal section of the tumor). The MHV entered into the tumor. *MHV* middle hepatic vein, *RPP* right posterior sectional pedicle

Mobilization of the Liver
(Figs. 78, 79, 80, 81, 82, 83, and 84)

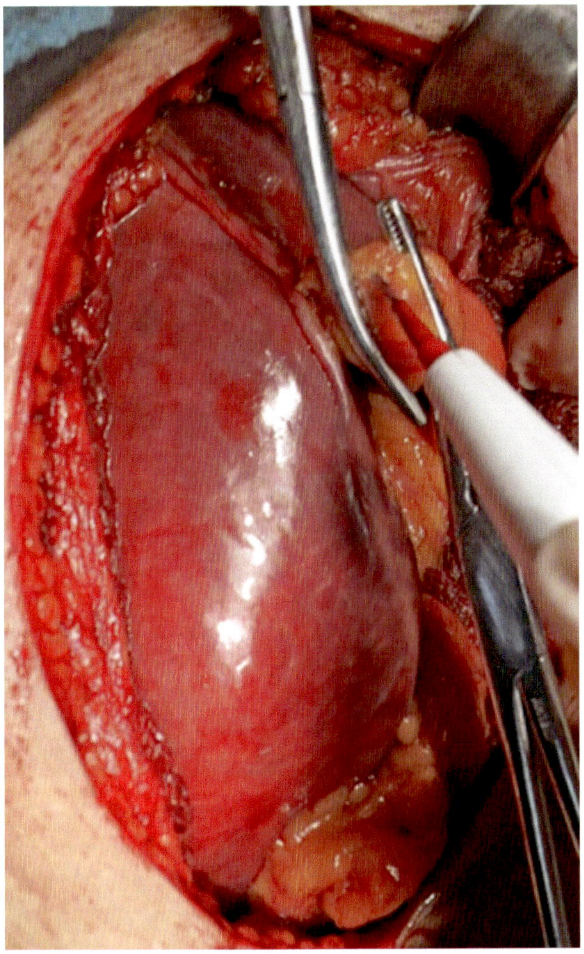

Fig. 78 The round ligament was divided and ligated

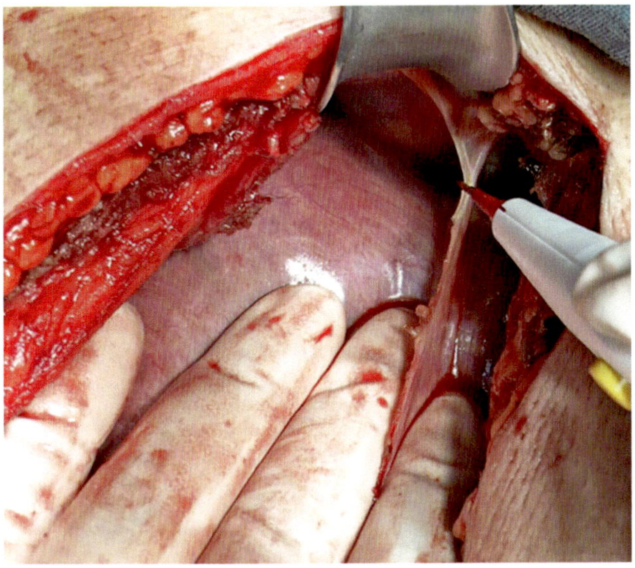

Fig. 79 The falciform ligament was divided with electrocautery

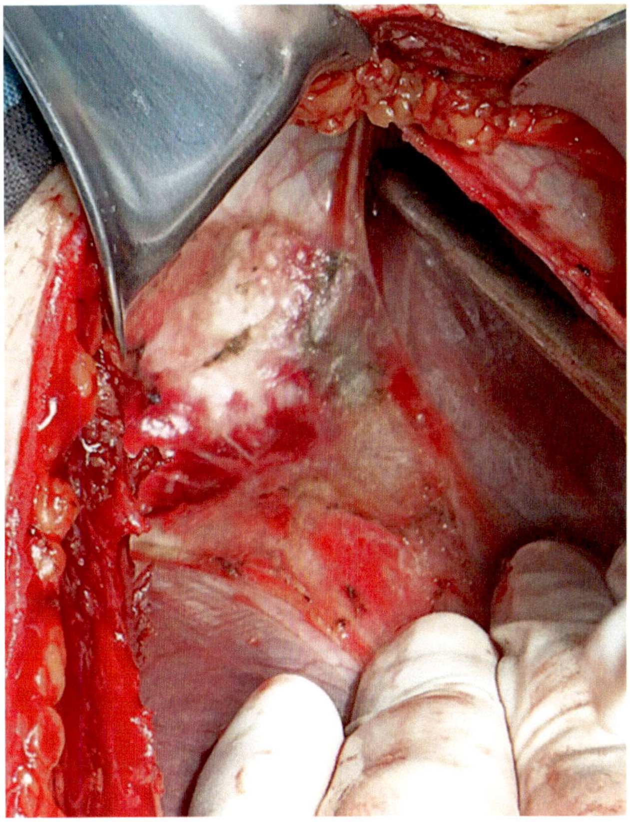

Fig. 80 Dissection of the anterior surface of the suprahepatic inferior vena cava was carried out

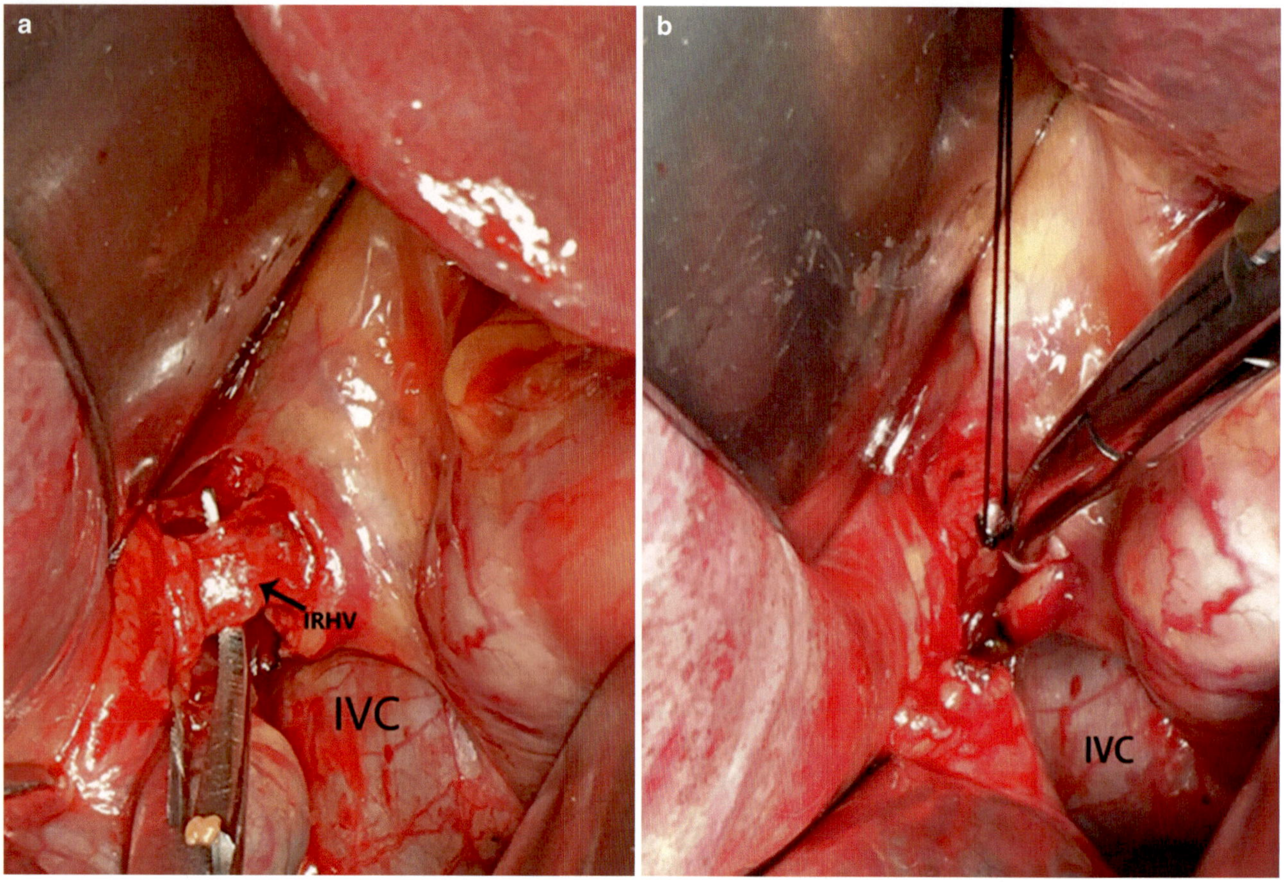

Fig. 81 (**a**, **b**) The inferior right hepatic vein (IRHV) was isolated, divided, and ligated. *IVC* inferior vena cava

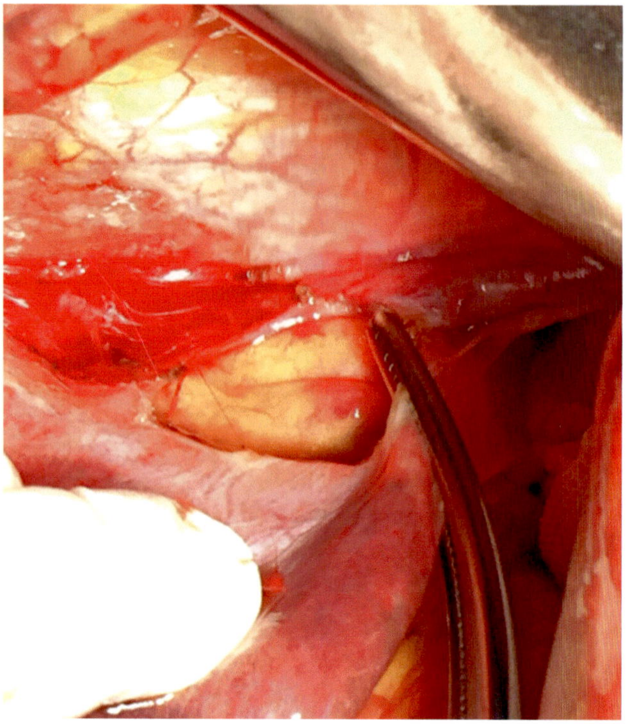

Fig. 82 The left triangular ligament was isolated, divided, and ligated

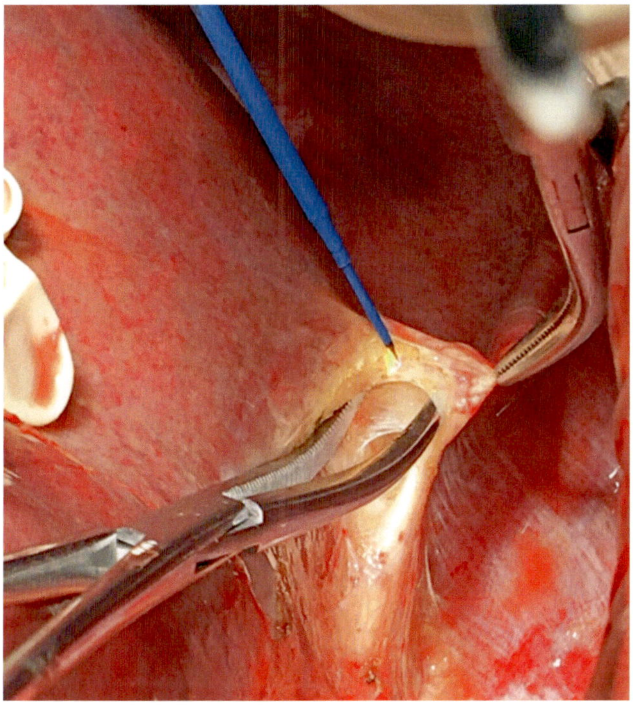

Fig. 83 The right coronary ligament was dissected

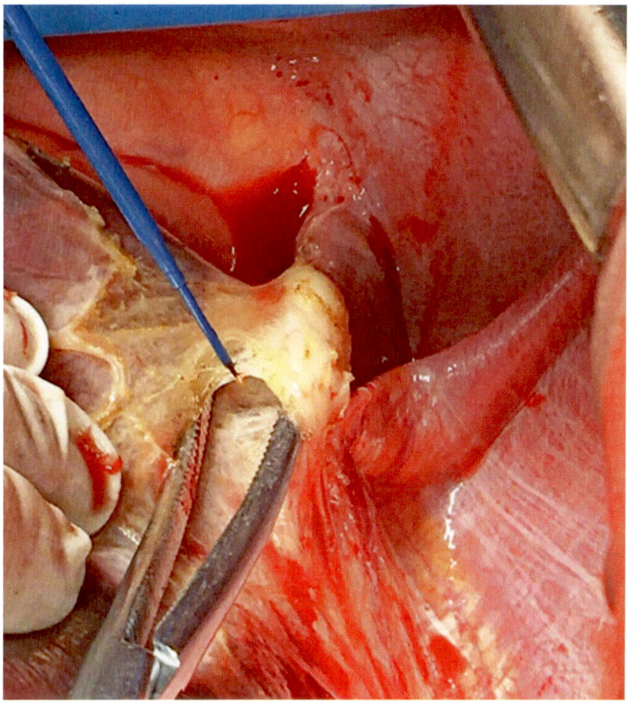

Fig. 84 The right triangular ligament was dissected with electrocautery

Preparation for Total Vascular Exclusion
(Figs. 85, 86, and 87)

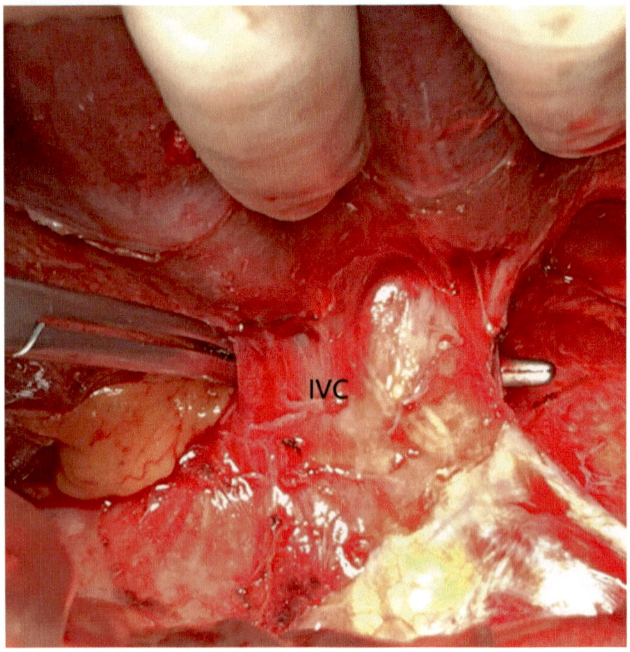

Fig. 85 The suprahepatic IVC was freed away from its surrounding tissues and isolated. *IVC* inferior vena cava

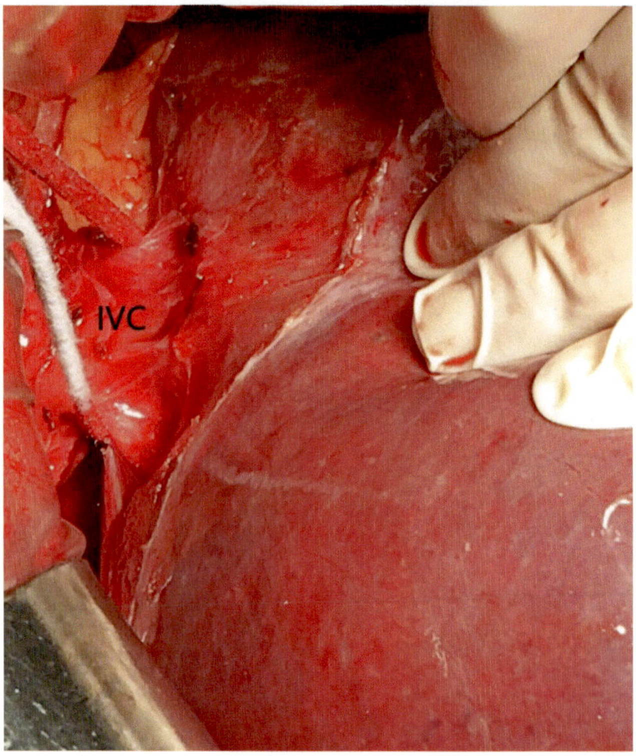

Fig. 86 The suprahepatic IVC was encircled with a vascular tape. *IVC* inferior vena cava

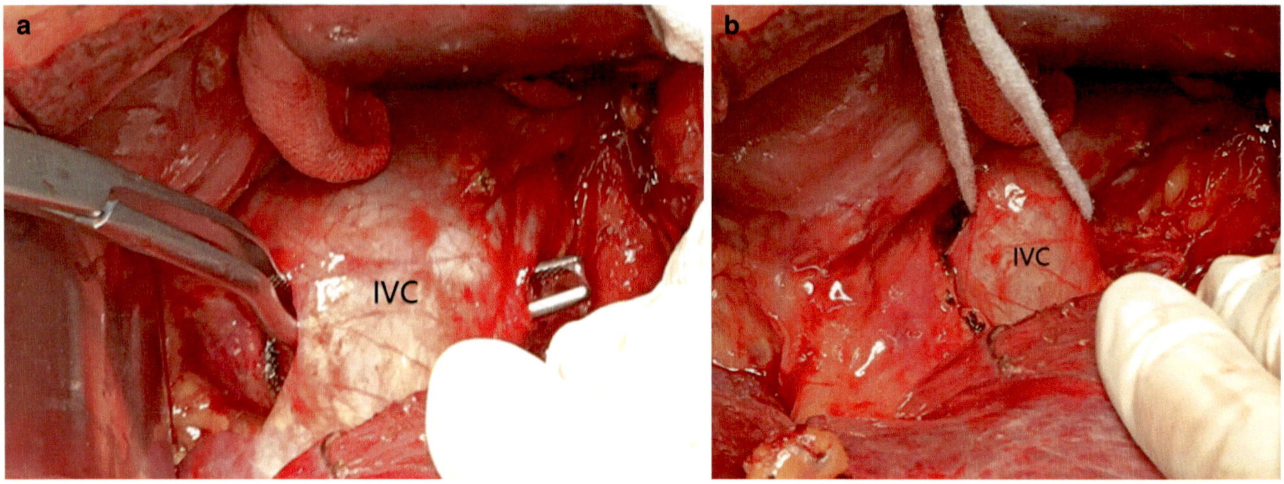

Fig. 87 (**a**, **b**) The infrahepatic IVC was isolated and encircled with a vascular tape. *IVC* inferior vena cava

Marking the Cut Line (Figs. 88 and 89)

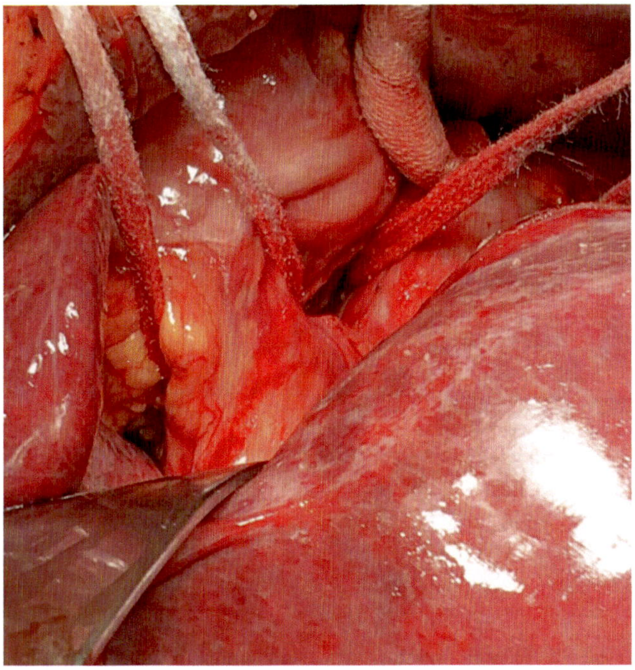

Fig. 88 The portal trial was also pre-placed with a vascular tape

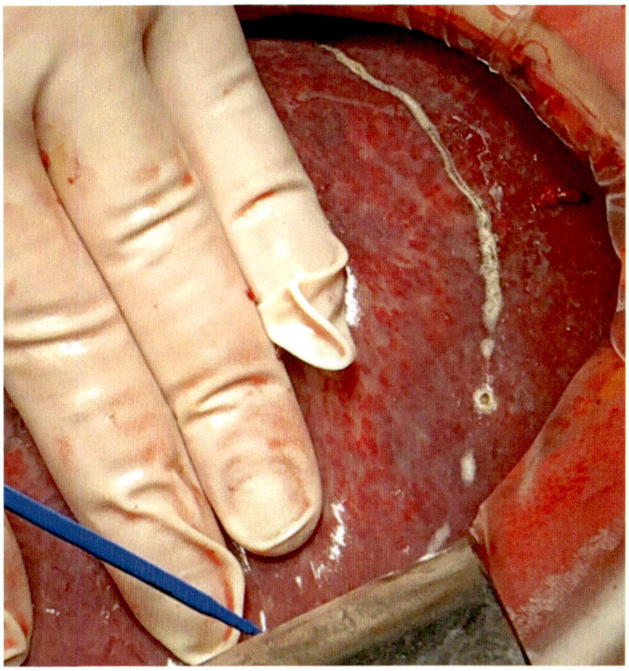

Fig. 89 The right and left hepatic parenchymal transection line was marked on the liver surface with electrocautery. The line runs 2 cm away from the edge of the tumor

Hepatic Parenchymal Transection

(Figs. 90, 91, 92, 93, and 94)

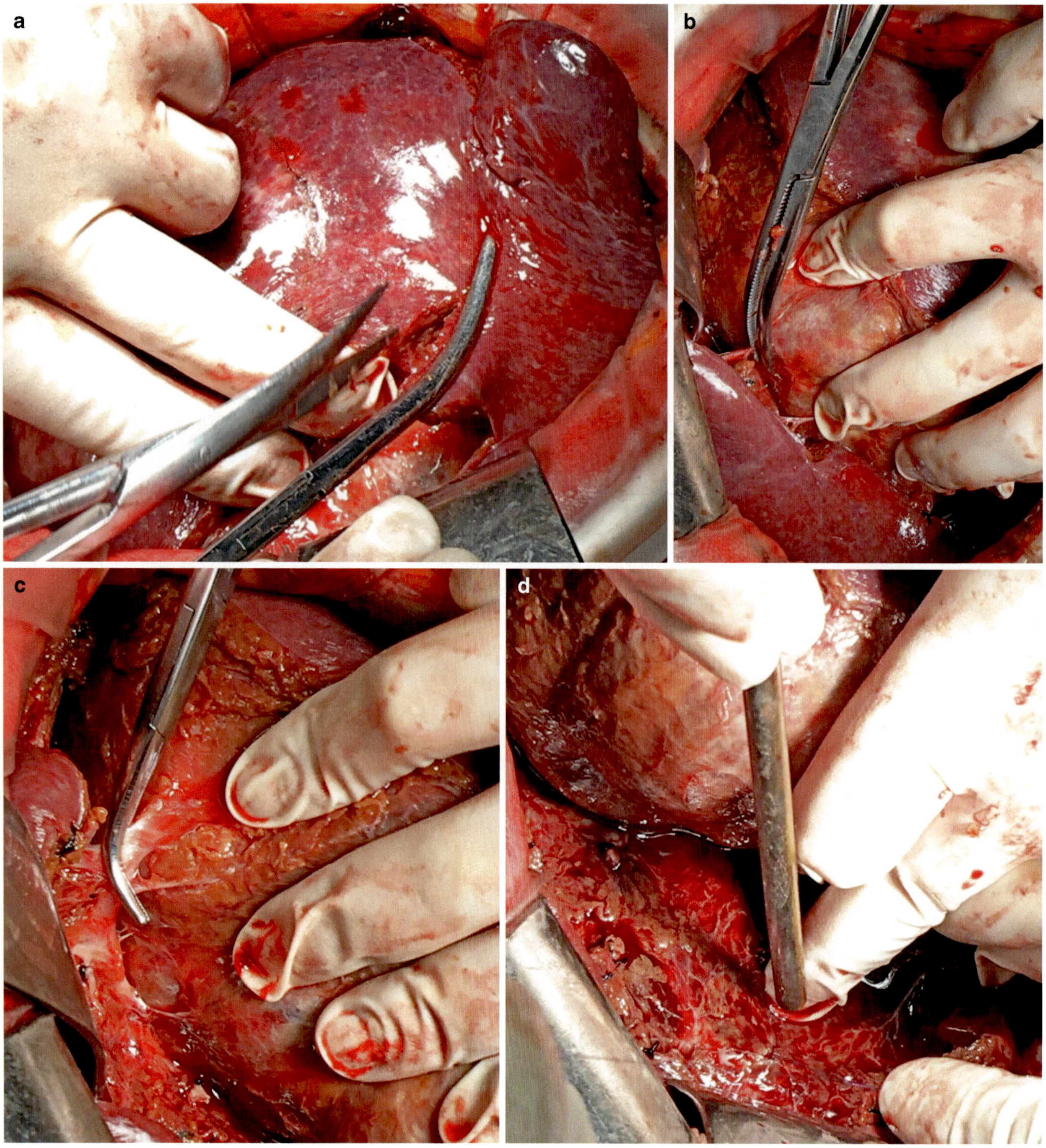

Fig. 90 (**a**–**d**) Having occluded the portal trial (Pringle maneuver) and the infrahepatic IVC, hepatic parenchymal transection was carried out along the cut line, using clamp crushing method. The right-side transection was initially begun cranial-caudally. During the transectional proceedings, all large vessels were divided and ligated, and small vessels were electrocauterized. Tiny holes on the trunks of the main vascular and biliary vessels were repaired with 4-0 or 5-0 polypropylene

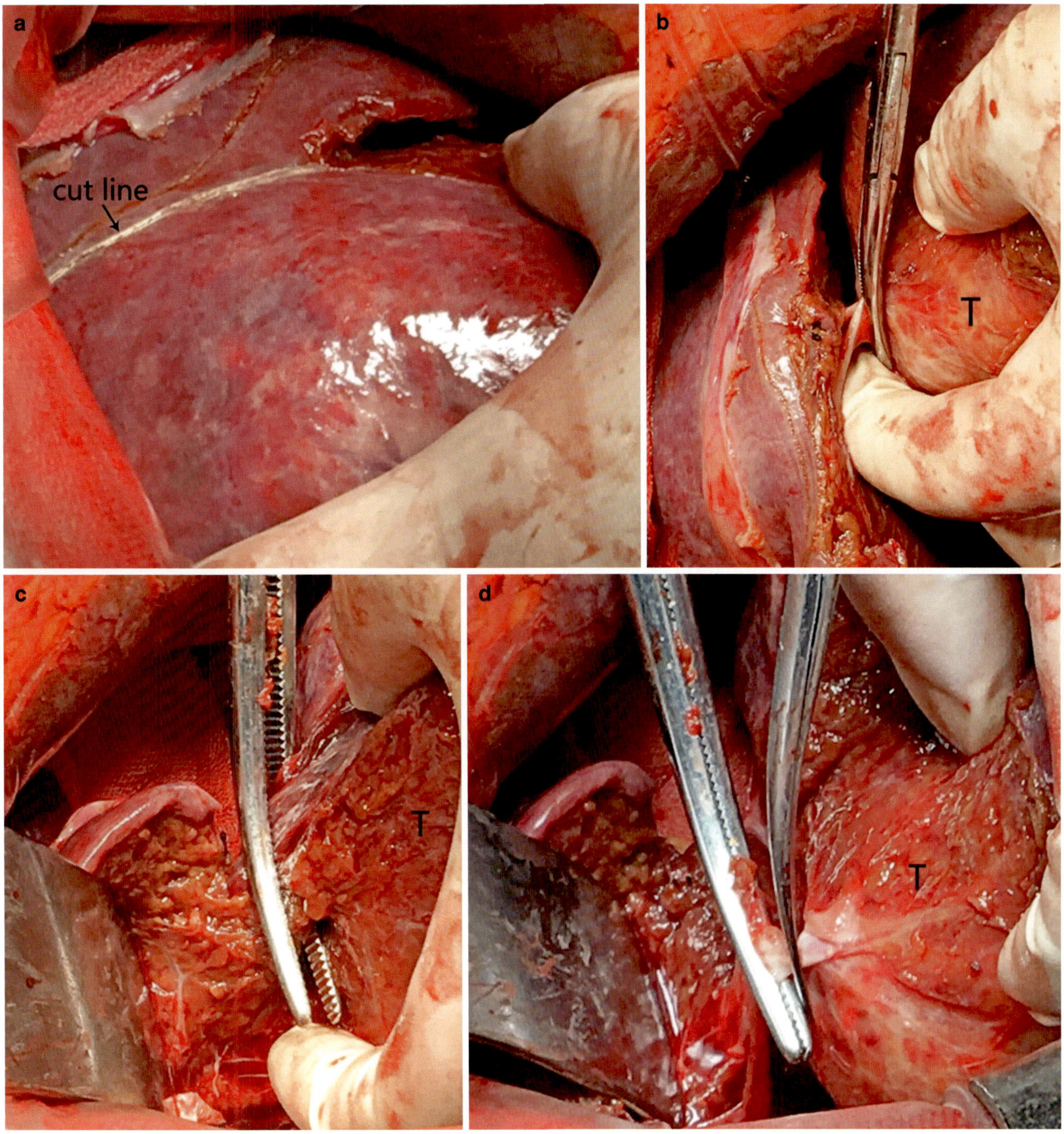

Fig. 91 (**a**–**d**) Left-side hepatic parenchymal transection was then performed caudal-cranially. Also, large branches of the main vascular and biliary vessels were divided and ligated, and small vessels were electrocauterized

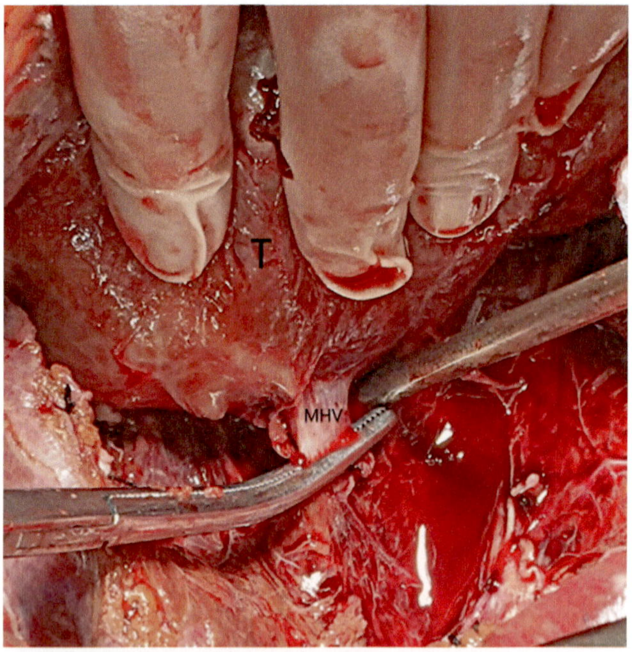

Fig. 92 The intrahepatic middle hepatic vein (MHV) was divided, and its proximal stump was suture-ligated

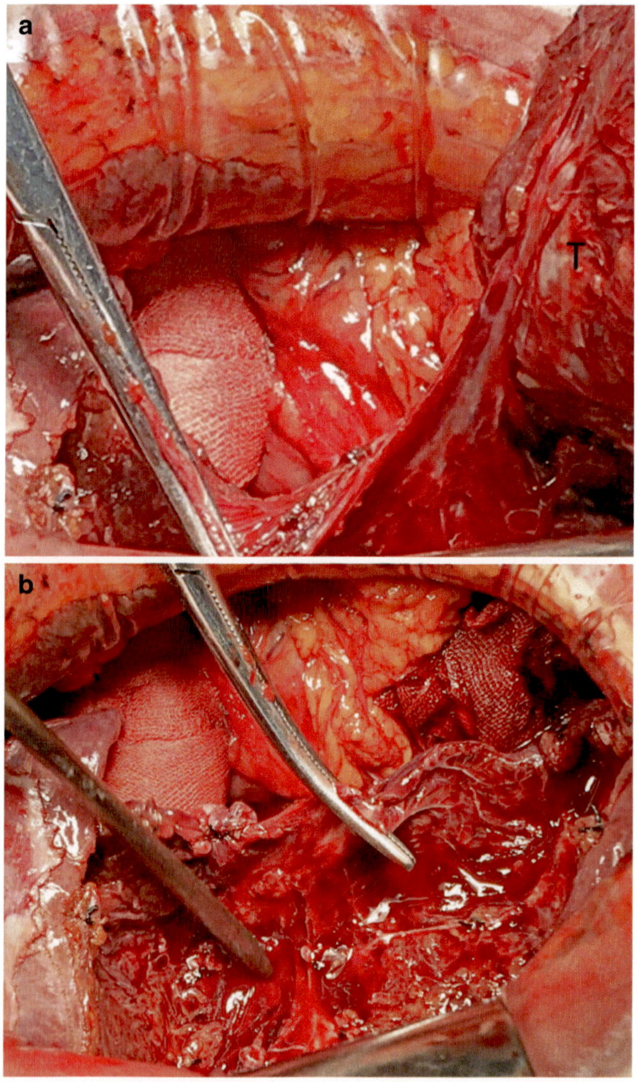

Fig. 93 (**a**, **b**) The pedicle of the tumor from the hepatic pedicle was isolated and divided, and its proximal stump was suture-ligated

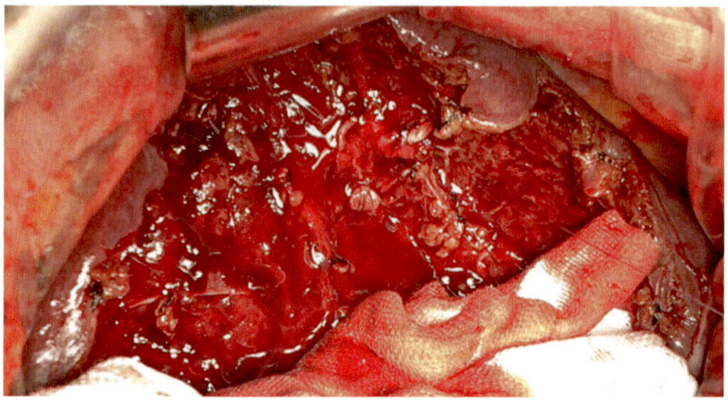

Fig. 94 The raw area of the residual liver. Oozing bleeding is lasting on the cut surface

Management of the Cut Surface of the Liver Remnant and the Specimen (Figs. 95 and 96)

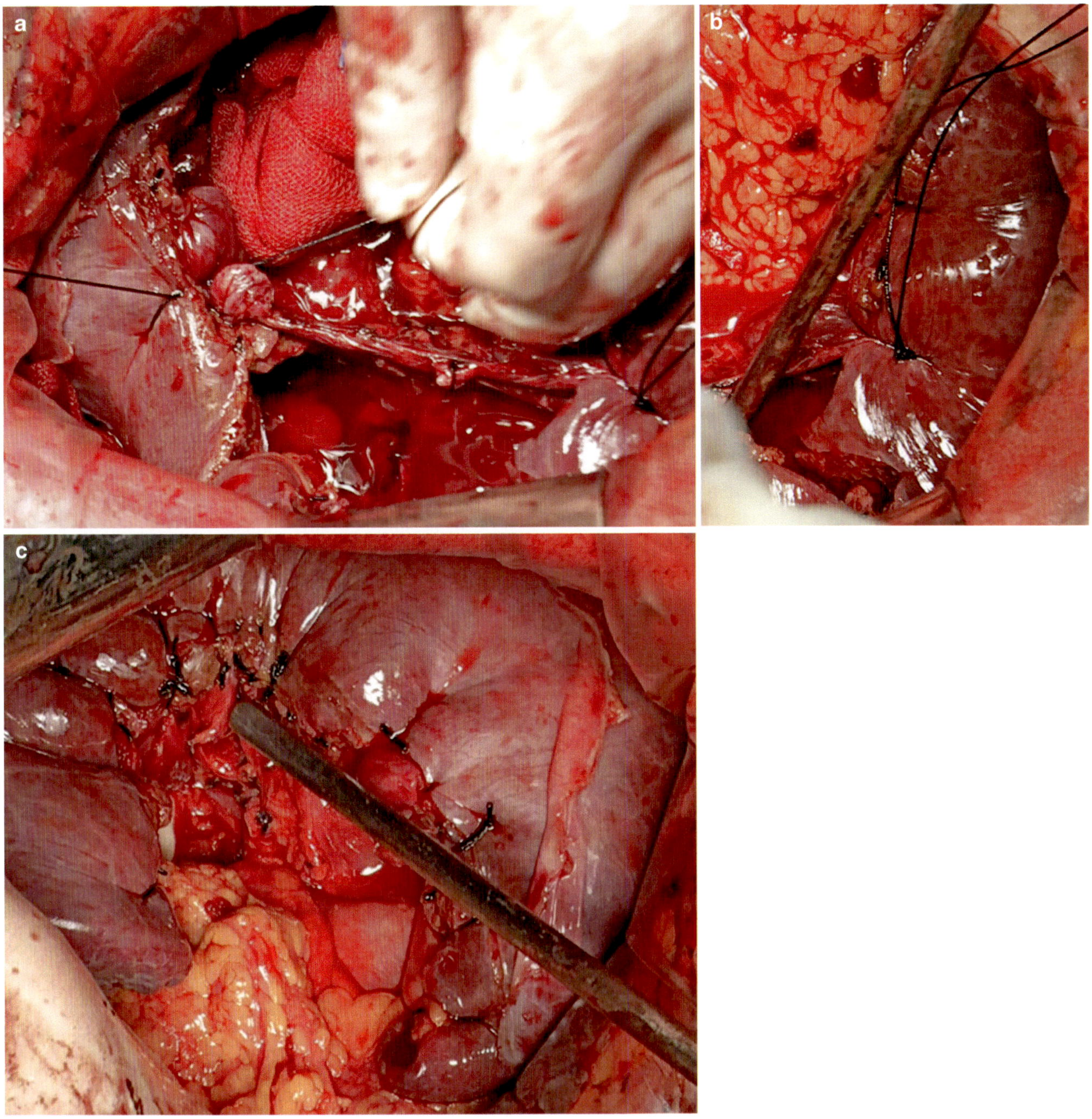

Fig. 95 (**a**–**c**) The residual liver was closely and intermittently sutured together to stop bleeding. Having performed this step, the color on the surface of the liver remnant was normal, which indicated inflow and outflow vascular system was maintained

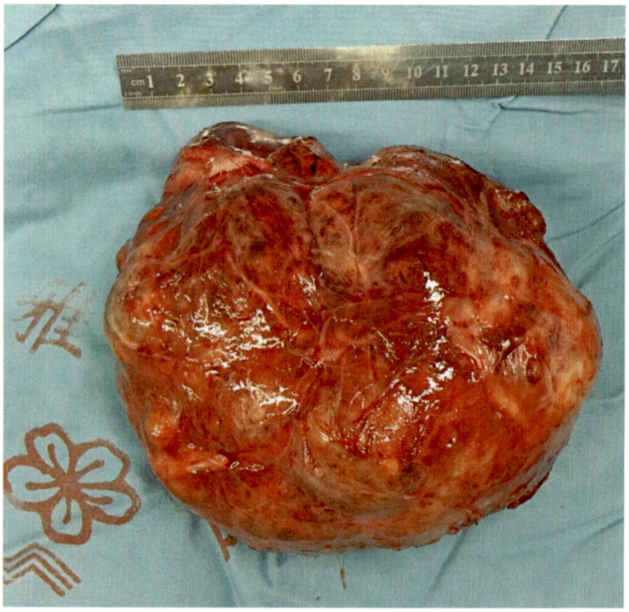

Fig. 96 The cut surface of the specimen. Surgical margin was macroscopically negative

Hepatic Resection for Hepatocellular Carcinoma with Bile Duct Tumor Thrombus

Jixiong Hu, Weidong Dai, and Tenglong Tang

Hepatocellular carcinoma (HCC) is often caused by hepatitis virus infection, cirrhosis, alcohol abuse, and obesity. Generally, HCC spreads intrahepatically by venous invasion. Thus, portal vein tumor thrombus is frequently observed in radiological imaging and resected specimen [61]. However, hepatocellular carcinoma with bile duct tumor thrombus (BDTT) is uncommon even in clinical practice. The incidence ranges from 1% to 12% in all HCC cases [62–67]. When bile duct tumor thrombus occurs in and obstructs the common hepatic duct or the common bile duct, jaundice often is the main and initial clinical presentation and can occasionally be misdiagnosed as a cholangiocarcinoma or choledocholithiasis [63, 68]. The first description of HCC with BDTT was reported in 1947 and was termed as "icteric-type hepatoma" [69]. BDTT is considered a risk factor of the prognosis of HCC patients and prognostic staging system such as the Liver Cancer Study Group of Japan (LCSGJ) staging system for HCC regards the presence of BDTT as an indicator of advanced stage, similar to macroscopic vascular invasion [70]. However, the pathological characteristics and prognostic implications of BDTT are less well defined [71]. These palliative treatment modalities, such as transcatheter arterial chemoembolization (TACE), internal biliary stenting, and radiotherapy, often bring about disencouraging outcomes. Although some studies have reported poor prognosis in HCC patients with BDTT [72, 73], other have reported acceptable postoperative survival [62, 74–77]. These conflicting reporters showed that the effectiveness and benefits of hepatic resection for long-term survival of HCC patients remain controversial [78, 79].

Surgical Indications

The routine preoperative imaging studies include abdominal ultrasound and high-resolution and contrast-enhanced computed tomography (CT). The most important component of preoperative imaging should be magnetic resonance cholangiopancreatography (MRCP). MRCP can clearly show the location and expanded extent of the BDTT. For patients with HCC with BDTT, anatomic hepatectomy was also preferred over nonanatomic resection, in combination with removal of the BDTT. With respect to the criterion for evaluation of liver function, Child-Pugh classification and ICGR15 were adopted. According to these main two values, appropriate type of liver resection was employed.

Operative Procedures	Technical Details
Laparotomy ↓	◀ A right subcostal incision was made and peritoneal exploration was performed.
Exploration of the extrahepatic bile duct and cholecystectomy ↓	◀ Cholecystectomy was performed. This common bile duct was obviously dilated.
Marking the cut line ↓	◀ Because this patient's ICGR15 is more than 25% and Child classification is Grade B, wedge resection was selected. The cut line away from the edge of the tumor was marked on the liver surface.
Remove the tumor embolus ↓	◀ The anterior wall of the common bile duct was cut open, and the tumor embolus was easily pulled out of the lumen of the common bile duct. Then, the lumen was lavished.
Hepatic parenchymal transection ↓	◀ Parenchymal transection was carried out along the cut line. During the surgical proceedings, large vessels were ligated.
T-tube drainage ↓	◀ A Gauze-22 rubber T-tube was inserted into the lumen of the common bile duct and was secured with surture-ligating.
Closure of the abdominal cavity and drainage	◀ A rubber tube was placed in the Winslow hole and secured.

Intraoperative Key Points

1. In case that preoperative ICGR15 and Child classification permits, anatomical hepatic resection should be adopted, because proper liver resection may offer an opportunity for a cure and favorable long-term survival [77, 80].
2. BDTT was not necessarily a contraindication for hepatectomy and do not imply advanced disease [81, 82].
3. Previous studies have demonstrated that BDTT can develop and grow even when the primary tumor was at an early stage [65, 83]. However, the mechanism underlying occurrence of BDTT is still obscure. In most instances, BDTT do not invade into the submucosa of large bile ducts and generally do not adhere to the bile duct wall and float up and down within the lumen of the bile duct [78, 84]. Consequently, the surgeons can easily pull the tumor thrombus out of the bile duct. In rare cases, the tumor is continuous with its main tumor and also invades into the bile duct. Under such a circumstance, it is required to resect the involved bile duct and reconstruct the biliary flow system by biliary-jejunal anastomosis.
4. Residual tumor thrombus debris must be avoided. If this cannot be achieved, early recurrence may very soon happen and obstructive jaundice must be once more managed (Fig. 97).

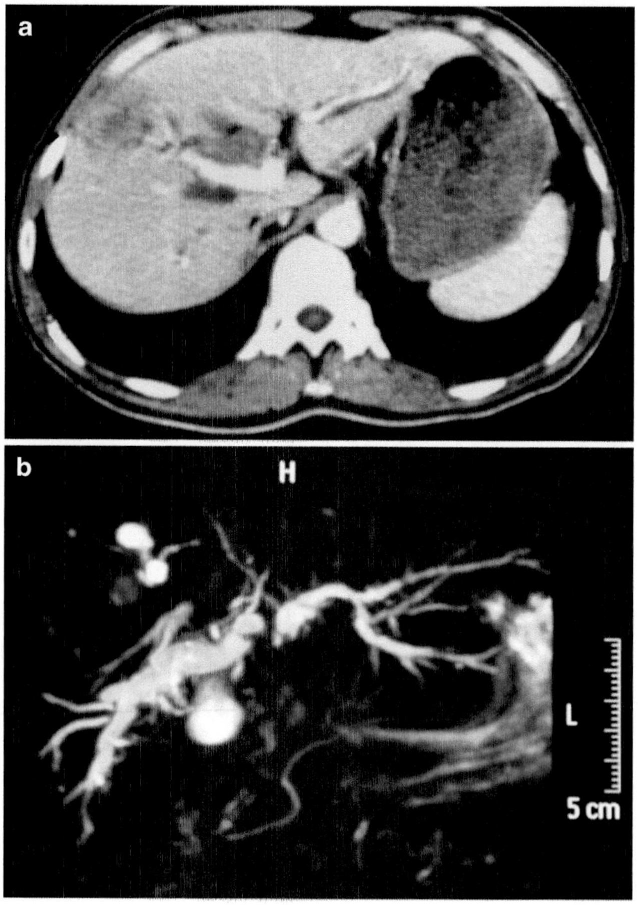

Fig. 97 (**a**) Preoperative CT (hepatic venous phase). The tumor, which appears heterogeneous enhancement, is located in the central segments. (**b**) MRCP shows that the intrahepatic ducts are dilated and the common bile duct is obstructed

Exploration of the Extrahepatic Bile Duct and Cholecystectomy (Fig. 98)

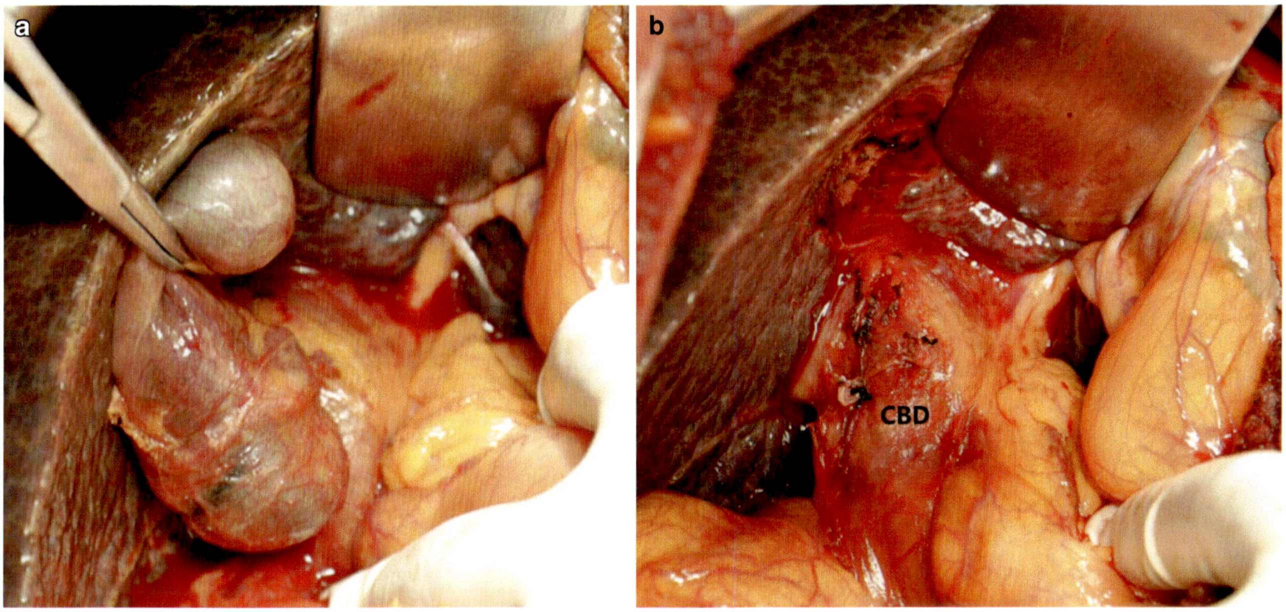

Fig. 98 (**a**, **b**) The liver obviously appeared cholestatic. Cholecystectomy was performed. The common bile duct (CBD) was dilated

Marking the Cut Line (Fig. 99)

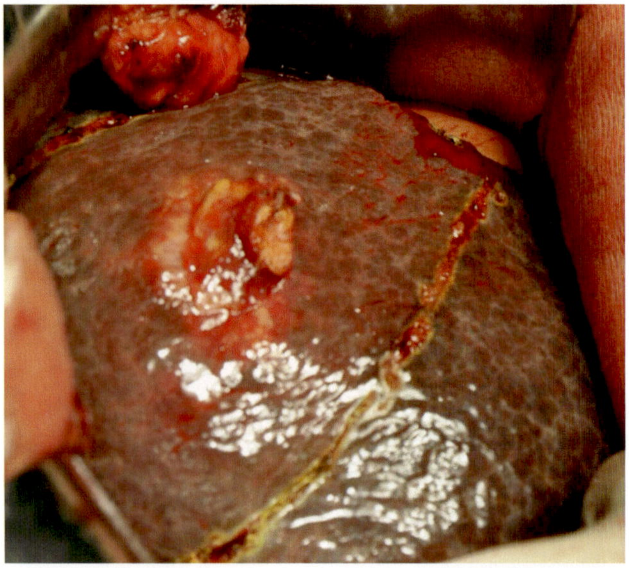

Fig. 99 The hepatic transection line was electrocauterized on the liver surface. The line runs 2 cm away from the edge of the tumor

Remove the Tumor Emboli Within the Common Bile Duct (Figs. 100, 101, 102, and 103)

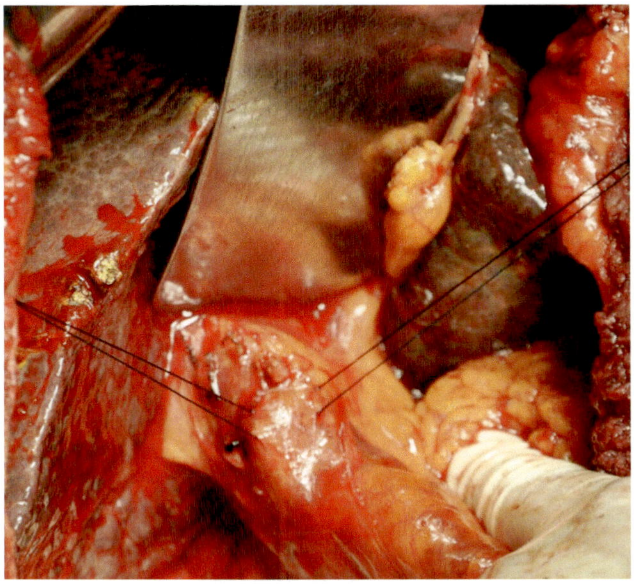

Fig. 100 The common bile duct (CBD) was hanging up

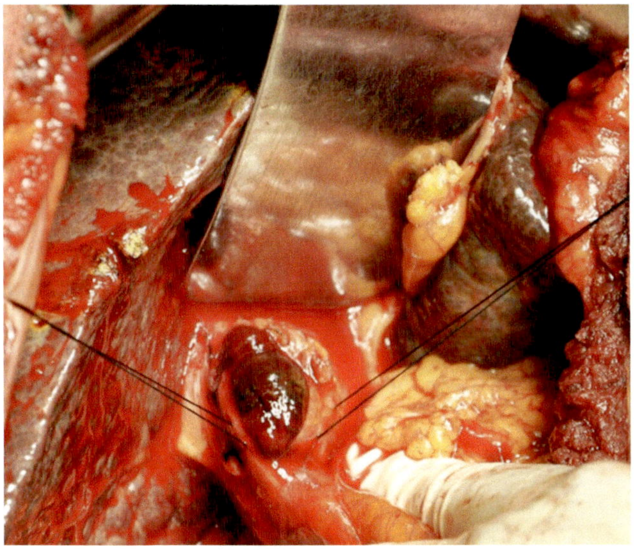

Fig. 101 The anterior wall of the common bile duct (CBD) was opened, and the tumor emboli within the lumen of the CBD were shown

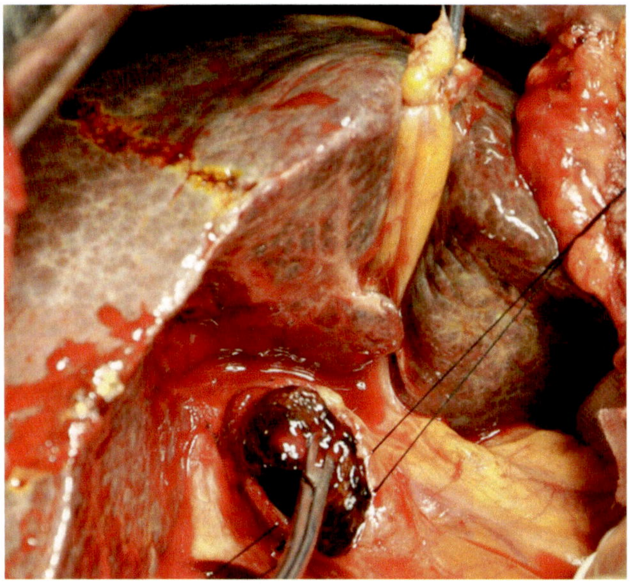

Fig. 102 The tumor emboli were pulled out of the lumen of the CBD

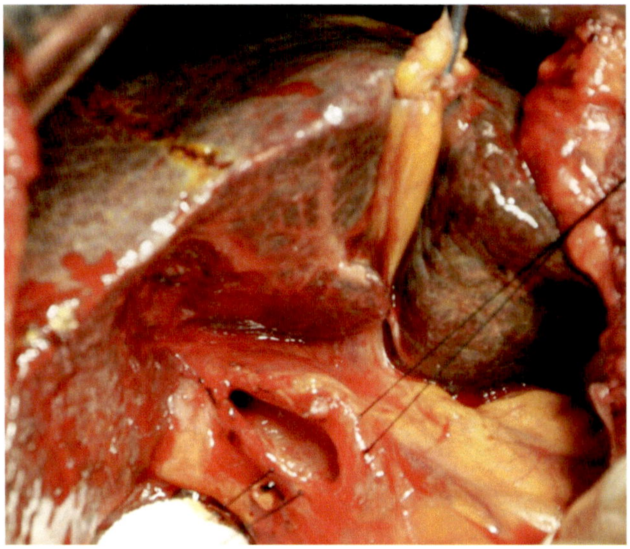

Fig. 103 The tumor emboli have been completely removed, and the lumen of the CBD was empty. Then, the lumen of the CBD was lavished with sterile saline

Hepatic Parenchymal Transection
(Figs. 104 and 105)

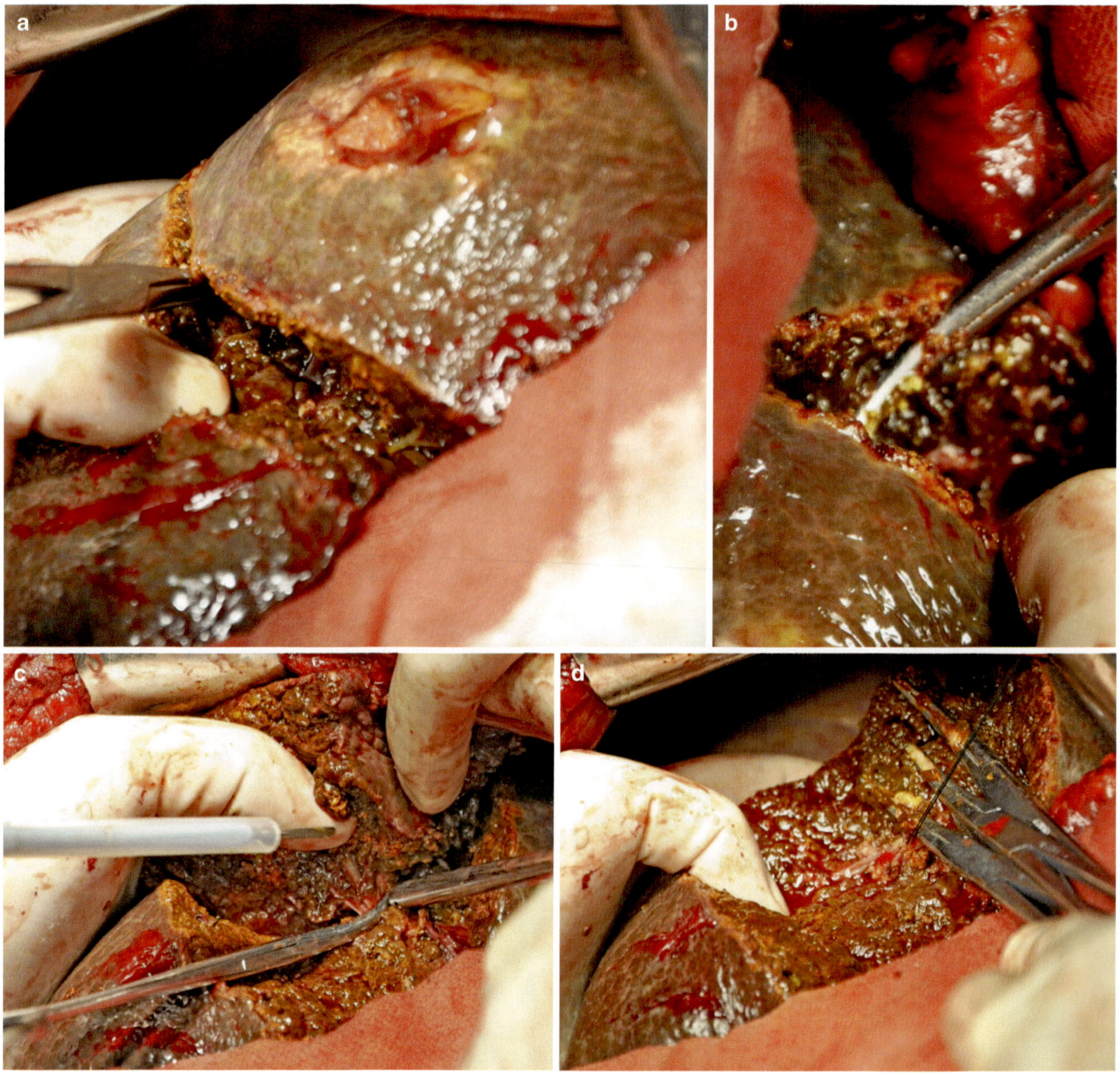

Fig. 104 (**a**–**d**) Hepatic parenchymal transection was undertaken along the cut line on the liver surface, using clamp crushing method. During the transectional proceedings, all large branches of the main vascular and biliary vessels were divided and ligated, and small branches were electrocauterized

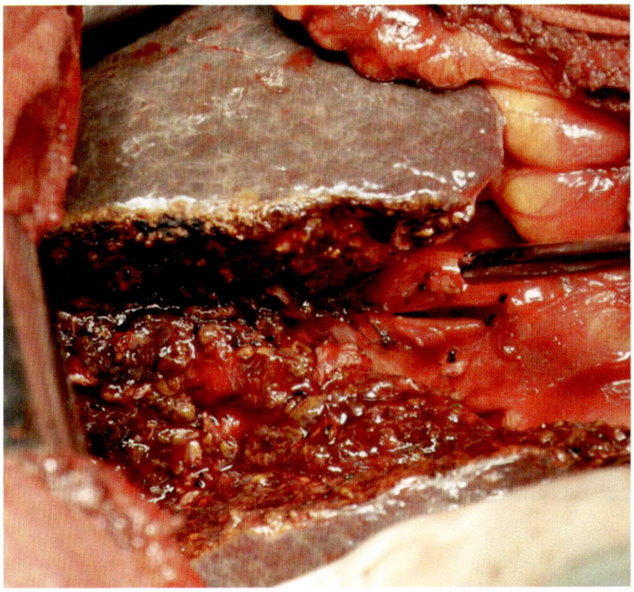

Fig. 105 Raw area of the residual liver

T-tube Drainage and the Specimen
(Figs. 106 and 107)

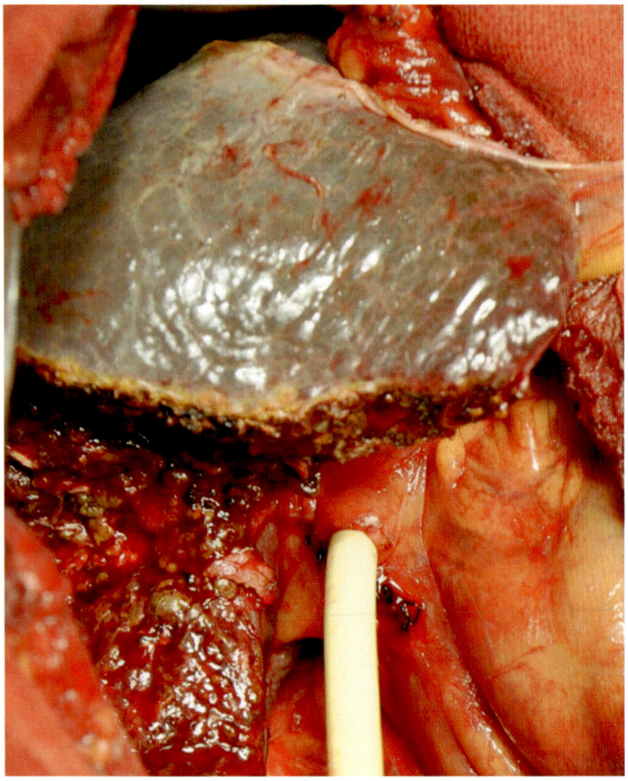

Fig. 106 A Gauze-22 T-tube was inserted into the CBD and secured with suture ligation

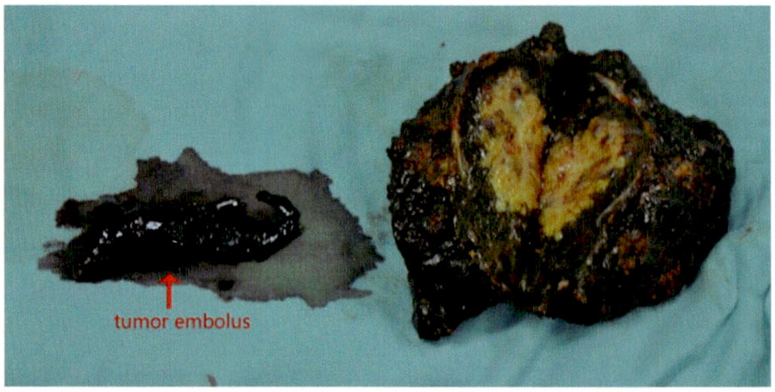

Fig. 107 Tumor emboli and the HCC tumor. Surgical margin was macroscopically negative

References

1. Abdel-Misih SRZ, Bloomston M. Liver anatomy. Surg Clin N Am. 2010;90(4):643–53.
2. Kumon M. Anatomy of the caudate lobe with special reference to portal vein and bile duct. Acta Hepatol Jpn. 1985;26(9):1193–9.
3. Cho A, Okazumi S, Takayama W, Takeda A, Iwasaki K, Sasagawa S, Natsume T, Kono T, Kondo S, Ochiai T, Ryu M. Anatomy of the right anterosuperior area (segment 8) of the liver: evaluation with helical CT during arterial portography. Radiology. 2000;214(2):491–5.
4. Sarmiento JM, Que FG, Nagorney DM. Surgical outcomes of isolated caudate lobe resection. A single series of 19 patients. Surgery. 2002;132(4):697–709.
5. Bartlett D, Fong Y, Blumgart LH. Complete resection of the caudate lobe of the liver: technique and results. Br J Surg. 1996;83(8):1076–81.
6. Elias D, Lasser PH, Desruennes E, Mankarios H, Jiang Y. Surgical approach to segment I for malignant tumors of the liver. Surg Gynecol Obstet. 1992;175(1):17–24.
7. Hu JX, Miao XY, Zhong DW, Dai WD, Liu W. Anterior approach for complete isolated caudate lobectomy. Hepatogastroenterology. 2005;52(66):1641–4.
8. Shimada M, Matsumata T, Maeda T, Yanaga K, Taketomi A, Sugimachi K. Characteristics of hepatocellular careinoma originating in the caudate lobe. Hepatology. 1994;19(4):911–5.
9. Fan J, Wu ZQ, Tang ZY, Zhou J, Qiu SJ, Ma ZC, Zhou XD, Yu YQ. Complete resection of the caudate lobe of the liver with tumor: technique and experience. Hepatogastroenterology. 2001;48(39):808–11.
10. Nagasue N, Kohno H, Yamanoi A, Vchida M, Yamaguchi M, Tachibana M, Kubota H, Ohmoir H. Resection of the caudate lobe of the liver for primary and recurrent hepatocellular carcinoma. J Am Coll Surg. 1997;184(1):1–8.
11. Yang MC, Lee PH, Sheu JC, Lai MY, Hu RH, Wei CK. Surgical treatment of hepatocellular carcinoma originating from the caudate lobe. World J Surg. 1996;20(5):562–6.
12. Dai WD, Huang JS, Hu JX. Isolated caudate lobe resection for huge hepatocellular carcinoma (10 cm or greater in diameter). Am Surg. 2014;80(2):159–65.
13. Ahanatha Pillai S, Sathyanesan J, Perumal S, Ulagendra Perumal S, Lakshmanan A, Ramaswami S, Ramasamy R, Palaniappan R, Rajagopal S. Isolated caudate lobe resection: technical challenges. Ann Gastroenterol. 2013;26(2):150–5.
14. Ochiai T, Ishii H, Toma A, Ishimoto T, Yamamoto Y, Morimura R, Ikoma H, Otsuji E. Modified high dorsal procedure for performing isolated anatomic total caudate lobectomy (with video). World J Surg Oncol. 2016;14(1):1–6.
15. Hiroshima Y, Matsuo K, Kawaguchi D, Kikuchi Y, Endo I, Koda K, Togo S, Hoffman RM, Tanaka K. Modified liver hanging maneuver for en-bloc right-sided hepatectomy combined with total caudate lobectomy for colon-cancer liver metastasis and hepatocellular carcinoma. Anticancer Res. 2016;36(4):1729–35.
16. Chaib E, Ribeiro MA Jr, Souza YE, D'Albuquerque LA. Anterior hepatic transection for caudate lobectomy. Clinics. 2009;64(11):1121–215.
17. Midorikawa Y, Takayama T. Caudate lobectomy (segmentectomy 1) (with video). J Hepatobiliary Pancreat Sci. 2012;19(1):48–53.
18. Sakoda M, Ueno S, Kubo F, Hiwatashi K, Tateno T, Kurahara H, Mataki Y, Shinchi H, Natsugoe S. Surgery for hepatocellular carcinoma located in the caudate lobe. World J Surg. 2009;33(9):1922–6.
19. Wang ZG, Lau W, Fu SY, Liu H, Pan ZY, Yang Y, Zhang J, Wu MC, Zhou WP. Anterior hepatic parenchymal transection for complete caudate lobectomy to treat liver cancer situated in or involving the paracaval portion of the caudate lobe. J Gastrointest Surg. 2015;19(5):880–6.
20. Nakaji S, Hirata N. Evaluation of the viability of hepatocellular carcinoma in the caudate lobe using contrast-enhanced endoscopic ultrasonography after transarterial chemoembolization. Endosc Ultrasound. 2016;5(6):390–2.
21. Hong DF, Liu YB, Peng SY, Pang JZ, Wang ZF, Cheng J, Shen GL, Zhang YB. Management of hepatocellular carcinoma rupture in the caudate lobe. World J Gastroenterol. 2015;21(26):8163–9.
22. Yamamoto T, Kubo S, Shuto T, Ichikawa T, Masao O, Hai S, Sakabe K, Tanaka S, Venishi T, Ikebe T, Tanaka H, Kaneda K, Hirohashi K. Surgical strategy for hepatocellalar carcinoma originating in the caudate lobe. Surgery. 2004;135(6):595–603.
23. Jin Y, Wang L, Yu YQ, Zhou DE, Liu DR, Yang JJ, Peng SY, Li JT. Anatomic isolated caudate lobectomy: is it possible to establish a standard surgical flow? World J Gastroenterol. 2017;23(41):7433–9.
24. Makuuchi M, et al. Chapter 14. Caudate lobectomy. In: Makuuchi M, editor. Makuuchi Kanzou Gekagaku (in Japanese)/(translated to Chinese by Yong Zeng). Beijing: People's Medical Publishing House; 2016. p. 110–21.
25. Yang JH, Gu J, Dong P, Chen L, Wu WG, Mu JS, Li ML, Wu XS, Zhao YL, Zhang L, Weng H, Ding Q, Ding QC, Liu YB. Isolated complete caudate lobectomy for hepatic tumor of the anterior transhepatic approach: surgical approaches and perioperative outcomes. World J Surg Oncol. 2013;11(1):197.
26. Huang JS, Dai WD, Miao XY, Zhong DW, Xiong SZ, Hu JX. Null-margin bisegmentectomy VII–VIII for hepatocellular carcinoma in cirrhotic patients. Hepatogastroenterology. 2012;59(118):1706–9.
27. Miao XY, Hu JX, Dai WD, Zhong DW, Xiong SZ. Null-margin mesohepatectomy for centrally located hepatocellular carcinoma in cirrhotic patients. Hepatogastroenterology. 2011;58(106):575–82.
28. Sakamoto Y, Nara S, Hata S, Yamamoto Y, Esaki M, Shimada K, Kosuge T. Prognosis of patients undergoing hepatectomy for solitary hepatocellular carcinoma originating in the caudate lobe. Surgery. 2011;150(5):959–67.
29. Thomas RL, Lordan JT, Devalia K, Quiney N, Fawcett W, Worthington TR, Karanjia ND. Liver resection for colorectal cancer metastases involving the caudate lobe. Br J Surg. 2011;98(10):1476–82.
30. Lee JW, Lee YJ, Park KM, Hwang DW, Lee JH, Song KB. Anatomical resection but not surgical margin width influence survival following resection for HCC, a propensity score analysis. World J Surg. 2016;40(6):1429–39.
31. Yanaga K, Matsumata T, Hayashi H, Shimada M, Urata K, Sugimachi K. Isolated hepatic caudate lobectomy. Surgery. 1994;115(6):757–61.
32. Wang Y, Zhang LY, Yuan L Sun FY, Wei TG. Isolated caudate lobe resection for hepatic tumor: surgical approaches and perioperative outcomes. Am J Surg. 2010;200(3):346–51.
33. Chaib E, Ribeiro MA Jr, Collet SF, Saad WA, Cecconello I. Caudate lobectomy: tumor location, topographic classification, and technique using right- and left-sided approaches to the liver. Am J Surg. 2008;196(2):245–51.
34. Liu P, Yang J, Niu W, Xie F, Wang Y, Zhou Y. Surgical treatment of huge hepatocellular carcinoma in the caudate lobe. Surg Today. 2011;41(4):520–5.
35. Shimada K, Sakamoto Y, Esaki M, Kosuge T. Role of a hepatectomy for the treatment of large hepatocellular carcinomas measuring 10 cm or larger in diameter. Langenbeck's Arch Surg. 2008;393(4):521–6.
36. Yamashita Y, Taketomi A, Shirabe K, Aishima S, Tsuijita E, Morita K, Kayashima H, Maehara Y. Outcomes of hepatic resection for huge hepatocellular carcinoma (≥10 cm in diameter). J Surg Oncol. 2011;104(3):292–8.
37. Shah SA, Wei AC, Cleary SP, Yang I, McGilvray ID, Gallinger S, Grant DR, Greig PD. Prognosis and results after resection of very large (≥10 cm) hepatocellular carcinoma. J Gastrointest Surg. 2007;11(5):589–95.

38. Couinaud C. Etudes anatomiques et chirurgicales. Paris: Mason; 1957. p. 3.
39. Muratore A, Conti P, Amisano M, Bouzari H. Bisegmentectomy 7-8 as alterative to more extensive liver resections. J Am Coll Surg. 2005;200(2):224–8.
40. Nakamura S, Tsuzuki T. Surgical anatomy of the hepatic veins and the inferior vena cava. Surg Gynecol Obstet. 1981;152(1):43–50.
41. Hirai I, Kimura W, Fuse A, Yamamoto T, Moriya T, Mizutani M. Evaluation of inferior right hepatic vein preserving hepatectomy with resection of the superior right hepatic vein. Hepatogastroenterology. 2006;53(70):516–20.
42. Makuuchi M, Hasegawa H, Yamazaki S, Takayasu K. Four new hepatectomy procedures for resection of the right hepatic vein and preservation of the inferior right hepatic vein. Surg Gyneeol Obstet. 1987;64(1):69–72.
43. Hata F, Hirata K, Murakami G, Mukaiya M. Identification of segments VI and VII of the liver based on the ramification patterns of the intrahepatic portal and hepatic veins. Clin Anat. 1999;12(4):229–44.
44. Mehran R, Schneider R, Franchebois P. The minor hepatic veins: anatomy and classification. Clin Anat. 2000;13(6):416–21.
45. Machado MAC, Herman P, Makdissi FF, Figueira ER, Bacchella T, Machado MC. Feasibility of bisegmentectomy 7–8 is independent of the presence of a large inferior right hepatic vein. J Surg Oncol. 2006;93(4):338–42.
46. Hu JX, Dai WD, Miao XY, Zhong DW, Huang SF, Wen Y, Xiong SZ. Anatomic resection of segment VIII of liver for hepatocellular carcinoma in cirrhotic patients based on an intrahepatic Glissonian approach. Surgery. 2009;146(5):854–60.
47. Hu JX, Dai WD, Miao XY, Zhong DW. Bisegmentectomy VII–VIII for hepatocellular carcinoma in cirrhotic livers. Hepatogastroenterology. 2007;54(77):1311–4.
48. Wu CC, Ho WL, Chen JT, Tang CS, Yeh DC, Liu TJ, P'eng FK. Mesohepatectomy for centrally located hepatocellular carcinoma: an appraisal of a rare procedure. J Am Coll Surg. 1999;188(5):508–15.
49. Lee JG, Choi SB, Kim KS, Choi JS, Lee WJ, Kim BR. Central bisectionectomy for centrally located hepatocellular carcinoma. Br J Surg. 2008;95(8):990–5.
50. Dai WD, Hu JX, Miao XY, Zhong DW, Wen Y, Xiong SZ. Intrahepatic glissonian access for mesohepatectomy in cirrhotic patients. Hepatogastroenterology. 2008;55(85):1153–7.
51. Miao XY, Hu JX, Dai WD, Zhong DW, Huang SF, Wen Y, Xiong SZ. Anatomic mesohepatectomy with extrahepatic control of hepatic veins. Hepatogastroenterology. 2009;56(96):1730–4.
52. Tanaka K, Shimada H, Matsumoto C, Matsuo K, Nagano Y, Endo I, Togo S. Anatomic versus limited nonanatomic resection for solitary hepatocellular carcinoma. Surgery. 2008;143(5):607–15.
53. Kang KJ, Ahn KS. Anatomical resection of hepatocellular carcinoma: a critical review of the procedure and its benefits on survival. World J Gastroenterol. 2017;23(7):1139–46.
54. Makuuchi M, Kosuge T, Takayama T, Yamazaki S, Kakazu T, Miyagawa S, Kawasaki S. Sugery for small liver cancers. Semin Surg Oncol. 1993;9(4):298–304.
55. Abdalla EK, Denys A, Chevalier P, Nemr RA, Vauthey JN. Total and segmental liver volume variations: implications for liver surgery. Surgery. 2004;135(4):404–10.
56. Seyama Y, Kokudo N. Assessment of liver function for safe hepatic resection. Hepatol Res. 2009;39(2):107–16.
57. Mise Y, Satou S, Shindoh J, Conrad C, Aoki T, Hasegawa K, Sugawara Y, Kokudo N. Three-dimensional volumetry in 107 normal livers reveals clinically relevant inter-segment variation in size. HPB. 2013;16(5):439.
58. Nakayama K, Oshiro Y, Miyamoto R, Kohno K, Fukunaga K, Ohkohchi N. The effect of three-dimensional preoperative simulation on liver surgery. World J Surg. 2017;41(7):1840–7.
59. You DD, Kim DG, Seo CH, Choi HJ, Yoo YK, Park YG. Prognostic factors after curative resection hepatocellular carcinoma and the surgeon's role. Ann Surg Treat Res. 2017;93(5):252–9.
60. Slotta JE, Kollmar O, Ellenrieder V, Ghadimi BM, Homayounfar K. Hepatocellular carcinoma: surgeon's view on latest findings and future perspectives. World J Hepatol. 2015;7(9):1168–83.
61. Moon DB, Hwang S, Wang HJ, Yun SS, Kim KS, Lee YJ, Kim KH, Park YK, Xu W, Kim BW, Lee DS, Lee DH, Kim HJ, Lim JH, Choi JS, Park YH, Lee SG. Surgical outcomes of hepatocellular carcinoma with bile duct tumor thrombus: a Korean multicenter study. World J Surg. 2013;37(2):443–51.
62. Zeng H, Xu LB, Wen JM, Zhang R, Zhu MS, Shi XD, Liu C. Hepatocellular carcinoma with bile duct tumor thrombus: a clinicopathological analysis of factors predictive of recurrence and outcome after surgery. Medicine. 2015;94(1):e364.
63. Huang JF, Wang LY, Lin ZY, Chen SC, Hsieh MY, Chuang WL, Yu MY, Lu SN, Wang JH, Yeung KW, Chang WY. Incidence and clinical outcome of icteric type hepatocellular carcinoma. J Gastroenterol Hepatol. 2002;17(2):190–5.
64. Kojiro M, Kawabata K, Kawano Y, Shirai F, Takemoto N, Nakashima T. Hepatocellular carcinoma presenting as intrabile duct tumor growth: a clinicopathologic study of 24 cases. Cancer. 1982;49(10):2144–7.
65. Qin LX, Ma ZC, Wu ZQ, Fan J, Zhou XD, Sun HC, Ye QH, Wang L, Tang ZY. Diagnosis and surgical treatments of hepatocellular carcinoma with tumor thrombosis in bile duct: experience of 34 patients. World J Gastroenterol. 2004;10(10): 1397–401.
66. Chen MF, Jan YY, Jeng LB, Hwang TL, Wang CS, Chen SC. Obstructive jaundice secondary to ruptured hepatocellular carcinoma into the common bile duct. Surgical experiences of 20 cases. Cancer. 1994;73(5):1335–40.
67. De Gaetano AM, Nure E, Grossi U, Frongillo F, Russo R, Vecchio FM, Lirosi MC, Sganga G, Felice C, Bonomo L, Agnes S. Fibrolamellar hepatocellular carcinoma with biliary tumor thrombus: an unreported association. Jpn J Radiol. 2013;31(10):706–12.
68. Ise N, Andoh H, Sato T, Yasui O, Kurokawa T, Kotanagi H. Three cases of small hepatocellular carcinoma presenting as obstructive jaundice. HPB. 2004;6(1):21–4.
69. Mallory TB, Castleman B, Parris E. Case records of the Massachusetts general hospital. N Engl J Med. 1947;237(11):673–6.
70. Minagawa M, Ikai I, Matsuyama Y, Yamaoka Y, Makuuchi M. Staging of hepatocellular carcinoma: assessment of the Japanese TNM and AJCC/UICC TNM systems in a cohort of 13,772 patients in Japan. Ann Surg. 2007;245(6):909–22.
71. Noda T, Nagano H, Tomimaru Y, Murakami M, Wada H, Kobayashi S, Marubashi S, Eguchi H, Takeda Y, Tanemura M, Umeshita K, Kim T, Wakasa K, Doki Y, Mori M. Prognosis of hepatocellular carcinoma with biliary tumor thrombi after liver surgery. Surgery. 2011;149(3):371–7.
72. Lai EC, Lau WY. Hepatocellular carcinoma presenting with obstructive jaundice. ANZ J Surg. 2006;76(7):631–6.
73. Wang HJ, Kim JH, Kim JH, Kim WH, Kim MW. Hepatocellular carcinoma with tumor thrombi in the bile duct. Hepatogastroenterology. 1999;46(28):2495–9.
74. Xin KY, Yee LS, Yong TT, Fui AC. Obstructive jaundice due to intraductal tumour thrombus in recurrent hepatocellular carcinoma: what is the optimal therapeutic approach? Hepatogastroenterology. 2014;61(135):1863–6.
75. Peng SY, Wang JW, Liu YB, Cai XJ, Deng GL, Xu B, Li HJ. Surgical intervention for obstructive jaundice due to biliary tumor thrombus in hepatocellular carcinoma. World J Surg. 2004;28(1):43–6.
76. Xiangji L, Weifeng T, Bin Y, Chen L, Xiaoqing J, Baihe Z, Feng S, Mengchao W. Surgery of hepatocellular carcinoma complicated

with cancer thrombi in bile duct: efficacy for criteria for different therapy modalities. Langenbeck's Arch Surg. 2009;394(1):1033–9.
77. Chotirosniramit A, Liwattanakun A, Lapisatepun W, Ko-Iam W, Sandhu T, Junrungsee S. A single institution report of 19 hepatocellular carcinoma patients with bile duct tumor thrombus. J Hepatocell Carcinoma. 2017;4:41–7.
78. Shao W, Sui C, Liu Z, Yang J, Zhou Y. Surgical outcome of hepatocellular carcinoma patients with biliary tumor thrombi. World J Surg Oncol. 2011;9(1):2.
79. Navadgi S, Chang CC, Bartlett A, McCall J, Pandanaboyana S. Systematic review and meta-analysis of outcomes after liver resection in patients with hepatocellular carcinoma (HCC) with and without bile duct thrombus. HPB. 2016;18(4):312–6.
80. Hu J, Pi Z, Yu MY, Li Y, Xiong S. Obstructive jaundice caused by tumor emboli from hepatocellular carcinoma. Am Surg. 1999;65(5):406–10.
81. Orimo T, Kamiyama T, Yokoo H, Wakayama K, Shimada S, Tsuruga Y, Kamachi H, Taketomi A. Hepatectomy for hepatocellular carcinoma with bile duct tumor thrombus, including cases with obstructive jaundice. Ann Surg Oncol. 2016;23(8):2627–34.
82. Rammohan A, Sathyanesan J, Rajendran K, Pitchaimuthu A, Perumal SK, Balaraman K, Ramasamy R, Palaniappan R, Govindan M. Bile duct thrombi in hepatocellular carcinoma: is aggressive surgery worthwhile? HPB. 2015;17(6):508–13.
83. Peng BG, Liang LJ, Li SQ, Zhou F, Hua YP, Luo SM. Surgical treatment of hepatocellular carcinoma with bile duct tumor thrombi. World J Gastroenterol. 2005;11(25):3966–9.
84. Narita R, Oto T, Mimura Y, Ono M, Abe S, Tabaru A, Yoshikawa I, Tanimoto A, Otsuki M. Biliary obstruction caused by intrabiliary transplantation from hepatocellular carcinoma. J Gastroenterol. 2002;37(1):55–8.

GPSR Compliance

The European Union's (EU) General Product Safety Regulation (GPSR) is a set of rules that requires consumer products to be safe and our obligations to ensure this.

If you have any concerns about our products, you can contact us on ProductSafety@springernature.com

In case Publisher is established outside the EU, the EU authorized representative is:

Springer Nature Customer Service Center GmbH
Europaplatz 3
69115 Heidelberg, Germany

Batch number: 10756367

Printed by Printforce, the Netherlands